AIDS

Contributors

James R. Allen
Peter Angritt
Donald Armstrong
John G. Bartlett
William A. Blattner
Michael R. Boyd
Edward N. Brandt, Jr.
Bruce Brew
Samuel Broder
Grace H. Christ
Don C. Des Jarlais
Maria L. De Vinatea
Roger Y. Dodd
Janie Eddy
Garth D. Ehrlich
Myron Essex
Judith Falloon
Chyang T. Fang
Anthony S. Fauci

Peter J. Fischinger
Margaret A. Fischl
Samuel R. Friedman
Alvin E. Friedman-Kien
Robert C. Gallo
Marianne Glasel
James J. Goedert
Scott Koenig
Joseph A. Kovacs
Robert L. Krigel
Barbara Laughon
Alexandra M. Levine
Zirimwabagangabo Lurhuma
Abe M. Macher
Henry Masur
Klaus Mayer
Kathleen McMahon
Rosemary T. Moynihan
Lawrence D. Papsidero

Johanna Pindyck
Philip A. Pizzo
James M. Pluda
Bernard J. Poiesz
Bruce Polsky
Richard W. Price
Thomas C. Quinn
Cheryl M. Reichert
Maryann Roper
Marc Rosenblum
S. Gerald Sandler
George M. Shaw
Karolynn Siegel
John J. Sninsky
M. Glenn Sutterer
Sylvana M. Tuur
Flossie Wong-Staal
Robert Yarchoan
Daniel Zagury

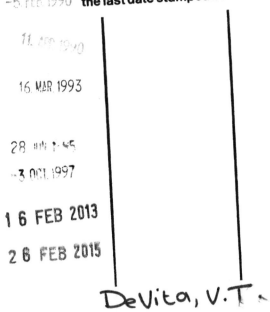

This book is to be returned on or before the last date stamped below.

-5. FEB 1990

11. APR 1990

16. MAR 1993

28 JUN 1995

-3 OCT 1997

1 6 FEB 2013

2 6 FEB 2015

DeVita, V.T.

AIDS

Etiology, Diagnosis, Treatment, and Prevention

Second edition

Edited by

Vincent T. DeVita, Jr., M.D.
Director, National Cancer Institute
Clinical Director, National Cancer Institute
Bethesda, Maryland
Professor of Medicine
George Washington University School of Medicine and Health Sciences
Washington, D.C.

Samuel Hellman, M.D.
Dean and Vice-President
Division of the Biological Sciences
Pritzker School of Medicine
Professor of Radiation Oncology
University of Chicago
Chicago, Illinois

Steven A. Rosenberg, M.D., Ph.D.
Chief of Surgery
National Cancer Institute
Professor of Surgery
Uniformed Services University of the Health Sciences School of Medicine
Bethesda, Maryland

J. B. Lippincott Company
Philadelphia / London / Mexico City / New York / St. Louis / São Paulo / Sydney

Developmental Editor: Richard Winters
Manuscript Editor: Patrick O'Kane
Indexer: Sandra King
Production Supervisor: Carol Florence
Production Coordinator: Caren Erlichman
Compositor: TAPSCO
Printer/Binder: Halliday

2nd Edition

Library of Congress Cataloging-in-Publication Data

AIDS: etiology, diagnosis, treatment, and prevention/edited by
  Vincent T. DeVita, Jr., Samuel Hellman, Steven A. Rosenberg.—2nd
  ed.
      p.   cm.
    Includes bibliographies and index.
    ISBN 0-397-50892-1
    1. AIDS (Disease) I. DeVita, Vincent T. II. Hellman, Samuel.
  III. Rosenberg, Steven A.
    [DNLM: 1. Acquired Immunodeficiency Syndrome.   WD 308 A2882]
    RC607.A26A346 1988
    616.97'92--dc19
    DNLM/DLC
    for Library of Congress   88-12771
                                                                 CIP

The authors and publisher have exerted every effort to ensure that drug
selection and dosage set forth in this text are in accord with current
recommendations and practice at the time of publication. However, in view of
ongoing research, changes in government regulations, and the constant flow of
information relating to drug therapy and drug reactions, the reader is urged to
check the package insert for each drug for any change in indications and
dosage and for added warnings and precautions. This is particularly important
when the recommended agent is a new or infrequently employed drug.

Contributors

James R. Allen, M.D., M.P.H.
Assistant Director for Medical Science
AIDS Program, Center for Infectious Diseases
Centers for Disease Control
Public Health Service
Atlanta, Georgia

Peter Angritt, MC, USA
Co-Director
Collaborator Center for the Investigation of AIDS
Co-Registrar
Registry of AIDS Pathology
Armed Forces Institute of Pathology
Washington, DC

Donald Armstrong, M.D.
Professor of Medicine
Cornell University Medical College
Chief, Infectious Disease Service
Director, Microbiology Laboratory
Memorial Sloan-Kettering Cancer Center
New York, New York

John G. Bartlett, M.D.
Professor of Medicine
Chief, Infectious Diseases
Department of Medicine
Johns Hopkins University School of Medicine
Baltimore, Maryland

William A. Blattner, M.D.
Chief, Viral Epidemiology Section
Environmental Epidemiology Branch
National Cancer Institute
Bethesda, Maryland

Michael R. Boyd, M.D., Ph.D.
Developmental Therapeutics Program
Division of Cancer Treatment
National Cancer Institute
Bethesda, Maryland

Edward N. Brandt, Jr., M.D., Ph.D.
Chancellor
Professor, School of Medicine
University of Maryland at Baltimore
Baltimore, Maryland

Bruce Brew, M.D., F.R.A.C.P.
Neurology Fellow
Memorial Sloan-Kettering Cancer Center
New York, New York

Samuel Broder, M.D.
Associate Director
Clinical Oncology Program
Division of Cancer Treatment
National Cancer Institute
Bethesda, Maryland

Grace H. Christ, A.C.S.W.
Director
Department of Social Work
Memorial Sloan-Kettering Cancer Center
New York, New York

v

Don C. Des Jarlais, Ph.D.
Coordinator of AIDS Research
New York State Division of Substance Abuse
    Service
New York, New York

Maria L. De Vinatea, M.D.
Staff Pathologist
Registry of AIDS Pathology
Armed Forces Institute of Pathology
Washington, DC

Roger Y. Dodd, Ph.D.
Head, Transmissible Diseases Laboratory
Biomedical Research and Development
Jerome Holland Laboratory
American Red Cross
Rockville, Maryland

Janie Eddy, R.N., M.S.N., C.P.N.P.
Research Nurse
Pediatric Branch
National Cancer Institute
National Institutes of Health
Bethesda, Maryland

Garth D. Ehrlich, Ph.D.
Research Instructor
SUNY Health Science Center
Syracuse, New York

Myron Essex, D.V.M., Ph.D.
Professor and Chairman
Department of Cancer Biology
Harvard School of Public Health
Boston, Massachusetts

Judith Falloon, M.D.
Medical Officer
Critical Care Medicine Department
Clinical Center
National Institutes of Health
Bethesda, Maryland

Chyang T. Fang
Coordinator, Quality Control Laboratory
Medical Operations
National Headquarters
American Red Cross
Rockville, Maryland

Anthony S. Fauci, M.D.
Director, National Institute of Allergy and
    Infectious Diseases
National Institutes of Health
Bethesda, Maryland

Peter J. Fischinger, M.D., Ph.D.
Deputy Director
National Cancer Institute
National Institutes of Health
Bethesda, Maryland

Margaret A. Fischl, M.D.
Associate Professor of Medicine
Department of Medicine
University of Miami School of Medicine
Miami, Florida

Samuel R. Friedman, Ph.D.
Narcotic and Drug Research, Inc.
New York, New York

Alvin E. Friedman-Kien, M.D.
Professor of Dermatology and Microbiology
New York University Medical Center
New York, New York

Robert C. Gallo, M.D.
Chief, Laboratory of Tumor Cell Biology
Division of Cancer Etiology
National Cancer Institute
National Institutes of Health
Bethesda, Maryland

Marianne Glasel, R.N., M.S., M.A.
Instructor in Clinical Nursing
Columbia University School of Nursing
Education Coordinator for Cancer Prevention and
    Sexual Health Care
Memorial Sloan-Kettering Cancer Center
New York, New York

James J. Goedert, M.D.
AIDS Coordinator
Virol Epidemiology Section
Environmental Epidemiology Branch
National Cancer Institute
National Institutes of Health
Bethesda, Maryland

Scott Koenig, M.D., Ph.D.
Senior Staff Fellow
Laboratory of Immunoregulation
National Institute of Allergy and Infectious
    Diseases
National Institutes of Health
Bethesda, Maryland

Joseph A. Kovacs, M.D.
Senior Investigator
Critical Care Medicine Department
Clinical Center
National Institutes of Health
Bethesda, Maryland

Robert L. Krigel, M.D.
Director of Hematology
Fox Chase Cancer Center
Assistant Professor of Medicine
Temple University School of Medicine
Philadelphia, Pennsylvania

Barbara Laughon, Ph.D.
Assistant Professor of Medicine
Johns Hopkins University School of Medicine
Baltimore, Maryland

Alexandra M. Levine, M.D.
Professor of Medicine
Executive Associate Dean
University of Southern California
School of Medicine
Los Angeles, California

Zirimwabagangabo Lurhuma
Professor and Chairman
University Clinic of Kinshasa
Chief, Department of Medicine
University Clinic Hospital
Kinshasa, Zaire

Abe M. Macher, M.D.
Director
Collaborative Center for the Investigation of AIDS
Registrar
Registry of AIDS Pathology
Armed Forces Institute of Pathology
Washington, DC

Henry Masur, M.D.
Critical Care Medicine Department
Clinical Center
National Institutes of Health
Bethesda, Maryland

Klaus Mayer, M.D.
Professor of Clinical Medicine
Cornell University Medical College
Associate Chairman for Clinical Laboratories
Department of Medicine
Memorial Sloan-Kettering Cancer Center
New York, New York

Kathleen McMahon, R.N., B.S.N., O.C.N.
AIDS Nurse Clinician
Memorial Sloan-Kettering Cancer Center
New York, New York

Sister Rosemary T. Moynihan, M.S.
Assistant Director
Department of Social Work
Memorial Sloan Kettering Cancer Center
New York, New York

Lawrence D. Papsidero, Ph.D.
Vice President for Research
Cellular Products, Inc.
Buffalo, New York

Johanna Pindyck, M.D.
Senior Vice President
New York Blood Center
Director
Greater New York Blood Program
New York, New York

Philip A. Pizzo, M.D.
Chief of Pediatrics
Head, Infectious Disease Section
Pediatric Branch
National Cancer Institute
National Institutes of Health
Bethesda, Maryland

James M. Pluda, M.D.
Medical Staff Fellow
Clinical Oncology Program
Division of Cancer Treatment
National Cancer Institute
National Institutes of Health
Bethesda, Maryland

Bernard J. Poiesz, M.D.
Professor of Medicine and Microbiology
SUNY Health Science Center and Veterans
  Administration Medical Center
Syracuse, New York

Bruce Polsky, M.D.
Instructor in Medicine
Cornell University Medical College
Clinical Assistant Physician
Infectious Disease Service
Memorial Sloan-Kettering Cancer Center
New York, New York

Richard W. Price, M.D.
Associate Professor of Neurology
Cornell University Medical College
Associate Member
Memorial Sloan-Kettering Cancer Center
Associate Attending Neurologist
Memorial Hospital
New York, New York

Thomas C. Quinn, M.D.
Associate Professor of Medicine
Johns Hopkins University School of Medicine
Baltimore, Maryland
Senior Investigator
National Institutes of Health
Bethesda, Maryland

Cheryl Reichert, M.D., Ph.D.
Department of Pathology
Columbus Hospital
Great Falls, Montana
Consultant
National Cancer Institute
National Institutes of Health
Bethesda, Maryland

Maryann Roper, M.D.
Acting Deputy Director
National Cancer Institute
Attending Physician
Pediatric Branch
National Cancer Institute
National Institutes of Health
Bethesda, Maryland

Marc Rosenblum, M.D.
Assistant Attending Pathologist and
    Neuropathologist
Memorial Sloan-Kettering Cancer Center
New York, New York

S. Gerald Sandler, M.D.
Associate Vice President
Medical Operations
National Headquarters
American Red Cross
Clinical Professor of Medicine
Georgetown University
School of Medicine
Washington, DC

George M. Shaw, M.D., Ph.D.
Associate Professor of Medicine and Biochemistry
University of Alabama at Birmingham
Birmingham, Alabama

Karolynn Siegel, Ph.D.
Director of Social Work Research

Memorial Sloan-Kettering Cancer Center
New York, New York

John J. Sninsky
Cetus Corporation
Emeryville, California

M. Glennon Sutterer, R.N.
Clinical Nurse III
Memorial Sloan-Kettering Cancer Center
New York, New York

Sylvana M. Tuur, M.D.
Staff Pathologist
Registry of AIDS Pathology
Armed Forces Institute of Pathology
Washington, DC

Flossie Wong-Staal, Ph.D.
Section Chief
Molecular Genetics of Hematopoietic Cells Section
Laboratory of Tumor Cell Biology
National Cancer Institute
National Institutes of Health
Bethesda, Maryland

Robert Yarchoan, M.D.
Senior Investigator
Clinical Oncology Program
Division of Cancer Treatment
National Cancer Institute
National Institutes of Health
Bethesda, Maryland

Daniel Zagury, M.D.
Professor and Chairman of Cell Physiology
University of Pierre and Marie Curie
Paris, France
Chief of Department of Immunology
Institut Jean Godinot
Reims, France

Foreword

It has been seven years since those first cases of "*Pneumocystis carinii* pneumonia in previously healthy young men" ushered in the epidemic—indeed, the global pandemic—of acquired immune deficiency syndrome, or AIDS.

Never before has so much been learned in so short a time about a devastating disease. Yet we know relatively little compared to what we would like to know. AIDS remains virtually 100 percent fatal and an effective vaccine and a therapeutic cure elude us; because of its long incubation and the variations in the manner in which the disease plays itself out, we still do not know the life history of the syndrome.

We have nothing at all to effectively stop the disease in its tracks except information and education. Polls seem to indicate that the public continues to be misinformed on how AIDS is *not* transmitted, and although they understand in general the modes of transmission by sexual contact and the sharing of equipment in the abuse of IV drugs, there is no indication that heterosexual behavior has changed. Indeed, the incidence of some other sexually transmitted diseases has risen remarkably in the past year. Homosexuals and bisexual men, who account for the majority of persons with AIDS, have apparently heard the health message and have altered sexual behavior, at least of the promiscuous, anonymous, variety.

There are three aspects of AIDS that color everything done and said about the disease: It is still something of a mystery, it is fatal, and most people get it by doing things that the majority of people don't do, and don't approve of other people doing either.

These three aspects of AIDS present the people of the United States, and elsewhere, a complex test of national character. In some ways, the scientific issues pale in comparison to the highly sensitive issues of law, ethics, economics, morality, and social cohesion that are beginning to surface—spored by those three aspects of AIDS.

We may already be at a sensitive stage in regard to the ethical foundation of health care itself as we hear of physicians, dentists, nurses, and other health personnel who refuse to treat persons with AIDS or even persons whom they *suspect* of having AIDS. They say they are afraid of catching the disease themselves. That certainly is understandable. But equally understandable is the fact that it is very unlikely that a health worker will catch the disease at all.

Thus far, of the five million persons in some kind of health work in this country, only ten have contracted AIDS on the job. In almost every case, the individual simply did not follow the routine instructions for self-protection that the Centers for Disease Control published early in 1986.

This remarkable text deals with the etiology, diagnosis, treatment, and prevention of AIDS. It is hoped that future developments built upon this foundation will bring us victory over the acquired immune deficiency syndrome. Yet it is probable that the final victory over this disease will not follow the patterns of other such victories—the one over smallpox, for example, or polio. This victory will probably not be the exclusive victory of scientific research and clinical practice. I believe it will also require the impelling force of compassionately committed, ethically motivated, and courageous men and women with little or no medical background at all

ix

who will tackle the current problems of the stigma associated with diagnosis, testing for the virus, and confidentiality of patient information.

This is not an easy time for us, even for those of us who have had the training and education and the professional commitment. How much more difficult, then, is it for our neighbors to be courageous, to be wise, and to be involved.

Sometimes those of us in Public Health will recognize a disease for which medicine itself can offer only a partial cure, while the social and spiritual strength of society must come up with the rest. I believe AIDS is such a disease and, therefore, we all have much work to do . . . together.

C. Everett Koop, M.D., Sc. D.
Surgeon General
United States Public Health
    Service and Director,
    Office of International Health

Preface

The first edition of this book was published in 1985. At that time, about 7,000 cases of AIDS had been reported in the United States and detailed studies of the viral pathogenesis of the disease were in their early stages. In the past three years, the understanding of all aspects of AIDS has increased substantially. Perhaps never before has so much been learned about a single disease in so short a time.

In preparing the second edition of this book we have attempted to provide a comprehensive source of information on all aspects of AIDS written by the clinicians and scientists who have made the central contributions in this field. All chapters in the book have been completely rewritten and 15 new chapters have been added.

The book has been divided into three major sections. The first section, "Basic Considerations," deals with the origins, etiology, epidemiology, and immunologic aspects of AIDS and considers, in detail, strategies for interfacing with retroviral replication and the development of vaccines to prevent AIDS.

The second section, "Clinical Aspects," considers the broad range of clinical presentation of patients in-fected with HIV, the diagnosis of AIDS, and malignancies in AIDS patients; detailed chapters cover each of the major organ system dysfunctions induced by HIV infection. Three chapters discuss current efforts to develop pharmacologic treatments for patients with AIDS, and a new chapter has been added on AIDS in pediatric populations.

The third section of the book, "Public Health Issues," has been expanded and deals with high-risk sexual practices in the transmission of AIDS, the problem of AIDS in drug addicts, and the prevention of AIDS during sexual intercourse. Other chapters of broad public health interest have been included that deal with the safety of blood products, safety precautions for health care personnel dealing with seropositive individuals, and screening programs for asymptomatic individuals.

We hope that this book will be useful as a comprehensive reference and can clarify many of the complex issues related to AIDS.

Vincent T. DeVita, Jr., M.D.
Samuel Hellman, M.D.
Steven A. Rosenberg, M.D., Ph.D.

Contents

PART III

Public Health Issues

AIDS

PART I

Basic Considerations

Origins of AIDS

Myron Essex

1

Acquired immune deficiency syndrome (AIDS) was first described as a new and distinct clinical entity in 1981.[1,2,3] The first cases were recognized because of unusual clustering of diseases such as Kaposi's sarcoma and pneumocystis pneumonia in young homosexual men. Although such syndromes were occasionally observed in different well-defined subgroups of the population, such as older men of Mediterranean origin in the case of Kaposi's sarcoma and severely impaired cancer patients in the case of pneumocystis pneumonia, the occurrence of these diseases in previously healthy young people was unprecedented. With the recognition that most of the first cases of this newly defined clinical syndrome to be described involved homosexual men, it was logical that the causes of this new syndrome might be related to a particular life-style unique to that population. In the 1960s and 1970s, the revolution in sexual permissiveness was accompanied by an enhanced societal acceptance of homosexuality. The commercial development of bathhouses and other outlets for homosexual contact increased promiscuity, and self-selected segments of the gay male population had increased numbers of sexual contacts, sometimes in anonymous situations. Because of this, it is not surprising that such factors as frequent exposure to sperm, rectal exposure to sperm, and/or amyl nitrate and butyl nitrate poppers, which were used to enhance sexual performance, were themselves considered potential causes of AIDS. Yet while it was apparent that AIDS was a new disease, most of the life-style factors had changed only in a relative, not in an absolute, sense.

Within a brief period of time AIDS cases were also reported in other populations, such as intravenous drug abusers[4] and hemophiliacs.[5–7] And although the latter groups would not necessarily be exposed to amyl and butyl nitrate poppers, or frequent doses of sperm by a rectal route, it was argued that they, like male homosexuals, would be exposed to frequent immunostimu-

latory doses of foreign proteins and tissue antigens. In the case of hemophiliacs, this would be associated with clotting factor preparations, which were prepared from the pooled blood of a huge number of donors. In the case of intravenous drug abusers, increased exposure to foreign tissue antigens might occur when recipients used dirty needles contaminated with small amounts of blood from previous users. Even independent of clinical AIDS, asymptomatic hemophiliacs and intravenous drug abusers were often found to have inverted T-lymphocyte helper to suppressor ratios, as did AIDS patients and a proportion of asymptomatic promiscuous homosexual men. In retrospect, it seems that in patients not infected with HIV this was more often due to an increase in the number of T-suppressor cells, as opposed to the decrease in T-helper cells seen in AIDS patients and HIV carriers with progressing disease. The increase in T-suppressor cells is presumably due to frequent antigenic stimulation.

Soon after, the first cases of blood-transfusion–associated AIDS were suspected. These were suspected because some individuals with clinical AIDS were found to lack any of the characteristics of the previously defined risk groups—homosexuality, hemophilia, or intravenous drug abuse—but were found to have a history of receiving blood transfusions within the preceding 3 to 5 years.

AN INFECTIOUS ETIOLOGY FOR AIDS

Although still dismissed by many, it seemed increasingly logical that an infectious etiology for AIDS had to be considered.[8] Subsequently, several studies were initiated to determine seroprevalence rates for exposure to numerous microorganisms, especially viruses, and to compare exposure to given agents in AIDS patients and controls.[9] High on the list of candidate viruses was cytomegalovirus, because it was already associated with less severe immunosuppression in kidney transplant patients; Epstein–Barr virus, presumably because it was a lymphotropic virus; and hepatitis B, because it was already known to occur at elevated rates in both homosexual men and recipients of blood or blood products. Yet, since AIDS was a new disease, it was difficult to imagine how it might be caused by a viral agent that was not itself new. If a virus such as hepatitis B, Epstein–Barr, or cytomegalovirus were to be etiologically involved, it would presumably have to be a newly mutated or recombined genetic variant.

At the same time, we, and independently Gallo and his colleagues and Montagnier and his colleagues, postulated that a variant T-lymphotropic retrovirus (HTLV) might be the etiologic agent of AIDS. Among the most compelling reasons for considering such a retrovirus was that the human T-lymphotropic retrovirus discovered as a cause of adult T-cell leukemia by Gallo and colleagues[10] was the only human virus known to infect T-helper lymphocytes, the cells that became impaired or eliminated in individuals with AIDS. Along with this cell tropism, HTLV was known to be transmitted by all the appropriate routes: sexual contact, with transmission apparently more efficient from males; transmission by blood; and transmission from mothers to newborn children.[11]

Another reason why it seemed logical to consider a retrovirus was the situation with the feline leukemia T-lymphotropic retrovirus (FeLV) of cats. Although FeLV was an important cause of leukemia in that species, it killed more animals by causing immunosuppression and the subsequent development of various other lethal infections.[12]

To determine if HTLV, the only human retrovirus known at the time, might also cause immune suppression, we examined individuals in an endemic region with various infectious diseases to determine if they had elevated rates of infection with HTLV. From seroepidemiologic studies conducted in southwestern Japan, it was apparent that individuals with conventional pneumonias, septicemias, encephalitis and other infections were antibody-positive for HTLV two or three times more often than healthy controls or individuals with nonlymphoid cancers.[13] Yet, although a segment of HTLV-infected individuals appeared to have an increased risk for certain infectious processes, they were ordinarily not the severe, irreversible and untreatable infections seen in AIDS patients. And clinical AIDS had not been observed in Japan or other areas endemic for HTLV. But, as in the case of other viruses considered possible candidates, a mutant variant had to be considered the most likely cause of this new disease.

Several approaches were taken to determine if a virus related to HTLV might be associated with AIDS, and enticing but inconclusive results were initially obtained. These included reports on the presence of antibodies cross-reactive with HTLV in one-third of AIDS patients,[14] related genomic sequences in cells taken from a few AIDS patients,[15] and retroviruses and HTLV-reactive antibodies in a few patients.[16,17] Further serologic studies using antigens of HTLV revealed high rates of antibodies in hemophiliacs[18] and in blood donors who donated to surgical patients who subsequently developed transfusion-associated AIDS.[19] Soon after, proof that the disease was linked to a T-lymphotropic retrovirus was obtained by Gallo and his colleagues.[20–23] Further characterization of the agent, now termed human immunodeficiency virus type 1 (HIV-1), revealed that it was only distantly related to HTLV but was the same as the isolate detected earlier by Montagnier and his colleagues.[24–27]

ORIGINS OF HUMAN RETROVIRUSES

HTLV, the first human retrovirus identified, was known to be present at elevated rates in regions such as southwestern Japan, the Caribbean basin, northern South America, and Africa, and at lower rates in most of North America and Europe. A proposal that this virus originated in Africa was initially suggested by Gallo, who cited early reports of Africans in southwestern Japan.[28] Miyoshi and his colleagues then identified a virus related to HTLV in Asian monkeys.[29] This virus, designated simian T-cell leukemia virus (STLV), was subsequently also found in African monkeys and apes[30,31] and associated with lymphoproliferative diseases in captive macaques.[32]

Seroepidemiologic studies in Old World primates from both Asia and Africa revealed that more than 30 species of monkeys and apes had widespread infection with an STLV.[33] However, on further molecular characterization it was recognized that the STLV viruses from Japanese macaques or related Asian species of primates were less related to HTLV than STLVs isolated from African primates such as chimpanzees and the African green monkey.[34] Thus, all isolates of HTLV, whether from Japanese, Caribbean, or African people were highly related to African strains of STLV but not as highly related to Asian strains of STLV. This suggested that all HTLVs thus far identified really evolved from a subgroup of STLV present in Africa but not in Asia. It also suggested quite clearly that the STLV/HTLV family of retroviruses had been present in numerous species of Old World monkeys for some time before moving to man from an African species of monkey or ape.

Genomic restriction enzyme analyses and nucleotide sequencing studies also indicated that different isolates of STLV/HTLV viruses were much more closely related to each other than different HIV-1 viruses.[35] Also, whereas HIV-1 viruses appear to cause AIDS or a related disease in a very high proportion of infected individuals, the STLV/HTLV viruses appear to cause disease in only a very small proportion of infected individuals. In the case of adult T-cell leukemia/lymphoma, this outcome is observed in only about 1 of 500 people who remain infected throughout adulthood. In the case of mild immunosuppression, this may occur at higher rates. Although not normally life-threatening, very rare cases of HTLV immunosuppression may progress to an AIDS-like illness.[36]

The high prevalence rates of infection with STLV in so many species of Old World monkeys also indicates that STLV only rarely causes lymphoma or other diseases under natural circumstances. Why STLV and HTLV are so limited in their pathogenicity is unclear, but it suggests that evolutionary pressure was exerted within the monkey species to select for virus that was not highly virulent. STLV that was of low virulence might then have been transmitted to man, where it remained a virus of limited virulence.

Whereas substantial genetic variation is seen among different isolates of HIV-1, particularly in the envelope gene, the same degree of variation is not seen in HTLV. Presumably, the rate of genetic drift seen in retroviruses is related to their rate of replication. While HIV-1 can replicate to high titers and be detected as free virus in serum or plasma, HTLV cannot. Because HTLV is apparently transmitted both between individuals and within the body only in a cell-associated manner, the rate of evolutionary diversion of this virus should be considerably less. Since STLV and its monkey host(s) had apparently undergone the host-parasite evolutionary selection process by fostering the development of a relatively attenuated virus—rather than just host immunity—when this virus was then transmitted to the human species it would remain a virus of low virulence. Very different and more rapid evolutionary development would apparently occur in the case of HIV-1.

ORIGIN OF HIV-1

Following the recognition that HIV-1 was the cause of AIDS it was soon apparent that this virus was new to western populations of people. This suggested that it either must have recently moved to western populations-at-risk from a different population of people in which AIDS had gone unrecognized, or the virus might have moved to people from an animal reservoir. In either case the possibility that HIV-1 or a related virus might have been present in either people or subhuman primates in Africa seemed worthy of consideration. Yet, if HIV-1 had been present in populations of people in Africa to the point of evolutionary equilibration as seen with HTLV, it probably would have been limited to isolated tribes of people, and would represent a situation in which selection for host immunity rather than selection of an avirulent virus would have occurred. This seemed essential because populations of Blacks in both the United States and Haiti seemed just as likely to develop clinical AIDS after exposure to HIV-1 as did Caucasians.

The possibility that HIV-1 or a related virus was present in human populations in central Africa at the same time or even before AIDS was diagnosed in the United States seemed even more likely when what was apparently the same syndrome was reported in Africans who presented in Europe for treatment. Subsequently it was recognized that HIV-1 infection and clinical AIDS were spreading in Central Africa.

Serum samples collected from Africans at earlier periods were also examined for the presence of antibodies reactive with HIV-1. In some cases, the examination of stored samples suggested high rates of infection in Africa during the period 1965–1975. Subsequently, it was revealed that most of those surveys were conducted with first stage tests that were imperfect, and the reactors were mostly false positives due to either contamination of the HIV antigen, or "sticky sera" containing antibodies that react nonspecifically because the sera were maintained under poor conditions with repeated freezing and thawing.

While examining sera taken from Africa in the period 1955–1965 we found one antibody-positive sample that was clearly positive in a specific manner.[37] When tested by radioimmunoprecipitation this sample contained high titers of antibodies that were reactive with virtually all the major antigens of HIV-1 detectable by this technique: gp160, gp120, p55, gp41, p27, p24, and p17. However, this sample represented only a rare positive reactor in a high-risk group of individuals exposed to venereal infections and AIDS-like illnesses in a region that is now known to have high rates of infection with HIV-1. Yet, only 1% or less of the individuals tested were positive from what is now classified as a region of moderate to high prevalence, Kinshasa, Zaire, suggesting that the virus was only rarely present at that time in places that would now be classified as cities within the AIDS belt of central and East Africa. Again, this suggested that HIV-1 or a virus very similar to it recently moved to the cities of this region of Africa, and we could speculate that either the virus moved from subhuman primates to people just prior to this time or that virus had been transmitted to the cities by migration of a few resistant carriers from a previously isolated tribe or tribes. It is recognized that population redistribution with movement of previously isolated people to newly expanding cities was occurring at this time. Still, it seems unlikely that HIV-1 would have been present as such for many generations in isolated tribal regions. If this were so, we might expect to find Africans who show greater resistance to infection and disease development due to evolutionary genetic development of the human species. In prospective studies conducted to date, exposed Africans appear to develop clinical AIDS and other signs and symptoms of HIV disease as rapidly as risk-group individuals in the United States or Europe.[38] Furthermore, recognizing the high rate of nucleotide variation seen in different HIV-1 viruses currently found in Africa,[35] projecting a similar rate of genetic drift prior to the last 10 to 20 years would suggest that a virus of this type was not present in people until perhaps 50 to 100 years ago. In the case of U.S. risk groups, no current evidence suggests infection prior to the last 10 to 15 years.

HIV-RELATED RETROVIRUSES OF MONKEYS

Still another reason to investigate the possibility that viruses related to HIV might already be present in Africa was the recognition that such viruses were found in selected species of Old World monkeys, both with and without disease. Soon after the recognition of clinical AIDS in people, several clinical reports described outbreaks of severe infections, wasting disease, and death in several colonies of Asian macaques housed at primate centers in the United States.[39,40] Such diseases were subsequently designated simian AIDS or SAIDS. As in the case of human AIDS, numerous causes were considered possible. Following the recognition that SAIDS appeared to be of infectious origin, cytomegalovirus of monkeys was also considered as a possible etiologic agent.

Recognizing that several other exogenous retroviruses had been found in subhuman primates, including the Mason–Pfizer type D virus of rhesus,[41] the gibbon ape leukemia virus[42] and related simian sarcoma virus found in a wooly monkey,[43] and the recently described STLV in numerous Old World species,[29-32] we investigated the possibility that rhesus and related species with SAIDS housed at the New England Regional Primate Research Center might be infected with T-lymphotropic retroviruses related to HIV. Seroepidemiologic screening revealed that a proportion of the SAIDS monkeys had antibodies that cross-reacted with HIV,[44] (Table 1-1). Such antibodies were not found in healthy rhesus.[45] While the antibodies cross-reacted with core antigens of HIV-1, they showed only very weak cross-reactivity with the envelope antigens. However, the same antibody positive rhesus sera reacted well with putative virus envelope antigens in reverse-transcriptase containing cultures of indicator human T4 cells co-cultivated with buffy-coat lymphocytes from antibody-positive monkeys.[44] Further characterization of the cultures revealed the presence of C virus-like particles, and antigens detectable with antibodies either from SAIDS monkeys or from human AIDS patients. The sizes of the protein antigens detected by radioimmunoprecipitation were similar to those of HIV-1. We initially called this primate virus STLV-3, because of its relationship to HIV-1 (which was then called HTLV-3 and/or LAV), and later simian immunodeficiency virus, SIV, or SIV-2.[46] When SIV antigens were tested with sera from human AIDS patients or healthy HIV carriers, virtually all sera had antibodies to the gp120 and gp160 antigens.

At the same time the studies were being done in rhesus monkey samples from a colony with SAIDS, we also examined wild-caught and colony-maintained African green monkeys (*Cercopithicus aethiops*) and other species of African subhuman primates, since rhesus are native to Asia, not Africa. In a serologic survey, from 20% to 70% of different groups of wild-caught African green monkeys were found positive.[47,48] These included monkeys from South Africa to Ethiopia in the Eastern region of sub-Saharan Africa, and Senegal in the western region of sub-Saharan Africa. Wild-caught African green

Table 1-1

*Presence of Antibodies Cross-Reactive with HIV
in Various Species of Old World Subhuman Primates*

Category	Status	Geographical Origin	Seropositivity Rate (%)
Healthy			
African green	Wild	Africa	40–50
African green	Captive	Africa	20–30
Baboon	Wild	Africa	<1
Baboon	Captive	Africa	<1
Chimpanzee	Wild	Africa	<1
Chimpanzee	Captive	Africa	<1
Patas	Captive	Africa	<1
Macaque	Wild	Asia	<1
Macaque	Captive	Asia	<1
Ill			
Macaque	Captive	Asia	20–30

monkeys were positive even more often than colony-maintained animals of the same species. Populations of other species of monkeys and apes from Africa were surprisingly negative. These included baboons, chimpanzees, and patas monkeys. However, species closely related to the African green (also termed genons and vervets), such as the mangabey, the diana monkey, and the mona monkey, were also infected with an agent that was serologically related to SIV.

Contrary to the association between SIV infection in captive rhesus and the occurrence of SAIDS, African green monkeys infected with SIV appeared to remain healthy. Captive African green monkeys infected with SIV revealed no disease symptoms, as did macaques. Also, up to half or more of the healthy wild-caught African green monkeys also showed evidence of exposure to SIV on the basis of antibodies. Although the possibility that SIV caused an unusual case of disease in this species obviously could not be ruled out, especially if the disease occurred after reproductive life, it seemed clear that SIV was not closely linked to an immunosuppressive syndrome in African green monkeys as it was in macaques. It was clear, for example, that the African green species was surviving very well despite the massive losses imposed by humans that use the animal as a source of food.

As in the case of STLV in monkeys and HTLV in people, the possibility that SIV might cause disease rarely in African green monkeys in advanced age could not be ruled out. Yet, it was clear that the situation in this species was one of evolutionary adaptation such that the virus did not cause severe disease as it did in rhesus monkeys and HIV-1 did in people. In the case of HTLV in people and STLV in monkeys it appeared that evolutionary adaptation had selected for a virus of low virulence. In the case of SIV in African green monkeys, it is more difficult to postulate why the virus apparently does not cause disease while the same or a closely related virus does cause disease in macaques. In fact, since wild macaques do not appear to be infected with SIV, and the virus is limited to a small set of African primates, it appears likely that the virus accidently infected captive rhesus quite recently. One possible explanation is that the African green species has evolved to manifest immune resistance while the virus itself has retained its virulence and this is manifested when it infects a species that has had no previous experience with the virus, such as the macaque. This is also compatible with the very widespread distribution of the virus in a high proportion of African green monkeys. However, it may seem surprising that a virus that had coexisted for this long with the African green species was not more widely distributed in numerous species of Old World primates. And in one species in which an SIV-related virus is present, humans in West Africa (see below), this virus does not appear to be associated with frequent and severe disease as it is in macaques.

HIV-2

Recognizing that a relative of the HIV-1 virus designated SIV had been found in wild African primates, and that SIV was only about 50% related to HIV-1 at the genetic level, we believed it logical to investigate the possibility that viruses more highly related to SIV might also be present in human populations. To address this question, serum samples from West African prostitutes were examined to determine if they had antibodies that were more highly cross-reactive with SIV than with HIV-1. West Africans were selected because at that time West Africa was largely free of HIV-1 and clinical AIDS, and female prostitutes were selected because they represent a group at high risk for amplification of prevalence rates for infection with a sexually transmitted virus. Since both HTLV-I and HIV-1 were sexually transmitted it appeared likely that any other human T-lymphotropic retroviruses would be transmitted in the same manner.

Using the procedure of Western blotting it was clear that a significant proportion of Senegalese prostitutes had antibodies that reacted very well with all the major antigens of SIV detected by this technique.[49] These included both the *gag* encoded p24 and the *pol* encoded p64/53 and p34 as well as the *env* gene encoded transmembrane protein p34. When the same SIV antigens are reacted by Western blotting with sera from conventional HIV-1 infected individuals of either European or central African origin, little or no reaction is seen with the transmembrane protein. Since the transmembrane protein of SIV is smaller than the comparable protein of HIV-1, this is usually manifested as the loss of reactivity where it might be expected at gp41 and the acquisition of reactivity with gp32, the carboxy terminus peptide of the *env* gene of SIV.[49] The class of reactivity seen with serum samples from West African prostitutes was in fact virtually indistinguishable from that seen with serum samples from African green monkeys or captive rhesus. Similar results were also obtained by radioimmunoprecipitation, except that this procedure readily detects the gp120 amino terminus *env* glycoprotein that is often missed by Western blotting. In this case serum samples from the West African prostitutes reacted very well with the gp120 and gp160 of SIV but only infrequently and quite weakly with the gp120 and gp160 of HIV-1.[50]

With the evidence that a virus more related to SIV was present in a number of Senegalese prostitutes, more extensive studies were undertaken to determine if the SIV-related virus was more widely distributed in Africa in general and in West Africa in particular. The screening of more than 2000 high-risk individuals from Central Africa, including many individuals with AIDS and other sexually transmitted diseases, revealed no evidence that a virus more related to SIV was present in that area.[51] Conversely, screening in West Africa revealed that 1% to 10% of the control adults in countries such as Senegal, Guinea Bissau, Burkina Faso, and Ivory Coast had evidence of infection while no such evidence was found in countries such as Guinea and Mauritania[52] (see Table 1-2). Even within Senegal, rates were substantially lower in cities in the northern region of their country and higher in the southern region of Casamance.

Infection with the SIV-related virus, which was first designated HTLV-4[49,50] and later LAV-2,[53,54] SBL-6669,[55] and West African Retrovirus and is now universally called HIV-2,[46] is also substantially higher in female prostitutes than in other population groups.[52] That seroprevalence rates were consistently 5 to 10 times higher in sexually

Table 1-2

Seroprevalence Rates for HIV-2 Infection in Risk Category and Control Populations in West and Central Africa

Region, Country	Health Status	Seropositivity Rate (%)
Central Africa		
Burundi	Healthy adults	<1
Burundi	Ill*	<1
Zaire	Healthy adults	<1
Zaire	Ill	<1
West Africa		
Burkina Faso	Healthy adults	1–4
Burkina Faso	Ill	1–10
Burkina Faso	Female prostitutes	15–25
Guinea Bissau	Healthy adults	5–15
Guinea Bissau	Ill	10–20
Guinea Bissau	Female prostitutes	60–70
Senegal	Healthy adults	1–4
Senegal	Ill	1–10
Senegal	Female prostitutes	10–20

* Ill category includes patients with AIDS or AIDS-like illnesses.

promiscuous groups indicated quite clearly that this virus was also sexually transmitted.

A more difficult issue to resolve, perhaps, is how closely infection with HIV-2 is related to development of AIDS. While this virus has been isolated from some patients with AIDS or AIDS-like diseases,[53,56] epidemiologic studies did not reveal a clear correlation between infection and AIDS development. Seropositive prostitutes also lacked evidence of lymphadenopathy, abnormal lymphocyte counts, or disease development.[57] Furthermore, since the AIDS diagnosis itself is not a pathognomonic clinical entity, many African patients with either "AIDS" or "AIDS-like illnesses" have diseases that are unrelated to either HIV-1 or HIV-2. The central question then is whether healthy individuals infected with HIV-2 have an elevated risk for developing AIDS, and if so, is the AIDS that is seen as frequent and severe as that seen in individuals infected with HIV-1. A conclusive answer to this question awaits further studies. Evidence obtained to date suggests that the likelihood for disease development with HIV-2 infection is substantially less than for HIV-1, and that when disease occurs it is less severe than is classical AIDS. Also, even individuals infected with HTLV-I have a somewhat elevated risk for development of various infectious diseases,[13] and a very small number of HTLV-I–infected individuals even develop classical AIDS.[58]

A determination of whether HIV-exposed West Africans show evidence of infection with either HIV-2 or HIV-1 is usually, but not always, straightforward. Although the two viruses share about 50% homology, this is unevenly distributed on the viral genome. Since the *gag* and *pol* gene products are more highly conserved, serologic tests such as ELISAs that are made primarily with viral core antigens of HIV-1 will detect most infections with HIV-2.[59] On the other hand, while many individuals infected with HIV-2 do not have detectable antibodies to the gp120 and gp41 of HIV-1, some do. In fact, about 40% of the amino acid sequences for the transmembrane proteins of HIV-1 and HIV-2 are common. This is even lower for the comparable gp120s, but several stretches of 25–40 amino acids are 35% to 45% identical. Even the 3'*orf* protein, often considered to be the least conserved, is 35% to 40% homologous for HIV-1 and HIV-2.

As a result of this homology, it is difficult to determine if individuals with detectable levels of antibodies to the gp120s of both HIV-1 and HIV-2 were actually infected with both viruses, or infected with only one virus but unusual in that they developed high-titers of cross-reactive antibodies to both. And if some individuals might have been exposed to both viruses at different times but persistent infection was maintained with one type while only transient infection with the other occurred, the possibility of cross-protective immunity and/or interference may be considered. While many consider that gp120 immunity is likely to be highly strain- or isolate-specific, even within HIV-1s, it seems clear that both HIV-1s and HIV-2s infect the same target cells through the same CD4 receptor. Thus, the theoretical possibility remains that an immune effector mechanism directed at preventing the binding of gp120 to the T4 cell receptor could be common not only for different HIV-1s but for HIV-2s as well.

Since HIV-2 and SIV seem highly related to each other and HIV-2 is apparently relatively restricted to West African people whereas SIV is present in green monkeys throughout Africa, the possibility that this virus moved from monkeys to people as a relatively recent event can obviously be considered. However, it is also surprising that SIV has not spread more rapidly to other species of sub-human primates.

CONCLUSIONS

Although SIV and HIV-2 are clearly highly related, and each is more than 50% related to HIV-1, none of these viruses is very closely related to other retroviruses. More distant relatives include lentiviruses such as equine infectious anemia and visna that share only a small amount of homology with the HIVs, and HTLV-I and II that share even less genomic homology but more biologic characteristics, such as T4 lymphocyte tropism. Accordingly, it seems less likely that SIV in African green monkeys was the immediate precursor of HIV-1, but highly likely that it did give rise to HIV-2. A more logical hypothesis might be that HIV-1 moved into people from a precursor virus in another species yet to be identified. Similarly, the postulated evolutionary virus progenitor that gave rise to both SIV and HIV-1 has not been identified. The identification of such progenitor viruses would be important only if the resulting information helps us understand the mechanisms by which viruses such as HIV-1 can be controlled.

REFERENCES

1. Gottlieb MS, Schroff R, Schranker HM et al: *Pneumocystis carinii* pneumonia and mucosal candidiasis in previously healthy homosexual men. N Engl J Med 305:1425, 1981
2. Masur H, Michelis MA, Greene JB et al: An out break of community-acquired *Pneumocystis carinii* pneumonia: Initial manifestation of cellular immune dysfunction. N Engl J Med 305:1431, 1985
3. Siegal FP, Lopez C, Hammer GS et al: Severe acquired immunodeficiency in male homosexuals, manifested by chronic perianal ulcerative *Herpes simplex* lesions. N Engl J Med 305:1439, 1981
4. Centers for Disease Control Task Force on Kaposi's Sarcoma and Opportunistic Infections. N Engl J Med 306:248, 1982
5. Davis KC, Horsburgh CR Jr, Hasiba U et al: Acquired immunodeficiency syndrome with hemophilia. Ann Intern Med 98:284, 1983
6. Poon M–C, Landay A, Prasthofer EF et al: Acquired immunodeficiency syndrome with *Pneumocystis carinii* pneumonia and *Mycobacterium avium-intracellulare* in-

```
```

fection in a previously healthy patient with classic hemophilia. Ann Intern Med 98:287, 1983

7. Elliot JL, Hoppes WL, Platt MS et al: The acquired immunodeficiency syndrome and *Mycobacterium avium-intracellulare* bacteremia in a patient with hemophilia. Ann Intern Med 98:290, 1983

8. Francis DP, Curran JW, Essex M: Epidemic acquired immune deficiency syndrome (AIDS): Epidemiologic evidence for a transmitted agent. J Natl Cancer Inst 71:1, 1983

9. Rogers MF, Morens DM, Stewart JA et al: National case-control study of Kaposi's sarcoma and *Pneumocystis carinii* pneumonia in homosexual men: Part 2, laboratory results. Ann Intern Med 99:151, 1983

10. Poiesz BJ, Ruscetti FW, Gazdar AF et al: Detection and isolation of type-C retrovirus particles from fresh and cultured lymphocytes of a patient with cutaneous T-cell lymphoma. Proc Natl Acad Sci 77:7415, 1980

11. Essex M: Adult T-cell leukemia/lymphoma: Role of a human retrovirus. J Natl Cancer Inst 69:981, 1982

12. Essex M: Horizontally and vertically transmitted oncornavirus of cats. Adv Cancer Res 21:175, 1975

13. Essex M, McLane MF, Tachibana N et al: Seroepidemiology of HTLV in relation to immunosuppression and the acquired immunodeficiency syndrome. In Gallo RC, Essex M, Gross L (eds): Human T-cell Leukemia Viruses, p 355. Cold Spring Harbor, NY, Cold Spring Harbor Press, 1984

14. Essex M, McLane MF, Lee TH et al: Antibodies to cell membrane antigens associated with human T-cell leukemia virus in patients with AIDS. Science 220:859, 1983

15. Gelmann EP, Popovic M, Blayney D et al: Proviral DNA of a retrovirus, human T-cell leukemia virus, in two patients with AIDS. Science 220:862, 1983

16. Gallo RC, Sarin PS, Gelmann EP et al: Isolation of human T-cell leukemia virus in acquired immune deficiency syndrome (AIDS). Science 220:865, 1983

17. Barre-Sinoussi F, Chermann JC, Rey F et al: Isolation of T-lymphotropic retrovirus from a patient at risk for acquired immune deficiency syndrome (AIDS). Science 220:868, 1983

18. Essex M, McLane MF, Lee TH et al: Antibodies to human T-cell leukemia virus membrane antigens (HTLV-MA) in hemophiliacs. Science 221:1061, 1983

19. Jaffe HW, Francis DP, McLane MF et al: Transfusion-associated acquired immunodeficiency syndrome: Serologic evidence of human T-cell leukemia virus infection of donors. Science 223:1309, 1984

20. Popovic M, Sarngadharan M, Read E et al: Detection, isolation, and continuous production of cytopathic retroviruses (HTLV-III) from patients with AIDS and pre-AIDS. Science 224:497, 1984

21. Gallo RC, Salahuddin SZ, Popovic M et al: Frequent detection and isolation of cytopathic retroviruses (HTLV-III) from patients with AIDS and at risk for AIDS. Science 224:500, 1984

22. Schüpbach J, Popovic M, Gilden RV et al: Serologic analysis of a subgroup of human T-lymphotropic retroviruses (HTLV-III) associated with AIDS. Science 224:503, 1984

23. Sarngadharan M, Popovic M, Bruch L et al: Antibodies reactive with human T-lymphotropic retroviruses (HTLV-III) in the serum of patients with AIDS. Science 224:506, 1984

24. Ratner L, Haseltine W, Patarca R et al: Complete nucleotide sequence of the AIDS virus, HTLV-III. Nature 313:277, 1985

25. Wain-Hobson S, Sonigo P, Danos O et al: Nucleotide sequence of the AIDS virus, LAV. Cell 40:9, 1985

26. Sanchez-Pescador R, Power M, Barr P et al: Nucleotide sequence and expression of an AIDS-associated retrovirus (ARV-2). Science 227:484, 1985

27. Muesing M, Smith D, Cabradilla C et al: Nucleic acid structure and expression of the human AIDS/lymphadenopathy retrovirus. Nature 313:450, 1985

28. Gallo RC, Sliski AH, de Noronha CMC et al: Origins of human T-lymphotropic viruses. Nature 320:219, 1986

29. Miyoshi I, Yoshimoto S, Fujishita M et al: Natural adult T-cell leukemia virus infection in Japanese monkeys. Lancet II:658, 1982

30. Saxinger WC, Linge-Wantzin G, Thomsen K et al: Human T-cell leukemia virus: A diverse family of related exogenous viruses of humans and Old World primates. In Gallo RC, Essex M, Gross L (eds): Human T-cell Leukemia Viruses, p 323. Cold Spring Harbor, NY, Cold Spring Harbor Press, 1984

31. Guo H, Wong-Staal F, Gallo RC: Novel viral sequences related to HTLV in T cells of a seropositive baboon. Science 223:1195, 1984

32. Homma T, Kanki PJ, King NW Jr et al: Lymphoma in Macaques: Association with exposure to virus of human T lymphotropic family. Science 225:716, 1984

33. Hayami M, Komuro A, Nozawa K: Prevalence of antibody to adult T-cell leukemia virus-associated antigens (ATLA) in Japanese monkeys and other non-human primates. Intl J Cancer 33:179, 1984

34. Watanabe T, Seiki M, Hirayama Y et al: Human T-cell leukemia virus type I is a member of the African subtype of simian viruses (STLV). Virology 148:385, 1986

35. Alizon M, Wain-Hobson S, Montagnier L et al: Genetic variability of the AIDS virus: Nucleotide sequence analysis of two isolates from African patients. Cell 46:63, 1986

36. Kobayashi M, Yoshimoto S, Fujishita M et al: HTLV-positive T-cell lymphoma/leukemia in an AIDS patient. Lancet I: 1361, 1984

37. Nahmias AJ, Weiss J, Yao X et al: Evidence for human infection with an HTLV-III/LAV-like virus in Central Africa, 1959. Lancet I:1278, 1986

38. Mann JM, Bila K, Colebunders RL et al: Natural history of human immunodeficiency virus infection in Zaire. Lancet II:707, 1986

39. Letvin NL, Eaton KA, Aldrich WR et al: Acquired immunodeficiency syndrome in a colony of Macaque monkeys. Proc Natl Acad Sci USA 80:2718, 1983

40. Henrickson RV, Maul DH, Osborn KG et al: Epidemic of acquired immunodeficiency in rhesus monkeys. Lancet I: 338, 1983

41. Chopra HC, Mason MM: A new virus in a spontaneous mammary tumor of a rhesus monkey. Cancer Res 30:2081, 1970

42. Kawakami TG, Huff SD, Buckley PM et al: C-type virus associated with gibbon lymphosarcoma. Nature, New Biol 235:170, 1972

43. Theilen GH, Gould D, Fowler M et al: C-type virus in tumor tissue of a woolly monkey (*Lagothrix spp.*) with fibrosarcoma. J Nat Cancer Inst 47:881, 1971

44. Kanki PJ, McLane MF, King NW Jr et al: Serologic identification and characterization of a Macaque T-lymphotropic retrovirus closely related to human T-lymphotropic retroviruses (HTLV) type III. Science 228:1199, 1985

45. Chou MJ, Kanki PJ, Essex M: Absence of natural STLV-3 infection in healthy Macaque monkeys. Submitted.

46. Biberfeld G, Brown F, Esparza J et al: WHO working group on characterization of HIV-related retroviruses: Criteria for

characterization and proposal for a nomenclature system. AIDS 1:189, 1987

47. Kanki PJ, Alroy J, Essex M: Isolation of T-lymphotropic retrovirus related to HTLV-III/LAV from wild-caught African green monkeys. Science 230:951, 1985

48. Kanki PJ, Kurth R, Becker W et al: Antibodies to simian T-lymphotropic virus type III in African green monkeys and recognition of STLV-III viral proteins by AIDS and related sera. Lancet I:1330, 1985

49. Barin F, M'Boup S, Denis F et al: Serological evidence for a virus related to Simian T-lymphotropic retrovirus III in residents of West Africa. Lancet II:1387, 1985

50. Kanki PJ, Barin F, M'Boup S et al: New human T-lymphotropic retrovirus related to Simian T-lymphotropic virus type III$_{AGM}$ (STLV-III$_{AGM}$). Science 232:238, 1986

51. Kanki PJ, Allan J, Barin F et al: Absence of antibodies to HIV-2/HTLV-4 in six Central African nations. AIDS Research and Human Retroviruses 3(3):317, 1987

52. Kanki PJ, M'Boup S, Ricard D et al: Human T-lymphotropic virus type 4 and the human immunodeficiency virus in West Africa. Science 236:827, 1987

53. Clavel F, Guetard D, Brun–Vezinet F et al: Isolation of a new human retrovirus from West African patients with AIDS. Science 233:343, 1986

54. Clavel F, Guyader M, Guetard D et al: Molecular cloning and polymorphism of the human immune deficiency virus type 2. Nature 324:691, 1986

55. Albert J, Bredberg U, Chiodi F et al: A new human retrovirus isolate of West African origin (SBL-6669) and its relationship to HTLV-IV, LAV-II, and HTLV-IIIB. AIDS Research and Human Retroviruses 3:3, 1987

56. Clavel F, Mansinho K, Chamaret S et al: Human immunodeficiency virus type 2 infection associated with AIDS in West Africa. N Engl J Med 316:1180, 1987

57. Marlink RG, Ricard D, M'Boup S et al: Clinical, hematologic, and immunologic cross-sectional evaluation of individuals exposed to human immunodeficiency virus type 2 (HIV-2). AIDS Research and Human Retroviruses (in press)

58. Miyoshi I: AIDS-like opportunistic infections in HTLV-I carriers. ARC International Symposium on Viruses and Cancers, Martinique, [abstr] Jan. 8, 1986

59. Denis F, Leonard G, Mounier M et al: Efficacy of five enzyme immunoassays for antibody to HIV in detecting antibody to HTLV-IV. Lancet I:324, 1987

Etiology of AIDS: Virology, Molecular Biology, and Evolution of Human Immunodeficiency Viruses

George M. Shaw
Flossie Wong-Staal
Robert C. Gallo

2

The acquired immunodeficiency syndrome (AIDS) was first recognized in 1981 as a clinical syndrome consisting of opportunistic infection and/or neoplasia associated with unexplained immunodeficiency.[1,2] As of January 1988, more than 50,000 cases of AIDS had been diagnosed in the United States alone, and an estimated 1 to 2 million more people in the United States were believed to be infected with the etiologic agent, human immunodeficiency virus type 1 (HIV-1).[3,4] It is now believed that approximately 25% to 35% of HIV-1–infected persons will develop full-blown AIDS by 7 years postinfection[4,5] and it is expected that they will have a mortality rate approaching 100% unless effective treatments are developed. Based on these projections, some 270,000 cumulative cases of AIDS will have been diagnosed in the United States by the year 1991. The outcome for the other 1 to 2 million infected individuals who have not by that time developed clinical immunodeficiency is less certain, although it is likely that a substantial proportion, if not all, will eventually go on to develop AIDS. From a worldwide perspective, it is estimated that the number of infected persons is currently in the millions and without effective intervention this number will rise.[6] The scientific community is challenged with defining the biology and pathogenesis of HIV infection, with guiding rational efforts to stop transmission, and with developing effective means of treatment and prevention. This chapter reviews the remarkable progress that has been made since the first description of AIDS in 1981 in elucidating the causative agent, defining its biologic and genetic properties, and understanding its evolutionary relationship to other retroviruses. It also focuses on emerging directions of basic research believed to be important for developing a better understanding of HIV disease and effective treatment and preventive measures.

HISTORY OF HUMAN RETROVIROLOGY

Human retrovirology is a young but rapidly advancing scientific discipline. The earliest descriptions of animal retroviruses came early in the 20th century from the work of Ellerman and Bang[7] and from Rous,[8] who showed that cell-free filtrates from leukemic chickens could induce leukemias and sarcomas in normal animals. Some 40 years later, Ludwik Gross isolated the first mammalian retrovirus from an inbred strain of mice infected with murine leukemia virus.[9] Shortly thereafter, other oncogenic retroviruses were identified in animals by Harvey and colleagues.[10] Although these studies had been done in inbred animals, subsequent studies by Jarrett[11] and by Essex and Hardy[12] showed that household cats were infected by a retrovirus (feline leukemia virus, FeLV) that caused lymphoproliferative disease and immunosuppression. Other outbred species found to have retrovirus-induced naturally occurring malignancies included chickens, mice, cattle, and certain primates. Despite an exhaustive search, however, the discovery of human retroviruses was slower to come.

In 1970, Temin and Mitzutani[13] and independently Baltimore[14] discovered the retroviral enzyme reverse transcriptase, and in 1971 the existence and integration of infectious proviral DNA of retroviruses was described by Hill and Hillova.[15] In 1970, after the discovery of reverse transcriptase, Gallo and co-workers began a search for human retroviruses by developing molecular biologic approaches for the detection of low-level expression of reverse transcriptase activity[16] and culture techniques for the long-term growth of various hematopoietic cells.[17] The rationale for this approach was that the identification of human retroviruses would likely require the cultivation of susceptible cell targets and the detection of low-level virus expression. Both concepts—the need for the long-term propagation of appropriate hematopoietic cells and the need to detect low-level virus expression—proved essential for the discovery first of the human leukemia viruses HTLV-I and HTLV-II, and subsequently the AIDS virus, HIV. The growth of mature human T cells in long-term suspension cultures was first made possible by the discovery of T-cell growth factor, or interleukin-2 (IL-2), by Gallo and co-workers in 1976.[17] As it turned out, the primary target cells of all known human retroviruses, including HTLV-I, HTLV-II, HIV-1, and HIV-2, possess receptors for IL-2 and require this factor for proliferation. In 1979, Gallo and associates[18,19] isolated and subsequently characterized the first human retrovirus, called human T-cell leukemia virus type I (HTLV-I). An enormous body of work subsequently defined HTLV-I as the causative agent of a form of human leukemia termed adult T-cell leukemia (ATL).[20,21] In 1982, Gallo and co-workers reported the discovery of the second human retrovirus, HTLV-II.[22] The intellectual and experimental developments leading to the discovery of HTLV-I and HTLV-II laid the critical scientific groundwork for the subsequent discovery of HIV-1 as the etiologic agent of AIDS.

DISCOVERY OF THE AIDS VIRUS

The original idea that AIDS might be caused by a retrovirus evolved from earlier studies on HTLV-I, HTLV-II, and FeLV, and from emerging epidemiologic evidence implicating a transmissible agent as the cause of the disease.[23] The AIDS epidemic was new in 1981. It first appeared in a limited geographic region and subsequently spread to other areas. The disease occurred in socially, economically, and geographically disparate groups, all of which shared a propensity for communicable diseases. Clusters of disease were found that were linked by common contacts, and recipients of blood products, heterosexual partners, and children of affected individuals developed AIDS despite having no other risk factors for the disease. Filtered Factor VIII coagulant transfused to individuals with hemophilia A resulted in transmission of disease. All of these facts argued strongly for a transmissible infectious agent as the cause of AIDS. A second line of evidence was the apparent selective loss of the helper T-lymphocyte population of blood cells. This suggested a restricted tropism for the putative agent highly reminiscent of infection with HTLV-I and HTLV-II. Third, the mode of transmission, including sexual, perinatal, and blood product exposures was also like that of the human leukemia viruses. Fourth, another animal retrovirus, FeLV, was well known to cause immunosuppression as well as lymphoproliferative disease. Finally, although the AIDS epidemic was first recognized in the United States and subsequently in Europe and Asia, it became apparent early on that the disease probably had originated in Africa, an area endemic for the human T-lymphotropic retroviruses.[24]

Because of this circumstantial evidence that a human T-lymphotropic retrovirus represented a likely cause of AIDS, investigative teams headed by Gallo and by Montagnier undertook to isolate such putative viruses from patients with AIDS and related conditions. Employing an experimental approach that included the use of IL-2 to stimulate growth of lymphoid cells and sensitive assays for reverse transcriptase activity to detect low-level expression of retrovirus, the Gallo group found as early as the fall of 1982 evidence for the existence of retrovirus in lymphocytes of AIDS patients.[23] However, unlike HTLV-I, which induced the proliferation and immortalization of lymphocytes, the agent in these AIDS cultures invariably killed the cells it infected. This greatly impeded progress in obtaining sufficient quantities of virus for characterization. Another investigative team led by Barré–Sinoussi, Chermann, and Montagnier independently reported the detection by reverse transcriptase activity, electron microscopy, and continuous passage in transient cultures of peripheral blood lymphocytes of a retrovirus in a patient with lymphadenopathy syndrome.[25] They also identified a putative major viral core protein, p25, not immunologically cross-reactive with the p24 of HTLV-I and detected by immunoprecipitation antibodies against this protein in two patients. The inability to propagate this virus to high titers and the lack of specific antiviral reagents at that time precluded the conclusion that this virus, termed lymphadenopathy-associated virus (LAV), was in fact the etiologic agent of AIDS. In late 1983, however, Popovic and others developed clones of a permanently growing T4 (CD4) positive cell line (HT) that were susceptible to infection by retroviruses from AIDS patients previously recognized only by transient elevations of reverse transcriptase in short-term lymphocyte cultures.[26] Single cell clones (H9 and H4) of this leukemic T-cell line were found to be highly susceptible to virus infection and partially resistant to its cytopathic effects. Infection of the H9 cell line by pooled blood samples from AIDS patients eventually led to the highly productive permanently producing cell line H9/HTLV-IIIb.[26] At the same time, 48 other AIDS virus isolates were obtained either in short-term lymphocyte culture or in cell lines.[27] The availability of continuous, high-titer producer cell lines allowed for the first time the development of highly purified and concentrated viral reagents necessary for the characterization of the virus and for the serologic detection of exposed individuals.[28,29] As sensitive serologic tests for exposure to the AIDS virus were developed, it became clear that essentially 100% of AIDS patients and a high proportion of individuals in high-risk populations were infected with this agent, which became known first as LAV or HTLV-III and then, by convention, HIV-1.[30] The repeated isolation[27,31] and serologic detection[4] of HIV-1 in patients with AIDS or risk factors for AIDS, and the cytopathic activity of biologically and molecularly cloned HIV-1 *in vitro,* argued convincingly for these early HTLV-III isolates as the causative agent of AIDS. Comparative analysis of HTLV-III and LAV showed the two viruses to be members of the same group (HIV-1),[34] and the etiology of AIDS was established.

OVERVIEW OF HIV-1 BIOLOGY

The discovery of HIV-1 as the causative agent of AIDS just 3 years after the initial description of the syndrome represented a remarkable scientific achievement. Initially, it was recognized that many parallels existed between HIV-1 and the human leukemia viruses, HTLV-I and HTLV-II, most notably the exquisite viral tropism for T4 (CD4)–bearing cells.[24] However, it soon became apparent that the AIDS virus was most closely related to the lentivirus subfamily of retroviruses.[35] These viruses derive their name from the slow course of infection that they cause. Like all retroviruses, HIV-1 is a single-strand plus-sense RNA virus slightly more than 100 nm in diameter. On electron microscopy, it has a characteristic dense, cylindrical nucleoid containing core proteins, genomic RNA, and reverse transcriptase surrounded by a lipid envelope (Fig. 2-1). The ultrastructural features of HIV-1 are virtually indistinguishable from another lentivirus, visna, and quite different from the human type C retroviruses, HTLV-I and HTLV-II.[35] The structural components of HIV-1 are shown diagrammatically in Figure 2-2. The RNA-dependent DNA polymerase, or reverse transcriptase, the *sine qua non* of retroviruses, is present in the virion in association with the RNA genome. In retroviruses, generally, the polymerase activity and the genomic RNA are found in close association with core protein structures. The major structural core protein of HIV-1 is the p24 protein. This, and the myristylated protein p18, comprise the major *gag* structural proteins. Surrounding the viral core is a lipid membrane derived from the outer membrane of the host cell. Studding the outer membrane of the virus are the envelope glycoproteins, gp120 and gp41.

The life cycle of HIV-1 is diagrammatically shown in Figure 2-3. Features of this life cycle distinguish retroviruses from all other viruses. The cell-free virion first binds to the target cell through a specific interaction between the viral envelope and the host cell membrane. The specificity of this interaction between virus and cell has been shown to be due to a high-affinity, specific interaction between the viral gp120 molecule and the target cell T4 (CD4) molecule. Following virus adsorption, fusion of the viral and cellular membranes is believed to occur, resulting in internalization of viral core components. Reverse transcription catalyzed by the viral RNA-dependent DNA polymerase generates a double-stranded DNA copy of the viral RNA genome, which may exist episomally or be integrated covalently within the host cell genome. Subsequent expression of viral DNA is controlled by a combination of viral and host cellular proteins interacting with viral DNA regulatory elements. Transcribed viral mRNA is translated into virus-specific proteins, and new virions are assembled at the cell surface where viral RNA, reverse transcriptase,

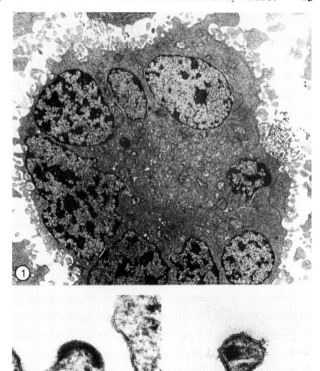

FIG. 2-1. Transmission electron micrograph of human lymphocyte syncytium infected with HIV-1. Panel 1 shows a syncytium of human lymphocytes expressing large numbers of HIV-1 virions. These can be seen as small dark particles around the surface of the cell and are enlarged in Panels 2A and 2B. The diameter of the virion shown in Panel 2B is approximately 110 nm. (Electron micrograph courtesy of S. Z. Salahuddin.)

structural and regulatory proteins, and envelope proteins are assembled in a highly organized fashion to produce infectious progeny.

Although HIV-1 was first cultured from peripheral blood lymphocytes and lymph node cells of infected patients, virus has subsequently been cultured from brain, cerebrospinal fluid, cell-free plasma, bone marrow, semen, vaginal secretions, intestinal epithelium, breast milk, saliva, and tears. It is likely that virus in certain of these tissues plays an important role in the pathophysiology of disease and in disease transmission, although it is equally clear that transmission of virus from casual contact with saliva and tears is extraordinarily unlikely and has never been documented.

One of the most prominent biologic features of HIV infection *in vitro* and *in vivo* relates to the cytopathic properties of the virus. The hallmark of HIV-1 infection in infected persons is a progressive depletion of T4 (CD4)–bearing lymphocytes, eventually leading to immunodeficiency and secondary infections and neo-

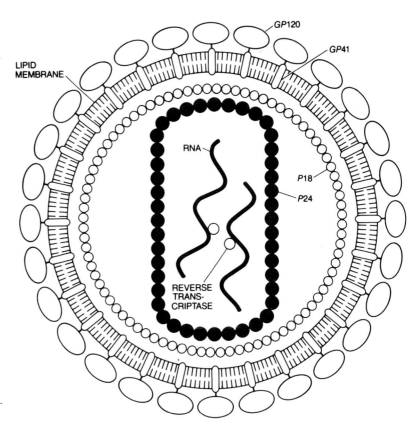

FIG. 2-2. Structure of HIV-1. See text for description.

LIFE CYCLE OF A RETROVIRUS

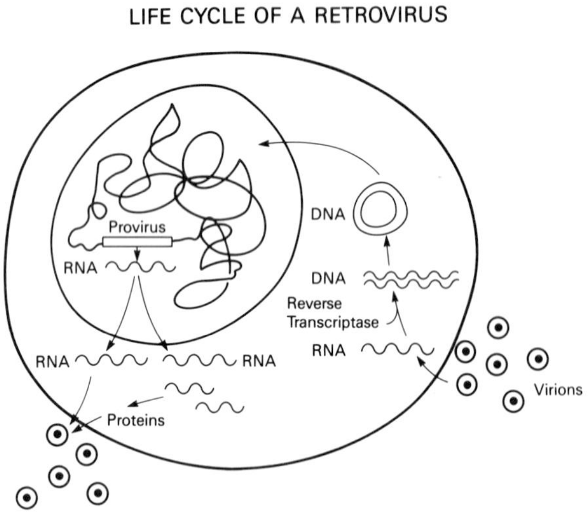

FIG. 2-3. Life cycle of HIV-1. See text for description.

plasms. *In vitro,* HIV-1 is highly cytopathic for T4 (CD4)–bearing lymphocytes and lymphoid cell lines and the typical cytopathic effect is demonstrated by generation of large syncytia representing the fusion of cells expressing the HIV-1 gp120 envelope glycoprotein and other cells expressing CD4 (Fig. 2-4). Fusion of infected cells and uninfected neighboring cells requires

the same high-affinity, specific interaction between viral gp120 (in this instance, expressed on the infected cell surface membrane) and cellular T4 (CD4), as occurs during virus infection.

The ultimate outcome of HIV-1 infection, *in vitro* and *in vivo,* is a reflection of the complex viral properties outlined here, and the remainder of this chapter examines the molecular basis of HIV structure, function, pathogenesis, and evolution.

MOLECULAR STRUCTURE AND FUNCTION OF HIV-1

The genomic organization of HIV-1 and the respective gene products are shown diagrammatically in Figure 2-5. HIV-1 is bounded by long-terminal repeat (LTR) elements and contains a series of genes found in other retroviruses as well as additional genes unique to HIV and its close relatives. The long-terminal repeat sequences of HIV-1 direct and regulate expression of the viral genome. Deletion mutant studies of the LTR[36,37] have identified four regions important for gene expression, including the promoter, where the polymerase binds and transcription is initiated (+1); a negative regulatory element (NRE) located between nucleotides −340 and −185, deletion of which increases the level of gene expression directed by the viral LTR by three to six times in both HIV-1–infected and HIV–uninfected

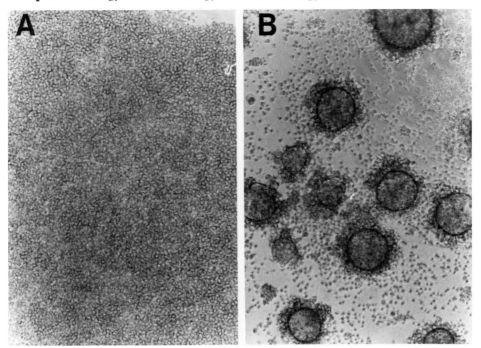

FIG. 2-4. Formation of syncytia by HIV-1. In this figure, cells infected with HIV-1 were co-cultured with uninfected cells expressing the CD4 molecule. Monoclonal antibody to OKT4A was included in the culture medium for Panel *A* but not for Panel *B.* HIV-1–infected cells that express the gp120 viral envelope glycoprotein on their surface form large syncytia with CD4-bearing uninfected lymphocytes (Panel *B*), a process that is blocked by pre-incubation of the CD4 positive cells with anti-OKT4A antibody (Panel *A*).

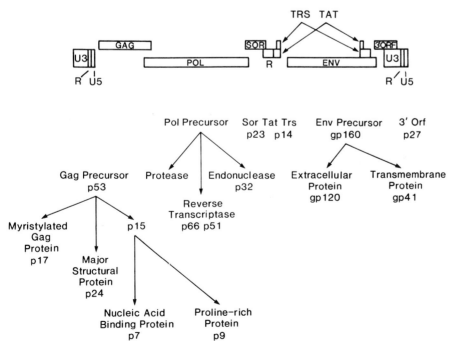

FIG. 2-5. Genomic map and protein products of HIV-1. See text for details.

cells; an enhancer located between nucleotides −137 and −17 that is also active in both infected and uninfected cells; and a *trans*-acting responsive region (TAR) located between nucleotides +1 and +80 that represents the putative binding region for the *tat* gene product (see below). The enhancer and promoter elements do not themselves respond to virus-associated *trans*-acting regulatory factors as does the TAR region. Other regulatory elements include three copies of an Sp1 consensus sequence, a TATA box, and a polyadenylation signal.[38] The *gag* gene encodes a precursor protein of 53 kilodaltons (pr53) that is cleaved into four smaller products with the linear order NH2-p17-p24-p7-p9-COOH.[38] These proteins constitute the core protein structure of the virus and also subserve nucleic acid and lipid membrane binding functions.[10] The *gag* proteins of HIV-1, as for other retroviruses, are synthesized as a polyprotein precursor that is subsequently cleaved during the maturation process. This facilitates the assembly of various components of a complex core structure in a three-dimensional configuration that when subsequently cleaved by specific proteases acquire specialized functions. The polymerase gene products are translated from the same genomic RNA message as the *gag* proteins but in a different overlapping reading frame as a result of ribosomal frameshifting.[39] The *pol* encodes three proteins that are cleaved from a larger precursor polypeptide. These genes include NH2-protease-reverse transcriptase (p66/p51)-endonuclease (p31)-COOH.[40] The HIV-1 protease plays a critical role in virus biology acting specifically to cleave *gag* and *pol* precursor polypeptides into functionally active proteins. The reverse transcriptase of HIV-1 has been shown to be a Mg^{2+} requiring RNA-dependent DNA polymerase that is responsible for replicating the RNA viral genome.[26] The endonuclease, or integrase, protein by analogy with other retroviruses is important in proviral integration, although it is noteworthy that visna virus, another lentivirus, has been reported to exist primarily as unintegrated episomal DNA.[41] The envelope gene (*env*) encodes a glycosylated polypeptide precursor (gp160) that is processed to form the exterior glycoprotein (gp120) and the transmembrane glycoprotein (gp41).[42] In comparison with the envelope proteins of other retroviruses, both of these proteins are unusually large and both contain many potential glycosolation sites. It is the viral envelope that possesses domains responsible for CD4 binding, fusion, and epitopes primarily involved in viral-host immune interactions.[43–51]

Within the HIV-1 genome, there are additional open reading frames (*orfs*) of various lengths in addition to those encoding the major structural proteins. These include *sor*, which is located between the *pol* and *env* genes; 3′ *orf*, located 3′ to the envelope gene and extending into the U3 region of the LTR; *tat*-3 and *art/trs*, both of which exist as two coding exons in the central and 3′ end of the virus; and R, which is located centrally (see Fig. 2-5). The *sor* gene encodes a protein product of 23kD that is recognized by the host immune system during natural infection and is synthesized in infected

cells.[52–54] Site-directed mutagenesis of the *sor* gene has shown this protein to be necessary for the production of fully infectious virions, and it is believed that the protein plays an important role in virus infectivity or in early postinfectivity events.[55–56] The 3′ *orf* protein has been identified as a p27 species in infected cells, and individuals infected with HIV-1 have antibodies against this product. Mutants defective in 3′ *orf* have been shown to replicate in higher titers and to be cytopathic for T cells *in vitro*,[57,58] and thus the 3′ *orf* product would appear to have some negative regulatory effect on virus replication. This gene product is conserved in different isolates of HIV-1 and in related viruses such as HIV-2 and SIV_{mac}, and its biologic function *in vivo* remains to be elucidated. Studies by Montagnier and associates have suggested that 3′ *orf* protein exhibits protein kinase activities.[59] The R open-reading frame also encodes a protein that is recognized immunologically by infected persons, but again the function of this protein is entirely unknown since deletion mutant studies of this gene indicate that virus replication and infectivity *in vitro* are not noticeably altered.[60]

Two other genes, *tat*-3 and *art/trs,* that were not originally recognized from nucleotide sequence analyses of HIV-1 have since been identified on the basis of functional mapping of deletion mutants defective in these regions. The existence of a *trans*-activator gene was first inferred when it was recognized that genes linked to the HIV-1 LTR were expressed at much higher levels in HIV-infected cells than in uninfected cells.[61] The apparent *trans*-activating function was subsequently mapped to a genetic locus now designated *tat*-3[62–64] and this function could be complemented using cDNA clones supplied in *trans.* The *tat*-3 gene is transcribed from two coding exons consisting of 256 base pairs, encoding an 86-amino-acid protein. The functional domain of the *tat* gene has been localized to the first exon that can be truncated to the first 58 amino acids without significant loss of activity.[65] The *tat*-3 gene product is specific for its own LTR and is not active for unrelated heterologous promoter enhancer sequences. The activation effect of this factor is significantly reduced in the presence of either antibodies to *tat*-3 or a DNA fragment containing the *tat*-3 responsive sequences, suggesting that *tat*-3 is indeed a transcriptional activator.[66] Direct mutagenesis of the *tat*-3 gene shows that an intact *tat* function is essential for the synthesis of viral mRNA.[67] There is, in addition, evidence to suggest that *tat*-3 also has a post-transcriptional enhancing effect at the level of message utilization, and less *tat*-3 appears to be required for optimal transcription than for optimal protein synthesis. Mutants expressing low levels of *tat*-3 have been shown to transcribe normal levels of viral mRNA but to synthesize viral proteins at a much reduced level.[68] The ability of *tat*-3 to affect both transcriptional and post-transcriptional events may be ascribed to its structure and the nature of its target sequences. The critical functional core of *tat*-3, based on mutagenesis studies as well as localization of conserved sequences within the *trans*-activator gene of the distantly related HIV-2/SIV genomes, contains two potential nucleic acid binding domains. The first, a cysteine-rich domain, is structurally analogous to the metal-binding fingers described for a class of DNA binding proteins that includes the transcription Factor IIIa (TFIIIa) of xenopus and some hormone receptors. The second is a highly basic domain. The TAR sequences for *tat-3* are located from +1 to +56 and contain a potential hairpin structure. Since these sequences are located in the DNA as well as in the transcribed RNA, it is conceivable that the protein could interact with both DNA and RNA and regulate both transcription and post-transcriptional processes.[37,69] Recent studies have suggested that the major action of *tat* in *trans*-activating HIV-1 transcription is due to the abolition of a specific block to transcriptional elongation within the TAR sequence.[70]

The existence of another viral gene that is critical for viral expression was discovered in the course of studies aimed at elucidating the function of *tat-3*. It was found that some mutants with deletions either within or near the two *tat-3* exons expressed low or undetectable levels of virus proteins. Unlike *tat-3* mutants, however, these defective genomes could not be complemented by functional *tat-3* cDNA clones.[68,70] A second open-reading frame overlapping extensively with *tat-3* coding sequences was identified, and mutants affecting only this gene (referred to as *trs* or *art* for *trans*-regulator of splicing and antirepressor *trans*-activator) could be constructed.[67] The *art/trs* mutants displayed an aberrant pattern of steady-state viral mRNA with a great reduction of genomic viral messages for *gag, pol,* and *env,* along with a concomitant increase in the multiply-spliced 1.8-kb to 2.0-kb messages. Thus, the primary activity of *art/trs* was inferred to be that of a facilitator of expression of mRNAs encoding structural proteins. There is also some evidence to suggest that *art/trs* may facilitate expression of structural protein mRNA at the translational level, and furthermore, *art/trs* may have some down-regulatory effect on overall mRNA transcription.[67] Both *tat-3* and *art/trs* are essential for expression of viral structural proteins and therefore for replication competence of the virus.

In summary, HIV-1 utilizes complex strategies for regulating viral expression. These operate at the level of transcription, mRNA processing, protein synthesis, and virus maturation. Although the specific functions of R and 3' *orf* are currently unknown, that they are highly conserved in evolutionarily divergent viruses argues that they are important in the biology of HIV *in vivo*.

Replication, Latency, and Persistence

Retroviral diseases are often characterized by restricted viral gene expression, latency, and persistence of virus in the face of substantial host immune responses. These features are characteristic of natural infections with visna virus in sheep, equine infectious anemia virus (EIAV) in horses, caprine arthritis encephalitis virus in goats, and both HTLV-I and HIV infection in humans.[71] Once

infected with HIV, persons are believed to be both infected and infectious for life, barring the development of effective treatment measures. Properties inherent to the retroviral life cycle contribute to this persistence. DNA replicated from the HIV genome is integrated into host cell chromosomes following infection,[72] and expression of the viral genome is down-regulated as it is in visna virus infection. This is supported by the observation that very few CD4+ lymphocytes express viral message at any one point in time[73] and that the general course of HIV-1 disease is characterized by a protracted, progressive T4 cell loss with an estimated mean period from time of infection to the development of clinical AIDS to be more than 5 years.[4] *In vitro,* infection of human peripheral blood lymphocytes and T4 positive cell lines by HIV-1 can result in an explosive lytic infection or in transient cytopathy followed by the outgrowth of virus-containing cells that either express very low levels of viral message or remain entirely latent until activated.[74,75] Activation signals include treatment with halogenated pyrimidines *in vitro* but can also include concomitant infections by other viruses such as Epstein–Barr virus (EBV), HTLV-I, cytomegalovirus (CMV), hepatitis-B virus, or herpes simplex virus, as well as activation signals inherent to the immune response.[76–81] For the HIV-infected individual, the wide range of antigenic stimuli to which one is normally exposed would be expected to serve as physiologically relevant cellular activators of virus expression. In this regard, it has been demonstrated that cultures of human lymphocytes, when exposed to HIV in the presence or absence of soluble antigen, such as tetanus toxoid or KLH, lead to virus production in cultures exposed to antigen but not in cultures lacking such stimulation.[77] Growth factors may also serve to stimulate virus expression, and recently GM-CSF was shown to induce expression of HIV in a chronically infected cloned promonocytic cell line that did not constitutively express virus.[78]

The cell types infected by HIV may also play an important role in dictating levels and patterns of virus expression. Monocytes and macrophages are known to harbor HIV-1 *in vivo* during natural infection and are likely to play an important role in disease pathogenesis.[82–85] Monocytes/macrophages are relatively resistant to the cytopathic effects of HIV and appear to be the major cell infected by HIV within the central nervous system of infected individuals.[86–88] For visna virus, the monocyte/macrophage has been shown to play a critical role in the dissemination of virus throughout multiple organ systems and in maintaining viral persistence.[89] At the present time, the multitude of viral and host factors that determine rates of viral replication, establishment of latency, and determinants of persistence are just beginning to be addressed.

Cell Tropism

The hallmark of AIDS is a selective depletion of CD4-bearing helper/inducer lymphocytes. This defect is believed to result largely from a selective tropism of HIV-

1 for this population of cells that is based on the affinity of the viral gp120 envelope protein for the CD4 molecule on the target cell. A structure–function representation of the HIV-1 envelope is shown in Figure 2-6.

Early studies of HIV-1 indicated that the virus appeared to replicate selectively in CD4[+] lymphocytes,[90] and subsequent studies showed that infection by HIV-1, and syncytia induction by HIV-1–bearing cells, could be blocked by monoclonal antibodies directed against specific epitopes of the OKT4 (CD4) molecule.[47-49] McDougal showed that binding of HIV-1 to CD4[+] cells involved the formation of a complex between the CD4 molecule and gp120, and immunoprecipitation of either molecule co-precipitated the other.[46] Subsequently, Maddon and colleagues demonstrated that HELA cells

(human cervical endothelial carcinoma cells) that do not normally express the CD4 antigen are resistent to HIV-1 infection, but when the CD4 gene is transfected into these cells and CD4 is expressed on the cell surface they become susceptible to HIV-1 infection.[50] Lasky and co-workers have gone on to show by direct measurements of affinity constants that the gp120 envelope protein and CD4 molecule form a high-affinity complex with a dissociation constant of approximately 4×10^{-9} M.[45] Following binding to the CD4 molecule, HIV is internalized and uncoded. The mechanism of virus entry into the target cell is presently unclear, although it was suggested that receptor-mediated endocytosis may play a role in this process.[50] More recently, it has been demonstrated that the pH-independent fusion of the HIV-1

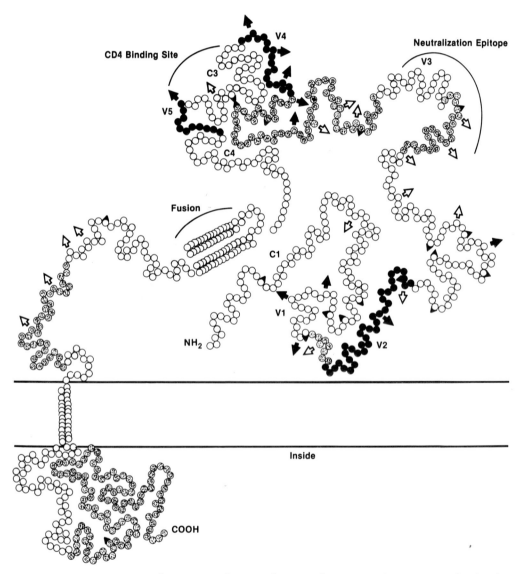

FIG. 2-6. Structure-function domains of HIV-1 envelope. See text for details.

envelope with the cell membrane is required for virus entry.[91] In addition, it has been shown that mouse cells that are transfected with the CD4 gene and express human CD4 on their surface are able to bind HIV-1 efficiently but do not become productively infected.[50] This suggests that other proteins expressed in the human cell are required for steps subsequent to virus binding.

A variety of cell types besides helper/inducer lymphocytes are now known to express the T4 (CD4) molecule. These include monocytes,[92] follicular dendritic cells,[93] Langerhans cells,[94] and possibly other cell types within the central nervous system.[50,95,96] These cells generally express smaller amounts of CD4 on their surface, and the corresponding cytopathic effect typically found with CD4[+] lymphocytes and lymphoid cell lines are not generally observed. In naturally infected individuals, it has been shown that their monocytes are infected with HIV-1 *in vivo*.[82,85] It has been speculated that HIV infection of monocytes and macrophages may result in defective chemotaxis; altered monokine production; enhanced release of interleukin-1 (IL-1), tumor necrosis factor (cachectin), or other pyrogens, and by this means lead to certain aspects of HIV infection including impaired pulmonary resistance to opportunistic disease and the wasting syndrome frequently present in end-stage diseases.

Within the central nervous system of affected humans, it appears that the predominant cell type infected with HIV is the monocyte/macrophage.[86–88,97] It was previously demonstrated by simultaneous *in situ* hybridization and immunohistochemical staining that HIV-1 mRNA was expressed selectively in multinucleated giant cells that also exhibited monocyte markers.[86] Other studies have also reported infection of mononuclear cells and multinucleated giant cells as well as endothelial cells and rarely astrocytes and neurons.[86–88,98–100] One possibility is that the virus enters the brain through infected monocytes and stimulates the release of monokines, enzymes, or other factors that are either toxic to neurons directly or lead to infiltration of brain with inflammatory cells. Interesting, but of unknown significance, is that the gp120 envelope glycoprotein of HIV has been shown to inhibit the growth of neurons in the presence of neuroleukin but not in the presence of nerve growth factor.[101] It was postulated, based on these experimental results and based on the observed partial sequence homology between gp120 and neuroleukin, that this inhibition of growth could be due to a competitive interaction by the HIV envelope.

Mechanisms of Cytopathicity

Although the hallmark of AIDS infection clinically is a progressive deterioration of immune competence due to progressive loss of CD4[+] helper/inducer lymphocytes,[23,102] and although HIV has been shown to have a direct cytopathic effect for these same cells *in vitro*[25,26,33] the precise mechanism(s) responsible for the cyto-

pathic, or cell killing, effects of HIV-1 in both instances are not entirely clear. Studies by Fisher and Wong–Staal using transfected HIV-1 proviral DNA have shown conclusively that the HIV-1 genome alone contains all necessary information to generate infectious, replication-competent, and profoundly cytopathic virus that is selective for CD4[+] cells.[33] Thus, there is no question that HIV-1 alone can have direct cytopathic activity on CD4[+] lymphocytes and lead to their destruction. It is also clear that envelope expression by the virus and CD4 expression by the target cell are critical determinants of cytopathicity. High-level HIV envelope expression on infected cells (manifest as cell-surface gp120) results in cell fusion with neighboring uninfected T4 cells by direct binding of a gp120–CD4 complex.[103–106] Such syncytia can be comprised of literally hundreds of infected and uninfected cells. Following the initial attachment phase mediated by the gp120–CD4 interaction, it is believed that the cell fusion process is mediated by a different domain on the HIV envelope, probably located in the transmembrane region. It has been shown that syncytia formation can occur when the envelope gene of HIV-1 alone is transfected and expressed on T4[+] cells.[106] It has also recently been shown that the carbohydrate moieties are required for this interaction.[103] Syncytia formation, however, is unlikely to be the major pathway for cell loss. Some cell lines (e.g., ATH8) do not form syncytia but are highly susceptible to the cytopathic effect. Conversely, cells infected by some mutant viruses undergo extensive syncytia without long-term cytopathology. gp120 and CD4 on the same cell surface or within the endoplasmic reticulum–golgi apparatus could bind and result either directly or indirectly in cell injury.[107]

In vivo, additional biologic mechanisms may be responsible for the T4 cell loss throughout the course of disease. It has been shown that only a very small proportion of circulating T4[+] lymphocytes (less than 1 in 1000) express HIV-1 mRNA or proteins at any one point in time during the course of disease, yet there is clearly a progressive and eventually total destruction of this cell type. While it has been speculated that a greater proportion of this cell type may actually be infected latently with HIV-1 (proviral infection without gene expression), this number cannot be very high since Southern blot hybridization studies that have a sensitivity of one viral DNA molecule detectable in 100 cells do not generally show evidence of HIV-1 DNA.[108] The progressive recruitment of T4 cells to form syncytia with HIV-1 expressing cells in blood, lymph node, and other tissues, as discussed above, could conceivably lead to substantial T4 cell loss. In addition, it has been shown that cell-free gp120 can adsorb to T4[+] cells and there serve as an effective antigen for mediating antibody-dependent cell-mediated cytotoxicity. A variety of other mechanisms for T4 cell-killing have also been postulated, including autoimmune phenomena directed against infected lymphocytes, terminal differentiation of infected lymphocytes, and increased susceptibility to other pathogens, although the importance of the processes remains to be demonstrated. An interesting possibility is that autoimmunization with MHC class-II-like antigens could lead to autoimmune recognition and destruction of host cells. This is because the CD4 molecule recognizes a portion of the class-II MHC complex during normal immune responses and since the HIV-1 envelope also binds to the CD4 molecule, it may mimic the configuration of a portion of the class-II MHC molecule. Antibodies and cytotoxic lymphocytes elicited against the HIV-1 envelope then could conceivably cross-react with class-II MHC antigens, thereby leading to autoimmunity against host cells. Again, the significance of this potential mechanism of lymphocyte destruction remains to be determined.

Genetic Variation of HIV-1

One of the most striking properties of the HIV-1 genome is the extent of variability that exists among independent virus isolates.[72,108–121] This property may be of considerable relevance to many aspects of the biology of HIV, including tissue and cell type specificity, clinical spectrum of disease pathogenesis, geographic and temporal distribution of virus, differential viral susceptibility to immune response, virulence, and importantly, the development of a broadly cross-reactive vaccine. Heterogeneity in the genomes of different HIV isolates has been assessed by several approaches: restriction enzyme analysis of uncloned DNA of infected cells or tissues from patients, restriction enzyme analysis of cloned viral genomes, heteroduplex analysis by electron microscopy, and nucleotide sequence comparisons. The first molecular descriptions of HIV-1 were based on Southern blot hybridizations of independent virus isolates.[72,108,114–116,120] It became clear from the earliest of these studies that isolates of HIV-1 from different individuals had restriction enzyme patterns that were distinguishable. Whereas the viral DNA molecules present in isolates of DNA from individuals from widely disparate geographic regions all hybridized to the same prototype HIV-1 viral DNA probe under conditions of high stringency, restriction endonuclease cleavage patterns of these viruses were quite distinct. Many of these independent virus isolates differed from each other by more than 50% of their restriction endonuclease cleavage sites. Once molecularly cloned proviruses were available, electron microscopic heteroduplex analysis was performed.[115] Full-length clones of two divergent HIV-1 viruses (BH10 and HAT3) were annealed under conditions of increasing stringency, and substitution loops first appeared in the envelope region of the heteroduplexed molecules. This was the first indication that the envelope gene of HIV-1 was more variable than other genes. Subsequently, nucleotide sequence determinations were obtained for a number of independent virus isolates, and these confirmed the nucleotide sequence divergence previously inferred from restriction enzyme analyses and heteroduplex studies.[72,108–121] Sequence comparisons demonstrated that the distribution of sequence differences among different viral genomes were not evenly distributed throughout the proviruses. For example, the extracellular envelope region of two HIV-1 isolates from the United States (BH10 and ARV2) differed by 11.4% in nucleotide sequence and 17.0% in amino acid sequence, whereas the *gag* regions of both viruses differed by only 5.6% in nucleotide sequence and 6.3% in amino acid sequence.[113] In general, the extracellular envelope region and the 3' *orf* region are more variable among independent virus isolates than are LTR, *gag, pol, sor,* R, *tat,* or *art/trs* regions. Not only are genes such as *gag* and *pol* more highly conserved generally, but the types of nucleotide and amino acid changes seen in these regions are different from those found in the envelope.[113] In *gag* and *pol,* most nucleotide sequence changes are due to point mutations, whereas in the envelope there are clustered changes involving in-frame deletions, insertions, and duplications. Furthermore, the majority of changes in *gag* and *pol* are in the third base pair position of codons. Within envelope, more than half of the single nucleotide changes occur in the first or second codon position, resulting in nonsilent mutations. Even third-position changes in envelope frequently lead to amino acid changes. These findings suggest two possible interpretations that are not mutually exclusive: first, there is stronger structure–function constraint for protein sequence conservation in *gag* and *pol* than in envelope, and second, there may be a positive selection for nonsilent nucleotide changes in envelope. Such a selective pressure could be immunologic or nonimmunologic in nature.

Despite the extreme variability of the HIV-1 envelope, there are regions that are highly conserved and presumed to play important biologic functions. All 18 cysteine residues located within the extracellular region of the envelope and most cysteines located in gp41 are conserved in most viruses.[122] This finding argues that the cysteine residues are necessary to maintain the envelope in proper three-dimensional structural configuration. There are also several highly conserved regions previously identified as C-1 through C-4 that are interspersed with regions of hypervariability (V1–V5) within the extracellular envelope region. Recently, Lasky and others have identified a region within the HIV-1 extracellular envelope protein defined by monoclonal antibodies that block gp120–CD4 binding that are involved directly in the interaction between CD4 and gp120.[45] Independently, Sodroski and associates[43] have utilized linker-insertion mutagenesis to identify three nonlinear regions within the HIV-1 gp120 envelope that are also involved in gp120–CD4 binding, and one of these includes the domain identified by Lasky. These findings argue that a conformational epitope comprised of domains within the carboxy-terminal third of the gp120 envelope molecule of HIV-1 is involved in CD4 binding. Rusche and colleagues[123] have also identified within the carboxy-terminal region of gp120 a major epitope that elicits fusion-inhibiting antibodies (neutralizing antibodies) that are type-specific in nature. These structures are illustrated diagrammatically in Figure 2-6. On-going studies relating structure to function within the HIV-1 envelope will continue to utilize parallel studies of envelope variability to identify biologically important domains.

In the last 2 years, considerable work has also been done examining the extent and nature of HIV-1 genetic variation in naturally infected individuals.[116] In one study, genetic variation of HIV-1 was ascertained by sequentially isolating virus from persistently infected individuals over a 2-year period and subjecting these virus isolates to Southern blot genomic analysis, molecular cloning, and nucleotide sequencing (Fig. 2-7). This study showed that nucleotide changes were detected throughout the genomes of viruses isolated from single individuals and consisted of isolated and clustered nucleotide point mutations as well as short deletions, insertions, and duplications. From genomic mapping studies and nucleotide sequence comparisons, it appeared that viruses isolated sequentially had actually evolved in parallel from common progenitor viruses. The rate of evolution of HIV-1 in these persistently infected patients was estimated to be at least 10^{-3} nucleotide substitutions per site per year for the envelope gene and 10^{-4} for the *gag* gene,[116] values similar to those recently obtained for visna virus and EIAV.[124,125,128]

There is thus considerable evidence for rapid genetic change of HIV-1 *in vivo* based on analysis of independent isolates of the virus and based on sequential isolates of HIV-1 from persistently infected persons. Notwithstanding these earlier studies of HIV-1 variation during natural infection, the spectrum of HIV-1 variation in chronically infected individuals, the mechanisms underlying this variation, and its biologic consequences still remain largely unknown. To address this question, Saag and co-workers have analyzed at a molecular level sequential virus isolates from two of the infected individuals (RJS and WMF) shown in Figure 2-7.[126] Recombinant λ phage libraries of one RJS isolate (RJS4) and two WMF isolates (WMF1 and WMF3) were prepared so that the viral DNA molecules that *in toto* comprise the hybridization patterns of the overall isolate DNA could be dissected and analyzed individually. Totals of 27, 17, and 18 full-length HIV-1 clones were obtained from the three libraries. A summary of the restriction patterns of distinguishable clones from one of these libraries is shown in Figure 2-8. Careful restriction enzyme mapping using 11 endonucleases revealed that 17 of the 27 RJS4 clones, 10 of the 17 WMF1 clones, and 13 of the 18 WMF3 clones were distinguishable by unique cleavage patterns. The remarkably large number of distinguishable viral clones within each isolate resulted from various combinations of restriction site polymorphisms distributed throughout the viral genomes.

Inspection of the genomic restriction patterns of the HIV-1 clones in Figure 2-8 showed that clones from

an individual virus isolate (RJS4a-q) were considerably more similar to other clones within that isolate than to unrelated clones such as HXB2, LAV-Mal, LAV-Eli, ARV2, and WMJ1. In order to quantify objectively the extent of similarity among the different viral clones, a pairwise comparison of the percentage of restriction site differences between each of the viral genotypes shown in Figure 1-8 was performed (Fig. 2-9). Such an analysis of restriction site differences among related clones is a valid means for estimating overall nucleotide sequence variability. Assuming the loss of a restriction site in otherwise highly related genomes results from a change in a single nucleotide, a 50% difference in restriction sites when using enzymes that recognize 6 base pair sequences corresponds to approximately 8% nucleotide sequence difference (i.e., 1 nucleotide change out of every 12 nucleotides sampled). This approach was used first to analyze clones of HIV-1 for which nucleotide sequence information is available, and the correlation between nucleotide sequence differences and restriction site differences was found to be quite good. For example, clone HXB2 differs from clones BH10, ARV2, and LAV-Eli by 13%, 41%, and 62% in restriction sites[116] (see Fig. 2-9). Based on these restriction site differences, the predicted nucleotide differences would be 2.2%, 6.8%, and 10.5%. The actual differences determined by nucleotide sequence comparisons are 1.6%, 5.8%, and 9.7%, respectively. Clones of LAV-Mal, LAV-Eli, and ARV2 differ from each other by 58% to 70% in restriction sites (see Fig. 2-9) and by 10.1% to 13.0% in nucleotide sequence. The viral DNA genomes comprising isolate RJS4 (and isolates WMF1 and WMF3, which are not shown) were considerably more similar to other viral genomes from within the same isolate than to viral genomes from unrelated (independent) isolates. For example, the 17 different RJS4 genotypes varied from each other by 3% to 28% (mean 13%), whereas the same clones varied from independent viruses by 41% to 70% (mean 55%; p < 0.0001).

The results summarized here indicate that genotypic variation of HIV-1 *in vivo* is rapid and extensive, that numerous variant viral forms coexist over time within the same patient, and that "isolates" of HIV-1 actually consist of complex mixtures of genotypically distinct, albeit related, viruses. The data also indicate that during natural infection by HIV-1, different viral genomes evolve in *parallel* and result in the emergence and persistence of multiple distinct genotypic forms. Importantly, while considerable genotypic diversity of viruses exists within a given isolate, these multiple distinguishable viral forms have all clearly evolved from one another, or from common precursor viruses, and do *not* represent concomitant infection by unrelated (independent) viruses. The possible molecular mechanisms underlying this extensive genetic variability of HIV-1 have been discussed.[113,116,117] A model for HIV-1 variation is shown in Figure 2-10.

Variation of HIV-1 has parallels in other lentiviral systems including EIAV, visna virus, and simian im-

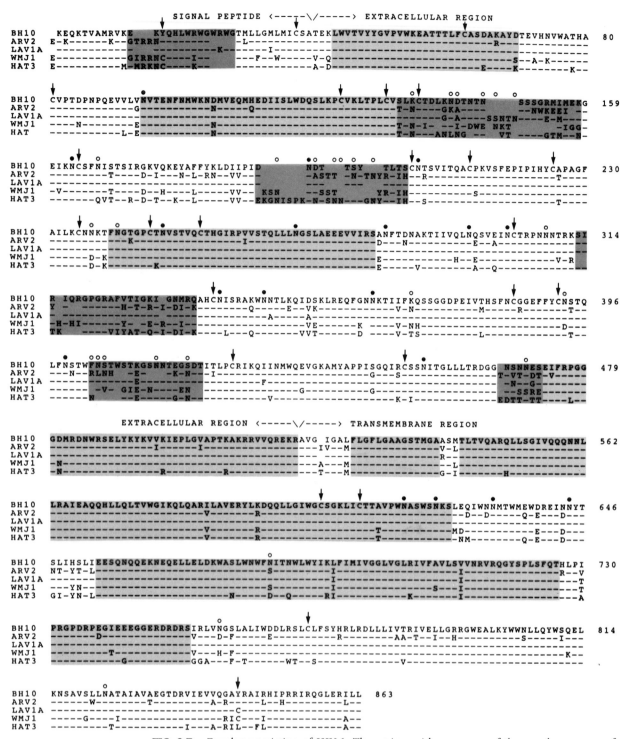

FIG. 2-7. Envelope variation of HIV-1. The amino acid sequences of the envelope genes of five independent AIDS virus isolates are shown. Alignment of sequences was performed pairwise with the assistance of PRTALN. Numbering of amino acids is from the first amino acid of BH10, and regions corresponding to the signal peptide, extracellular envelope glycoprotein (gp120), and transmembrane glycoprotein (gp41) are shown. *Dashes* indicate amino acid identity with BH10 and spaces indicate the absence of that amino acid. *Arrows* denote cysteine residues and *solid* or *open circles* denote conserved and non-conserved sites of potential *N*-linked glycosyla-

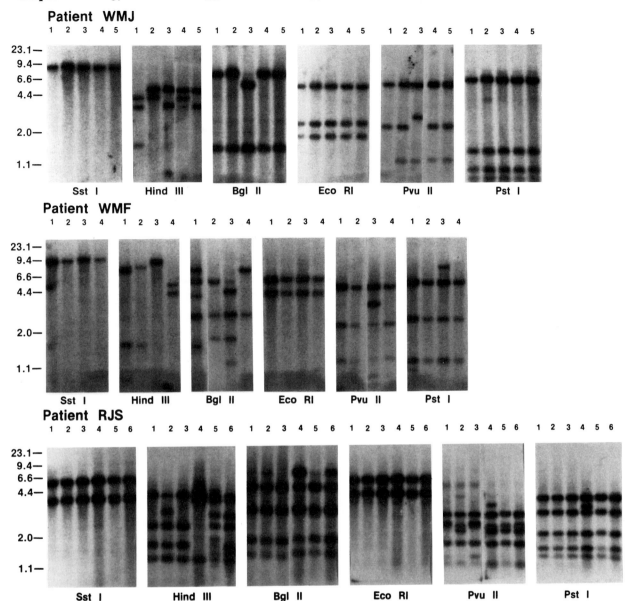

FIG. 2-8. Southern blot hybridization analysis of sequential HIV-1 isolates. Virus was isolated from mononuclear cells from peripheral blood and propagated in tissue culture. The sequential virus isolates were obtained from patients WMJ, WMF, and RJS over a 1- to 2-year period. (Figure reproduced with permission from Hahn BH, Shaw GM, Taylor ME, et al: Genetic variation in HTLV-III/LAV over time in patients with AIDS or at risk for AIDS. Science 232:1548, 1986)

tion, respectively. Darkly shaded regions within the extracellular envelope glycoprotein correspond to regions of hypervariability. Lightly shaded regions correspond to areas that are relatively highly conserved. (Figure reproduced with permission from Starcich BR, Hahn BH, Shaw GM, et al: Identification and characterization of conserved and variable regions in the envelope gene of HTLV-III/LAV, the retrovirus of AIDS. Cell 45:637, 1986)

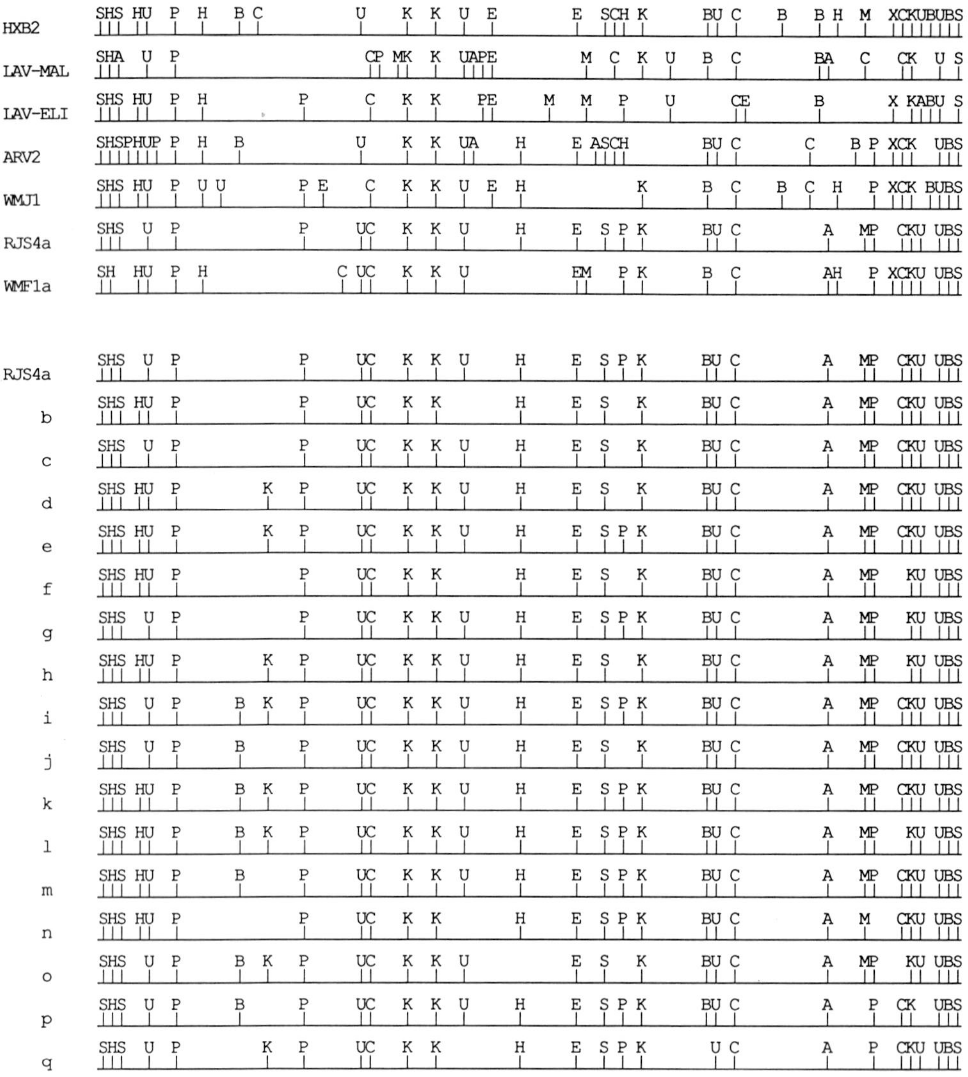

FIG. 2-9. Restriction endonuclease cleavage patterns for seven independent HIV-1 viral clones (HXB2; LAV/MAL; LAV/ELI; ARV2; WMJ1; RJS4a; WMF1a) and for seventeen distinguishable clones from isolate RJS4. The restriction enzymes mapped include E-EcoRI; S-SstI; X-XhoI; B-BglII; U-PvuII; H-HindIII; P-PstI; K-KpnI; M-BamHI; C-CvnI; A-XbaI. See text for details.

munodeficiency virus (SIV).[127–130] For EIAV, it is clear that genotypic changes are responsible for biologically important alterations in viral antigenicity that allow the virus to elude host immune defenses.[127–129] For visna, the significance of antigenic variation is less clear.[130] In the SIV system, a virus strain has recently been isolated from a pigtailed macaque that possesses altered biologic and antigenic properties leading to a broader host range and a rapid, fatal immunodeficiency syndrome several weeks after inoculation.* There are indications that genotypic variation in HIV-1 is similarly associated with potentially important biologic differences among variant forms. These findings are especially intriguing in light of recent findings by Mullins and associates[31] who showed that the envelope/LTR region of a replication-defective variant of FeLV, when introduced into a replication-competent construct of FeLV, was responsible for inducing a highly reproducible fatal immunodeficiency illness in cats. Furthermore, Gartner and Popovic have shown that some isolates of HIV-1 preferentially replicate in mononuclear phagocytes, whereas others show preference for T-lymphocytes,[85] and Koyanagi and Chen have identified genotypically distinct viral forms of HIV-1 in a patient with pronounced central nervous system dysfunction that could be distinguished by their replicative activity in mononuclear phagocytes and brain

* Fultz P: Personal communication

	HXB2	LAV-MAL	LAV-ELI	ARV2	WMJ1	RJS4 a	b	c	d	e	f	g	h	i	j	k	l	m	n	o	p	q
HXB2	—	63	62	41	49	46																
LAV-MAL	63	—	58	68	63	61																
LAV-ELI	62	58	—	70	58	67																
ARV2	41	68	70	—	55	49																
WMJ1	49	63	58	55	—	49																
RJS4 a	46	61	67	49	49	—	11	04	11	07	15	04	15	07	07	10	14	07	12	18	08	15
b						11	—	08	07	11	04	15	11	07	11	11	14	17	11	08	18	22	19
c						04	08	—	11	11	12	12	11	11	04	14	17	11	15	15	15	19
d						11	07	11	—	04	11	14	04	10	11	07	10	10	14	14	21	18
e						07	11	11	04	—	14	11	07	07	14	03	07	07	11	17	17	14
f						15	04	12	11	14	—	12	08	21	15	17	14	14	12	19	25	22
g						04	15	12	14	11	12	—	11	11	11	14	11	11	15	15	15	19
h						15	11	11	04	07	08	11	—	14	14	10	07	14	18	11	24	21
i						17	17	11	10	07	21	11	14	—	07	03	07	07	11	11	11	14
j						07	11	04	11	14	15	11	14	07	—	10	14	07	18	11	11	21
k						10	14	07	03	17	14	10	03	10	—	03	03	14	14	14	17
l						14	17	17	10	07	14	11	07	07	14	03	—	07	17	11	17	21
m						07	11	11	10	07	14	11	14	07	07	03	07	—	11	17	11	21
n						12	08	15	14	11	12	15	18	17	18	14	17	11	—	28	21	19
o						18	18	15	14	17	19	15	11	11	14	11	17	28	—	21	25
p						08	22	15	21	17	25	15	24	11	11	14	17	11	21	21	—	19
q						15	19	19	18	14	22	19	21	14	21	17	21	21	19	25	19	—

FIG. 2-10. Analysis of variation among viral DNA clones of HIV-1 isolate RJS4 and the independent virus isolates HXB2, LAV/MAL, LAV/ELI, ARV2, WMJ1, and RJS. Each of the different viral clone patterns depicted in Figure 2-9 was compared pairwise to every other clone pattern, and the percentage difference in restriction endonuclease cleavage sites between each pair was calculated as follows:

$$\frac{A + B}{C} \times 100 = \% \text{ restriction site differences}$$

where *A* equals the number of restriction sites present in one clone (*X*) that are missing in the other clone (*Y*); *B* equals the number of restriction sites in clone *Y* that are missing in clone *X*; *C* equals the total number of restriction sites present in clones *X* and *Y* combined with identical sites in the pair counted only once. See text for details.

glioma explant cultures.[132] The results of studies of HIV-1 variation demonstrate the extreme plasticity of the HIV-1 genome as a genetic substrate for important biologic variation, including cell tropism, virulence, and antigenicity. The observation that HIV-1 "isolates" generally consist of complex mixtures of genotypically distinct viruses is in keeping with the general concept of RNA viruses as "quasi-species."[133] Experiments examining the genetic, biologic, and immunologic properties of HIV-1 will need to account for this extensive genotypic heterogeneity, and in some instances may require the use of biologically or molecularly cloned viruses.

HUMAN IMMUNODEFICIENCY VIRUS TYPE 2

HIV-1 is the etiologic agent of epidemic AIDS in Central Africa, Europe, the United States, and most other countries worldwide. The geographic origin of HIV-1, and of the current AIDS epidemic, is believed to be Central Africa since clinical syndromes indicative of AIDS were retrospectively recognized there as early as the mid-1970s and serum samples taken in Africa at that time and before contained antibodies reactive with HIV-1.[4,6,134] Although genetic variability of HIV-1, especially in its envelope gene, is recognized as a characteristic property of the virus, it is clear that independent isolates of HIV-1 from Central Africa, Europe, and the United States all constitute a single viral species, distinct from other retroviruses. Evidence for a second major group of human immunodeficiency–associated retroviruses came from a report by Barin and others that human populations, like wild-caught African green monkeys, had serum antibodies that reacted more strongly with a simian immunodeficiency virus than with HIV-1[135-137] Reasoning that human immunodeficiency viruses could be phylogenetically related to simian viruses, these investigators used immunoblot and radioimmunoprecipitation techniques to screen sera from human and monkey populations for a reactivity to HIV-1 and to a related simian retrovirus, SIV_{mac}, discovered earlier in captive rhesus monkeys (*Macaca mulatta*) with AIDS-like illness.[138] Wild-caught African green monkeys and Senegalese people who had increased risk for sexually transmitted disease showed strong serologic reactivity to a virus more closely related to SIV_{mac} than to HIV-1. Subsequently, these investigators reported the isolation of T-lymphotropic retroviruses from healthy Senegalese West Africans (HTLV-4) and from African green monkeys (STLV-3).[136,139] Considerable controversy has surrounded these early studies since the viruses isolated from co-cultures of human and African green monkey blood were genetically indistinguishable from previous isolates of SIV_{mac} (in particular, isolate SIV_{mac}-251). It is now generally recognized that these early "HTLV-4" and "STLV-3/AGM" isolates represent laboratory contaminations with SIV_{mac}-251.[140] Nonetheless, the results of the serologic studies of West African populations using the SIV_{mac} antigen preparations identified correctly patients who were infected with what has subsequently been shown to be a T-lymphotropic human virus related to SIV (HIV-2). Working independently, Clavel and co-workers reported the isolation of a retrovirus termed HIV-2 from patients in Guinea Bissau and Cape Verde.[141-143] Antigenically, the HIV-2 virus was cross-reactive with HIV-1 only in the major core protein p24/p25 and slightly in the polymerase protein, whereas it was considerably more related to SIV_{mac}. At the level of nucleotide sequence, HIV-2 was also shown to be more related to SIV_{mac} than to HIV-1. HIV-2 and SIV_{mac} share approximately 75% overall nucleotide sequence homology, and each is only distantly related to HIV-1, sharing approximately 40% homology.[144,145]

Like HIV-1 and SIV_{mac}, HIV-2 is bounded by terminally redundant LTR sequences and contains *gag, pol,* and *env* genes. (Fig. 2-11). Like the other two viruses, HIV-2 also contains open reading frames for *tat, art/trs, sor, 3' orf,* and R. However, unlike HIV-1, both HIV-

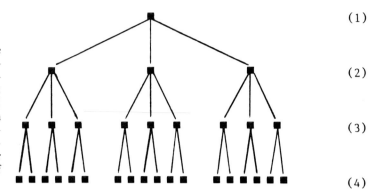

FIG. 2-11. Model of genetic variation of HIV-1. The experimental observation that individuals are persistently infected by a group of highly related yet distinguishable and changing viral genotypes[126] suggests that individuals are naturally infected by only a very limited number of viruses that undergo substantial variation in their genomic sequences over time. That host factors, including immunologic responses, may exert selective pressures for genetic and biologic change over time is currently a hypothesis relevant to studies of disease pathogenesis and vaccine development.

2 and SIV$_{mac}$ contain an additional reading frame within their central region termed X. This potential open-reading frame overlaps the *sor* gene on its 5′ end. The X open-reading frame is 336 nucleotides long and could encode a protein of 112 amino acids. Although not present in HIV-1, the X regions in HIV-2 and SIV$_{mac}$ are very highly conserved, having 94 of 112 deduced amino acids conserved. Recent studies using X-specific heteroantisera have shown that the X open-reading frame does in fact encode a protein of approximately 12 kD to 14 kD that is expressed in infected cells and is present in mature virions.[146,147] Whereas the function of the novel X protein is currently unknown, the function of the other open-reading frames in HIV-2 that are also present in HIV-1 is expected to be analogous.

Interestingly, there are some reports that the HIV-2 group of viruses, although clearly a causative agent of some cases of fatal immunodeficiency, may be less pathogenic in some populations than is HIV-1.[137] This conclusion has been based on large-scale seroepidemiologic studies that failed to link HIV-2 seropositivity with signs and symptoms of clinical immunodeficiency. Interestingly, a recent isolate of HIV-2 (ST) has been shown to be attenuated in its cytopathicity in comparison with prototype strains of HIV-1 and HIV-2,[148] suggesting that naturally occurring forms of human immunodeficiency viruses may exist that have attenuated virulence and be associated with less severe forms of immunodeficiency in certain patient populations. Consistent with this is the observation that HIV-2 does not appear to be spreading within at-risk populations as rapidly as has HIV-1. On the other hand, there is an increasing number of reports identifying HIV-2 viruses as the cause of fatal immunodeficiency in West Africa and other countries, and thus the true spectrum of HIV-2 virulence patterns remains to be determined.

EVOLUTION OF HUMAN IMMUNODEFICIENCY VIRUSES

The evolutionary origins of human immunodeficiency viruses are currently not known. The rapid accumulation of nucleotide sequence information from immunodeficiency viruses originating in simian and human species, however, promises to provide important insight into the phylogeny of these important viral pathogens. Clinically, AIDS was first recognized in the United States in 1981 some years after the virus was introduced into the population, and blood samples collected in the United States and Europe before the mid-1970s generally lacked evidence of anti-HIV-1 antibodies. On the other hand, the earliest serologic response to HIV-1 found in stored blood is from samples from Zaire dating to 1959.[134] Serologic and clinical evidence suggests that HIV-1 infection began to spread epidemically in urban areas of Central Africa during the mid and late 1970s, and in retrospect, cases of AIDS in African individuals from that period are now recognized.[6,149–151] In contrast, the spread of HIV-1 in rural areas of Africa appears not to have changed substantially during that same time period. For example, there was a ten-fold increase in HIV-1 seroprevalence documented in pregnant women in an urban area of Zaire (Kinshasha) between 1970 and 1980, but the prevalence of HIV-1 antibodies in a rural area of the same country remained unchanged at 0.8% between the years 1976 and 1986.[152] This is strong evidence that HIV-1 has existed in Central Africa for a long time, that the rate of HIV-1 transmission is related to social and economic factors and the disruption of traditional life-styles, and that once introduced into populations where individuals were likely to have multiple sexual partners or be exposed to blood products, the virus spread rapidly and became clinically apparent.

Nucleic acid sequence comparisons of independent isolates of HIV-1 obtained from Africa, Haiti, Europe, and the United States, and from sequential virus isolations from individual patients, has demonstrated the rate of evolution of the virus to be on the order of 10^{-3} nucleotide substitutions per site per year.[116] Similar rates of variation have been documented for other retroviruses such as visna[125] and EIAV.[128] Two other immunodeficiency viruses, HIV-2 and SIV$_{mac}$, have also been examined at the nucleotide sequence level and shown to be approximately 75% similar to each other, whereas each is approximately 40% similar to HIV-1.[144,145] That HIV-2 and SIV$_{mac}$ are nearly equally divergent from HIV-1 and more similar to each other in genomic organiza-

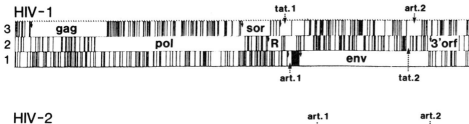

FIG. 2-12. Comparative genomic organization of HIV-1, HIV-2, and SIV$_{mac}$. See text for details.

tion (Fig. 2-12) suggests that HIV-2 and SIV$_{mac}$ evolved from a common ancestral virus, which in turn had common origins with HIV-1. Comparison of independent isolates of HIV-2 indicates that they are as divergent as different HIV-1 isolates.[148,153] Preliminary studies on isolates and clones of SIV obtained from wild-caught African green monkeys suggest that SIV$_{agm}$ is evolutionarily quite divergent from SIV$_{mac}$, HIV-2, and HIV-1 providing further complexity to the study of the evolution of these viruses.[153] Isolation of additional related viruses from human and simian populations and characterization of their genomes and biologic properties will aid considerably the elucidation of the phylogeny of these important human pathogens. Another question still to be answered is what will be the long-range biologic consequences of high mutational rates of human immunodeficiency viruses that continue to spread epidemically in many populations throughout the world.

REFERENCES

1. Gottlieb MS, Schroff R, Schanker HM et al: Pneumocystis carinii pneumonia and mucosal candidiasis in previously healthy homosexual men: Evidence of a new acquired cellular immunodeficiency. N Engl J Med 305:1425, 1981
2. Pneumocystis pneumonia. Los Angeles. Morbid Mortal Week Rept 30:250, 1981
3. Coolfont report: A PHS plan for prevention and control of AIDS and the AIDS virus. Public Health Report 101:341, 1986
4. Curran JW, Jaffe WH, Hardy AM et al: Epidemiology of HIV infection and AIDS in the United States. Science 239:610, 1988
5. Hessol, NA: Presentation at the Third International Conference on AIDS, Washington, DC, June 1987
6. Piot P, Plummer LFA, Mhalu FS et al: AIDS: An international perspective. Science 239:573, 1988
7. Ellerman V, Bang O: Experimentelle leukemie bei Huhnern. Zentralbl Bakteriol Mikrobiol Hyg 46:595, 1908
8. Rous P: A sarcoma of the fowl transmissible by an agent separable from the tumor cells. J Exp Med 13:397, 1911
9. Gross L: "Spontaneous" leukemia developing in C3H mice following inoculation, in infancy, with AK-leukemic extracts, or AK-embryos. Proc Soc Exp Biol Med 78:27, 1951
10. Weiss R, Teich N, Varmus H et al: (eds): RNA Tumor Viruses, 2nd ed. Cold Spring Harbor, NY, Cold Spring Harbor Laboratory, 1982
11. Jarrett W, Crawford E, Martin W et al: Leukaemias in the cat: A virus-like particle associated with leukaemia (lymphosarcoma). Nature 202:567, 1964
12. Hardy WD, Geering G, Old LJ et al: Feline leukemia virus: Occurrence of viral antigen in the tissues of cats with lymphosarcoma and other diseases. Science 166:1019, 1969
13. Temin HM, Mitzutani S: RNA-directed DNA polymerase in virions of Rous sarcoma virus. Nature 226:1211, 1970
14. Baltimore D: RNA-dependent DNA polymerase in virions of RNA tumor viruses. Nature 226:1209, 1970
15. Hill M, Hillova J: C r Acad Sci Paris 272D:3094, 1971
16. Sarngadharan MG, Allandeen HS, Gallo RC: Reverse transcriptase of RNA tumor viruses and animal cells. Meth Cancer Res 12:3, 1976
17. Morgan DA, Ruscetti FW, Gallo RC: Selective in vitro growth of T-lymphocytes from normal human bone marrows. Science 193:1007, 1976
18. Poiesz BJ, Ruscetti FW, Gazdar AF et al: Detection and isolation of type C retrovirus particles from fresh and cultured lymphocytes of a patient with cutaneous T-cell lymphoma. Proc Natl Acad Sci USA 77:7415, 1980
19. Poiesz BJ, Ruscetti FW, Reitz MS et al: Isolation of a new

type-C retrovirus (HTLV) in primary uncultured cells of a patient with Sezary T-cell leukemia. Nature 294:268, 1981

20. Gallo RC: Human T-cell leukaemia-lymphoma virus and T-cell malignancies in adults. Cancer Surv 3:113, 1984
21. Gallo RC: The first human retrovirus. Sci Am 255:88, 1986
22. Kalyanaraman VS, Sarngadharan MG, Robert–Guroff M et al: A new subtype of human T-cell leukemia virus (HTLV-II) associated with a T-cell variant of hairy cell leukemia. Science 218:571, 1982
23. Gallo RC: The AIDS virus. Sci Am 256:46, 1987
24. Wong–Staal F, Gallo RC: Human T-lymphotropic retroviruses. Nature 317:395, 1985
25. Barre-Sinoussi F, Chermann JC, Rey F et al: Isolation of a T-lymphotropic retrovirus from a patient at risk for acquired immune deficiency syndrome (AIDS). Science 220:868, 1983
26. Popovic M, Sarngadharan MG, Read E et al: Detection, isolation, and continuous production of cytopathic retroviruses (HTLV-III) from patients with AIDS and pre-AIDS. Science 224:497, 1984
27. Gallo RC, Salahuddin SZ, Popivic M et al: Frequent detection and isolation of cytopathic retroviruses (HTLV-III) from patients with AIDS and at risk for AIDS. Science 224:500, 1984
28. Sarngadharan MG, Popovic M, Bruch L et al: Antibodies reactive with a human T lymphotropic retrovirus (HTLV-III) in the sera of patients with acquired immune deficiency syndrome. Science 224:506
29. Schupbach J, Popovic M, Gilden R et al: Serologic analysis of a new type of human T-lymphotropic retrovirus (HTLV-III) associated with AIDS. Science 224:504, 1984
30. Coffin JM, Haase A, Levy JA et al: Human immunodeficiency viruses. Science 232:697, 1986
31. Salahuddin SZ, Markham PD, Popovic M et al: Isolation of infectious human T-cell leukemia/lymphotropic virus type III (HTLV-III) from patients with acquired immunodeficiency syndrome (AIDS) or AIDS-related complex (ARC) and from healthy carriers: A study of risk groups and tissue sources. Proc Natl Acad Sci USA 82:5530, 1985
32. Safai B, Sargadharan MG, Groopman JE et al: Seroepidemiological studies of HTLV-III in AIDS. Lancet 1:1438, 1984
33. Fisher AG, Collalti E, Ratner L et al: A molecular clone of HTLV-III with biological activity. Nature 316:262, 1985
34. Ratner L, Gallo RC, Wong–Staal F: HTLV-III, LAV, ARV are variants of same AIDS virus. Nature 313:636, 1985
35. Gonda MA, Braun MJ, Clements JE et al: Human T-cell lymphotropic virus type III shares sequence homology with a family of pathogenic lentiviruses. Proc Natl Acad Sci USA 83:4007, 1986
36. Rosen CA, Sodroski JG, Haseltine WA: The location of cis-acting regulatory sequences in the human T cell lymphotropic virus type III (HTLV-III/LAV) long terminal repeat. Cell 41:813, 1985
37. Patarca R, Heath C, Goldenberg GJ et al: Transcription directed by the HIV long terminal repeat in vitro. AIDS Res Hum Retroviruses 3:41, 1987
38. Ratner L, Haseltine W, Patarca R et al: Complete nucleotide sequence of the AIDS virus, HTLV-III. Nature 313:277, 1985
39. Jacks T, Power MD, Masiary FR et al: Characterization of ribosomal frameshifting in HIV-1 gag-pol expression. Nature 331:280, 1988
40. Veronese F, Copeland T, DeVico AL et al: Characterization

of highly immunogenic p66/p51 as the reverse transcriptase of HTLV-III/LAV. Science 231:1289, 1986
41. Harris JD, Blum H, Scott J et al: Slow virus visna: reproduction in vitro of virus from extra chromosomal DNA. Proc Natl Acad Sci USA 81:7212, 1984
42. Veronese F, DeVico AL, Copeland TD et al: Characterization of gp41 as the transmembrane protein coded by the HTLV-III/LAV envelope gene. Science 229:1402, 1985
43. Kowalski M, Potz J, Basiripour L et al: Functional regions of the envelope glycoprotein of human immunodeficiency virus type 1. Science 237:1351, 1987
44. Lasky LA, Groopman JE, Fennie CW et al: Neutralization of the AIDS retrovirus by antibodies to a recombinant envelope glycoprotein. Science 233:209, 1986
45. Lasky LA, Nakamura G, Smith DH et al: Delineation of a region of the human immunodeficiency virus type 1 gp120 glycoprotein critical for interaction with the CD4 receptor. Cell 50:975, 1987
46. McDougal JS, Kennedy MS, Sligh JM et al: Binding of HTLV-III/LAV to T4+ T cells by a complex of the 110K viral protein and the T4 molecule. Science 231:382, 1986
47. McDougal JS, Mawle A, Cort SP et al: Cellular tropism of the human retrovirus HTLV-III/LAV-I. Role of T cell activation and expression of the T4 antigen. J Immunol 135:3151, 1985
48. Klatzmann D, Champagne E, Chamaret S et al: T-lymphocyte T4 molecule behaves as the receptor for human retrovirus LAV. Nature 312:767, 1984
49. Dalgleish AG, Beverly PCL, Clapham PR et al: The CD4 (T4) antigen is an essential component of the receptor for the AIDS retrovirus. Nature 312:763, 1984
50. Maddon PJ, Dalgleish AG, McDougal JS et al: The T4 gene encodes the AIDS virus receptor and is expressed in the immune system and the brain. Cell 47:333, 1986
51. Allan JS, Coligan JE, Barin F et al: Major glycoprotein antigens that induce antibodies in AIDS patients are encoded by HTLV-III. Science 228:1091, 1985
52. Lee TH, Coligan JE, Allan JS et al: A new HTLV-III/LAV protein encoded by a gene found in cytopathic retroviruses. Science 231:1546, 1986
53. Kan NC, Franchini G, Wong–Staal F et al: Identification of HTLV-III/LAV sor gene product and detection of antibodies in human sera. Science 321:1553, 1986
54. Sodroski J, Goh WC, Rosen C et al: Replicative and cytopathic potential of HTLV-III/LAV with sor gene deletions. Science 231:1549, 1986
55. Fisher AG, Ensoli B, Ivanoff L et al: The sor gene of HIV-1 is required for efficient virus transmission in vitro. Science 237:888, 1987
56. Strebel K, Daugherty D, Clouse K et al: The HIV 'A' (sor) gene product is essential for virus infectivity. Nature 328:728, 1987
57. Fisher AG, Ratner L, Mitsuya H et al: Infectious mutants of HTLV-III with changes in the 3' region and markedly reduced cytopathic effects. Science 233:655, 1986
58. Luciw PA, Cheng–Mayer C, Levy JA: Mutational analysis of the human immunodeficiency virus: The orf-B region down-regulates virus replication. Proc Natl Acad Sci USA 84:1434, 1987
59. Guy B, Kieny MP, Riviera Y et al: HIV F/3' orf encodes a phosphorylated GTP-binding protein resembling an oncogene product. Nature 330:267, 1987
60. Wong–Staal F, Chanda P, Ghrayeb J: Human immunodeficiency virus: The eighth gene. AIDS Res Hum Retrovirol 3:33, 1987

61. Sodroski J, Rosen C, Wong–Staal F et al: *Trans*-acting transcriptional regulation of human T-cell leukemia virus type III long terminal repeat. Science 227:171, 1985

62. Sodroski J, Patarca R, Rosen C et al: Location of the *trans*-activating region on the genome of human T-cell lymphotropic virus type III. Science 229:74, 1985

63. Rosen CA, Sodroski JG, Goh WC et al: Post-transcriptional regulation accounts for the *trans*-activation of the human T-lymphotropic virus type III. Nature 319:555, 1986

64. Arya SK, Guo C, Josephs SF et al: *Trans*-activator gene of human T-lymphotropic virus type III (HTLV-III). Science 229:69, 1985

65. Seigel LJ, Ratner L, Josephs SF et al: Transactivation induced by human T-lymphotropic virus type III (HTLV III) maps to a viral sequence encoding 58 amino acids and lacks tissue specificity. Virology 148:226, 1986

66. Okamoto T, Wong–Staal F: Demonstration of virus-specific transcriptional activator(s) in cells infected with HTLV-III by an in vitro cell-free system. Cell 47:29, 1986

67. Sadaie R, Benter T, Wong–Staal F: Site-directed mutagenesis of two *trans*-regulatory genes (tat-3, trs) of HIV-1. Science 239:910, 1988

68. Feinberg MB, Jarrett RF, Aldovini A et al: HTLV-III expression and production involve complex regulation at the levels of splicing and translation of viral RNA. Cell 46:807, 1986

69. Patarca R, Haseltine WA: Letter. AIDS Res Hum Retroviruses 3:1, 1987

70a. Sodroski J, Goh WC, Rosen C et al: A second post-transcriptional *trans*-activator gene required for HTLV-III replication. Nature 321:412, 1986

70b. Kao S–Y, Colman AF, Luciw P et al: Anti-termination of transcription within the long terminal repeat of HIV-1 by tat gene product. Nature 330:489, 1987

71. Haase AT: Pathogenesis of lentivirus infections. Nature 322:130, 1986

72. Wong–Staal F, Shaw GM, Hahn BH et al: Genomic diversity of human T-lymphotropic virus type III (HTLV-III). Science 229:759, 1985

73. Harper ME, Marselle LM, Gallo RC et al: Detection of lymphocytes expressing human T-lymphotropic virus type III in lymph nodes and peripheral blood from infected individuals by in situ hybridization. Proc Natl Acad Sci USA 83:772, 1986.

74. Hoxie JA, Haggarty BS, Rackowski JL et al: Persistent noncytopathic infection of normal human T lymphocytes with AIDS-associated retrovirus. Science 229:1400, 1985

75. Folks T, Powell DM, Lightfoote MM et al: Induction of HTLV-III/LAV from a nonvirus-producing T-cell line: Implications for latency. Science 231:600, 1986

76. Gendelman HE, Phelps W, Feigenbaum L et al: *Trans*-activation of the human immunodeficiency virus long terminal repeat sequence DNA viruses. Proc Natl Acad Sci USA 83:9759, 1986

77. Margolick JB, Volkman DJ, Folks TM et al: Amplification of HTLV-III/LAV infection by antigen-induced activation of T cells and direct suppression by virus of lymphocyte blastogenic responses. J Immunol 138:1719, 1987

78. Folks TM, Justement J, Kinter A et al: Cytokine-induced expression of HIV-1 in a chronically infected promonocyte cell line. Science 238:800, 1987

79. Schnittman SM, Lane HC, Higgins SE et al: Direct polyclonal activation of human B lymphocytes by the acquired immune deficiency syndrome virus. Science 233:1084, 1986

80. Pahwa S, Pahwa R, Good RA et al: Stimulatory and inhibitory influences of human immunodeficiency virus on normal B lymphocytes. Proc Natl Acad Sci USA 83:9124, 1986

81. Pahwa S, Pahwa R, Saxinger C et al: Influence of the human T-lymphotropic virus/lymphadenopathy-associated virus on functions of human lymphocytes: Evidence for immunosuppressive effects and polyclonal B-cell activation by banded viral preparations. Proc Natl Acad Sci USA 82:8198, 1985

82. Ho DD, Rota TR, Hirsch MS: Infection of monocyte/macrophages by human T lymphotropic virus type III. J Clin Invest 77:1712, 1986

83. Nicholson JKA, Gross GD, Callaway CS et al: In vitro infection of human monocytes with human T-lymphotropic virus type III/lymphadenopathy-associated virus (HTLV-III/LAV). J Immunol 137:323, 1986

84. Salahuddin SZ, Rose RM, Groopman JE et al: Human T lymphotropic virus type III infection of human alveolar macrophages. Blood 68:281, 1986

85. Gartner S, Markovits P, Markovitz DM et al: The role of mononuclear phagocytes in HTLV-III/LAV infection. Science 233:215, 1986

86. Koenig S, Gendelman HE, Orenstein JM et al: Detection of AIDS virus in macrophages in brain tissue from AIDS patients with encephalopathy. Science 233:1089, 1986

87. Wiley CA, Schrier RD, Nelson JA et al: Cellular localization of human immunodeficiency virus infection within the brains of acquired immune deficiency syndrome patients. Proc Natl Acad Sci USA 83:7089, 1986

88. Gabuzda DH, Ho DD, De la Monte SM et al: Immunohistochemical identification of HTLV-III antigen in brains of patients with AIDS. Ann Neurol 20:289, 1986

89. Gendelman HE, Narayan O, Kennedy–Stoskopg S et al: Tropism of sheep lentiviruses for monocytes: Susceptibility to infection and virus gene expression increases during maturation of monocytes to macrophages. J Virol 58:67, 1986

90. Klatzmann D, Barré-Sinoussi F, Nugeyre MT et al: Selective tropism of lymphadenopathy associated virus (LAV) for helper–inducer T lymphocytes. Science 225:59, 1984

91. Stein BS, Gowda SD, Lifson JD et al: pH-Independent HIV entry into CD4-positive T cells via virus envelope fusion to the plasma membrane. Cell 49:659, 1987

92. Talle MA, Rao PE, Westberg E et al: Patterns of antigenic expression on human monocytes as defined by monoclonal antibodies. Cell Immunol 78:83, 1983

93. Biberfeld P, Chayt KJ, Marselle LM et al: HTLV-III expression in infected lymph nodes and relevance to pathogenesis of lymphadenopathy. Amer J Pathol 125:436, 1986

94. Tschachler E, Groh V, Popovic M et al: Epidermal langerhans cells—a target for HTLV-III/LAV infection. J Invest Dermatol 88:233, 1987

95. Cheng–Mayer C, Rutka JT, Rosenblum ML et al: Human immunodeficiency virus can productively infect cultured human glial cells. Proc Natl Acad Sci USA 84:3526, 1987

96. Chiodi F, Fuerstenberg S, Gidlund M et al: Infection of brain-derived cells with the human immunodeficiency virus. J Virol 61:1244, 1987

97. Price RW, Brew B, Sidtis J et al: The brain in AIDS: Central nervous system HIV-1 infection and AIDS dementia complex. Science 239:586, 1988

98. Stoler MH, Eskin TA, Benn S et al: Human T-cell lym-

photropic virus type III infection of the central nervous system: A preliminary in situ analysis. JAMA 256:2360, 1986

99. Gyorkey F, Melnick JL, Gyorkey P: Human immunodeficiency virus in brain biopsies of patients with AIDS and progressive encephalopathy. J Infect Dis 155:870, 1987

100. Funke I, Hahn A, Rieber EP et al: The cellular receptor (CD4) of the human immunodeficiency virus is expressed on neurons and glial cells in human brain. J Exp Med 165:1230, 1987

101. Lee MR, Ho DD, Gurney ME: Functional interaction and partial homology between human immunodeficiency virus and neuroleukin. Science 237:1047, 1987

102. Fauci AS: The human immunodeficiency virus: Infectivity and mechanisms of pathogenesis. Science 239:617, 1988

103. Lifson J, Courtre S, Huang E et al: Role of envelope glycoprotein carbohydrate in human immunodeficiency virus (HIV) infectivity and virus-induced cell fusion. J Exp Med 164:2101, 1986

104. Lifson JD, Feinberg MB, Reyes GR et al: Induction of CD4-dependent cell fusion by the HTLV-III/LAV envelope glycoprotein. Nature 323:725, 1986

105. Lifson JD, Reyes GR, McGrath MS, Stein BS et al: AIDS retrovirus induced cytopathology: Giant cell formation and involvement of CD4 antigen. Science 232:1123, 1986

106. Sodroski J, Goh WC, Rosen C et al: Role of the HTLV-III/LAV envelope in syncytium formation and cytopathicity. Nature 322:470, 1986

107. Hoxie JA, Alpers JD, Rackowski J et al: Alterations in T4 (CD4) protein and mRNA synthesis in cells infected with HIV. Science 234:1123, 1986

108. Shaw GM, Hahn BH, Arya SK et al: Molecular characterization of human T-cell leukemia (lymphotropic) virus type III in the acquired immune deficiency syndrome. Science 226:1165, 1984

109. Alizon M, Wain–Hobson S, Mantagnier L et al: Genetic variability of the AIDS virus: Nucleotide sequence analysis of two isolates from African patients. Cell 46:63, 1986

110. Srinivasan A, Anand R, York D et al: Molecular characterization of human immunodeficiency virus from Zaire: Nucleotide sequence analysis identifies conserved and variable domains in the envelope gene. Gene 52:71, 1987

111. Willey RL, Rutledge RA, Dias S et al: Identification of conserved and divergent domains within the envelope gene of the acquired immunodeficiency syndrome retorvirus. Proc Natl Acad Sci USA 83:5038, 1986

112. Wain–Hobson S, Sonigo P, Danos O et al: Nucleotide sequence of the AIDS virus, LAV. Cell 40:9, 1985

113. Starich BR, Hahn BH, Shaw GM et al: Identification and characterization of conserved and variable regions in the envelope gene of HTLV-III/LAV, the retrovirus of AIDS. Cell 45:637, 1986

114. Hahn BH, Shaw GM, Arya SK et al: Molecular cloning and characterization of the HTLV-III virus associated with AIDS. Nature 312:166, 1984

115. Hahn BH, Gonda MA, Shaw GM et al: Genomic diversity of the acquired immune deficiency syndrome virus HTLV-III: different viruses exhibit greatest divergence in their envelope genes. Proc Natl Acad Sci USA 82:4813, 1985

116. Hahn BH, Shaw GM, Taylor ME et al: Genetic variation in HTLV-III/LAV over time in patients with AIDS or at risk for AIDS. Science 232:1548, 1986

117. Coffin JM: Genetic variation in AIDS viruses. Cell 46:1, 1986

118. Muesing MA, Smith DH, Cabradilla CD et al: Nucleic acid structure and expression of the human AIDS/lymphadenopathy retrovirus. Nature 313:450, 1985

119. Sanchez–Pescador R, Power MD, Barr PJ et al: Nucleotide sequence and expression of an AIDS-associated retrovirus (ARV-2). Science 227:484, 1985

120. Benn S, Rutledge R, Folks T et al: Genomic heterogeneity of AIDS retroviral isolates from North America and Zaire. Science 230:949, 1985

121. Desai SM, Kalyanaraman VS, Casey JM et al: Molecular cloning and primary nucleotide sequence analysis of a distinct human immunodeficiency virus isolate reveal significant divergence in its genomic sequences. Proc Natl Acad Sci USA 83:8380, 1986

122. Modrow S, Hahn BH, Shaw GM et al: Secondary structure analysis of the envelope amino acid sequences of 7 isolates of HTLV-III/LAV. J Virol 61:570, 1987

123. Rusche JR, Javaherian K, McDanol C et al: Antibodies that inhibit fusion of HIV infected cells bind a 24 amino acid sequence of the viral envelope, gp 120. Proc Natl Acad Sci USA (in preparation)

124. Salinovich O, Payne SL, Montelaro RC et al: Rapid emergence of novel antigenic and genetic variants of equine infectious anemia virus during persistent infection. J Virol 57:71, 1986

125. Braun MJ, Clements JE, Gonda MA: The visna virus genome: Evidence for a hypervariable site in the env gene and sequence homology among lentivirus envelope proteins. J Virol 61:4046, 1987

126. Saag M, Hahn B, Li Y et al: Extensive variation of HIV-1 in vivo. Nature (in press) 1988

127. Payne S, Salinovich O, Nauman S et al: Course and extent of variation of equine infectious anemia virus during parallel persistent infections. J Virol 61:1266, 1987

128. Payne SL, Fang FD, Liu CP et al: Antigenic variation and lentivirus persistence: Variations in envelope gene sequences during EIAV infection resemble changes reported for sequential isolates of HIV. Virology 161:321, 1987

129. Montelaro RC, Parekh B, Orrego A et al: Antigenic variation during persistent infection by equine infectious anemia virus, a retrovirus. J Biol Chem 259:10539, 1984

130. Thormar H, Barshatzky MR, Arnesen K et al: The emergence of antigenic variants is a rare event in long-term visna virus infection in vivo. J Gen Virol 64:1427, 1983

131. Overbaugh J, Donahue PR, Quackenbush SL et al: Molecular cloning of a feline leukemia virus that induces fatal immunodeficiency disease in cats. Science 239:906, 1988

132. Koyanagi Y, Miles S, Mitsuyasu RT et al: Dual infection of the central nervous system by AIDS viruses with distinct cellular tropisms. Science 236:819, 1987

133. Steinhauer DA, Holland JJ: Ann Rev Microbiol 41:409, 1987

134. Nahmias AJ, Weiss J, Yao X et al: Evidence for human infection with an HTLV-III/LAV-like virus in Central Africa. Lancet I:1279, 1986

135. Barin F, M'Boup S, Denis F et al: Serological evidence for virus related to simian T-lymphotropic retrovirus III in residents of West Africa. Lancet 2:1387, 1985

136. Kanki PJ, Barin F, M'Boup S et al: New human T-lymphotropic retrovirus related to simian T-lymphotropic virus type III (STLV-III$_{AGM}$). Science 232:238, 1986

137. Kanki PJ, M'Boup S, Ricard D et al: Human T-lympho-

tropic virus type 4 and the human immunodeficiency virus in West Africa. Science 236:827, 1987

138. Daniel MD, Letvin NL, King NW et al: Isolation of T-cell tropic HTLV-III-like retrovirus from macaques. Science 228:1201, 1985

139. Kanki PJ, Alroy J, Essex M: Isolation of T-lymphotropic retrovirus related to HTLV-III/LAV from wild-caught African green monkeys. Science 230:951, 1985

140. Kestler HW, Li Y, Naidu YM et al: Comparison of simian immunodeficiency virus isolates. Nature 331:619, 1988

141. Clavel F, Guetard F, Brun–Vezinet F et al: Isolation of a new human retrovirus from West African patients with AIDS. Science 233:343, 1986

142. Clavel F, Guyader M, Guetard D et al: Molecular cloning and polymorphism of the human immune deficiency virus type 2. Nature 324:691, 1986

143. Clavel F, Mansinho K, Charmaret S et al: Human immunodeficiency virus type 2 infection associated with AIDS in West Africa. N Engl J Med 316:1180, 1987

144. Guyader M, Emerman M, Sonigo P et al: Genome organization and transactivation of the human immunodeficiency virus type 2. Nature 326:662, 1987

145. Chakrabarti L, Guyader M, Alizon M et al: Sequence of simian immunodeficiency virus from macaque and its relationship to other human and simian retroviruses. Nature 328:543, 1987

146. Kappes J, Morrow C, Hahn BH et al: (Submitted)

147. Franchini G, Kusche J, O'Keefe T et al: (Submitted)

148. Kong L, Lee S–W, Kappes J et al: West African HIV-2 related human retrovirus with attenuated cytopathicity. Science (in press) 1988

149. Quinn TC, Mann JM, Curran JW et al: AIDS in Africa: An epidemiologic paradigm. Science 234:955, 1986

150. Bygbjerg C: Letter. Lancet 1:925, 1983

151. Vandepitte J, Verwilghen R, Zachee P: AIDS and cryptococcosis (Zaire, 1977). Lancet 1:925, 1983

152. Nzilambi N, DeCock KM, Forthal DN et al: The prevalence of infection with HIV over a 10-year period in rural Zaire. N Engl J Med 318:276, 1988

153. Zagury JF, Franchini G, Reitz M et al: The genetic variability between HIV-2 isolate is comparable to the variability among HIV-1. Proc Nat Acad Sci (In press)

154. Ohta Y, Masuda T, Tsujimoto H et al: Isolation of simian immunodeficiency virus from African green monkeys and seroepidemiologic survey of the virus in various nonhuman primates. Int J Cancer 41:115, 1988

The Epidemiology and Natural History of Human Immunodeficiency Virus

James J. Goedert
William A. Blattner

3

Human immunodeficiency virus (HIV) is a sexual and blood-borne pathogen that infects and, in most persons, gradually destroys a critical component of immunity, the population of helper–inducer lymphocytes identified by the CD4+ (T4+) surface epitope.[1,2] Because CD4+ cells coordinate the entire cellular immune response, HIV infection can have myriad manifestations, ranging from subclinical laboratory abnormalities to the opportunistic infections and malignancies that define the acquired immunodeficiency syndrome (AIDS). Recent evidence indicates that HIV also infects monocytes, macrophages, and certain glial cells of the central nervous system, which helps to explain the pathogenesis and some of the clinical features of HIV infection.[3–5] This chapter reviews the modes of transmission of HIV, its natural history, various subclinical and clinical manifestations, and the implications for the course of the epidemic and prevention of the disease.

In tracking the natural history of HIV infection, time is a critical (and sometimes overlooked) parameter of the epidemiology. This oversight has contributed to erroneous suggestions that most persons infected with HIV will remain asymptomatic or that homosexual men have a higher incidence of AIDS following HIV than do other individuals. Issues such as these can be studied in proper perspective only by considering that AIDS is an increasing worldwide epidemic that apparently did not exist in any population prior to the mid-1970s and that the manifestations of HIV in individuals may be highly dynamic. Similar cautions must be applied to related human retroviruses as they are discovered[6,7] and to any pathogen that is newly introduced into a population.

DEFINITIONS

Any investigation of epidemiology or natural history must clearly define both the exposure and outcome parameters. Exposure measures for HIV are often complex and specific to each study. These may include sexual activities, contraceptive practices, drug use patterns, obstetric history, cultural factors, nosocomial injuries, and serologic or other laboratory measures. Because of their diversity and complexity, these exposure factors are considered later in this chapter. In contrast, the diseases and other outcome measures of HIV infection are defined more uniformly.

HIV Infection

Currently there are four means of defining HIV infection: isolating the virus by culturing cellular or body fluid samples, usually by noting high levels of reverse transcriptase and HIV proteins in susceptible target cells; identification of HIV-specific nucleic acid sequences in cellular materials; identification of HIV-specific antigens in body fluids; and identification of HIV antibodies in serum or other body fluids. Only the last of these, the HIV antibody assays, have been investigated for sensitivity, specificity, and predictive value.[8] In practical terms, virtually all of the relevant epidemiologic and natural history data derive from studies employing antibody assays. It is likely, however, that HIV-antigen and -nucleic-acid assays will become more widely applied during the next few years.

For most epidemiologic studies, HIV infection has been defined as a clearly positive HIV antibody assay, usually the enzyme-linked immunosorbent assay (ELISA) confirmed by demonstrating antibodies against the full array of HIV proteins or, at a minimum, against the HIV envelope glycoproteins (gp41 and/or gp120) or core proteins (p24 and p55). The use of antibody positivity to define HIV infection appears to be well substantiated by the finding from several laboratories that HIV can be isolated from the majority of antibody-positive individuals,[9,10] particularly in the context that retroviruses become permanently incorporated as proviral DNA in the host cell genome.

Young children with HIV antibodies are a special case, as the vast majority are born with passively acquired antibodies from their HIV-infected mothers. During at least the first 6 months of life, and in many children up to 15 months of age, conventional HIV ELISA and Western blot tests cannot define HIV infection, unless there is unequivocal evidence that HIV antibody levels are increasing or that new HIV antibody specificities are appearing over time on Western blots run in tandem. Figure 3-1 shows an example of this approach to diagnosis, in which prospectively collected sera were frozen and later tested simultaneously by the Western blot method. By 6 months of age, active HIV infection of the baby in pair 1 is strongly suggested by increases in the levels of immunoglobulin G (IgG) antibodies against the p24 and p17 core proteins and reappearance of antibodies against p55, which is the precursor of p24. In contrast, the IgG Western blots on the baby in pair 2 show the waning of maternal antibodies by 6 months of age. Pair 3 is a negative control that also demonstrates the caution required to interpret unproven diagnostic methods, such as anti-HIV immunoglobulin M (IgM) Western blots. Because IgM antibodies are not transferred from mother to baby *in utero,* the presence of specific IgM antibodies in a baby would be diagnostic of infection. Neonatal rubella infection, for example, is identified by the presence of IgM rubella antibodies. Unfortunately, other IgM assays have lacked sensitivity and/or specificity, including prototype HIV IgM Western

blots, as shown in Figure 3-1. The baby in pair 1 is clearly infected with HIV, not only by IgG Western blots but also by the later development of HIV-related illnesses. Baby 1's IgM Western blots, however, were nondiagnostic, with only a faint band at p24. Similar p24 IgM bands are noted in the baby in pair 3, who is clearly not infected, indicating that current, investigational IgM Western blots have problems with specificity and sensitivity. Thus, as a general rule, HIV infection in very young children can be defined only by direct identification of live virus, HIV-specific nucleic acids, or HIV-specific antigens, in addition to cases indirectly defined by virtue of AIDS or another condition that is closely linked to HIV (see below).

AIDS

The term AIDS should be reserved for a person with at least one well defined life-threatening clinical condition that is clearly linked to HIV-induced immunosuppression. The surveillance definition of AIDS, developed by the United States Centers for Disease Control (CDC) prior to the discovery of HIV, recently has been revised in order to improve surveillance sensitivity and specificity by incorporating HIV data (Table 3-1).[11] Histologically identified or culture-proven *Pneumocystis carinii* pneumonia, other life-threatening opportunistic infections, and Kaposi's sarcoma still define most AIDS cases

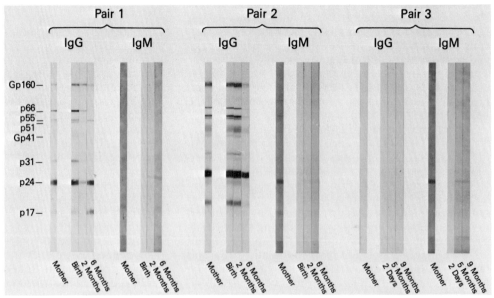

FIG. 3-1. HIV antibody Western blots (biotin–avidin method) using disrupted whole virus, developed with monospecific antisera against IgG or IgM. Sera were collected from three pregnant women and from their babies at ages 0 to 9 months. All sera were stored at −70°C, and all four sera from a mother–baby pair were tested on a single tray. IgG blots show decay of maternal antibodies in babies 1 and 2, with reappearance or increases in several anti-HIV specificities in baby 1 at age 6 months. Mother–baby pair 3 is an uninfected negative control, demonstrating false-positive p24 band on mother and baby 3's IgM blots.

Table 3-1
AIDS—Revised Surveillance Definition of the Centers for Disease Control

HIV Status Positive, Negative,* or Unknown†

One or more of the following diagnoses proven by microscopy or culture:

Pneumocytis carinii pneumonia
Candidiasis of the esophagus, trachea, bronchi, or lungs
Extrapulmonary *Mycobacterium avium* complex or *M. kansasii* infection
Herpes simplex virus infection causing bronchitis, pneumonitis, or esophagitis or a mucocutaneous ulcer persisting > 1 month‡
Cytomegalovirus infection of an internal organ other than liver‡
Toxoplasmosis of an internal organ‡
Cryptosporidiosis with diarrhea persisting > 1 month
Extraintestinal strongyloidiasis
Progressive multifocal leukoencephalopathy
Kaposi's sarcoma (<60 years of age)
Primary lymphoma of the brain (<60 years of age)
Pulmonary lymphoid hyperplasia or lymphoid interstitial pneumonitis (<13 years of age)

HIV Status Positive

One or more of the following diagnoses proven by microscopy or culture:

Kaposi's sarcoma (at any age)
Primary lymphoma of the brain (at any age)
B-cell non-Hodgkin's lymphomas of the small non-cleaved (Burkitt-like) or immunoblastic sarcoma (large cell lymphoma, diffuse histiocytic or undifferentiated lymphoma, reticulum cell sarcoma, or high-grade lymphoma) types
HIV dementia complex
HIV wasting syndrome (enteropathic AIDS, "slim" disease)
Extrapulmonary or disseminated tuberculosis or other noncutaneous mycobacterial infection other than leprosy
Extrapulmonary or disseminated histoplasmosis
Extrapulmonary or disseminated coccidioidomycosis
Isosporiasis with diarrhea persisting > 1 month
Nocardiosis
Salmonella septicemia
Two or more bacterial infections within 2 years of the following types in a child < 13 years of age not predisposed by chronic lung disease: septicemia, pneumonia, meningitis, or brain abscess caused by *Legionella, Hemophilus, Streptococcus* (including pneumococcus), or another pyogenic bacterium

One or more of the following diagnoses not proven by microscopy or culture:

Pneumocytis carinii pneumonia
Toxoplasmosis of an internal organ‡
Esophageal candidiasis
Extrapulmonary or disseminated mycobacterial infection (acid-fast bacilli of undetermined species)
Progressive multifocal leukoencephalopathy
Kaposi's sarcoma
Pulmonary lymphoid hyperplasia or lymphoid interstitial pneumonitis (<13 years of age)

* AIDS is not excluded by negative HIV serology in patients with *Pneumocystis carinii* pneumonia or a T4 (T-helper) lymphocyte count < 400/µl, since in some patients with advanced immune deficiency hypogammaglobulinemia may supervene with reversion to HIV-antibody negative.
† If HIV status is unknown or negative, the following causes of immunodeficiency must be excluded: systemic corticosteroid, immunosuppressive, or cytotoxic therapy within 3 months; Hodgkin's disease, non-Hodgkin's lymphoma (other than primary brain lymphoma), lymphocytic leukemia, multiple myeloma, other cancer of lymphoreticular or histiocytic tissue, or angioimmunoblastic lymphadenopathy within 3 months; any genetic, congenital, or acquired immunodeficiency syndrome atypical of HIV infection.
‡ Over 1 month of age
(Revision of the CDC surveillance definition for acquired immunodeficiency syndrome. Morbid Mortal Weekly Rep (suppl) 36:1S–15S, 1987)

in the United States, irrespective of HIV status. Primary lymphoma of the brain and pulmonary lymphoid hyperplasia/lymphoid interstitial pneumonia in children have been added to this list. Under the revisions, patients are included as AIDS cases if they have serologic evidence of HIV infection and one or more other conditions associated with immunodeficiency, including B-cell non-Hodgkin's lymphomas, the HIV dementia complex, the HIV wasting syndrome (enteropathic AIDS), tuberculosis, and multiple life-threatening bacterial infections in children. Finally, the revised case definition counts HIV-positive patients who may have another cause of immunodeficiency (such as renal failure or immunosuppressive therapy) and those with clinically but not microscopically diagnosed classical AIDS conditions, such as Pneumocystis carinii pneumonia. Pediatric AIDS is no longer a separately defined condition, as provisions for the different manifestations

of AIDS in children are provided in the surveillance definition.

Because laboratory facilities in many developing countries are insufficient to allow reliable diagnoses of many opportunistic infections and malignant disorders, the World Health Organization (WHO) has developed a provisional clinical case definition of AIDS for purposes of surveillance.[12] These clinically defined cases of AIDS include patients with disseminated Kaposi's sarcoma, cryptococcal meningitis, or a combination of major and minor signs and symptoms of HIV infection (Table 3-2). The major signs are weight loss greater than 10% of body weight; chronic diarrhea for longer than one month; fever (intermittant or constant) for longer than one month. The minor signs are persistent cough for longer than one month (excluding patients with tuberculosis); general lymphadenopathy (excluding patients with tuberculosis); general pruritic dermatitis;

history of herpes zoster during the previous five years; oropharyngeal candidiasis; chronic progressive and disseminated herpes simplex infection. It is likely that there will be further modifications of this WHO provisional definition as its predictive value is tested in on-going field studies.

AIDS-Related Complex (ARC)

Persistent generalized lymph node enlargement, often referred to as PGL or lymphadenopathy syndrome (LAS), is strongly associated with HIV seropositivity.[13,14] However, lymph node enlargement can occur during the acute phase of initial HIV infection[15] or several years later, concurrent with HIV-induced immunosuppression.[16] Thus, even when the various other causes of lymphadenopathy are excluded, cohorts of PGL include a spectrum ranging from asymptomatic, immunologically normal subjects to those with imminent AIDS. In addition, lymphadenopathy per se is a benign condition, provided that it is symmetrical and not rapidly progressive.[17] AIDS-related complex (ARC) is a heterogeneous condition with a variety of definitions, most often including those with at least two AIDS-related clinical conditions (such as lymphadenopathy, persistent fevers, weight loss, or oral candidiasis) plus one or more AIDS-related laboratory abnormalities (such as a low number of T4 lymphocytes or an inverted ratio of T4:T8 lymphocytes). Although the many studies of patients with PGL, LAS, and ARC do provide useful clinical information, the heterogeneous definitions make comparative data nearly impossible.

DEMOGRAPHY OF AIDS

North America

AIDS is a true pandemic, with cases reported from virtually every country on earth. Nonetheless, the majority of reported cases are from North America, particularly the United States (Table 3-3). As of September 21, 1987, 42,182 cases had been reported to the CDC.[18] An additional 10% to 20% are believed to have been missed by the surveillance system, because of adherence to a strict definition (see above), reporting delays, missed diagnoses, and purposeful underreporting to avoid an embarrassing diagnosis. Of the 41,602 adults reported with AIDS to the CDC, 27,483 (66%) are homosexual or bisexual men not known to have used intravenous drugs, 6,853 (16%) are heterosexual intravenous drug users, 3,129 (8%) are male homosexual intravenous drug users, 379 (1%) are patients with hemophilia and related disorders, 1644 (4%) are probably acquired by heterosexual contact, 882 (2%) are recipients of transfusions, and 1,232 (3%) are undetermined due to death or refusal to be interviewed, cases still under investigation, men

Table 3-2
AIDS—Provisional Clinical Surveillance Definition of the World Health Organization

AIDS is defined as:*

Disseminated Kaposi's sarcoma
or

Cryptococcal meningitis
or

At least two major signs:	Plus	At least one minor sign:
Weight loss > 10%		Cough > 1 month†
Diarrhea > 1 month		General lymphadenopathy†
Fever > 1 month		General pruritic dermatitis
		History of herpes zoster within 5 years
		Oropharyngeal candidiasis
		Chronic and progressive herpes simplex

* Excluding patients with other known causes of immunosuppression.
† Excluding patients with proven tuberculosis.
(Colebunders R, Mann JM, Francis H et al: Evaluation of a clinical case-definition of acquired immunodeficiency syndrome in Africa. Lancet 1:492, 1987)

reporting contact with prostitutes, and patients with no specific risk factor identified.[18] Among the 580 reported children meeting the surveillance definition of AIDS, the vast majority (456, 79%) are offspring of a parent with AIDS or at high risk of AIDS (discussed in more detail below). The remaining pediatric AIDS cases include 31 (5%) with hemophilia, 70 (12%) transfusion recipients, and 23 (4%) as yet undetermined. By racial and ethnic group, Black non-Hispanics represent 24% of the adults and 54% of the children with AIDS, and Hispanics represent 14% of the adults and 24% of the children. Of total cases, 88% are aged 20–49 years, with only 243 (0.58%) aged 5 to 19 years.

The number of AIDS cases reported to the CDC continues to increase in all groups in the United States (Figs. 3-2 and 3-3), with one noteworthy exception. In children, transfusion-associated AIDS declined steadily during 1986 (Fig. 3-3). Undoubtably this decline can be attributed to the universal screening of donated blood, started in the spring of 1985, and to the relatively short incubation period, often 12 months or less, for transfusion-associated AIDS in children.[19,20] Declines in adults with transfusion-associated AIDS cannot be anticipated until at least 1989, since the average incubation period is at least 4.5 years.[20,21]

Among the other high-incidence groups, homosexual men and parenteral drug users account for the largest proportion of cases, although the rate of increase is less steep than it was during the early 1980s (Fig. 3-2). Overall, the doubling time for the number of new cases has increased from less than 9 months to nearly 14 months. Over the past 2 years the most rapid increases

Table 3-3
Cumulative AIDS Cases Reported to the World Health Organization

Country	Total Cases	Rate per Million	Date of Report	Country	Total Cases	Rate per Million	Date of Report
Canada	1,233	48.5	9/87	Eastern Mediterranean Reg.	30	0.4	4/87
United States	41,366	165.5	8/87	Hong Kong	4	0.7	12/86
Total North America	38,510			India	9	0.0	5/87
				Indonesia	1	0.0	4/87
Andean group	352	4.2	9/87	Israel	38	9.0	3/87
Brazil	2,013	14.8	9/87	Japan	43	0.4	6/87
Caribbean	628	87.8	3–9/87	Lebanon	3	1.2	6/87
Central American Isthmus	142	5.1	6–9/87	Malaysia	1	0.1	4/87
Latin Caribbean	1,116	41.6	3–9/87	Qatar	9	30.0	5/87
Mexico	534	6.6	6/87	Republic of Korea	1	0.0	4/87
Southern cone	181	3.7	6–9/87	Singapore	1	0.4	4/87
Total South and Central				Sri Lanka	2	0.1	4/87
Americas	4,966			Thailand	6	0.1	4/87
Austria	72	9.6	3/87	Turkey	21	0.4	6/87
Belgium	230	23.2	3/87	Total Asia	175		
Czechoslovakia	7	0.4	3/87				
Denmark	150	29.4	3/87	Algeria	5	0.2	6/87
Finland	19	3.9	3/87	Angola	6	0.7	9/86
France	1,632	29.9	3/87	Benin	3	0.8	5/87
German Democratic Rep.	3	0.2	3/87	Botswana	12	10.9	5/87
Germany (Federal Rep.)	1,089	17.9	5/87	Burundi	128	27.2	3/87
Greece	41	4.1	3/87	Cameroon	25	2.6	3/87
Hungary	3	0.3	3/87	Central African Rep.	254	4.3	10/86
Iceland	4	20.0	3/87	Chad	1	0.2	11/86
Ireland	19	5.3	3/87	Congo	250	147.1	11/86
Italy	850	14.8	6/87	Ethiopia	5	0.1	5/87
Luxembourg	7	17.5	3/87	Gabon	2	1.8	4/87
Malta	5	16.7	3/87	Gambia	14	23.3	3/87
Netherlands	260	17.9	3/87	Ghana	145	10.7	5/87
Norway	45	11.0	3/87	Ivory Coast	118	12.0	11/86
Poland	2	0.1	3/87	Kenya	625	30.3	7/87
Portugal	54	5.3	3/87	Lesotho	1	0.7	11/86
Romania	2	0.1	3/87	Liberia	2	0.5	6/87
Spain	357	9.3	3/87	Malawi	13	1.9	11/86
Sweden	129	15.5	7/87	Mozambique	1	0.1	12/86
Switzerland	266	42.2	6/87	Nigeria	5	0.1	5/87
United Kingdom	935	16.7	7/87	Rwanda	705	117.5	2/87
United Soviet Social. Rep.	58	0.2	6/87	South Africa	77	2.1	7/87
Yugoslavia	10	0.4	3/87	Swaziland	7	11.7	7/87
Total Europe	6,249			Tanzania	1,130	50.4	4/87
				Tunisia	2	0.3	5/86
Australia	562	35.8	7/87	Uganda	1,138	73.9	2/87
New Zealand	45	13.6	6/87	Zambia	395	59.8	6/87
Total Oceania	607			Zimbabwe	57	6.6	1/87
China	2	0.0	4/87	Total Africa	5,126		
China (Taiwan)	1	—	1/86				
Cyprus	3	5.0	6/87	Total Cases	58,753		

(Laboratory Center for Disease Control Update: "AIDS" in Canada, September 1987; Pan American Health Organization: Aids in the Americas: The Situation. September 21, 1987)

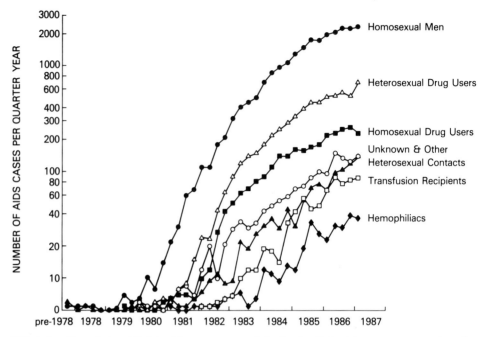

FIG. 3-2. Cumulative AIDS incidence among adults in the United States as reported to the Centers for Disease Control (provisional data through July 1987) by quarter year of diagnosis for seven exposure groups. The plots suggest that AIDS incidence has been leveling off among the most severely affected groups (homosexual men and drug users) and has been increasing most rapidly among heterosexual contacts.

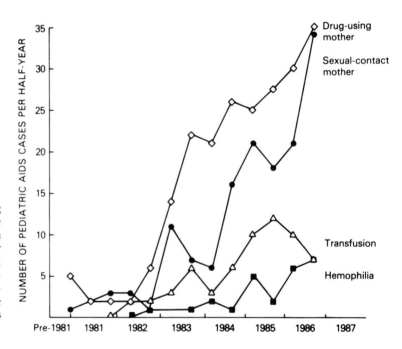

FIG. 3-3. Cumulative AIDS incidence among children in the United States as reported to the Centers for Disease Control (provisional data through July 1987) by half-year of diagnosis for four exposure groups. Children born to drug-using or sexual-contact mothers are at highest and increasing risk, whereas transfusion-associated pediatric AIDS has been decreasing since the screening of donated blood for HIV antibodies was initiated in the spring of 1985.

have been among adults with heterosexually acquired AIDS (see Fig. 3-2) and among children whose mothers use parenteral drugs or who are sexual partners of high-incidence men (see Fig. 3-3).

AIDS cases have been reported from all 50 states and the District of Columbia. During the 12 months ending September 21, 1987, New York and California reported about half of all cases (51.5%), with 19.0% from Florida, Texas, and New Jersey, and the remaining 29.4% from the other 46 areas.[18] Although AIDS appeared at later times in central areas of the United States, the rates of increase have been remarkably parallel nationwide (Fig. 3-4). On a per capita basis, some metropolitan areas have been severely affected, including smaller and middle-sized cities that receive little notice, such as Jersey City, New Jersey and Ft. Lauderdale, Florida (Table 3-4).

The proportion of cases reported with an initial diagnosis of only Kaposi's sarcoma has declined over time (Fig. 3-5), but in 10% of the new cases reported during the first half of 1987 Kaposi's sarcoma was the only AIDS diagnosis. An additional 6% of the new cases had both Kaposi's sarcoma and an opportunistic infection. AIDS-associated Kaposi's sarcoma occurs predominantly among homosexual men, but cases of Kaposi's sarcoma have also been reported in all other high-incidence

groups, including eight cases among children with AIDS.

Canada reported 1,233 cases of AIDS as of September 8, 1987.[22] The demographic profile of AIDS in Canada closely resembles the disease in the United States, although only five Canadian drug users have been reported with AIDS (0.4% of all cases). AIDS has been reported in all 11 Canadian provinces and territories.

South and Central Americas

Among the nations of South America and Central America, Brazil has the largest number of AIDS cases with 1,695 reported (see Table 3-3). Some of the smaller island nations of the Latin Carribean, particularly Haiti, and the Caribbean, particularly Trinidad and Tobago, have a much higher per capita rate of AIDS. In Haiti, most of the cases appear to be attributable to heterosexual activity, whereas homosexual and bisexual men account for most of the cases in other Central and South American nations. However, there is an emerging trend for increasing rates among heterosexually active populations which may reflect transmission of HIV infection from bisexual men whose initial exposure resulted from homosexual contact.

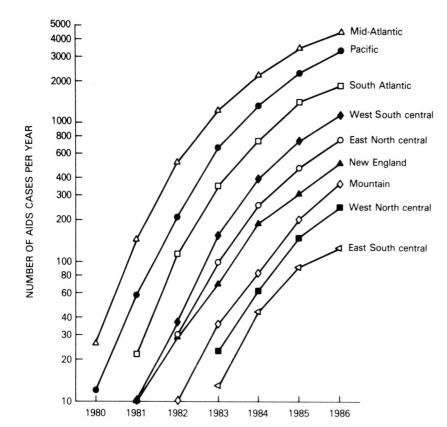

FIG. 3-4. Cumulative AIDS incidence for all nine geographic areas of the United States as reported to the Centers for Disease Control by year of diagnosis. Plots are generally parallel and have a leveling off trend in all regions.

Africa

Africa, of all the continents, presents the greatest diversity and probably the greatest challenges with regard to AIDS. The diversity is easily apparent, in that the largely Arab nations of North Africa have noted very few cases, whereas the sub-Saharan nations, particularly in central and east Africa, have recorded many patients with AIDS (Fig. 3-6). Within these nations, as in the United States, AIDS has been largely an urban disease. Zaire, for example, has one of the highest AIDS incidence rates in the world in the capital city of Kinshasa, with 500 to 1000 cases per million people in early 1985.[23] In contrast, remote areas of eastern Zaire, as in many less-urbanized areas of Africa, had no or few AIDS cases or HIV seropositives.[24–26]

Age- and sex-specific rates of AIDS incidence in Kinshasa and of HIV antibody prevalence in Lusaka, Zambia, show that the infection and disease peak in the sexually active years, particularly women aged 20 to 39 and men aged 30 to 49.[23,27] Other sexually transmitted diseases are quite common among persons with AIDS and HIV infection, and relatively few adolescents or elderly persons with either AIDS or HIV infection have been noted.[23,27] HIV antibodies and AIDS have been noted among African infants and young children,[28,29] but as in the United States the scope of pediatric AIDS in Africa has not been fully characterized.

The clinical picture of AIDS in Africa is similar to that elsewhere, with some exceptions.[26] First, there appear to be relatively fewer pulmonary diseases but more cases of the diarrhea–wasting syndrome referred to as AIDS enteropathy or "slim disease."[30] In addition, AIDS is superimposed on a number of endemic diseases in Africa, including tuberculosis and endemic Kaposi's sarcoma.[26] AIDS-related, or epidemic, Kaposi's sarcoma is much more aggressive than the endemic variety[31–33] and can be distinguished by HIV serology.[33,34]

In addition to sexual activity and urban centers, mobility is a common thread among persons with AIDS or HIV infection in central and east Africa. This includes the recruitment of young female prostitutes from the countryside to large capitals and port cities that are frequented by traveling businessmen and sailors, respectively. It also includes cities and towns that serve as inland trading or military posts. These patterns thus serve to spread HIV first into major urban areas, gradually into the secondary cities and towns, and finally into rural areas. Because HIV seroprevalence data from outside the urban centers are nearly nonexistent, the magnitude of the epidemic for the whole of Africa cannot be estimated with any degree of certainty. Within the few urban areas that have been studied, however, including Kinshasa, Lusaka, Kigali, Kampala, and to a lesser extent Nairobi, the problem rivals that in certain high-risk subpopulations in the United States.[26] With HIV seroprevalence rates of 6% or more noted in healthy blood donors in some urban populations, projections for morbidity and mortality, with the potential for substantial

Table 3-4
Density of Reported Aids Cases in the United States, as of September 21, 1987

Standard Metropolitan Statistical Area	1980 Census Population	Cumulative AIDS Cases	AIDS Cases per Million
San Francisco, CA	3.25	4,098	1,261
New York, NY	9.12	10,961	1,201
Jersey City, NJ	0.56	468	836
Miami, FL	1.63	1,180	724
Ft. Lauderdale, FL	1.02	543	532
Newark, NJ	1.97	973	494
Los Angeles, CA	7.48	3,595	481
Houston, TX	2.91	1,346	463
Washington, DC	3.06	1,225	400
Atlanta, GA	2.03	683	336
New Orleans, LA	1.19	361	303
San Diego, CA	1.86	530	285
Seattle, WA	1.61	408	253
Dallas, TX	2.97	796	268
Boston, MA	2.76	663	240
Denver, CO	1.62	370	228
Nassau-Suffolk, NY	2.61	515	197
Anaheim, CA	1.93	348	180
Philadelphia, PA	4.72	818	173
Chicago, IL	7.10	1,010	142
Rest of U.S.	168.72	11,291	67
Total	230.11	42,182	183

(Center for Disease Control: AIDS Weekly Surveillance Report. Sept 21, 1987)

social impact, mirrors the severity of the problem in some areas of the United States and elsewhere.[27,35,36]

Europe

AIDS in Europe has three patterns, each reflecting economic and cultural relationships with other countries. First is the division between Eastern and Western block nations. AIDS has been virtually nonexistent in eastern Europe (see Table 3-3, Fig. 3-6), undoubtably reflecting the few opportunities for sexual contact with persons from the United States, other western countries, or Africa. Second is the on-going relationship between countries of Western Europe with their former colonies in central Africa. Thus, the vast majority of patients with AIDS first noted in Belgium were current or former residents of Zaire or Rwanda.[37] In addition to former African emigrants, AIDS has also been noted in Europeans who lived in Africa and had sexual contacts there.[38,39] Finally, the North American pattern of AIDS has become dominant in western Europe, with homosexual men in the vast majority, large numbers of drug users with AIDS in certain cities, and an overrepresentation of hemophiliacs

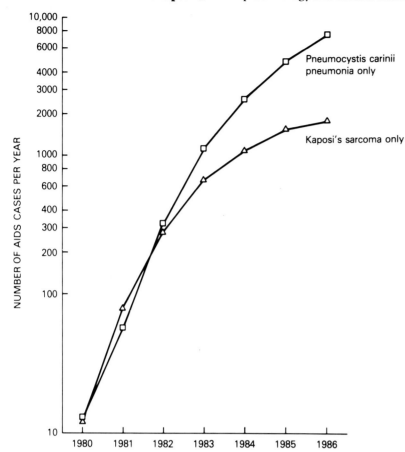

FIG. 3-5. Cumulative number of AIDS cases in the United States as reported to the Centers for Disease Control with an initial diagnosis of only *Pneumocystis carinii* pneumonia or Kaposi's sarcoma. Plots show a continuing rapid increase in the incidence of *Pneumocystis pneumonia* and a leveling off of Kaposi's sarcoma.

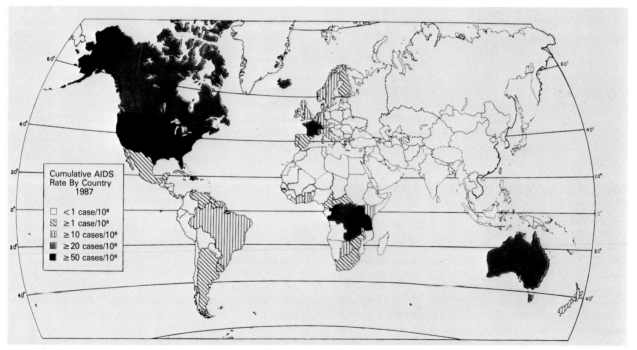

FIG. 3-6. Population-based cumulative AIDS incidence by early 1987 as reported to the World Health Organization[22] or as studied in Zaire.[23] Although AIDS cases have been noted in virtually every nation in the world, map demonstrates that reported AIDS is most concentrated in North America, Australia, and areas of central Africa and western Europe.

with AIDS.[40] Studies of homosexual men and hemophiliacs in Europe clearly point to the United States as the primary source of AIDS in these populations.[41,42] No country in Europe has reached the very high cumulative AIDS incidence rates noted in the United States, Haiti, or central Africa (see Table 3-3, Fig. 3-6).

Middle and Far East

Although few cases of AIDS thus far have been reported in the Middle and Far East (see Table 3-3), the presence of even a few cases strongly suggests that HIV is likely to be present in these populations. Studies in Europe and North America have shown that early in the AIDS epidemic, prior to the implementation of educational activities, screening of blood donors, and other intervention activities, the ratio of asymptomatic HIV infection to AIDS cases was 10:1 to 300:1. With early, aggressive intervention, it may be possible for the nations of these regions to reduce the impact of AIDS. Even with intervention, particularly to stem sexual transmission, several thousand cases of AIDS are likely to be diagnosed in Asia during the coming years. Without such intervention, more rapid spread of HIV in these areas can be anticipated, which would result in many thousands of cases of AIDS before the end of the 20th century.

Australia and Oceania

Australia and New Zealand, with strong ties to Europe and North America, have each had a relatively large number of patients with AIDS (Table 3-3). The vast majority thus far have been homosexual men, with several cases of transfusion-associated AIDS also noted. Thus, as noted elsewhere in the world, travelers appear to have acquired HIV infection in other countries, most likely in the United States, and transmitted it to the local population through sexual activity and blood donation. AIDS also has been noted in several of the tiny island nations of the Pacific.

PREVALENCE OF HIV IN THE UNITED STATES

Population Studies

Most of the published HIV seroprevalence data in the United States are from six highly selected groups, homosexual men, parenteral drug users, female prostitutes, hemophilia patients, military recruit applicants, and volunteer blood donors (Table 3-5). A few general themes are evident in the seroprevalence data. First, HIV antibodies were present in 4% of one group of San Francisco homosexual men in 1978 and in a similar small portion of hemophiliacs in Pennsylvania in the same year. Second, the seroprevalence rate increased rapidly during the first half of the 1980s among homosexual men in San Francisco, New York City, and Washington, DC, and among hemophiliacs in many areas of the United States. Third, HIV prevalence among drug users was very heterogeneous, with high rates during 1984 among drug users in or close to New York City but much lower rates in many other cities, including Chicago and San Francisco. HIV prevalence rates among female prostitutes, many of whom are parenteral drug users, also have a wide range (1% or less to 57%). Because the clients of these women may travel extensively, however, the potential for widespread heterosexual transmission is clear. Fourth, and perhaps most important since homosexual men have accounted for the vast majority of AIDS cases, studies in 1984 and 1985 in San Francisco show that volunteers for the hepatitis B cohort study, with a seroprevalence of 67% to 68%, markedly overestimate the seroprevalence rate, 49% to 51%, among a population-based sample of homosexual men in San Francisco census tracts with the highest AIDS rates (see Table 3-5). These data suggest that true seroprevalence rates among all homosexual men in entire cities may be 50% lower than the rates among homosexual men who participate in research studies. The principal implication is that widely quoted estimates of more than 1 million Americans infected with HIV[63] may be too high, because they are driven by estimates of the male homosexual population and their seroprevalence. Self-selection can, of course, also lead to underestimates of the HIV prevalence in the United States. Blood donors, for example, not only tend to be very healthy but since 1983 have been instructed not to donate if they are homosexual men, drug users, and others possibly at risk of AIDS. The prevalence of 0.04% in this highly selected population indicates the high degree of safety of the American blood supply but clearly would underestimate the HIV prevalence in the nation as a whole. Military recruit applicants, with a prevalence of 0.15%, are less self-selected, although the military also turns away openly homosexual men and drug users prior to serologic testing. The magnitude of underestimates derived from military recruit applicant data is unknown. An accurate estimate of HIV prevalence could be obtained by careful statistical sampling of the nation, although the high cost of such a project might be better spent in other ways.

Race

Female prostitutes and parenteral drug users who are Black or Hispanic have higher HIV prevalence rates than those of other races. Specifically, among female prostitutes who also use parenteral drugs, HIV prevalence among Blacks or Hispanics was 31 of 124 (25%) compared with 16 of 157 (10%) among drug-using female prostitutes of other races.[57] HIV prevalence was also higher among non–drug-using female prostitutes who were Black or Hispanic, 12 of 156 (8%), compared with

Table 3-5
Published HIV Seroprevalence Rates in Selected Populations in the United States

Population	Year	No. Positive/Total	% Positive
A. Homosexual men			
1. New York City[13,43,44]	1982	35/66	53
	1983	39/64	61
	1985	55/85	65
2. Washington, DC[43,44]	1982	19/158	12
	1985	70/160	44
3. Boston[45]	1983–84	34/160	21
4. San Francisco			
a. Hepatitis B cohort[46,47]	1978	13/290	4
	1979	11/87	12
	1980	7/29	24
	1984	293/435	67
	1985	247/361	68
b. Matched controls[48]	1983–84	148/300	49
c. Random sample of selected	1984	388/799	49
census tracts[49,50]	1985	404/799	51
	June 1986	411/799	51
B. Parenteral drug users			
1. New York City[51,52]	1981–82	26/56	46
	1984	162/273	68
2. New Jersey—total[53]	1984	280/740	38
<5 miles from Manhattan		136/231	59
5–9 miles from Manhattan		75/166	45
10–25 miles from Manhattan		68/283	24
100 miles from Manhattan		1/60	2
3. Boston[54]	1982–83	29/69	42
4. Chicago[55]	1984	4/35	11
5. San Francisco[55]	1984	5/53	9
6. New Orleans[53,56]	1985	2/216	1
C. Female prostitutes[57]	1986		
1. Northern New Jersey		32/56	57
2. Miami		47/252	19
3. San Francisco		9/146	6
4. Los Angeles		8/184	4
5. Colorado Springs		1/71	1
6. Atlanta		1/92	1
7. Las Vegas		0/34	0
D. Hemophilia patients			
1. Pittsburgh, PA[58]	1978	7/112	6
	1981	2/26	8
	1982	8/40	20
	1983	20/44	46
	1984	49/80	61
2. Worcester, MA[59]	1983–84	33/50	66
3. Hershey, PA[16]	1983–84	52/69	75
4. Georgia[60]	1985	187/269	70
E. Volunteer blood donors[61]	1985	333/868,000	0.04
F. Military recruit applicants[62]	1985	400/270,000	0.15

3 of 127 (2%) who were of other races.[57] Similarly, among drug users in treatment programs, Blacks or Hispanics had higher HIV seroprevalence rates than Whites in Manhattan (54% vs 42%), New Jersey (45% vs 31%), and San Francisco (14% vs 6%)[56,64,65]. More dramatic racial differences have been noted in prevalence of anti-bodies against the prototype human retrovirus, human T-lymphotropic virus type I (HTLV-I), including, in New Jersey, 30% of Black drug users compared with 9% of non-Black drug users and, in New Orleans, fully 49% of Black drug users compared with only 6% of non-Black drug users.

RISK FACTORS FOR HIV INFECTION

Male Homosexual Activity

Our original reports that numerous homosexual partners and frequent receptive anal intercourse accounted for virtually all prevalent HIV-seropositive homosexual men in Manhattan and Denmark[13,41] have been independently confirmed by several larger studies.[49,66,67] In addition, the Multicenter AIDS Cohort Study evaluated 2,507 homosexual men for seroconversion from HIV-negative to HIV-positive.[68] 95 (3.8%) of these men seroconverted during 6 months of follow-up, including 58 (10.6%) of the 548 who reported receptive anal intercourse with two or more partners. As in the seroprevalence risk factor studies,[13,49,66,67] multiple logistic regression analysis showed that number of homosexual partners and frequency of receptive anal intercourse were the only statistically significant risk factors for HIV seroconversion.[68] The only three men to seroconvert without reported receptive anal intercourse within 12 months were among those 344 men who reported anal intercourse as the insertive partner only—a six-month seroconversion rate of 0.9%. This study demonstrates that relatively inefficient modes of transmission, for example to the insertive partner, can be detected only with large cohorts because of the overriding efficiency of receptive anal intercourse.

Female Homosexual Activity

Two brief case reports have suggested that intimate sexual contact between women may be able to transmit HIV.[69,70] In both cases, oral exposure to vaginal fluid or menses was suggested as the possible mode of transmission, and in one case the partners had vaginal bleeding as a result of traumatic sexual activities.

Parenteral Drug Use

The population of parenteral drug users appears to be far less mobile than the population of homosexual men, resulting in striking differences in the HIV seroprevalence by geography. For example, in New Jersey during 1984, within 5 miles of central Manhattan 59% of parenteral drug users had HIV antibodies, but the prevalence fell to 45% 5 to 9 miles from Manhattan, 24% 10 to 25 miles from Manhattan, and only 2% among New Jersey drug users who were 100 miles from Manhattan (see Table 3-5).[53] Likewise in Glasgow, Scotland during 1985, only 27 (4.5%) of 606 drug users had HIV antibodies, and 20 (74%) of these were from the city of Edinburgh.[71] Once HIV seroprevalence reaches 10% to 15%, however, infection appears to accelerate, resulting in spread to the majority within that community.

Among drug users, the risk of being infected with HIV is closely linked to both the frequency of drug injection and the sharing of needles or injection with previously used needles in "shooting galleries."[64,65] These factors are analogous to frequent receptive anal intercourse and numerous homosexual partners.

Heterosexual Activity

HIV has been isolated from semen and cervical secretions[72-74] and appears to be efficiently transmitted to either partner by heterosexual vaginal intercourse. In some communities in the United States, heterosexually acquired HIV is evident, and the prevalence of HIV is reaching a critical level. A population-based serologic survey in Belle Glade, Florida, has shown that 3.6% of adult men and 2.8% of adult women are infected with HIV.[75] Risk factor analysis has shown that seropositivity is related to the number of heterosexual partners, to prostitution, and/or to heterosexual partners having AIDS or HIV antibodies. No adult over age 60 years and no child aged 2 to 10 years was HIV seropositive. Other assays performed on the Belle Glade sera showed that HIV seropositivity correlated with antibodies to hepatitis B virus and syphilis and not to five arboviruses prevalent in the area.[75]

The principal mode by which HIV is likely to enter American heterosexual communities is by male customers of female prostitutes. During 1986, the HIV antibody prevalence among female prostitutes was 57.1% in northern New Jersey, 18.7% in Miami, 6.2% in San Francisco, 4.3% in Los Angeles, 1.4% in Colorado Springs, 1.1% in Atlanta, and none of 34 in Las Vegas (see Table 3-5).[57] With all cities combined, HIV seropositivity was higher in prostitutes who reported using intravenous drugs (16.7%), but HIV seroprevalence was also substantial in those who did not use drugs (5.3%) and appeared to be particularly related to not using condoms with husbands or boyfriends.[57] Case-control studies of AIDS among Haitians have strongly pointed to heterosexual transmission of the disease,[76] with sexual contact with prostitutes in the United States being the strongest single risk factor for Haitian men.[76]

Central Africa illustrates heterosexual transmission of HIV on a wide scale. During August 1985 a hospital-based survey in Lusaka, Zambia, found that 189 (17.5%) of 1,078 subjects had HIV antibodies.[27] HIV prevalence was low before 20 or after 60 years of age, with peak prevalences of 32.9% in men aged 30 to 35 years and 24.4% in women aged 20 to 25 years. Among patients, the prevalence was highest in those attending sexually transmitted disease clinics (37.3% in repeat attenders and 22.8% in first-time attenders) and relatively low, but still substantial, among antenatal women (8.7%) and orthopedic patients (9.3%). Blood donors and hospital workers in Lusaka had HIV prevalence rates of 18.4% and 19.0%, respectively.[27]

By early 1985, very high HIV infection rates also were present in other heterosexual populations in central Africa, including 6% of hospital workers and 31% of female prostitutes in Kinshasa, Zaire,[77,78] 15.5% of blood donors and 80% of non–drug-using female prostitutes in Kigali, Rwanda,[36,79,80] and 31% to 66% of non–drug-using female prostitutes in Nairobi, Kenya.[81] Among seronegative women in the latter group, the 2-year HIV seroconversion rate was 56%,[82] suggesting that nearly all female prostitutes in Nairobi may soon be infected with HIV.

Genital ulcer disease appears to increase the risk of HIV transmission in Africa, not only in prostitutes and their customers,[82] but also in married couples.[83] In the one carefully studied population in the United States, adult hemophiliacs and their wives or steady female sexual partners in whom genital ulcers and other sexually transmitted diseases have not been noted, extreme immune deficiency in the man was associated with transmission to the woman, suggesting that increased infectiousness occurs late in the pathogenic process.[84] Use of condoms clearly reduces, but does not eliminate, the risk of heterosexual transmission of HIV.[85,86] One report has suggested that heterosexual transmission may occur through oral sexual contact,[86] while two other investigations indicated that anal intercourse may facilitate heterosexual HIV transmission.[87,88] Although heterosexual transmission clearly occurs, estimates of the rate and efficiency of transmission are limited by the paucity of carefully designed large-scale prospective studies.

Transmission from Mother to Baby

At least some cases of HIV infection in children, and probably the majority, occur by transplacental passage of HIV in pregnant, infected women, as demonstrated by two reports of AIDS or HIV infection in babies born by cesarian section[89,90] and two in which HIV has been isolated from 15- to 20-week fetuses.[91,92] Two recent reports of HIV IgM antibodies in cord blood[93] or sera of newborns[94] also point to the likelihood of *in utero* transmission. As noted near the beginning of this chapter (see Fig. 3-1), however, such IgM assays are not well standardized, as illustrated by widely divergent rates of IgM seroprevalence (17% to 46%) in the three recent studies.[93–95] In addition, an astute physician noted that a mother infected with HIV by a postpartum transfusion probably transmitted the virus to her baby by breast-feeding.[96] HIV has been isolated from breast milk,[97] and nursing is a primary mode of transmission of the prototype human retrovirus, human T-lymphotropic virus type I.[98]

Studies to quantify the risk of a mother infecting her baby by any route are incomplete, because no sensitive and specific assays are available to distinguish neonatal infection. The majority of babies still have maternal antibodies at 10 months of age, and approximately 25% will have HIV seropositivity beyond 12 months of age.[99] Estimates of the HIV infection rate in babies born to seropositive women range from 25%, when the mothers are largely asymptomatic,[99,100] to 65%, when the mothers have had a previous baby with AIDS.[101]

Some reports suggest that the risk of perinatal transmission is higher when the mother has a low CD4:CD8 (helper:suppressor) T-cell ratio,[94] which is analogous to the increased risk of heterosexual transmission when the infected partner has severe immune deficiency.[84]

Transfusion and Related Therapies

The first report of AIDS in hemophiliacs[102] provided persuasive evidence that the cause of AIDS was almost certainly a very small infectious agent such as a virus that not only was transmitted by intimate sexual contact but that also had contaminated the blood and plasma supply. In retrospect, hemophiliacs first became infected in the late 1970s and early 1980s[16,58] through concentrated plasma products, particularly commercial Factor VIII concentrate that had been pooled from many thousands of American donors. In our original serosurvey of hemophiliacs,[103] we noted a much higher prevalence of HIV antibodies among recipients of Factor VIII concentrate (51/69, 74%) than among patients with the rarer hemophilia type B (Christmas disease) who had received Factor IX concentrate (0/12). Subsequent studies have confirmed that the likelihood of becoming infected is related to the dose of commercial Factor VIII concentrate,[42] which is highest among patients with severe hemophilia A (Table 3-6). It is unclear why virtually 100% of Factor VIII concentrate recipients did not become infected with HIV. The prevalence of serologic markers for hepatitis B virus, for example, is nearly universal among such patients, and this is true even with eliminating blood and plasma that is positive for hepatitis B surface antigen.[104] Of 33 patients with hemophilia A, 18 (55%) became infected with HIV from a single batch of Scottish Factor VIII concentrate.[105,106] None of 10 recipients of Factor IX concentrate made from the same batch of plasma became infected. In the follow-up report, only the number of bottles of implicated Factor VIII that the patients used distinguished seroconverters from seronegative hemophiliacs, with all those who received more than 30 bottles becoming infected.[107] There was no evidence of a predisposition to seroconvert based on total or annual dose of Factor VIII, total number of T4 cells, or T4:T8 ratios. It could be that the lower prevalence of HIV antibodies among recipients of Factor IX concentrate, particularly those with hemophilia B (see Table 3-5), is also simply related to dose, with hemophilia B patients requiring less intensive treatment. However, we have also postulated that HIV may sediment preferentially into the cryoprecipitate, which is made into Factor VIII concentrate, rather than into the cryosupernate, which is made into Factor IX concentrate.[103]

Two procedures have reduced markedly the risk of additional hemophiliacs becoming infected. The first of these is heat treatment of commercial clotting factor concentrates, originally designed to reduce the risk of hepatitis B virus transmission. With the report that HIV

Table 3-6
Prevalence of HIV Antibodies During 1986 by Type and Severity of Clotting Disorder

Clotting Disorder	Severity	No. HIV-Positive/No. Tested	Prevalence (%)
Hemophilia A	Severe	404/531	76
	Moderate	24/53	45
	Mild	35/121	29
Hemophilia B	Severe	28/67	42
	Moderate	2/13	15
	Mild	5/25	20
Von Willebrand's	Severe	3/14	21
	Moderate	0/5	0
	Mild	0/7	0
Other	Any	0/15	0

(Goedert JJ et al: National Cancer Institute study of AIDS in hemophiliacs. Unpublished data.)

was heat labile, most hemophilia treatment centers switched their patients to heat-treated plasma products shortly after they became available—Factor VIII concentrate in late 1984 and early 1985 and Factor IX concentrate in late 1985. The second procedure is screening of donated blood and plasma for HIV antibodies, which began in the spring of 1985. The use of heat-treated products greatly reduced but did not eliminate HIV seroconversions among hemophiliacs.[107-109] The added step of eliminating HIV-positive plasma from the donor pool probably has reduced HIV transmission through these products to virtually nil.

HIV has been transmitted by transfusion of whole blood, red blood cells, platelets, and plasma.[110-113] Some 89% of the recipients of HIV-positive blood components have become infected.[113] In Kinshasa, Zaire, where the background prevalence of HIV appears to be very high, 40 (3.8%) of 1,046 children presenting to the hospital were HIV-positive; and there was a strong dose-response association between blood transfusions and HIV seropositivity.[35] Malaria was the primary indication for transfusion. Among heavily transfused patients in the United States, the prevalence of HIV antibodies is 8% among those with leukemia in New York City[114] and 6% with congenital anemias from several cities combined.[113] Among the leukemia patients, the estimated risk of becoming infected appeared to decrease in parallel with the HIV prevalence in the donor pool. Based on data shown in Table 3-7, it has been estimated that approximately 10,000 to 12,000 people now living in the United States acquired transfusion-associated HIV infection between 1978 and 1984.[114]

Prior to the initiation of HIV screening of donated blood and plasma in the spring of 1985, the HIV seroprevalence among donors (with risk-group deferral programs in place) ranged from 0.01% in cities such as Peoria, Illinois, where there were few cases of AIDS, to 0.1% to 0.2% in large American cities with a high incidence of AIDS.[61] During the first year of HIV screening,

Table 3-7
Prevalence of Transfusion-Associated HIV Infection Among Patients with Leukemia in New York City

Year of Specimen	No. HIV-Positive/ No. Tested	Risk per Component (%)*
1978–1980	0/86	0.00%
1981–1983	9/77	0.07%
1984–1986†	7/41	0.10%
Total	16/204	0.05%

* Estimated risk based on an average of 164 components per recipient.
† Transfused before screening of blood began in March 1985.
(Centers for Disease Control: Human immunodeficiency virus infection in transfusion recipients and their family members. Morbid Mortal Weekly Rep 36:137, 1987)

the overall prevalence among American Red Cross donors in the United States has declined from 0.04% to 0.02%.[115] Only one case of HIV transmission by an antibody-negative donor has been reported in the United States,[115] but this case emphasizes the need for continued vigilance in maximizing voluntary deferral by donors who might have been infected recently and not yet developed antibodies. Three steps to improve voluntary deferral of possibly infected donors have been taken. First, the time frame for self-deferral of men with homosexual contact was expanded back from 1979 to 1977, and even men with a single homosexual contact are included. Second, most collection centers now enable donors to confidentially indicate that their blood should be used for "research only" and not for transfusion. Finally, most collection agencies now recognize the real threat of heterosexually acquired HIV infection and request that women who have engaged in prostitution and men who have used prostitutes voluntarily refrain from donating blood.[116-118]

As a general rule, blood products with a high risk of transmitting hepatitis B virus[104] are also likely to transmit HIV. In addition to clotting factor concentrates, another noteworthy example is the unorthodox "immunoaugmentive therapy" derived from human serum proteins that was given to cancer patients by a clinic in the Bahamas.[119] At the opposite end of the spectrum, correctly pasteurized human albumin preparations have an unblemished safety record with regard to virus transmission, and HIV could not be recovered from albumin preparations that were made from HIV-spiked plasma.[120] With regard to licensed, commercial immunoglobulin preparations, the risk of HIV transmission is either very low or zero. HIV antibodies can be detected in a variety of immunoglobulin preparations,[121] but virtually all HIV appears to be removed during the plasma fractionation process.[122-124] In addition, six healthy volunteers were given HIV-positive intravenous immune globulin, none of whom seroconverted to HIV or developed immunologic or clinical abnormalities.[124] Likewise, 16 patients treated with HIV-positive hepatitis-B immune globulin developed low levels of passively acquired HIV antibodies, but all 16 were seronegative within 6 months.[125] In addition, attempts to isolate HIV from intravenous gamma globulin have been unsuccessful, and the vast majority of patients treated with intravenous gamma globulin have no evidence of HIV infection or disease.[126] Nonetheless, non-A, non-B hepatitis has been transmitted by intravenous gamma globulin, and HIV was identified in two patients treated with intravenous gamma globulin.[127] Finally, there is no evidence that HIV has been or could be transmitted by plasma-derived hepatitis B vaccine, including both the preparation made in the United States (Heptavax-B)[128] and that made in France (HEVAC).[129]

Transplantation and Dialysis

HIV has been transmitted from HIV-infected donors by transplantation of kidneys[130-133] and by artificial insemination.[134] It is likely that HIV could also be transmitted in other donated organs and tissues. Thus, it has been recommended that all potential organ, tissue, and semen donors be tested for HIV antibodies.[135] Donors to milk banks are not included, although consideration should be given to screening such women or to pasteurization of donated breast milk.[136,137] Despite screening precautions, at least one HIV-infected cadaver was missed by initial HIV screening, which resulted in HIV infections in the two recipients of his kidneys.[138] Despite this tragic mishap, sera from cadavers generally yield very high sensitivity and specificity with the standard HIV ELISA kits.[139]

HIV does not appear to have been transmitted by dialysis.[133,140] Nonetheless, patients with AIDS and related conditions often require dialysis,[141] placing HIV-negative dialysis patients and health care workers at potential risk. Although published guidelines from the United States Centers for Disease Control (CDC) state that "standard blood and body fluid precautions and disinfection and sterilization strategies routinely practiced in dialysis centers are adequate to prevent transmission" of HIV,[142] others have recommended the additional step of segregating HIV-positive patients during dialysis sessions as is done with patients positive for hepatitis B surface antigen.[143] With either strategy, the risk appears to be low but warrants monitoring in sufficiently large cohorts to detect minimal risk exposure.

Exposures to Needles, Arthropods, and Body Fluids

Studies of more than 2,000 nurses and other health care workers with intensive exposure to AIDS patients and their body fluids have demonstrated no HIV seroconversions except as a consequence of parenteral injuries with contaminated needles or other sharp instruments.[144-149] Although fewer than 10 such seroconversions have been reported, careless handling and disposal of sharp instruments is widespread,[145-149] which could result in many more accidental HIV infections. To minimize these events, hospital safety policies must be emphasized and procedures enforced, particularly with an aim to eliminate recapping of needles. Recommended biosafety precautions have been published.[150-155]

With regard to nonparenteral exposure to blood and other body fluids as a risk factor for HIV infection, case reports of six subjects need to be considered.[156-160] Four of the cases[156,157] are well documented and appear to represent HIV seroconversions. One case was a mother who provided intensive, prolonged nursing care for her HIV-infected baby, which included repeated exposures to blood, urine, feces, and gastric contents. A second was a phlebotomist who was splashed in the face and mouth with blood from an HIV-infected patient. The third had her hands and arms covered with blood that spilled from an apheresis machine, while the fourth assisted in an unsuccessful attempt at cardiopulmonary resuscitation, during which she had blood on her index finger for 20 minutes. A fifth case reported AIDS in a woman whose only apparent risk factor was prolonged home-care nursing for a man with AIDS.[158] This woman and three of the four above reportedly had eczema or other potential ports of entry on the skin of their hands. The final case is an HIV-seropositive older brother of a boy who died from transfusion-associated AIDS.[159] The authors speculated that a nonpenetrating bite by the younger boy with AIDS may have been the mode of transmission. Put in the context of the large, carefully performed studies of health care workers[144-149] and families of patients with AIDS, ARC, and HIV seropositivity,[160-163] a handful of such cases, particularly in the universe of intensively exposed health care workers, is not unexpected. With these reports, broader use of gloves, masks, and protective garments by hospital personnel and/or mandatory HIV screening of patients may be appropriate. Clearly dentists and dental hygienists must wear gloves during all procedures to protect themselves and their patients and should also wear masks and protective eyewear to protect themselves during certain procedures.[152] It is reassuring that the only case of possible household transmission is anecdotal,[159] although additional follow-up of exposed family members in cohorts of sufficient size will be needed to quantify these extremely rare events.

Recently, HIV infections have been reported in two laboratory workers involved in the production of large quantities of HIV for blood test kits and research work.*,[164] One case involved exposure from a cannula used to clean potentially infectious material from an apparatus that resulted in a penetrating cut of a gloved hand. The other case had no obvious episode of exposure but may have been infected by the culture-proven HTLV-IIIb laboratory strain through undetected skin exposure or possibly by aerosol exposure. The estimated risk in this setting (0.48 per 100 person-years) approximates that for health care workers experiencing a parenteral needle stick exposure.[164] The findings in these cases, as in the health care setting, stress the need for strict adherence to current biosafety guidelines.[164a]

Repeated medical injections appear to be related to HIV seropositivity among children in Kinshasa, Zaire, who have HIV-negative mothers.[28] This observation was not confirmed in Kigali, Rwanda,[165] and could simply be a spurious association of HIV-positive children receiving more injections because they were already ill. However, given the clear association of HIV seropositivity among parental drug users with number of injections and exposure to "shooting galleries" where needles and syringes are reused,[64,65] it is likely that medical injections with reused, unsterilized equipment in a high-prevalence area could transmit HIV. Injection of a child with AIDS followed by injection of his older brother appears to have transmitted HIV in one family.[166]

Hypothetically, biting insects could transmit HIV either by serving as a stage in the HIV life cycle, with replication and growth of the virus within the insect, or simply as "flying syringes" carrying minute amounts of HIV-infected undigested blood from person to person. There is no evidence for either hypothesis, although an unmeasurably low risk by the latter mechanism cannot be excluded.[167-169] The possibility of arthropod-borne HIV was specifically ruled out in Belle Glade, Florida;[75] and several studies in Africa have noted that children and elderly adults, all of whom are frequently bitten by insects, have a remarkable absence of HIV infections.[23,26-29] On the other hand, experimental studies with related animal retroviruses document the potential for biting flies to be vectors for transmission under certain limited conditions.

---

* National Institutes of Health, unpublished data.

NATURAL HISTORY OF HIV INFECTION

AIDS Incidence

Incidence is the measure of risk made by dividing the number of cases that occur by the number of people in the population who are at risk. With AIDS, cumulative rather than annual incidence rates are generally most informative for counseling and planning resource allocation. Mistakes in estimating the denominator, the number of persons at risk, can lead to gross underestimates in AIDS incidence for those who are truly at risk. The denominator can be determined only by testing the population for HIV antibodies. Those persons who have HIV antibodies at the first evaluation are termed prevalent positives and can be compared to other prevalent positive persons with caution.[43,170] Among prevalent cohorts, the 3-year incidence of AIDS ranged from a low of 8% among homosexual men in Denmark to a high of 34% among homosexual men in Manhattan.[43] The incidence of AIDS was intermediate among prevalent cohorts of homosexual men in Washington, DC, parenteral drug users in Queens, New York, and hemophiliacs in Hershey, Pennsylvania.[43] The 5-year incidence of AIDS in these prevalent cohorts was 15% among the Hershey hemophiliacs, 39% among the Washington homosexual men, and 45% among the Manhattan homosexual men (Fig. 3-7).[171]

AIDS incidence among parenteral drug users is complicated by difficult prospective follow-up and missed diagnosis. Mortality attributed to drug overdose can, in fact, be due to AIDS.[171a] Moreover, while 5-year cumulative AIDS incidence among prevalent HIV-infected drug abusers is a substantial 17%, simultaneous mortality among these HIV-infected drug abusers is nearly 50%, five times higher than among HIV-negative drug abusers (Fig. 3-8). This strongly suggests that underascertainment of AIDS in drug abusers is substantial. There appears to be similar difficulty with the one study that examined the risk of AIDS in prevalent HIV-infected African hospital employees.[77] Specifically, there were serious illnesses and deaths in the cohort that may have been missed AIDS diagnoses. In addition, the African data are not comparable with the data cited above, because all of the African workers who enrolled with any clinical manifestations of HIV were excluded from prospective analysis.

A more accurate picture of the natural history of HIV is obtained in incident seroconverters, rather than prevalent seropositives, particularly because almost no cases of AIDS occur in adults during the first 2 years after infection (Figs. 3-9, 3-10).[43,47,171,173] Cumulative AIDS incidence reaches 30% 7 to 8 years after seroconversion, at least in homosexual men. AIDS incidence among persons infected through blood transfusions is likely to be as high as or higher than in homosexual men, but follow-up is not yet sufficient to be certain of this (Fig. 3-9). AIDS incidence appears to be slightly

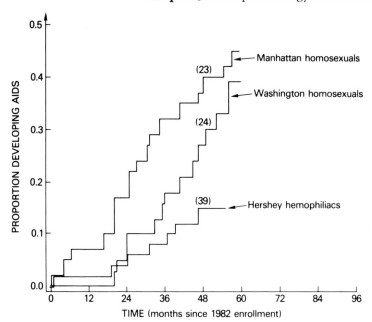

FIG. 3-7. Cumulative AIDS incidence among individuals with HIV antibodies detected in 1982 (Kaplan–Meier survival method). Plots show that nearly 5 years (60 months) after enrollment AIDS incidence was 45% among homosexual men in Manhattan, New York, 39% among homosexual men in Washington, DC, and 15% among persons with hemophilia in Hershey, Pennsylvania.

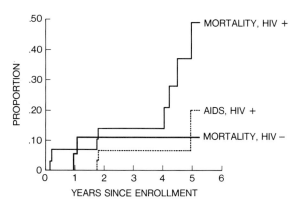

FIG. 3-8. Five-year cumulative mortality and AIDS incidence among parenteral drug users enrolled in a prospective cohort study in late 1981. Among drug users with HIV antibodies (HIV+) at enrollment, 5-year AIDS incidence was 17%, but mortality was nearly 50%. Among drug users without HIV antibodies (HIV−), no AIDS cases occurred and cumulative mortality was 12%. With a substantial excess of HIV-associated mortality, plots suggest that many AIDS cases among drug users were undiagnosed or unreported.

lower among hemophiliacs than homosexual men, an observation that is discussed in greater detail below.

Factors Predicting or Modifying AIDS Risk

Four articles have examined markers of increased AIDS risk and whether cofactors exist that increase or decrease AIDS risk.[44,173–175] All showed that the total number of CD4+ cells (T4 count) is strongly predictive of AIDS, particularly in the ensuing year if the count is below 300 CD4+ cells/μl. In one paper,[174] an increased number of CD8+ cells was predictive of AIDS, but this measure had no predictive value in the other studies.[44,173,175] Two of the studies noted an increased risk of AIDS with thrombocytopenia;[174,175] and in one or more there were similar associations with anemia, monocytopenia, high levels of immunoglobulins G, A, or M, high levels of cytomegalovirus antibodies, or low levels of HIV antibodies.[173,174] Lymphadenopathy had no effect on AIDS risk in any of the three studies in which it could be evaluated,[44,173,174] but AIDS risk was clearly increased in subjects who reported fever, unintentional weight loss, or, to a lesser extent, diarrhea.[44,174,175] Oral candidiasis has also been shown to be strongly associated with AIDS risk.[177] Detection of α interferon in serum, particularly at high levels, appears to be a useful marker for AIDS;[178,179] and three preliminary studies suggest that detection of HIV core (p24) antigen in serum may be strongly predictive of AIDS.*,[180,181]

To date no unequivocal cofactors have been found that modify the AIDS incidence among HIV-infected individuals. However, in the one study that examined the issue in a cohort of incident seroconverting hemophiliacs, the risk of AIDS was substantially lower for those who seroconverted during childhood compared to seroconversion during adulthood. (Fig. 3-10).[173] The precise mechanism by which children would tolerate HIV infection better and have a lower risk of AIDS than adults is unclear, but it has been speculated that chronic

* Goedert JJ, Eyster ME: Unpublished data.

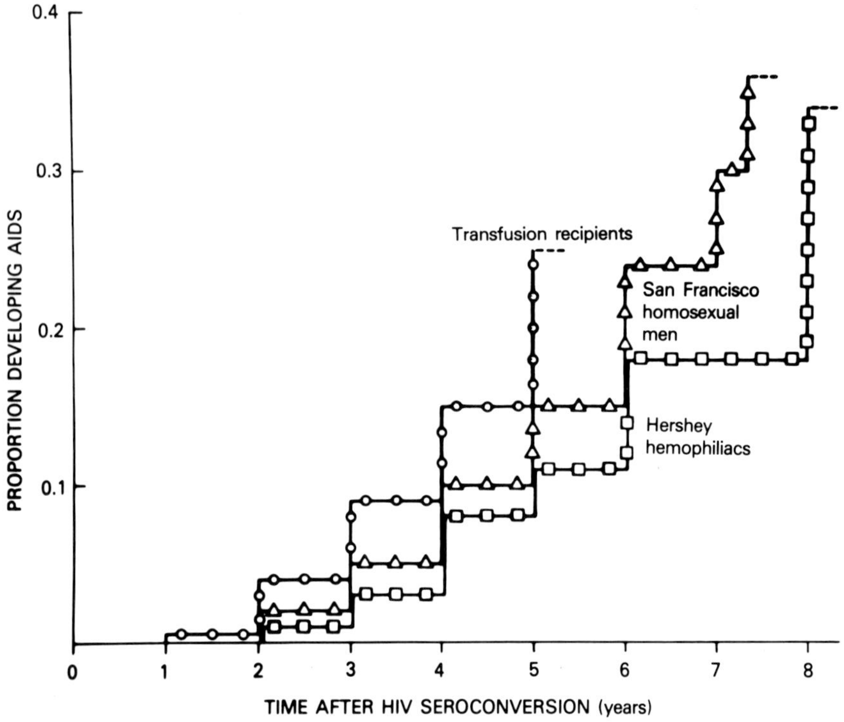

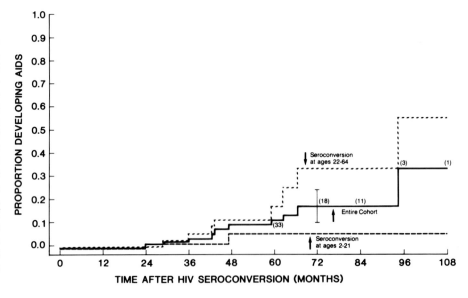

FIG. 3-9. Cumulative AIDS incidence (Kaplan–Meier method) among three cohorts from the known or estimated date of HIV infection. Time for the transfusion recipients is measured from the date of transfusion with HIV antibody-positive blood. Time for the San Francisco homosexual men and adults with hemophilia in Hershey, Pennsylvania, is measured from the midpoint between the last HIV-seronegative and first HIV-seropositive specimens. Plots show that the AIDS experience for all three groups is similar, with few cases occurring during the first 2 years after HIV infection and AIDS incidence rates of about 20% 5 to 7 years after infection.

FIG. 3-10. Cumulative AIDS incidence (Kaplan–Meier method) in 84 hemophiliacs from their estimated dates of HIV antibody seroconversion. Numbers in parentheses indicate the number of patients still in follow-up at years 5 through 9 after seroconversion. Vertical bar at 72 months (6 years) indicates one standard error. Plots show that adults with hemophilia are at significantly higher risk of AIDS than are children (p = 0.03). (Eyster ME, Gail MH, Ballard JO et al: Natural history of human immunodeficiency virus (HIV) infections in hemophiliacs: Effects of T-cell subsets, platelet counts and age. Ann Intern Med 107: 1, 1987)

liver disease may increase the risk in adult hemophiliacs.[173]

The two studies of homosexual men with prevalent HIV infections[44,174] noted very weak increases in AIDS risk with numerous homosexual partners and no effect of race, nitrite inhalant use, or several other factors on the risk of Kaposi's sarcoma, opportunistic infections, or total AIDS. There was an increased risk of AIDS among those who had sex with someone who developed

AIDS, an observation that has not been independently confirmed but that raises the possibility of relatively aggressive strains of HIV.[174] Independent work has noted that some strains of HIV may be non-cytocidal for $CD4^+$ cells.[182]

Two general classes of host factors have been evaluated with regard to AIDS risk, human leukocyte antigen (HLA) types and group-specific component (Gc) types. The early report that HLA-DR5 was associated with Kaposi's sarcoma[183] has not been replicated in other large studies, except among persons of Mediterranean heritage known to have a high frequency of this specificity.[184-187] More recently, an increased risk of AIDS has been noted among prevalent HIV-infected homosexual men with HLA-DR1.[188] One study noted that AIDS risk appeared to be related to Gc types,[189] but no such association was found in five other investigations.[190-194] Thus, the relationship between host factors and AIDS is largely unsettled.

Staging Systems

Two general staging systems for HIV disease have been proposed (Table 3-8), but it is unclear that either system has any advantage over simply measuring the total number of CD4$^+$ cells in an HIV-infected individual. The Walter Reed system[195] is soundly based on the pathobiology of HIV but is rather cumbersome, particularly in an outpatient setting, since it requires not only a physical examination, an HIV antibody assay, and T-cell testing, but also delayed hypersensitivity testing with a battery of skin test antigens that must be read by a trained examiner 48 hours after application. Although some HIV-infected persons may be hard to stage because of CD4$^+$-counts that vary above and below the arbitrary level of 400 cells/μl that distinguishes stages WR1 and 2 from WR3, investigators in Frankfurt have shown that the majority of individuals appears to progress to higher stages in a similar system.[196] The proportions of each WR stage that progress to WR6 (i.e., AIDS with a life-threatening opportunistic infection) have not been precisely quantified.

In contrast to the *in vitro* and *in vivo* measures of cellular immunity required by the Walter Reed system, the CDC system[197] is almost entirely clinical, with particular focus on the many infectious diseases and other clinical conditions that occur in persons with HIV infection (see Table 3-8). Also unlike the Walter Reed system, the CDC system has little or no relationship to pathobiology or prognosis. For example, individuals in CDC group II (Asymptomatic Infection) may be much closer to extreme immune deficiency and death than those in group III (Persistent Generalized Lymphadenopathy). Likewise, within CDC group IV (Other Disease) are those with AIDS (Subgroup C-1) and those with relatively mild abnormalities such as idiopathic thrombocytopenia (Subgroup E). The value of the CDC system for prognosis or other purposes remains to be seen.

Table 3-8
Staging Systems for Conditions Related to HIV

Walter Reed Classification System[195]

Stage	HIV Antibody or Culture	Chronic Lymphadenopathy	CD4+ Cell Count/μl	Cutaneous Anergy	Thrush	Opportunistic Infection
WR0	−	−	>400	None	−	−
WR1	+*	−	>400	None	−	−
WR2	+*	+*	>400	None	−	−
WR3	+*	±	<400*	None	−	−
WR4	+*	±	<400*	Partial*	−	−
WR5	+*	±	<400	Complete or partial	+*	−
WR6	+*	±	<400	Complete or partial	±	+*

Centers for Disease Control (CDC) Classification System[197]

Group	Description
I	Acute infection
II	Asymptomatic infection
III	Persistent generalized lymphadenopathy
IV	Other disease
Subgroup A	Constitutional disease
Subgroup B	Neurologic disease
Subgroup C	Secondary infectious diseases
Category C-1	Specified secondary infectious diseases listed in the CDC surveillance definition for AIDS†
Category C-2	Other specified secondary infectious diseases
Subgroup D	Secondary cancers, including those within the CDC surveillance definition for AIDS†
Subgroup E	Other conditions

* Indicates critical features of each Walter Reed (WR) stage.
† See Table 3-1 for the CDC surveillance definition for AIDS.

Sublethal Conditions Related to HIV

As illustrated by the problems with the CDC staging system described above, no rational system has been developed for categorizing the many sublethal conditions that can and do occur in HIV-infected individuals. For example, a minority of individuals have an acute mononucleosis-like syndrome coincident with HIV seroconversion[198] that may be accompanied by severe neurologic complications including encephalitis.[15] Nonetheless, there are no clinical sequelae, except for residual lymph node enlargement in some individuals, and no suggestion of adverse long-term prognosis compared to individuals with asymptomatic initial HIV infection.

A general problem is to separate conditions that are actually related to HIV or HIV-related immune deficiency from those that occur in HIV-infected individuals by coincidence. This process has begun for malignancies in HIV-infected individuals and is described below. Other conditions, such as herpes zoster in homosexual men and unexplained oral candidiasis, are well known to occur in the setting of defective cellular immunity and also have been shown to be highly predictive of AIDS.[177,199] Persistent unexplained vaginal candidiasis may fall into the same category.[200]

A second group of conditions probably occurs in HIV-infected individuals by coincidence, but their natural history or required treatments are altered by HIV-induced immune deficiency. Tuberculosis, for example, has been noted disproportionately in patients with AIDS, particularly among Blacks, and the reported incidence of tuberculosis in the United States is no longer declining.[201-203] Although standard antituberculosis regimens are effective in many HIV-infected patients, more aggressive treatment has been recommended.[204] A similar approach has been advocated for aggressive treatment of syphilis in persons with HIV infection,[205] as it appears that tertiary neurosyphilis may emerge as a persistent problem.[206,207]

A myriad of conditions, ranging from oral hairy leukoplakia[208-210] to Addison's disease,[211] have been noted in patients with or at high risk of AIDS. Many of these, such as the two just mentioned, appear to be manifestations of chronic viral infections. Except for bacterial pneumonias in patients with AIDS,[212] the pathogenic mechanisms have not been elucidated for most of the other conditions coincident with AIDS, such as immune thrombocytopenia,[213-218] Reiter's syndrome,[219] pyomyositis,[220] congestive cardiomyopathy,[221] and several dermatologic conditions, particularly seborrheic dermatitis.[222-224]

HIV Disease in Children

HIV disease is more complicated in infants than in adults, due at least in part to significant functional abnormalities in humoral as well as cell-mediated immunity.[225,226] Thus, infants with HIV infection may develop not only pneumocystis pneumonia and other manifestations of adult AIDS but also repeated life-threatening infections with encapsulated bacteria including species of *Hemophilus* and *Streptococcus.*[227-230] They also have a high incidence of lymphoid interstitial pneumonitis, which may be caused by HIV infection of pulmonary mononuclear cells.[231] These features of pediatric AIDS have been incorporated in the revision of the CDC surveillance definition of AIDS (see Table 3-1). Newborns are also susceptible to congenital or perinatal transmission of several life-threatening infectious diseases in the absence of HIV, including vital organ involvement by *Toxoplasma,* herpes simplex virus, or cytomegalovirus. HIV serology, if negative, will help to rule out AIDS in such cases, but is unhelpful if positive due to passive transfer of maternal antibodies (see Definitions, above). In children who are infected with HIV, the impact on the neurologic system may be profound, including severe impairments in both cognitive and motor development.[232] Finally, one group has noted unusual facies in HIV-infected infants, suggesting that HIV may be teratogenic *in utero.*[233] This observation has not been independently confirmed.

Cancers, Including Kaposi's Sarcoma

As is true with the nonmalignant conditions described above, many different types of cancer have been noted in patients with or at high risk of AIDS. Biggar and associates have developed a method for systematically determining which tumor types are part of the AIDS epidemic, by using the United States population-based surveillance, epidemiology, and end results (SEER) tumor registry system.[234,235] With particular focus on young, never-married men, a surrogate population for the largest AIDS risk group, homosexual men, the authors have shown that Kaposi's sarcoma increased 2,479 times between 1978 and 1984 in San Francisco and 182 times elsewhere.[235] Significant increases were also noted within San Francisco for non-Hodgkin's lymphomas (4.2 times, p < 0.0001), particularly Burkitt-like lymphomas (11.2 times, p = 0.003) or lymphomas of the central nervous system. These findings thus provide independent statistical confirmation and quantification of the large series of homosexual men with non-Hodgkin's lymphomas that has been reported.[236] Biggar et al also noted non-significant increases in single young men in San Francisco with Hodgkin's disease (p = 0.13) and hepatoma (p = 0.08); and, *a posteriori,* noted increases in urinary tract tumors and acute lymphoblastic leukemia. Additional investigation will be needed to determine whether these are simply chance associations.

The group of malignancies that deserve the closest observation are those associated with viruses, as it is clear that persistent viral infections are a hallmark of AIDS. In addition to Burkitt-like lymphomas and hepatoma, which are closely associated with Epstein–Barr virus and hepatitis B virus, respectively, close attention should be paid to anorectal and cervical carcinomas, which have been linked to certain types of papilloma virus, and to adult T-cell leukemia, the malignant manifestation of human T-lymphotropic virus type I (HTLV-I).[237-240]

AIDS IN THE FUTURE

Mathematical projections suggest that the cumulative number of patients diagnosed with AIDS will reach 135,000 to 270,000 or more by the end of 1991.[63,241] The AIDS epidemic beyond that point will depend on at least two issues—the emergence of related viruses and the success or failure of intervention strategies.

HIV-2 and Other Retroviruses

A new human retrovirus, termed HIV-2, has been identified in areas of West Africa by teams at the Pasteur Institute in Paris and at Harvard University in Boston.[6,7] Patients with AIDS or AIDS-related complex who were infected with HIV-2, but not HIV-1, have been noted.[242-249] It has been suggested, however, that HIV-2 may be somewhat less cytotoxic to target $CD4^+$ cells both *in vivo* and *in vitro*.[7,249,250] Nonetheless, given that HIV-2 can induce serious disease and potentially be missed by current serologic assays, modifications to current assays are being developed to detect HIV-2 and/or HIV-1.[251-255] Seroprevalence surveys[6,7,242-250,256] indicate that HIV-2 is relatively common, particularly among female prostitutes, in some West African countries, particularly former Portugese colonies. HIV-2 also has been noted in a few Europeans with links to these former colonies.[257-260] No Americans with HIV-2 infection have yet been noted, but there can be little doubt that this will occur.

The retrovirus that is more likely to cause increasing disease in the United States is the prototype, human T-lymphotropic virus type I (HTLV-I). HTLV-I is the etiologic agent of adult T-cell leukemia and also appears to cause a multiple-sclerosis–like neurodegenerative disease, termed tropical spastic paraparesis.[261,262] Until recently, HTLV-I was thought to be tightly concentrated in areas of southern Japan, the Caribbean, and perhaps Africa and to be quite rare in the United States.[144] However, Weiss et al recently noted very high seroprevalence rates for HTLV-I among parenteral drug users in northern New Jersey and New Orleans.[56] The findings were particularly striking among Black drug users, with 30% of those in New Jersey and 49% of those in New Orleans infected with HTLV-I but not HIV. Of particular concern, given that HIV may potentiate the replication rate or leukemogenic effect of HTLV-I, 16% of the Black drug users in New Jersey were co-infected with HTLV-I and HIV. An HTLV-related virus also has been noted in areas of Italy.[263] Thus, although only a small portion (perhaps 1%) of persons infected with HTLV-I are thought to pro-gress to adult T-cell leukemia, co-infection with HIV could readily increase the incidence of both HTLV-I infections and leukemia cases. Studies are in progress to assess this possibility.

Intervention Strategies

Public health strategies (covered in detail in Part III of this volume) involve complex issues of medicine, psychology, sociology, education, economics, and the law. Despite these complexities, some considerations are straightforward. First, HIV causes serious disease and death in a large portion of infected individuals. Second, virtually all HIV infections occur by sexual contact, by sharing needles, from mother to fetus or newborn, or by transfusion of infected blood; as a corollary, virtually all of these infections can be prevented by a combination of serologic testing and behavior modification. Third, given the serious morbidity and mortality caused by HIV and the ability to avoid infection, intervention strategies ought to be direct in their use of the two tools available, serologic testing and education, while providing adequate safeguards against unfounded discrimination or other abuses of legitimate rights.

A specific proposal to eliminate the sexual transmission of HIV has been published.[85] Briefly, truly safe sex is defined as a monogamous relationship by a non-drug using couple, both of whom are proven to be negative for HIV antibodies, or mutual masturbation by individuals who have not been tested, abuse parenteral drugs or have a partner who does, are not monogamous, or are dichotomous on HIV antibody testing. This approach, which defines "safe" as elimination of risk, has been applied to donated blood since antibody screening was added to education and voluntary deferral in the spring of 1985. Similar approaches can be developed by testing parenteral drug users and exhorting the seronegative individuals to eliminate needle sharing or inadvertent reuse of needles. Likewise, perinatal transmission could be virtually eliminated by the use of effective contraception by HIV-infected women. Although in some instances HIV testing may be mandatory, such as in blood donors, the behavior modification to actually eliminate HIV transmission is likely always to be voluntary. Thus, coercion or actual quarantine must always be viewed as extreme, last-resort measures that would be administered only in highly selected, recalcitrant cases.

The prospects for successful control of HIV and AIDS are unknown. Particularly in the developing nations of the world, much will depend on the development of safe and effective vaccines or chemotherapies that prevent viral replication, release, or attachment to receptors. However, even with the arrival of such modalities, factors that influence sexual activities and other personal behaviors are likely to have major effects on the worldwide prevalence and incidence of human retroviruses, AIDS, and their associated conditions.

REFERENCES

1. Popovic M, Sarngadharan MG, Read E et al: Detection, isolation, and continuous production of cytopathic retroviruses (HTLV-III) from patients with AIDS and pre-AIDS. Science 224:497, 1984
2. Melbye M: The natural history of human T lymphotropic virus-III infection: The cause of AIDS. Br Med J 292:5, 1986
3. Gartner S, Markovits P, Markovitz DM et al: The role of mononuclear phagocytes in HTLV-III/LAV infection. Science 233:215, 1986
4. Koenig S, Gendleman HE, Orenstein JM et al: Detection of AIDS virus in macrophages in brain tissue from AIDS patients with encephalopathy. Science 233:1089, 1986
5. Gabuzda DH, Hirsh MS: Neurologic manifestations of infection with human immunodeficiency virus: Clinical features and pathogenesis. N Engl J Med 107:383, 1987
6. Clavel F, Guetard D, Brun–Vezinet F et al: Isolation of a new human retrovirus from West African patients with AIDS. Science 233:343, 1986
7. Kanki PJ, Barin F, M'Boup S et al: New human T-lymphotropic retrovirus related to simian T-lymphotropic virus type III (STLV-IIIagm). Science 232:238, 1986
8. Goedert JJ: Testing for human immunodeficiency virus. Ann Intern Med 105:609, 1986
9. Salahuddin SZ, Markham PD, Popovic M et al: Isolation of human T leukemia lymphotropic virus type III (HTLV-III) from patients with acquired immunodeficiency syndrome (AIDS) or AIDS-related complex (ARC) and from healthy carriers: A study of risk groups and tissue sources. Proc Natl Acad Sci USA 82:5530, 1985
10. Levy JA, Shimabukuro J: Recovery of AIDS-associated retrovirus from patients with AIDS or AIDS-related conditions and from clinically healthy individuals. J Infect Dis 152:734, 1985
11. Centers for Disease Control: Revision of the CDC surveillance definition for acquired immunodeficiency syndrome. Morbid Mortal Weekly Rep (suppl) 36:1S, 1987
12. Colebunders R, Mann JM, Francis H et al: Evaluation of a clinical case-definition of acquired immunodeficiency syndrome in Africa. Lancet 1:492, 1987
13. Goedert JJ, Sarngadharan MG, Biggar RJ et al: Determinants of retrovirus (HTLV-III) antibody and immunodeficiency conditions in homosexual men. Lancet 2:711, 1984
14. Bayer H, Bienzle U, Schneider J et al: HTLV-III antibody frequency and severity of lymphadenopathy. Lancet 2:1347, 1984
15. Biggar RJ, Johnson BK, Musoke SS et al: Severe illness associated with appearance of antibody to HIV in an African. Br Med J 293:1210, 1986
16. Eyster ME, Goedert JJ, Sarngadharan MG et al: Development and early natural history of HTLV-III antibodies in persons with hemophilia. JAMA 253:2219, 1985
17. Abrams DI: AIDS-related lymphadenopathy: The role of biopsy. J Clin Oncol 2:126, 1986
18. Centers for Disease Control: AIDS Weekly Surveillance Report. September 21, 1987
19. Peterman TA, Jaffe HW, Getchell JP et al: Transfusion-associated acquired immunodeficiency syndrome in the United States. JAMA 254:2913, 1985
20. Medley GF, Anderson RM, Cox DR et al: Incubation period of AIDS in patients infected via blood transfusion. Nature 328:719, 1987
21. Lui KJ, Lawrence DN, Morgan WM et al: A model-based approach for estimating the mean incubation period of transfusion-associated acquired immunodeficiency syndrome. Proc Natl Acad Sci USA 83:3051, 1986
22. Laboratory Centers for Disease Control: Update: "AIDS" in Canada. September 1987; Pan American Health Organization. AIDS in the Americas: The situation. September 21, 1987
23. Mann JM, Francis H, Quinn T et al: Surveillance for AIDS in a central African city: Kinshasa, Zaire. JAMA 255:3255, 1986
24. Biggar RJ, Melbye M, Kestens L et al: Seroepidemiology of HTLV-III antibodies in a remote population of eastern Zaire. Br Med J 290:808, 1985
25. Biggar RJ, Gigase PL, Melbye M et al: ELISA HTLV retrovirus antibody reactivity associated with malaria and immune complexes in healthy Africans. Lancet 2:520, 1985
26. Biggar RJ: The AIDS problem in Africa. Lancet 1:79, 1986
27. Melbye M, Njelesani EK, Bayley A et al: Evidence for heterosexual transmission and clinical manifestations of human immunodeficiency virus infection and related conditions in Lusaka, Zambia. Lancet 2:1113, 1986
28. Mann JM, Francis H, Davachi F et al: Risk factors for human immunodeficiency virus seropositivity among children 1–24 months old in Kinshasa, Zaire. Lancet 2:654, 1986
29. Mann JM, Francis H, Davachi F et al: Human immunodeficiency virus seroprevalence in pediatric patients 2 to 14 years of age at Mama Yemo Hospital, Kinshasa, Zaire. Pediatrics 78:673, 1986
30. Serwadda D, Mugerwa RD, Serwankambo NK et al: Slim disease: A new disease in Uganda and its association with HTLV-III infection. Lancet 2:849, 1985
31. Bayley AC: Aggressive Kaposi's sarcoma in Zambia (1983). Lancet 1:1318, 1984
32. Downing RG, Eglin RP, Bayley AC: African Kaposi's sarcoma and AIDS. Lancet 1:478, 1984
33. Biggar RJ, Melbye M, Kestems L et al: Kaposi's sarcoma in Zaire is not associated with HTLV-III infection. N Engl J Med 311:1051, 1984
34. Bayley AC, Downing RG, Cheingsong–Popov R et al: HTLV-III serology distinguishes atypical and endemic Kaposi's sarcoma in Africa. Lancet 1:359, 1985
35. Greenberg AE, Nguyen–Dinh P, Mann JM et al: The association between HIV seropositivity, blood transfusions, and malaria in a pediatric population in Kinshasa, Zaire. Third International Conference on AIDS, Washington, DC, p 6. 1987
36. VandePerre P, Munyambuga D, Zissis G et al: Antibody to HTLV-III in blood donors in central Africa. Lancet 1:336, 1985
37. Clumeck N, Sonnet J, Taelman H et al: Acquired immunodeficiency syndrome in African patients. N Engl J Med 310:492, 1984
38. Tauris P, Black FT: Heterosexuals importing HIV from Africa. Lancet 1:325, 1987
39. Vittecoq D, May T, Roue RT et al: Acquired immunodeficiency syndrome after traveling in Africa: An epidemiological study in seventeen Caucasian patients. Lancet 1:612, 1987
40. Centers for Disease Control. Update: acquired immunodeficiency syndrome—Europe. Morbid Mortal Weekly Rep 35:35, 43, 1986
41. Melbye M, Biggar RJ, Ebbesen P et al: Seroepidemiology

of HTLV-III in Danish homosexual men: Prevalence, transmission, and disease outcome. Br Med J 289:573, 1984

42. Melbye M, Froebel KS, Madhok R et al: HTLV-III seropositivity in European haemophiliacs exposed to factor VIII concentrate imported from the USA. Lancet 2:1444, 1984

43. Goedert JJ, Biggar RJ, Weiss SH et al: Three-year incidence of AIDS in five cohorts of HTLV-III–infected risk group members. Science 231:992, 1986

44. Goedert JJ, Biggar RJ, Melbye M et al: Effect of T4 count and cofactors on the incidence of AIDS in homosexual men infected with human immunodeficiency virus. JAMA 257:331, 1987

45. Groopman JE, Mayer KN, Sarngadharan MG et al: Seroepidemiology of human T-lymphotropic virus type III among homosexual men with acquired immunodeficiency syndrome or generalized lymphadenopathy and among asymptomatic controls in Boston. Ann Intern Med 102:334, 1985

46. Jaffe HW, Darrow WW, Echenberg DF et al: The acquired immunodeficiency syndrome in a cohort of homosexual men: A six year follow-up study. Ann Intern Med 103:210, 1985

47. Hessol NA, Rutherford GW, O'Malley PM et al: The natural history of human immunodeficiency virus infection in a cohort of homosexual and bisexual men: A 7-year prospective study. Third International Conference on AIDS. Washington, DC, p 1. 1987

48. Moss AR, Osmond D, Bachetti P et al: One year follow-up of men exposed to AIDS in San Francisco. International Conference on AIDS, Atlanta, April 17, 1985

49. Winkelstein W, Jr, Lyman DM, Padian N et al: Sexual practices and risk of infection by the human immunodeficiency virus: The San Francisco Men's Health Study. JAMA 257:321, 1987

50. Winkelstein W, Jr, Samuel M, Padian NS et al: The San Francisco Men's Health Study: III. Reduction in human immunodeficiency virus transmission among homosexual/bisexual men, 1982–86. Am J Pub Health 77:685, 1987

51. Weiss SH, Goedert JJ, Sarngadharan MG et al: Screening test for HTLV-III (AIDS agent) antibody: Specificity, sensitivity and applications. JAMA 253:221, 1985

52. Cohen N, Marmor M, Des Jarlais D et al: Behavioral risk factors for HTLV-III/LAV seropositivity among intravenous drug users. International Conference on AIDS, Atlanta, April 16, 1985

53. Weiss SH, Ginzburg HM, Goedert JJ et al: Risk factors for HTLV-III infection among parenteral drug abusers (PDU). Proc Am Soc Clin Oncol 5:3, 1986

54. Craven DE, Kunches LM, Groopman JE et al: Prevalence of antibodies to human T-cell leukemia (lymphotropic) virus type III (HTLV-III) in parenteral drug abusers (PDA's) attending a methadone clinic. International Conference on AIDS, Atlanta, April 17, 1985

55. Spira TJ, Des Jarlais DC, Bokos D et al: HTLV-III/LAV antibodies in intravenous (IV) drug abusers: comparison of high and low risk areas. International Conference on AIDS, Atlanta, April 17, 1985

56. Weiss SH, Ginzberg HM, Saxinger WC et al: Emerging high rates of human T-cell lymphotropic virus type I (HTLV-I) and HIV infection among U.S. drug abusers (DA). Third International Conference on AIDS. Washington, DC, p 211. 1987

57. Centers for Disease Control: Antibody to human immu-

nodeficiency virus in female prostitutes. Morbid Mortal Weekly Rep 36:157, 1987

58. Ragni MV, Tegtmeier GE, Handwerk–Leber C et al: Prevalence and seroconversion rate of human T-lymphotropic retrovirus (HTLV-III) antibody in patients with hemophilia. International Conference on AIDS, Atlanta, April 17, 1985

59. Kitchen LW, Baren F, Sullivan JL et al: Antibodies to HTLV-III in asymptomatic hemophiliacs and in hemophiliac AIDS cases. International Conference on AIDS, Atlanta, April 17, 1985

60. Jason J, McDougal JS, Holman RC et al: Lymphadenopathy-associated virus (LAV) antibody in persons with hemophilia. International Conference on AIDS, Atlanta, April 17, 1985

61. Schorr JB, Berkowitz A, Cumming PD et al: Prevalence of HTLV-III antibody in American blood donors. N Engl J Med 313:384, 1985

62. Burke DS, Brundage JF, Herbold JR et al: Human immunodeficiency virus infections among civilian applicants for United States military service, October 1985 to March 1986: Demographic factors associated with seropositivity. N Engl J Med 317:131, 1987

63. Coolfont report: A PHS plan for prevention and control of AIDS and the AIDS virus. Public Health Rep 101:342, 1986

64. Marmor M, DesJarlais DC, Cohen H et al: Risk factors for infection with human immunodeficiency virus among intravenous drug abusers in New York City. AIDS 1:39, 1987

65. Chiasson RE, Moss AR, Onishi R et al: Human immunodeficiency virus infection in heterosexual intravenous drug users in San Francisco. Am J Pub Health 77:169, 1987

66. Darrow WW, Echenberg DF, Jaffe HW et al: Risk factors for human immunodeficiency virus (HIV) infections in homosexual men. Am J Pub Health 77:479, 1987

67. Moss AR, Osmond D, Bacchetti P et al: Risk factors for AIDS and HIV seropositivity in homosexual men. Am J Epidemiol 125:1035, 1987

68. Kingsley LA, Detels R, Kaslow R et al. Risk factors for seroconversion to human immunodeficiency virus among male homosexuals: Results from the Multicenter AIDS Cohort Study. Lancet 1:345, 1987

69. Marmor M, Weiss LR, Lyden M et al: Possible female-to-female transmission of human immunodeficiency virus. Ann Intern Med 105:969, 1986

70. Monzon OT, Capellan JMB: Female-to-female transmission of HIV. Lancet 2:40, 1987

71. Follett EA, McIntyre A, O'Donnell B et al: HTLV-III antibody in drug abusers in the west of Scotland: The Edinburgh connection. Lancet 1:446, 1986

72. Wofsy CB, Cohen JB, Hauer LB et al: Isolation of AIDS-associated retrovirus from genital secretions of women with antibodies to the virus. Lancet 1:527, 1986

73. Vogt MW, Witt DJ, Craven DE et al: Isolation of HTLV-III/LAV from cervical secretions of women at risk for AIDS. Lancet 1:525, 1986

74. Vogt MW, Witt DJ, Craven DE et al: Isolation patterns of the human immunodeficiency virus from cervical secretions during the menstrual cycle of women at risk for the acquired immunodeficiency syndrome. Ann Intern Med 106:380, 1987

75. Castro KG, Lieb S, Jaffe HW et al: Transmission of HIV in Belle Glade, Florida: Lessons for other communities in the United States. Science 239:193, 1988

76. The Collaborative Study Group of AIDS in Haitian-Americans: Risk factors for AIDS among Haitians residing in the United States: evidence for heterosexual transmission. JAMA 257:635, 1987

77. Mann JM, Bila K, Colebunders RL et al: Natural history of human immunodeficiency virus infection in Zaire. Lancet 2:707, 1986

78. Mann J, Quinn TC, Piot P et al: Condom use and HIV infection among prostitutes in Zaire. N Engl J Med 316: 345, 1987

79. Clumeck N, Robert–Guroff M, VandePerre P et al: Seroepidemiological studies of HTLV-III antibody prevalence among selected groups of heterosexual Africans. JAMA 254:2599, 1985

80. VandePerre P, Clumeck N, Carael M et al: Female prostitutes: A risk group for infection with human T-cell lymphotropic virus type III. Lancet 2:524, 1985

81. Kreiss JK, Koech D, Plummer FA et al: AIDS virus infection in Nairobi prostitutes: Spread of the epidemic to East Africa. N Engl J Med 314:414, 1986

82. Plummer FA, Simonsen JN, Ngugi EN et al: Incidence of human immunodeficiency virus (HIV) infection and related disease in a cohort of Nairobi prostitutes. Third International Conference on AIDS. Washington, DC, p 6. 1987

83. Katzenstein DA, Latif A, Bassett MT et al: Risks for heterosexual transmission of HIV in Zimbabwe. Third International Conference on AIDS. Washington, DC, p 6. 1987

84. Goedert JJ, Eyster ME, Biggar RJ, Blattner WA: Heterosexual transmission of human immunodeficiency virus: Association with severe depletion of T-helper lymphocytes in men with hemophilia. AIDS Res (in press).

85. Goedert JJ: What is safe sex? Suggested standards linked to testing for human immunodeficiency virus. N Engl J Med 316:1339, 1987

86. Fischl MA, Dickinson GM, Scott GB, et al: Evaluation of heterosexual partners, children, and household contacts of adults with AIDS. JAMA 257:640, 1987

87. Melbye M, Ingerslev J, Biggar RJ et al: Anal intercourse as a possible factor in heterosexual transmission of HTLV-III to spouses of hemophiliacs. N Engl J Med 312:857, 1985

88. Padian N, Marquis L, Francis DP et al: Male-to-female transmission of human immunodeficiency virus. JAMA 258:788, 1987

89. Lapointe N, Michaud J, Pekovic D et al: Transplacental transmission of HTLV-III virus. N Engl J Med 312:1325, 1985

90. Cowan MJ, Hellman D, Chudwin D et al: Maternal transmission of acquired immunodeficiency syndrome. Pediatrics 73:382, 1984

91. Jovaisas E, Koch MA, Schafer A et al: LAV/HTLV-III in a 20-week fetus. Lancet 2:1129, 1985

92. Sprecher S, Soumenkoff G, Puissant F, Degueldre M: Vertical transmission of HIV in 15-week fetus. Lancet 2:288, 1986

93. Braddick M, Kreiss JK, Quinn T et al: Congenital transmission of HIV in Nairobi, Kenya. Third International Conference on AIDS. Washington, DC, p 158. 1987

94. Nzilambi N, Ryder RW, Behets F et al: Perinatal transmission in two African hospitals. Third International Conference on AIDS. Washington, DC, p 158. 1987

95. Landesman S, Mendez H, Biggar R et al: Evaluation of HIV IgM and antigen assays for determination of perinatal infection with HIV. Third International Conference on AIDS. Washington, DC, p 175. 1987

96. Ziegler JB, Cooper DA, Johnson RO et al: Postnatal transmission of AIDS-associated retrovirus from mother to infant. Lancet 1:896, 1985

97. Thiry L, Sprecher–Goldberger S, Jonckheer T et al: Isolation of AIDS virus from cell-free breast milk of three healthy virus carriers. Lancet 2:891, 1985

98. Hino S, Sugiyama H, Doi H et al: Breaking the cycle of HTLV-I transmission via carrier mothers' milk. Lancet 2: 158, 1987

99. Mok JQ, Giaquinto C, DeRossi A et al: Infants born to mothers seropositive for human immunodeficiency virus: Preliminary findings from a multicentre European study. Lancet 1:1164, 1987

100. Thomas PA, Lubin K, Enlow RW et al: Comparison of HTLV-III serology, T-cell levels, innercity mothers in New York. International Conference on AIDS, Atlanta, April 17, 1985

101. Scott GB, Fischl MA, Klimas N et al: Mothers of infants with the acquired immunodeficiency syndrome. JAMA 253:363, 1985

102. Centers for Disease Control: *Pneumocystis carinii* pneumonia among persons with hemophilia A. Morbid Mortal Weekly Rep 31:365, 1982

103. Goedert JJ, Sarngadharan MG, Eyster ME et al: Antibodies reactive with human T cell leukemia viruses in the serum of hemophiliacs receiving Factor VIII concentrate. Blood 65:492, 1985

104. Gerety RJ, Aronson DL: Plasma derivatives and viral hepatitis. Transfusion 22:347, 1982

105. Ludlam CA, Tucker J, Steel CM et al: Human T-lymphotropic virus type III (HTLV-III) infection in seronegative haemophiliacs after transfusion of factor VIII. Lancet 2: 233, 1985

106. Ludlam CA, Cuthbert RJG, Beatson D et al: HIV infection in the Edinburgh haemophiliac cohort. Third International Conference on AIDS. Washington, DC, p 102. 1987

107. White GC II, Matthews TJ, Weinhold KJ et al: HTLV-III seroconversion associated with heat-treated factor VIII concentrate. Lancet 1:611, 1986

108. van den Berg W, ten Cate JW, Breederveld C et al: Seroconversion to HTLV-III in haemophiliac given heat-treated factor VIII concentrate. Lancet 1:803, 1986

109. Centers for Disease Control: Survey of non-U.S. hemophilia treatment centers for HIV seroconversions following therapy with heat-treated factor concentrates. Morbid Mortal Weekly Rep 36:121, 1987

110. Peterman TA, Jaffe HW, Feorino PM et al: Transfusion-associated acquired immunodeficiency syndrome in the United States. JAMA 254:2913, 1985

111. Esteban JI, Shih J W-K, Tai C-C et al: Importance of Western blot analysis in predicting infectivity of anti-HTLV-III/LAV positive blood. Lancet 2:1083, 1985

112. Ward JW, Deppe DA, Samson S et al: Risk of human immunodeficiency virus infection from blood donors who later developed the acquired immunodeficiency syndrome. Ann Intern Med 106:61, 1987

113. Mosley JW, the Transfusion Safety Study Group: The Transfusion Safety Study. Third International Conference on AIDS. Washington, DC, p 160. 1987

114. Centers for Disease Control: Human immunodeficiency virus infection in transfusion recipients and their family members. Morbid Mortal Weekly Rep 36:137, 1987

115. Centers for Disease Control: Transfusion-associated hu-

man T-lymphotropic virus type III/lymphadenopathy-associated virus infection from a seronegative donor: Colorado. Morbid Mortal Weekly Rep 35:389, 1986

116. Goedert JJ: Blood donation by persons at high risk of AIDS. N Engl J Med 312:1190, 1985

117. Centers for Disease Control: Update: Revised Public Health Service definition of persons who should refrain from donating blood and plasma: United States. Morbid Mortal Weekly Rep 34:547, 1985

118. Kalish RI, Cable RG, Roberts SC: Voluntary deferral of blood donations and HTLV-III antibody positivity. N Engl J Med 314:1115, 1986

119. Centers for Disease Control: Isolation of human T-lymphotropic virus type III/lymphadenopathy-associated virus from serum proteins given to cancer patients: Bahamas. Morbid Mortal Weekly Rep 34:489, 1985

120. Cuthbertson B, Rennie JG, Aw D et al: Safety of albumin preparations manufactured from plasma not tested for HIV antibody. Lancet 2:41, 1987

121. Piskiewicz D, Mankarikous S, Holst S et al: HIV antibodies in commercial immune globulins. Lancet 1:1327, 1986

122. Wood CC, Williams AE, McNamara JG et al: Antibody against the human immunodeficiency virus in commercial intravenous gammaglobulin preparations. Ann Intern Med 105:536, 1986

123. Wells MA, Wittek AE, Epstein JS et al: Inactivation and partition of human T-cell lymphotropic virus, type III, during ethanol fractionation of plasma. Transfusion 26:210, 1986

124. Hein R, McCue J, Mozen MM et al: Elimination of human immunodeficiency virus from immunoglobulin preparations. Lancet 1:1217, 1986

125. Tedder RS, Uttley A, Cheingsong–Popov R: Safety of immunoglobulin preparation containing anti-HTLV-III. Lancet 1:815, 1986

126. Zuck TF, Preston MS, Tankersley DL et al: More on partitioning and inactivation of AIDS virus in immune globulin preparations. Lancet 1:1454, 1986

127. Webster ADB, Dalgleish AG, Malkovsky M et al: Isolation of retroviruses from two patients with "common variable" hypogammaglobulinemia. Lancet 1:581, 1986

128. Francis DP, Feorino PM, McDougal S et al: The safety of the hepatitis B vaccine: Inactivation of the AIDS virus during routine vaccine manufacture. JAMA 256:869, 1986

129. Muylle L, Vranckx P, Peetermans ME: No HTLV-III antibodies after HBV vaccination. N Engl J Med 314:581, 1986

130. L'age-Stehr J, Schwarz A, Offermann G et al: HTLV-III infection in kidney transplant recipients. Lancet 2:1361, 1985

131. Kumar P, Pearson JE, Martin DH et al: Transmission of human immunodeficiency virus by transplantation of a renal allograft, with development of the acquired immunodeficiency syndrome. Ann Intern Med 106:244, 1987

132. Margreiter R, Fuchs D, Hausen A et al: HIV infection in renal allograft recipients. Lancet 2:398, 1986

133. Neumayer H–H, Wagner K, Kresse S: HTLV-III antibodies in patients with kidney transplants or on haemodialysis. Lancet 1:497, 1986

134. Stewart GJ, Tyler JPP, Cunningham AL et al: Transmission of human T-lymphotropic virus type III (HTLV-III) virus by artificial insemination by donor. Lancet 2:581, 1985

135. Centers for Disease Control: Testing donors of organs, tissues, and semen for antibody to human T-lymphotropic

virus type III/lymphadenopathy-associated virus. Morbid Mortal Weekly Rep 34:294, 1985

136. Eglin RP, Wilkinson AR: HIV infection and pasteurisation of breast milk. Lancet 1:1093, 1987

137. Lucas A: AIDS and human milk bank closures. Lancet 1:1092, 1987

138. Centers for Disease Control: Human immunodeficiency virus infection transmitted from an organ donor screened for HIV antibody: North Carolina. Morbid Mortal Weekly Rep 36:306, 1987

139. Pepose JS, Pardo FS, Quinn TC: HTLV-III ELISA testing of cadaveric sera to screen potential organ transplant donors. JAMA 256:864, 1986

140. Morrison AJ, Freer CV, Poole CL et al: Prevalence of human T-lymphotropic virus type III antibodies among patients in dialysis programs at a university hospital. Ann Intern Med 104:805, 1986

141. Rao TKS, Friedman EA, Nicastri AD: The types of renal disease in the acquired immunodeficiency syndrome. N Engl J Med 316:1062, 1987

142. Centers for Disease Control: Recommendations for providing dialysis treatment to patients infected with human T-lymphotropic virus type III/lymphadenopathy-associated virus. Morbid Mortal Weekly Rep 35:376, 1986

143. Favero MS: Recommended precautions for patients undergoing hemodialysis who have AIDS or non-A non-B hepatitis. Infect Control 6:301, 1985

144. Weiss SH, Biggar RJ: The epidemiology of human retrovirus-associated illnesses. Mt Sinai J Med 53:579, 1986

145. Weiss SH, Saxinger WC, Rechtman MH et al: HTLV-III infection among health care workers: Association with needle-stick injuries. JAMA 254:2089, 1985

146. McCray E, the cooperative needlestick surveillance group: Occupational risk of the acquired immunodeficiency syndrome among health care workers. N Engl J Med 314:1127, 1986

147. Hirsh MS, Wormser GP, Schooley RT et al: Risk of nosocomial infection with human T-cell lymphotropic virus III (HTLV-III). N Engl J Med 312:1, 1985

148. Gerberding JL, Bryant–LeBlanc CE, Nelson K et al: Risk of transmitting the human immunodeficiency virus, cytomegalovirus, and hepatitis B virus to health care workers exposed to patients with AIDS and AIDS-related conditions. J Infect Dis 156:1, 1987

149. Henderson DK, Saah AJ, Zak BJ et al: Risk of nosocomial infection with human T-cell lymphotropic virus type III/lymphadenopathy-associated virus in a large cohort of intensively exposed health care workers. Ann Intern Med 104:644, 1986

150. Conte JE: Infection with human immunodeficiency virus in the hospital: Epidemiology, infection control, and biosafety considerations. Ann Intern Med 105:730, 1986

151. Centers for Disease Control: Recommendations for preventing transmission of infection with human T-lymphotropic virus type III/lymphadenopathy-associated virus during invasive procedures. Morbid Mortal Weekly Rep 35:221, 1986

152. Centers for Disease Control: Recommended infection-control practices for dentistry. Morbid Mortal Weekly Rep 35:237, 1986

153. Hay A: Laboratory safety and HIV. Lancet 1:1094, 1987

154. Gerberding JL, University of California San Francisco Task Force on AIDS. Recommended infection-control policies for patients with human immunodeficiency virus infection: An update. N Engl J Med 315:1562, 1986

155. Centers for Disease Control: Human T-lymphotropic virus type III/lymphadenopathy-associated virus: Agent summary statement. Morbid Mortal Weekly Rep 34:540, 1986

156. Centers for Disease Control: Apparent transmission of human T-lymphotropic virus type III/lymphadenopathy-associated virus from a child to a mother providing health care. Morbid Mortal Weekly Rep 35:76, 1986

157. Centers for Disease Control: Update: Human immunodeficiency virus infections in health-care workers exposed to blood of infected patients. Morbid Mortal Weekly Rep 36:285, 1987

158. Grint P, McEvoy M: Two associated cases of the acquired immunodeficiency syndrome (AIDS). Commun Dis Rep 42:4, 1985

159. Wahn V, Kramer HH, Voit T et al: Horizontal transmission of HIV infection between two siblings. Lancet 2:694, 1986

160. Friedland GH, Saltzman BR, Rogers MF et al: Lack of transmission of HTLV-III/LAV infection to household contacts of patients with AIDS or AIDS-related complex with oral candidiasis. N Engl J Med 314:344, 1986

161. Berthier A, Chamaret S, Fauchet R et al: Transmission of human immunodeficiency virus in haemophilic and non-haemophilic children living in a private school in France. Lancet 2:598, 1986

162. Madhok R, Gracie JA, Lowe GDO et al: Lack of HIV transmission by casual contact. Lancet 2:863, 1986

163. Goedert JJ, Eyster ME, Bodner AJ et al: A search for HTLV-III and its antibodies in hemophilic families. International Conference on AIDS, Atlanta, April 17, 1985

164. Weiss SH, Goedert JJ, Gartner S et al: Risk of human immunodeficiency virus (HIV-1) infection among laboratory workers. Science 239:68, 1988

164a. United States Public Health Service: Biosafety in Microbiological and Biomedical Laboratories. HHS Publication No. (CDC) 84-8395, Washington, U.S. Government Printing Office, 1984

165. Lepage P, VandePerre P, Carael M et al: Are medical injections a risk factor for HIV infection in children? Lancet 2:1103, 1986

166. Koenig RE, Gautier T, Levy JA: Unusual intrafamilial transmission of human immunodeficiency virus. Lancet 2:627, 1986

167. Srinivasan A, York D, Bohan C: Lack of HIV replication in arthropod cells. Lancet 1:1094, 1987

168. Zuckerman AJ: AIDS and insects. Br Med J 292:1094, 1986

169. Booth W: AIDS and insects. Science 237:355, 1987

170. Brookmeyer R, Gail MH, Polk BF: The prevalent cohort study and the acquired immunodeficiency syndrome. Am J Epidemiol 126:14, 1987

171. Goedert JJ, Landesman SH, Eyster ME et al: AIDS incidence in pregnant women, their babies, homosexual men and hemophiliacs. Third International Conference on AIDS. Washington, DC, p 71. 1987

171a. Macher AM, De Vinatea ML, Parisi JE et al: AIDS case for diagnosis, 1986: Military medicine. Military Med 151: M33, 1986

172. Weiss SH, Margolis IB, Zelnick R et al: Mortality, AIDS incidence and immunologic abnormalities among intravenous drug abusers (IVDA) in New York City (NYC): A 5-year prospective study. Third International Conference on AIDS. Washington, DC, p 77. 1987

173. Eyster ME, Gail MH, Ballard JO et al: Natural history of human immunodeficiency virus (HIV) infections in hemophiliacs: Effects of T-cell subsets, platelet counts and age. Ann Intern Med 107:1, 1987

174. Polk BF, Fox R, Brookmeyer R et al: Predictors of the acquired immunodeficiency syndrome developing in a cohort of seropositive homosexual men. N Engl J Med 316:61, 1987

175. Schechter MT, Boyko WJ, Weaver MS et al: Progression to AIDS, predictors of AIDS, and seroconversion in a cohort of homosexual men: results of a four year prospective study. Third International Conference on AIDS. Washington, DC, p 2. 1987

176. Ward JW, Deppe D, Perkins H et al: Risk of disease in recipients of blood from donors later found infected with human immunodeficiency virus (HIV). Third International Conference on AIDS. Washington, DC, p 2. 1987

177. Klein RS, Harris CA, Butkus Small C et al: Oral candidiasis in high-risk patients as the initial manifestation of the acquired immunodeficiency syndrome. N Engl J Med 311: 354, 1984

178. Eyster ME, Goedert JJ, Poon M–C et al: Acid-labile alpha interferon: A possible preclinical marker for the acquired immunodeficiency syndrome in hemophilia. N Engl J Med 309:583, 1983

179. Eyster ME, Preble OT, Goedert JJ et al: Prospective study of AIDS in hemophiliacs with elevated interferon alpha levels. Third International Conference on AIDS. Washington, DC, p 21. 1987

180. Allain J–P, Laurian Y, Paul DA et al: Prognostic value of HIV antigen capture assay in a long-term prospective study of seropositive hemophiliacs. Third International Conference on AIDS. Washington, DC, p 17. 1987

181. Osmond D, Chaisson R, Leuther M et al: Serum HIV antigen (HIV-Ag) as a predictor of progression to AIDS and ARC in homosexual men. Third International Conference on AIDS. Washington, p 24. 1987

182. Hoxie JA, Haggarty BS, Rackowski JL et al: Persistent noncytopathic infection of normal human T lymphocytes with AIDS-associated retrovirus. Science 229:1400, 1985

183. Friedman–Kien AE, Laubenstein LJ, Rubenstein P et al: Disseminated Kaposi's sarcoma in homosexual men. Ann Intern Med 96:693, 1982

184. Pollack MS, Safai B, Myskowski PL et al: Frequencies of HLA and Gm immunogenetic markers in Kaposi's sarcoma. Tissue Antigens 21:1, 1983

185. Pollack MS, Safai B, Dupont B et al: HLA-DR5 and DR2 are susceptibility factors for acquired immunodeficiency syndrome with Kaposi's sarcoma in different ethnic subpopulations. Disease Markers 1:135, 1983

186. Pollack MS, Gold J, Metroka CE et al: HLA-A, B, C and DR antigen frequencies in acquired immunodeficiency syndrome (AIDS) patients with opportunistic infections. Human Immunol 11:99, 1984

187. Scorza Semeraldi R, Fabio G, Lazzarin A et al: HLA-associated susceptibility to acquired immunodeficiency syndrome in Italian patients with human-immunodeficiency-virus infection. Lancet 2:1187, 1986

188. Mann DL, Murray C, Goedert JJ et al: HLA phenotypes are possible risk factors for development of AIDS. Third International Conference on AIDS. Washington, DC, p 206. 1987

189. Eales L–J, Nye KE, Parkin JM et al: Association of different allelic forms of group specific component with susceptibility to and clinical manifestation of human immunodeficiency virus infection. Lancet 1:999, 1987

190. Thymann M, Dickmeiss E, Svejgaard A et al: AIDS and the Gc protein. Lancet 1:1378, 1987

191. Nixon DF, Eglin RP, Westwood SA et al: Group-specific component and HIV infection. Lancet 2:39, 1987
192. Constans J, Smilovici W, Ducos J et al: Group-specific component and HIV infection. Lancet 2:40, 1987
193. Gilles K, Louie L, Newman B et al: Genetic susceptibility to AIDS: Absence of an association with group-specific component (Gc). N Engl J Med 317:630, 1987
194. Daiger SP, Brewton GW, Rios AA et al: Genetic susceptibility to AIDS: Absence of an association with group-specific component (Gc). N Engl J Med 317:631, 1987
195. Redfield RR, Wright DC, Tramont EC: The Walter Reed staging classification for HTLV-III/LAV infection. N Engl J Med 314:131, 1986
196. Brodt HR, Helm EB, Werner A et al: Spontanverlauf der LAV/HTLV-III-infektion: verlaufsbeobachtungun bei personen aus AIDS-risikogruppen. Deutsche Medizinische Wodenschrift 111:1175, 1986
197. Centers for Disease Control: Classification system for human T-lymphotropic virus type III/lymphadenopathy-associated virus infections. Morbid Mortal Weekly Rep 35:334, 1986
198. Cooper DA, Gold J, Maclean P et al: Acute AIDS retrovirus infection: Definition of a clinical illness associated with seroconversion. Lancet 1:537, 1985
199. Melbye M, Grossman RJ, Goedert JJ et al: Risk of AIDS after herpes zoster. Lancet 1:728, 1987
200. Rhoads JL, Wright C, Redfield RR et al: Chronic vaginal candidiasis in women with human immunodeficiency virus infection. JAMA 257:3105, 1987
201. Centers for Disease Control: Tuberculosis—United States, 1985—and the possible impact of human T-lymphotropic virus type III/lymphadenopathy-associated virus infection. Morbid Mortal Weekly Rep 35:74, 1986
202. Centers for Disease Control: Tuberculosis and acquired immunodeficiency syndrome: Florida. Morbid Mortal Weekly Rep 35:587, 1986
203. Centers for Disease Control: Tuberculosis and AIDS: Connecticut. Morbid Mortal Weekly Rep 36:133, 1986
204. Centers for Disease Control: Diagnosis and management of mycobacterial infection and disease in persons with human T-lymphotropic virus type III/lymphadenopathy-associated virus infection. Morbid Mortal Weekly Rep 35:448, 1986
205. Tramont EC: Syphilis in the AIDS era. N Engl J Med 316:1600, 1987
206. Johns DR, Tierney M, Felsenstein D: Alteration in the natural history of neurosyphilis by concurrent infection with the human immunodeficiency virus. N Engl J Med 316:1569, 1987
207. Berry CD, Hooton TM, Collier AC et al: Neurologic relapse after benzathine penicillin therapy for secondary syphilis in a patient with HIV infection. N Engl J Med 316:1587, 1987
208. Greenspan D, Greenspan JS, Conant M et al: Oral "hairy" leukoplakia in male homosexuals: Evidence of association with both papillomavirus and a herpes-group virus. Lancet 2:831, 1984
209. Friedman–Kien AE: Viral origin of hairy leukoplakia. Lancet 2:694, 1986
210. Newman C, Polk BF: Resolution of oral hairy leukoplakia during therapy with 9-(1,3-dihydroxy-2-propoxymethyl) guainine (DHPG). Ann Intern Med 107:348, 1987
211. Guenthner EE, Rabinowe SL, VanNiel A et al: Primary Addison's disease in a patient with the acquired immunodeficiency syndrome. Ann Intern Med 100:847, 1984

212. Polsky B, Gold JWM, Whimbey E et al: Bacterial pneumonia in patients with the acquired immunodeficiency syndrome. Ann Intern Med 104:38, 1986
213. Morris L, Distenfeld A, Amorosi E et al: Autoimmune thrombocytopenic purpura in homosexual men. Ann Intern Med 96:714, 1982
214. Walsh CM, Nardi MA, Karpatkin S: On the mechanism of thrombocytopenic purpura in sexually active homosexual men. N Engl J Med 311:635, 1984
215. Stricker RB, Abrams DI, Corash L et al: Target platelet antigen in homosexual men with immune thrombocytopenia. N Engl J Med 313:1375, 1985
216. Abrams DI, Kiprov DD, Goedert JJ et al: Antibodies to human T-lymphotropic virus type III and development of acquired immunodeficiency syndrome in homosexual men presenting with immune thrombocytopenia. Ann Intern Med 104:47, 1986
217. Walsh C, Krigel R, Lennett E et al: Thrombocytopenia in homosexual patients: Prognosis, response to therapy, and prevalence of antibody to the retrovirus associated with the acquired immunodeficiency syndrome. Ann Intern Med 103:542, 1985
218. Holzman RS, Walsh CM, Karpatkin S: Risk for acquired immunodeficiency syndrome among thrombocytopenic and nonthrombocytopenic homosexual men seropositive for the human immunodeficiency virus. Ann Intern Med 106:383, 1987
219. Winchester R, Bernstein DH, Fischer HD et al: The co-occurrence of Reiter's syndrome and acquired immunodeficiency syndrome. Ann Intern Med 106:19, 1987
220. Watts RA, Hoffbrand BI, Paton DF et al: Pyomyositis associated with human immunodeficiency virus infection. Br Med J 294:1524, 1987
221. Cohen IS, Anderson DW, Virmani R et al: Congestive cardiomyopathy in association with the acquired immunodeficiency syndrome. N Engl J Med 315:628, 1986
222. Eisenstat BA, Wormser GP: Seborrheic dermatitis and butterfly rash in AIDS. N Engl J Med 311:189, 1984
223. Perniciaro C, Peters MS: Tinea faciale mimicking seborrheic dermatitis in a patient with AIDS. N Engl J Med 314:315, 1986
224. Johnson TM, Duvic M, Rapini RP et al: AIDS exacerbates psoriasis. N Engl J Med 313:1415, 1985
225. Ammann AJ, Schiffman G, Abrams D et al: B-cell immunodeficiency in acquired immunodeficiency syndrome. JAMA 251:1447, 1984
226. Lane HC, Masur H, Elgar LC et al: Abnormalities of B-cell activation and immunoregulation in patients with the acquired immunodeficiency syndrome. N Engl J Med 309:453, 1983
227. Rubenstein A, Sicklick M, Gupta A et al: Acquired immunodeficiency with reversed T4/T8 ratios in infants born to promiscuous and drug-addicted mothers. JAMA 249:2350, 1983
228. Oleske J, Minnefor A, Cooper R et al: Immune deficiency syndrome in children. JAMA 249:2345, 1983
229. Scott GB, Buck BE, Leterman JG et al: Acquired immunodeficiency syndrome in infants. N Engl J Med 310:76, 1984
230. Pahwa S, Kaplan M, Fikrig S et al: Spectrum of human T-cell lymphotropic virus type III infection in children. JAMA 255:2299, 1986
231. Chayt KJ, Harper ME, Marselle LM et al: Detection of HTLV-III RNA in lungs of patients with AIDS and pulmonary involvement. JAMA 256:2356, 1986

232. Epstein LG, Sharer LR, Joshi VV et al: Progressive encephalopathy in children with acquired immunodeficiency syndrome. Ann Neurol 17:488, 1985

233. Marion RW, Wiznia AA, Hutcheon G et al: Human T-cell lymphotropic virus type III (HTLV-III) embryopathy: A new dysmorphic syndrome associated with intrauterine HTLV-III infection. Am J Dis Child 140:638, 1986

234. Biggar RJ, Horm J, Lubin JH et al: Cancer trends in a population at risk of acquired immunodeficiency syndrome. J Natl Cancer Inst 74:793, 1985

235. Biggar RJ, Horm J, Goedert JJ et al: Cancer in a group at risk of acquired immunodeficiency syndrome (AIDS) through 1984. Am J Epidemiol 126:578, 1987

236. Ziegler JL, Beckstead JA, Volberding PA et al: Non-Hodgkin's lymphoma in 90 homosexual men: Relation to generalized lymphadenopathy and the acquired immunodeficiency syndrome. N Engl J Med 311:565, 1984

237. Frazer IH, Medley G, Crapper RM et al: Association between anorectal dysplasia, human papillomavirus, and human immunodeficiency virus infection in homosexual men. Lancet 2:657, 1986

238. Grunebaum A, Webber C, Minkoff H et al: Prevalence of human papillomavirus infection in pregnant women with human immunodeficiency virus infection. Proc Soc Perinatal Obstet 1987 (in press).

239. Harper ME, Kaplan MH, Marselle LM et al: Concomitant infection with HTLV-I and HTLV-III in a patient with T8 lymphoproliferative disease. N Engl J Med 315:1073, 1986

240. Bartholomew C, Clark JW, Saxinger WC et al: Transmission of HTLV-I and HIV among homosexuals in Trinidad. JAMA 257:2604, 1987

241. Brookmeyer R, Gail MH. Minimum size of the acquired immunodeficiency syndrome (AIDS) epidemic in the United States. Lancet 2:1320, 1986

242. Brun–Vezinet F, Rey MA, Katalama C et al: Lymphadenopathy-associated virus type 2 in AIDS and AIDS-related complex: Clinical and virological features in four patients. Lancet 1:128, 1987

243. Clavel F, Mansinho K, Chamaret S et al: Human immunodeficiency virus type 2 infection associated with AIDS in West Africa. N Engl J Med 316:1180, 1987

244. Molbak K, Lauritzen E, Fernandes D et al: Antibodies to HTLV-IV associated with chronic, fatal illness resembling "slim" disease. Lancet 2:1214, 1986

245. Brucker G, Brun–Vezinet F, Rosenheim M et al: HIV-2 infection in two homosexual men in France. Lancet 1:223, 1987

246. Biberfeld G, Bottiger B, Bredberg–Raden U et al: Findings in four HTLV-IV seropositive women from West Africa. Lancet 2:1330, 1986

247. Saimot AG, Coulaud JP, Mechali D et al: HIV-2/LAV-2 in Portuguese man with AIDS (Paris, 1978) who had served in Angola in 1968–1974. Lancet 1:688, 1987

248. Ancelle R, Bletry O, Baglin AC et al: Long incubation period for HIV-2 infection. Lancet 1:688, 1987

249. Kanki PJ, M'Boup S, Ricard D et al: Human T-lymphotropic virus type 4 and the human immunodeficiency virus in West Africa. Science 236:827, 1987

250. Barin F, M'Boup S, Denis F et al: Serological evidence for virus related to simian T-lymphotropic retrovirus III in residents of West Africa. Lancet 2:1387, 1985

251. Rey MA, Girard PM, Harzic M et al: HIV-1 and HIV-2 double infection in French homosexual male with AIDS-related complex (Paris, 1985). Lancet 1:388, 1987

252. Foucault C, Lopez O, Jourdan G et al: Double HIV-1 and HIV-2 seropositivity among blood donors. Lancet 2:165, 1987

253. Karpas A, Hayhoe FGJ, Hill F et al: Use of Karpas HIV cell test to detect antibodies to HIV-2. Lancet 2:132, 1987

254. Rey F, Salaun D, Lasbordes JL et al: HIV-I and HIV-II double infection in Central African Republic. Lancet 2:1391, 1986

255. Denis F, Leonard G, Mounier M et al: Efficacy of five enzyme immunoassays for antibody to HIV in detecting antibody to HTLV-IV. Lancet 1:324, 1987

256. Denis F, Barin F, Gershy–Damet G et al: Prevalence of human T-lymphotropic retrovirus type III (HIV) and type IV in Ivory Coast. Lancet 1:408, 1987

257. Werner A, Staszewski S, Helm E–B et al: HIV-2 (West Germany, 1984). Lancet 1:868, 1987

258. Kroegel C, Hess G, Meyer zum Buschenfelde K–H: Routes of HIV-2 transmission in Western Europe. Lancet 1:1150, 1987

259. Vittecoq D, Ferchal F, Charmaret S et al: Routes of HIV-2 transmission in Western Europe. Lancet 1:1150, 1987

260. Courouce A–M: HIV-2 in blood donors and in different risk groups in France. Lancet 1:1151, 1987

261. Gessain A, Vernant JC, Maurs L et al: Antibodies to human T-lymphotropic virus type-I in patients with tropical spastic paraparesis. Lancet 2:1211, 1985

262. Rodgers–Johnson P, Gajdusek DC, Morgan St C et al: HTLV-I and HTLV-III antibodies and tropical spastic paraparesis. Lancet 2:1247, 1985

263. Manzari V, Gismondi A, Barillari G et al: HTLV-V: A new human retrovirus isolated in a Tac-negative T cell lymphoma/leukemia. Science 238:1581, 1987

AIDS: Immunopathogenesis and Immune Response to the Human Immunodeficiency Virus

Scott Koenig
Anthony S. Fauci

4

The acquired immunodeficiency syndrome (AIDS) is unique among the clinical disorders caused by defects of the immune system. While patients with AIDS may share certain clinical and laboratory features with individuals with primary immunodeficiencies, especially the severe combined immunodeficiencies (SCID), the pathophysiology and spectrum of immunologic defects of AIDS is unparalleled (Table 4-1). Since the first description of patients with this disorder,[1-3] 43,000 cases have been reported and 20,000 individuals have died in this country alone as a result of AIDS.[4] The etiologic agent of AIDS, the human immunodeficiency virus (HIV),[5-8] causes a relentless depletion of the helper/inducer subset of T lymphocytes, phenotypically defined by the expression of the CD4 molecule on their surface, and undermines the generation and regulation of the immune response (Table 4-2). Two major forms of HIV have been described, HIV-1[5-7] and HIV-2.[9-10] Immunologic changes associated with AIDS have been primarily derived from studies of individuals infected with HIV-1, which is widely disseminated throughout the world. Despite the marked heterogeneity in envelope structure[11] and ability to propagate HIV-1 isolates *in vitro*,[12] the immunologic abnormalities seen in individuals infected with different HIV-1 serotypes appear similar. HIV-2 has a more restricted geographic distribution and has been mostly isolated from individuals in western Africa, as well as from several patients in Europe and South America. The clinical manifestations in patients infected with HIV-2 are identical to their HIV-1 counterparts, and the immunologic changes, as yet not thoroughly delineated, are likely to be comparable to HIV-1.[13]

Although all compartments of the immune system are at least indirectly affected in patients with AIDS, impaired T-cell–mediated responses appear to have the greatest clinical consequences. As a result, AIDS patients are particularly prone to develop opportunistic infections and neoplasms.[1-3,14-16] *Pneumocystis carinii* pneumonia (PCP) is the predominant opportunistic infection and the immediate cause of death in the majority of AIDS patients. The aggressive form of Kaposi's sarcoma,[17] which is found characteristically in AIDS patients, may be due in part to a T-cell defect. However, other conditions besides immunosuppression must influence its development, since it preferentially occurs in homosexual men and is rarely found in other immunocompromised risk groups. In addition, it is sometimes seen in HIV-infected individuals with little or no immunologic impairment. An increased susceptibility to certain bacterial pathogens is seen in AIDS patients, particularly within the pediatric population.[18,19] As many of these bacterial infections affect the respiratory and gastrointestinal systems, defects in cell-mediated and humoral mucosal immunity are likely. While the neurologic manifestations of AIDS cannot be directly attributed to an immune defect, an unregulated replication of HIV within cells of the immune system that are transported to the brain, namely macrophages, may be responsible for the pathogenesis of certain HIV-related central nervous system disorders.

In addition to the immunologic abnormalities induced by HIV itself, other organisms concomitantly infecting these patients may depress immune function.[20] This may contribute to the morbidity and mortality of patients, especially at the later stages of their illness. Apart from their effects on the immune system, persistence of pathogens other than HIV may alter the clinical course of HIV infected individuals. For example, some DNA viruses that frequently are harbored by AIDS patients have been shown to enhance the transcription of HIV *in vitro*.[21,22] As a result, in patients coinfected with these viruses, HIV viremia may be amplified and depletion of $CD4^+$ cells may be accelerated.

QUANTITATIVE T-CELL ABNORMALITIES

One of the earliest laboratory abnormalities recognized in patients with AIDS was the alteration in the T4 to T8 cell ratio of circulating T cells. In patients with AIDS, this is primarily the result of depletion of $CD4^+$ lymphocytes.[23-33] Depression of the T4 to T8 ratio and depletion of the $CD4^+$ population correlates somewhat with the severity of the disease. Asymptomatic individuals and patients with AIDS-related complex (ARC) generally have higher T4 counts than either patients with Kaposi's sarcoma alone or AIDS patients manifesting opportunistic infections.[32] In fact, in HIV-seropositive individuals, low T4 cell counts (less than 200/mm³) is often an indication of the imminent development of AIDS with an opportunistic infection.[33-35] The rate of depletion of T4 cells varies among patients. After an initial fall, many may maintain a level of $CD4^+$ cells that is relatively normal or slightly lower than normal for prolonged periods followed by precipitous declines. In several patients, this rapid loss has coincided with marked increases in circulating HIV antigen.* Others may experience a progressive, unremitting decline in $CD4^+$ cell counts, with an accelerated and unfavorable clinical course.[36,37] Inconsistent changes in selective depletion of subpopulations of $CD4^+$ have been reported. One group found that healthy seropositive individuals and lymphadenopathy patients had proportional decreases in the $CD4^+Leu8^+$ and $CD4^+Leu8^-$ populations,[38] and others have noted that the $CD4^+Leu8^+$ subset is preferentially depleted in the lymphadenopathy patients.[39,40] Some of the discrepant results in earlier studies may be due to inaccurate assignment of patients to the various clinical groups before HIV serologic testing was available.

Changes in numbers of $CD8^+$ cells also occur in HIV-infected individuals. Many healthy HIV-seropositive individuals, in addition to those with lymphadenopathy syndromes—ARC and progressive generalized lymphadenopathy (PGL)—were found to have elevated levels of $CD8^+$ cells. Subpopulations of $CD8^+$ cells, particularly the $CD8^+Leu7^{+41}$ and the $CD8^+Leu8^{-38}$ subsets have been reported to be substantially increased in HIV-seropositive individuals. The expansion of the $CD8^+$ population may represent the generation of cytotoxic responses against HIV or other pathogens; alternatively, $CD8^+$ suppressor cells may be stimulated to down-modulate other immune responses such as the polyclonal activation of B cells that is present in seropositive patients. It was reported that HIV isolation could be achieved more easily from peripheral blood cell cultures of seropositive individuals if $CD8^+$ cells were eliminated. The addition of these $CD8^+$ cells back to the cultures suppressed HIV propagation.[42] It seems likely, therefore, that the expanded $CD8^+$ population functions

---

* Lane HC: Unpublished observations.

Table 4-1
Immunologic Abnormalities in AIDS

T cells
 CD4$^+$ cell depletion*
 Decreased proliferation to soluble antigens*
 Decreased helper response for PWM-induced immunoglobulin synthesis*
 Impaired delayed-type hypersensitivity*
 Decreased γ-interferon production in response to antigens*
 Decreased proliferation to T-cell mitogens alloantigens and to anti-CD3
 Decreased AMLR response
 Decreased cell-mediated cytotoxicity to virally infected cells
 Decreased IL-2 production
 Lymphopenia
B cells
 Polyclonal activation with hypergammaglobulinemia (IgG, IgA, and IgD), increased spontaneous plaque forming cells, and proliferation*
 Decreased humoral response to immunization*
 Circulating autoantibodies
Macrophage/monocytes
 Decreased chemotaxis*
Natural killer cells
 Decreased cytotoxicity*
Other humoral responses
 Increased acid-labile γ-interferon production
 Increased soluble immune complexes
 Decreased α₁-thymosin

* Characteristic disorders

Table 4-2
Cell Types Infected by HIV

Consistently observed
 CD4$^+$ T cells
 Monocytes/macrophages (CNS, peripheral blood, lung)
 Transformed B cells
 Dendritic cells (lymph node and peripheral blood)
 Microglial cells
Occasional reports
 Endothelial cells
 Astrocytes and oligodendrocytes
 Transformed colon cells
 Neurons
 CD8$^+$, CD4$^-$ cells

in part to suppress HIV replication *in vivo,* even in symptomatic individuals.

Late in the course of their disease, AIDS patients with opportunistic infections are often depleted of all lymphoid cells, including the $CD8^+$ population.[32] The mechanism for this depletion is unclear but may be caused by severe bone marrow suppression.

Mechanisms of T4 Cell Depletion

HIV and CD4 as a Receptor

The pathophysiology of CD4[+] cell depletion is a consequence of the high affinity of the HIV envelope for the CD4 molecule, which appears to be the cellular receptor for HIV. In early studies it was observed that HIV could be propagated exclusively in CD4[+] cells,[43–46] and monoclonal antibodies to CD4 could prevent infection.[47,48] Certain epitopes of the CD4 molecule are important for viral binding, since antibodies to CD4 exhibited differential capacities for blocking infection.[48–50] Specifically, antibody to T4A but not T4 could prevent the binding of HIV to the CD4 molecule and cells bearing T4A but not T4 could be infected *in vitro*.[51,52] The human HELA line, which is CD4[−] was transfected with the cloned CD4 gene, resulting in the expression of the CD4 protein and consequent susceptibility to HIV infection.[53] In contrast, murine cells expressing the human CD4 molecule could not be infected with HIV but could support HIV replication after they were transfected with the HIV genome. This suggests that other surface receptors may facilitate HIV entry. It has been proposed that the HLA-DR molecule may serve as another receptor for HIV. HLA-DR expression has been found to decrease transiently after viral exposure in association with a more persistent loss of CD4[+] expression from the same cells.[54] Further characterization of the role of HLA-DR in the infective process is actively being explored.

Cytopathic Mechanisms

Although some of the conditions for viral entry have been elucidated, the mechanisms by which cells are destroyed by HIV are unclear. It has been suggested that the cytopathic effect of HIV in CD4[+] cells is a function of the density of the CD4 molecule on the surface of cells. The cell lines with the highest density were found to be the most susceptible to cell death, and it was speculated that the complex of CD4 and the envelope protein of HIV in the cytoplasm may be cytopathic for cells.[55,56] However, there is recent evidence of marked cytopathic effects in HIV, even in cell lines that bear only modest amounts of membrane-expressed CD4.* The formation of syncytia as a result of fusion of HIV infected cells with CD4-bearing cells has been observed *in vitro* and has been proposed as a mechanism for T4 lymphocyte depletion *in vivo*.[57,58] Multinucleated giant cells have been observed in the brain of HIV-infected patients, but it is unclear whether they form as a result of cell fusion.[59] Similar forms have been observed in lymph nodes of infected patients.[60] The large amounts of unintegrated viral DNA that are found in HIV-infected cells but not in cells infected with other transforming retroviruses has been proposed to be responsible for the cytopathic effects of this virus.[61] Although this is an

attractive hypothesis, no experimental evidence has implicated this finding in HIV cytotoxicity.

In addition to the direct cytopathic effects of HIV, depletion of CD4[+] lymphocytes *in vivo* may be caused in part by immune-mediated responses.[62,63] For instance, as part of immune surveillance, HIV-infected cells that express viral antigens on their surface could be eliminated by HLA-restricted and -unrestricted cytotoxic cells. Although in a given specimen of peripheral blood, a small percentage of cells appears to be actively producing virions,[64] significant cell losses could occur over time due to viral persistence, reactivation of latent virus, and progressive dissemination to uninfected cells. A likely prerequisite for lymphodepletion, however, would be concomitant failure of hematopoietic organs to regenerate the depleted lymphocytes. In support of this notion, AIDS patients have a decreased capacity to generate T-cell colonies.[65] Also, colony formation of granulocytes–macrophages (CFU–GM) and erythrocytes (BFU-E) from bone marrow of AIDS patients is inhibited when cultured in the presence of their sera. HIV can be isolated from some of these cultures as well.[66] Autoimmune mechanisms may also be partially responsible for CD4 cell depletion. These processes may entail the recognition of novel activation antigens or viral antigens that cross-react with physiologic epitopes. For example, an 18,000 MW antigen was found to be expressed on HIV-infected CD4[+] cells as well as on lectin-stimulated cells and was recognized by antibodies in the sera of HIV-infected individuals. These auto-antibodies reacted with the activated CD4[+] cells but not CD8[+] cells. Other lymphocytotropic autoantibodies have been described in patients by other investigators but have not been as well characterized.[67–72] In addition, since CD4 serves as a receptor for both HIV and Class II molecules, an immune response against HIV may result in a cross-reactive response against Class II-bearing cells as well as an anti-idiotypic response against cells expressing CD4.[63] In support of this model, a septamer generated from the amino acid sequence that is shared between a conserved region of the Class II and the gp41 of HIV could block the binding of anti-CD4 antibodies to CD4[+] cells.[73] However, two recent studies have localized the regions involved in the binding of HIV envelope to CD4 within the gp120 portion of the molecule.[74,75] There remains the possibility that several other regions within the envelope, including gp41, may participate in binding to CD4.

HIV Infection of Other Cell Types in the Immune System

Besides the depletion of CD4[+] lymphocytes, early studies suggested that other cell types may be eliminated by HIV infection as well. AIDS patients were found to have reduced numbers of Langerhans' cells in their skin.[76] This cell serves in antigen presentation and expresses both Class II and CD4 on its surface. It was found that purified Langerhans' cells could be infected

---

* Rabson A: Personal communication.

in vitro, and HIV could be identified by electron microscopy in some Langerhans' cells from AIDS patients.[77] Follicular dendritic cells that reside in lymph nodes and probably arise from fibroblastic reticulum cells, was one of the first cell types observed to contain HIV *in vivo.*[78] Bone-marrow–derived dendritic cells, which are found in the circulation and the paracortical regions of lymph nodes, are important in antigen presentation. These cells have been found capable of replicating virus *in vitro.*[79] By virtue of their location and function, they may play a pivotal role in the initial spread of HIV to lymphoid cells. Likewise, monocytes, macrophages, and promonocytic tumor cells that express CD4 have also been found to be infected by HIV *in vitro* and in monocytes *in vivo.*[80–90] These cells may be important as a reservoir for infection and in the pathogenesis of some of the clinical disorders associated with AIDS. For example, HIV has been detected primarily in monocytes, macrophages, and microglial cells in the brains of patients with encephalopathy, suggesting that these cells play a key role in the encephalopathic process (Fig. 4-1).[85–89] It has been observed that the AIDS viral envelope protein can inhibit the *in vitro* growth of neurons stimulated by neuroleukin.[91] As these two proteins share a common sequence, HIV envelope probably competes for binding to the growth factor receptor on neurons. Thus, the release of high concentrations of envelope in the central nervous system by macrophages may be inhibitory to neuron growth *in vivo.* Reactive glial cells often appear to be in intimate contact with macrophages in the brains of AIDS patients. Because glial cells may be permissive for HIV replication,[92,93] infected macrophages may be the primary source of HIV for these cells.

An issue of current debate in the virology of AIDS is whether or not individuals harbor several forms of HIV that can be exclusively tropic for particular cell types *in vivo.* It was first reported that some HIV isolates obtained from the trypsin-resistent, adherent cells of the brain and lung of AIDS patients exhibit a selective tropism for monocytes. These isolates infected T cells inefficiently.[84] Conversely, HIV isolates from peripheral blood that were passaged *in vitro* through T cells were unable to infect monocytes. Recent studies from another group support these observations using a culture system that enhances the growth of macrophages *in vitro.** Of note, CD4 could not be detected on the surface of these monocytes, suggesting that another receptor may serve to permit viral entry into monocytes. In another report,[94] two structurally dissimilar isolates were obtained from the frontal cortex and cerebrospinal fluid of a single patient with encephalopathy. In contrast to the other studies, both of these viruses were isolated and passaged in lectin-stimulated lymphocytes. The isolate derived from the cortex infected macrophages as well, whereas the other strain infected glioma cells but not macrophages. Selective cell tropism of viral isolates is either coded by genes for viral-specific sequences or acquired

---

* Gendelman HE: Personal communication.

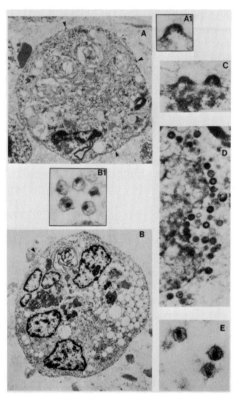

FIG. 4-1. Transmission electron micrographs of budding HIV virions from mononucleated and multinucleated monocytes from an AIDS patient with encephalopathy. (Koenig S, Gendelman HE, Orenstein JM et al: Detection of AIDS virus in macrophages in brain tissue from AIDS patients with encephalopathy. Science 233:1089, 1986)

through integration of the receptor on the host cell membrane in the viral envelope during the budding process. The molecular cloning of these biologically different isolates should provide insight into this issue.

Reports of other cell types that have been noted to be infected with HIV include transformed B cells,[95] endothelial cells,[86] transformed colon cells,[96] and normal CD8+CD4− lymphocytes.[97] Some but not all of these cell types have been shown to express CD4 mRNA or protein. It is unclear whether infection of these cells *in vitro* has any physiologic significance or can account for any of the pathologic and immunologic changes seen in AIDS patients.

IMMUNE FUNCTION

T Cells

With regard to functional changes within the immune system, immune defects have been observed in CD4+ and CD8+ T-lymphocytes, B cells, monocytes, and natural killer cells. Studies of bulk populations of T cells have shown modest increases in spontaneous proliferation with profound decreases in responses to mitogens, alloantigens, and soluble antigens.[98-100] The degree of functional changes that transpire in a given individual will vary, although AIDS patients with opportunistic infections appear in general to have more depressed T-cell functions than individuals with other HIV associated conditions.[32] The primary functional T-cell defect is intimately related to T-cell depletion. For instance, the reconstitution of a mitogenic response to pokeweed mitogen (PWM) or phytohemagglutinin (PHA) can be achieved by increasing the absolute numbers of CD4+ lymphocytes in cultures of cells from AIDS patients to levels comparable to those seen in cells of uninfected individuals.[98] In one study, exposure of PBMC from normal donors to purified gp120 was reported to selectively inhibit mitogenic responses to PHA, but not to Concanavalin A (Con A), PWM, or allogeneic cells.[101] This induced defect for a select mitogen has not been reported with patient's cells. However, concentrations of envelope protein that were used *in vitro* may not be achieved during the natural infection.

Beyond the quantitative T-cell defect in cells derived from AIDS patients, there appears to be a qualitative deficiency in the response to soluble protein antigens. Purified populations of CD4+ lymphocytes are unable to proliferate to soluble antigen *in vitro*.[98] The defect appears to be intrinsic to the T cells and not due to an accessory cell defect since the addition of syngeneic monocytes from healthy seronegative identical twins to cultures of T4-lymphocytes from AIDS patients cannot reconstitute this response (Fig. 4-2). The site of this selective defect is unclear. Theoretically, suppressed function may be due to soluble lymphokine mediators, viral proteins, latent infection with HIV, or changes within the structure or function of the antigen-specific receptor. Alternatively, loss of the subpopulations responsive to particular antigens may occur through recurrent *in vivo* priming and activation. Since HIV propagates best in activated cells, this may explain the selective sensitivity of these subsets of cells to infection with the virus and their ultimate elimination.[43,102,103] The loss of proliferative responses to soluble antigen is often one of the first impaired laboratory parameters observed in healthy seropositive individuals.

In addition to the deficiencies in the proliferative responses to antigen, AIDS patients have impaired cell-mediated cytotoxic responses. For example, HLA Class I restricted cytotoxic T-lymphocyte responses against influenza and cytomegalovirus (CMV) were reported depressed in patients in the early stages of their disease.[104-107] Since these responses are mediated by CD8+ cells, which usually are not infected with HIV, alternative mechanisms must be responsible for their depressed function. Because the generation of Class I CTL activity is characteristically dependent on intact T4 cell-inducer function, the observed impairment of this response may be the consequence of the T4 cell dysfunction. Thus, it is implied that T4 cell reconstitution should

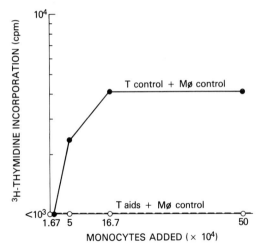

FIG. 4-2. Inability of normal monocytes to reconstitute the proliferative response of T cells from an AIDS patient to tetanus toxoid. Graded numbers of enriched monocytes (AET-SRBC depleted cells) from a healthy HIV-seronegative twin patient were added to autologous purified T cells (5 × 10⁴ AET-SRBC rosetted cells) and to purified T cells from his twin brother with AIDS. Cells were cultured in RPMI 1640 with 10% fetal calf serum for 6 days. Each data point represents the mean ³H-thymidine incorporation (12 μCi/ml) of quadruplicate cultures following a 4-hour pulse.

ameliorate this cytotoxic defect if the effector function of CD8+ cells is intact. In support of this concept, *in vitro* T-cell–mediated cytotoxicity to CMV was restored with IL-2, possibly by bypassing the usual CD4+ inductive signals.[108] Likewise, CD8+ cytotoxic responses against alloantigens appear to be relatively preserved in AIDS patients since it is thought that these alloreactive responses may not require CD4+ cells for induction.[109]

IL-2

In the generation of a specific immune response, T-cell activation and the expansion of the T cell pool is contingent upon the production of IL-2 and the expression of high affinity IL-2 receptors.[110] The state of activation is maintained by autocrine stimulation of T-cell IL-2 receptors by the IL-2 secreted by T cells. Most activated T cells will elaborate γ-interferon that amplifies the immune response by activating macrophages, B cells, and natural killer cells. Therefore, it is not surprising that IL-2 and γ-interferon production has been found to be reduced in the circulation of many patients with AIDS and in cultures of their cells,[111-115] since this may be a reflection of their quantitative T-cell losses. In one study, under conditions when equivalent numbers of T cells from AIDS and control patients have been tested for IL-2 production by mitogen stimulation, comparable levels were measured.[98] Similarly, when tumor cell lines were examined for IL-2 mRNA expression after HIV infection, the constitutive expression of IL-2 mRNA could be enhanced with PHA and phorbol-12 myristate acetate (PMA).[117] In a recent study, however, decreased IL-2 mRNA expression was seen in Jurkat cells infected with HIV. This suggests that decreased mRNA IL-2 expression may be responsible for some of the observed immune defects and decreased survival of HIV infected cells.* IL-2 receptor expression may be depressed in some clinical groups,[118] but has not been observed categorically in HIV-infected individuals. It is unlikely, therefore, that decreased IL-2 receptor expression plays a significant role in the immunopathogenesis of HIV infection.

Efforts to reconstitute *in vitro* immune function with IL-2 have had variable success.[119-121] One group reported that impaired *in vitro* γ-interferon production by lymphocytes from AIDS patients can be restored by addition of IL-2 to cultures.[115] Others have shown that impaired natural killer cell function can be reconstituted by *in vitro* culture in the presence of IL-2.[108] In clinical trials with IL-2, mild improvement in CD4+ lymphocyte counts were seen in association with eosinophilia in patients who received 2 million units by continuous infusion, although other laboratory and clinical parameters were not dramatically improved.[122] Although IL-2 is disappointing as a single therapeutic agent for immune reconstitution, it may have some efficacy when used in conjunction with antiviral and other immunomodulatory agents.

Suppressor Substances

There have been numerous reports of the suppressive effects on T-cell responses of sera and plasma obtained from AIDS patients.[123-126] One of the first studies[123] demonstrated that both PHA and mixed-lymphocyte proliferative responses were suppressed by AIDS sera. The antiproliferative activity could be removed by absorption of sera with sheep red blood cells (SRBC), suggesting the presence of antibody activity against T cells. Absorption of the same sera with allogeneic mononuclear cells removed the antiproliferative activity only in the mixed-lymphocyte response, implying that suppression in this latter assay may be directed against major histocompatibility determinants. Another substance derived from patients' plasma was able to suppress antigen- and mitogen-induced proliferative responses, as well as IL-2 and IL-2 receptor expression, and did not bind to an immunoglobulin affinity column.[124] Similar observations were made by other investigators with a heat, acid, and alkali-stable factor from sera that suppressed mitogen induced IL-2 production by peripheral blood mononuclear cells.[125]

In vitro induced suppressive factors have been produced in cultures of T cells from AIDS patients that have been stimulated with Con A.[126] These factors could inhibit pokeweed mitogen-induced plaque-forming cell

responses and tetanus toxoid proliferative responses, but not Epstein–Barr Virus (EBV) induced proliferative responses. T-cell hybridomas generated from peripheral blood cells of AIDS patients produced factors of about 47,000 daltons with activities similar to those found in the Con A–stimulated culture supernatants.[127]

Although suppressor substances can be found in sera and can be induced *in vitro*, the issue of whether or not excessive suppressor cell activity contributes significantly to immune suppression in AIDS patients is unresolved. Some investigators have reported increased suppressor activity directed against PWM-induced immunoglobulin production in unfractionated populations of PBMC.[128,129] In a limited study others have not corroborated these results using enriched T8+ populations.[130] Suppression in an unfractionated population from a given individual may demonstrate some enhanced suppressive activity, but this may merely reflect an increase in the proportion of that cell type in the population.

Monocytes and Macrophages

While some functional abnormalities have been observed in monocytes from HIV-seropositive individuals, the majority of activities appear to be preserved.[131-139] Chemotaxis is the monocyte function that is most consistently observed to be impaired in AIDS and lymphadenopathy patients.[131,132] This defect is not specific for HIV infection since other chronically ill patients also have depressed chemotactic responses. Impaired monocyte respiratory burst activity was seen in AIDS patients after prolonged intravenous courses of γ-interferon.[140] Monocyte candicidal activity has been noted to be depressed in one study,[137] although normal fungicidal activity against *Aspergillus fumigatus, Cryptococcus neoformans,* and *Thermoascus crustaceus* has been found by others.[133] Cytotoxicity against *Toxoplasma gondii* and *Chlamydia psittaci* generated in response to γ-interferon was found normal in monocytes from AIDS patients,[134] and antibody-dependent cytotoxicity,[132] tumoricidal activity,[135] and phagocytic function[133] was generally found to be intact as well. Macrophages from AIDS patients function reasonably well in soluble antigen presentation in both syngeneic* and Class II compatible systems,[136] despite a report indicating decreased Class II expression on patients' monocytes.[141] The accessory cell function required for proliferative responses of T cells to anti-T3 could be augmented in lymphadenopathy patients when normal allogeneic macrophages were added to culture, suggesting that a partial functional defect existed in this system.[142] IL-1 production and secretion by monocytes appears to be maintained, although inhibitors to this lymphokine may be present in the circulation of AIDS patients.[139]

---

* Lane HC: Personal communication.

* Koenig S: Unpublished observations.

B Cells and Immunoglobulin Production

Humoral immunity is severely compromised in patients with AIDS. Apart from the consequences of the absence of CD4[+] T-helper cells in initiating specific antibody production, intrinsic B-cell physiology is abnormal in HIV-seropositive individuals. B cells from patients are typically in a perpetual state of polyclonal activation.[1–3,130,143–147] Spontaneous proliferation, increased hemolytic plaque forming cells (PFC), and hypergammaglobulinemia is seen in the majority of symptomatic individuals (Fig. 4-3). In affected adults, serum levels of IgG, IgA, and IgD are increased,[27,130,143,144] although IgM levels are relatively normal.[147] IgM hypergammaglobulinemia may be seen in children with AIDS.

In sharp contrast to this spontaneous hyperactivity, antigen-specific and nonspecific B-cell responses are impaired in AIDS patients.[130] Decreased *in vitro* proliferative responses to antigen and mitogen, as well as decreased PWM-induced immunoglobulin synthesis, are seen. AIDS patients have poor responses to primary and secondary immunizations with protein and polysaccharide antigens.[130,147]

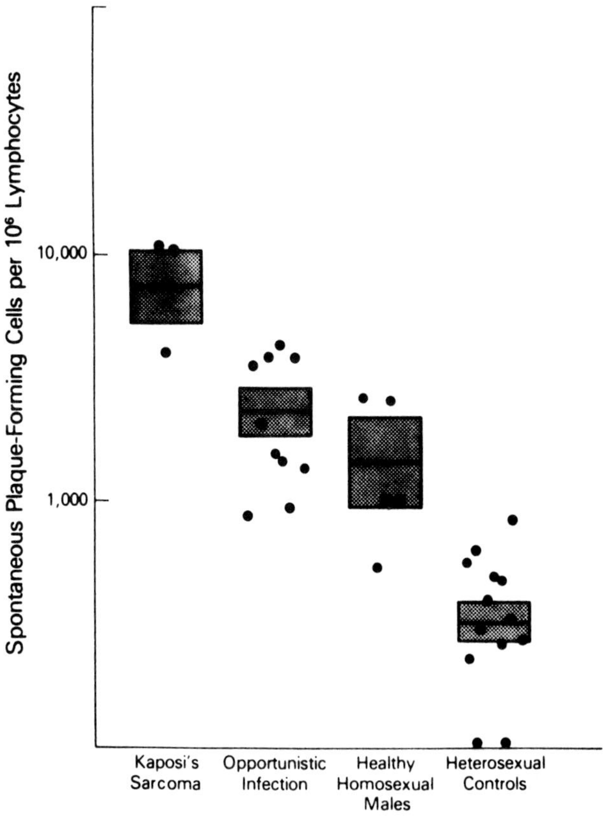

The enhanced *in vitro* transformation of B cells of AIDS patients by EBV[148] may be secondary to impaired immune surveillance by T cells and natural killer (NK) cells, and not related to intrinsic B cell dysfunction. The increased incidence of lymphomas in these individuals is probably associated with the increased transformation by EBV and not infection with HIV. Despite the ability to infect EBV-transformed B cells *in vitro* with HIV, there is no evidence that HIV integration occurs in the lymphomas of AIDS patients.

Although there is no current indication that nontransformed B cells can be infected with HIV, the effects of viral proteins on B-cell activity may account for some of the changes observed *in vivo*. Both intact and disrupted viral particles were found to induce polyclonal activation of normal B cells, achieving levels of proliferation and immunoglobulin production comparable to other B-cell mitogens (Fig. 4-4).[149–151] These responses may be due to effects solely on the B cells or may require the presence of T cells to "present" concentrated virions or to secrete soluble factors. In contrast to the stimulatory properties of viral particles on B cells, one group has also reported that HIV could suppress EBV-induced PFC formation by purified B cells.[152] The mechanism by which this is achieved is unclear.

Natural Killer Cells

A number of phenotypically distinct cell types have been associated with the functional properties of natural killer (NK) cells. The majority of these cells comprise a small population of circulating large granular lymphocytes (LGL). Monoclonal antibodies have been used to characterize subsets of LGL with NK activity (HNK-1, NKH-1, anti-CD16). A smaller circulating population of CD16[−] cells expressing the product of the γ-δ T-cell receptor gene has been shown to have NK activity.[153] NK cells have been presumed to perform the function of immunosurveillance by virtue of their ability to kill virally infected cells, tumor cells, and allogeneic cells in an HLA unrestricted manner.

NK cell function, as measured in unfractionated populations of mononuclear cells of AIDS patients, is depressed as compared with cells from healthy HIV seronegative controls.[108,154–158] The number of circulating NK cells does not appear to be diminished in AIDS patients, and these cells are capable of binding to appropriate target cells.[159] When activated by IL-2 (Fig. 4-5), Con A, or phorbol ester and calcium ionophore *in vitro*,[154,160] their function can be enhanced or restored to normal levels. It seems that NK cells from AIDS patients cannot deliver an adequate transmembrane "signal" for activation when in contact with an appropriate target, but are intrinsically intact to execute cytolysis once activation is accomplished by another pathway.

FIG. 4-3. Increased spontaneous hemolytic plaque-forming cells in patients with AIDS. (Lane HC, Masur H, Edgar LC et al: Abnormalities of B-cell activation and immunoregulation in patients with the acquired immunodeficiency syndrome. N Engl J Med 309:453, 1983)

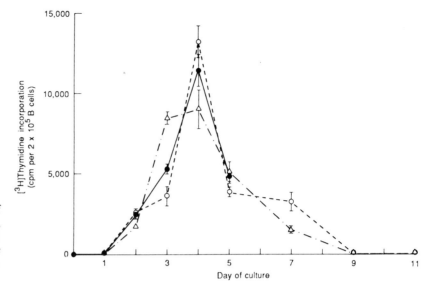

FIG. 4-4. HIV-induced proliferation of normal B cells *in vitro*. (Schnittman SM, Lane HC, Higgins SE et al: Direct polyclonal activation of human B lymphocytes by the aquired immune deficiency syndrome virus. Science 233:1084, 1986)

Other Humoral Abnormalities

Elevated levels of acid labile α-interferon,[161,162] α_1-thymosin,[163] and β_2-microglobulin[164] have been reported in patients with AIDS and are of unknown clinical consequence. Antibodies to α_1-thymosin appear to cross-react with p17 and may be effective in viral neutralization.[165] Increases in circulating immune complexes have been observed in AIDS patients[166,167] and may be responsible for certain of the mild constitutional symptoms in patients, although classical diseases resulting from immune complex deposition have not occurred with an increased frequency in AIDS.

IMMUNE RESPONSES TO HIV

Multiple factors influence the outcome of a person's exposure to HIV. Conditions such as the route of viral entry, the number of contacts, the virulence of the isolate, the size of the viral inoculum, the presence of co-infecting pathogens, and the nutritional state and the response of the immune system of the exposed individual may determine whether or not he or she will become infected with HIV or manifest symptoms of AIDS. A resistence to infection based on HLA association has not been observed. There are a number of individuals who practice high risk behavior, including homosexuals and intravenous drug abusers, who remain uninfected despite engaging in activities that are infectious to others. One study[168] has found an association between an individual's group-specific component (Gc) type and the resistence or susceptibility to infection and disease progression he or she exhibits. In a cohort of homosexual men, persistently seronegative individuals were more

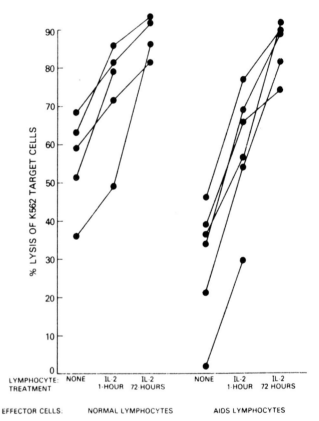

FIG. 4-5. Enhancement of depressed natural killer cytotoxicity in AIDS patients by pre-incubation of cells with IL-2. (Rook AH, Masur H, Lane HC et al: Interleukin-2 enhances the depressed natural killer and cytomegalovirus-specific cytotoxic activities of lymphocytes from patients with the acquired immune deficiency syndrome. J Clin Invest 72:398, 1983)

often found to carry a Gc-2 subtype while those who progressed to AIDS were more often of a Gc-1 fast type. The underlying mechanism to explain these observations remains elusive at present. It should be pointed out that subsequent studies by others have not corroborated these original observations.[169,170]

It is estimated that 30% of all asymptomatic HIV infected individuals will develop AIDS within 5 years of infection.[171] It is unclear what proportion of infected individuals will develop AIDS over a longer time frame. It would seem likely that the success of the immune system in containing or eliminating the virus would be a principal determinant of clinical outcome. The conditions necessary for inducing effective immunity in an exposed or infected individual have not been established. For most individuals, HIV infection is associated with lifelong seroconversion and viral persistence. Rare healthy individuals have been reported to lose HIV seroreactivity in the absence of disease, and under these unusual circumstances, a person may be free of the virus.

Multiple arms of the immune system could participate in a protective immune response to HIV. Antibodies with neutralizing or cytolytic activity may be produced and the complement cascade may be activated to kill free and cell bound virions. Antibody-dependent cytotoxic cells and NK cells may mediate HLA-non-restricted lysis of infected cells. HLA Class I and Class II restricted cytotoxic T lymphocytes (CTL) could be stimulated and provide long lived immunity for some individuals.

Neutralizing Antibodies

Antibodies with neutralizing capacity have been detected in seropositive individuals at all stages of clinical illness. Neutralizing antibodies are generally of low titer and in the majority of studies their *in vitro* effects have not correlated with their ability to prevent progressive disease.[172-175] However, one group reported rising titers in those with clinically stable disease.[176] By convention, neutralization is considered type or group specific depending on the ability of the sera to inhibit structurally similar or heterogeneous HIV isolates. Both patterns of neutralizing activity have been seen but neither confers a particular protective advantage to the individual. Sera from patients can be fractionated to yield neutralizing activity with either type or group specificity. In one study,[175] serum passaged over an affinity column of recombinant gp120 resulted in the adherence of the type-specific activity to the gp120 with group-specific activity contained in the effluent fraction. A pattern of preferential neutralization of autologous isolates has been observed in some patients.[173,174]

Attempts to stimulate neutralizing antibodies experimentally in uninfected animals and humans with different recombinant and purified proteins have been successful.[177-182] Glycosylation of these proteins is not required to induce antibodies with neutralizing capa-

bility,[178-179] although theoretically it may yield some qualitative advantages. Not all of the experimentally induced antibodies are neutralizing. In particular, antibodies generated against the amino-terminal half of gp120 and p41 could bind but not neutralize HIV.[178] Also, there may be a dichotomy in the regions that can induce antibody formation and T-cell proliferation. Virally induced antibodies found in the sera of patients reacted strongly with recombinant proteins from the carboxy-terminus of gp120, but bound weakly to proteins from the amino-terminus of gp120. Conversely, T cells from these same patients proliferated well to the latter proteins, but poorly to the carboxy-terminus gp120.[183] Specific sequences have been predicted as being immunogenic based on their location within the amphipathic α-helical regions of envelope. Cells from mice that were immunized with purified envelope proteins proliferated to such a 16-amino acid residue, but it is not yet known if neutralizing antibodies are produced to this peptide.[184]

There is a suggestion that even if high-titered neutralizing antibodies could be stimulated in uninfected individuals, the biologic properties of HIV (and other retroviruses) may preclude protection against infection. HIV has the propensity to mutate rapidly in its envelope region, resulting in the frequent creation of new variants. Neutralizing antibodies may hasten this selection process, as has been seen *in vitro*[185] and in other lentiviral diseases *in vivo*.[186] The recent attempt to immunize chimpanzees with purified gp120 was disappointing, since despite the formation of neutralizing antibodies in these animals, they became infected after viral challenge.

Cell-Mediated Cytotoxicity

The development of a cellular cytotoxic immune response may be more important than neutralizing antibody formation in providing protection against retroviruses. It was shown in a murine system that the development of cell-mediated cytotoxic responses to Friend leukemia virus protected animals against the development of leukemia, whereas animals that developed only neutralizing antibodies succumbed to leukemia.[187] Protective cell-mediated responses against HIV may include ADCC, CTL, and NK responses.

Antibody-Dependent Cellular Cytotoxicity

Several studies have demonstrated that sera from seropositive patients can mediate antibody-dependent cellular cytotoxicity (ADCC) (Fig. 4-6).[188-190] The activity of sera appears to correlate roughly with the clinical condition of the individual from whom they are derived; healthy seropositive individuals tend to have more activity than AIDS patients.[188] In one study, there did not seem to be a correlation between ADCC-specific anti-

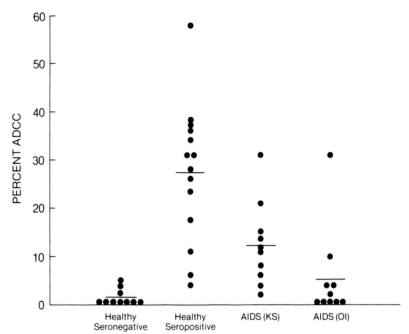

FIG. 4-6. Antibody-dependent cytotoxicity against HIV-infected target cells with sera from healthy HIV-seropositive individuals and patients with AIDS. (Rook AH, Lane HC, Folks T et al: Sera from HTLV-III/LAV antibody-positive individuals mediate antibody-dependent cellular cytotoxicity against HTLV-III/LAV-infected T cells. J Immunol 138:1064, 1987)

body titer and anti-HIV antibody titer as tested in an ELISA assay.[190] However, absence of antibody to a particular viral protein may be more important than total anti-HIV antibody titers. ADCC activity seemed to correlate best with the presence of anti-p24 in one of the studies,[188] whereas in a more recent report[190] activity was present in sera without anti-p24 activity, but was undetectable when anti-envelope activity was absent. Examination of a large group of sera for both neutralizing and ADCC activities in either a prospective or retrospective manner to see if one or both activities correlate with clinical progression may provide insight into the clinical relevance of these *in vitro* responses. In a prospective study of a cohort of healthy seropositive homosexuals over a 3-year period, those individuals who remained healthy had more substantial anti-p24 activity;[191] there were no significant differences in neutralizing activity between those who became symptomatic and those who remained healthy. ADCC activity was not examined in this study.

Natural Killer Cells

Purified populations of LGLs from seronegative individuals have been shown to have minimal activity against HIV infected cells, and this activity could be markedly bolstered by culture in the presence of IL-2.[192] Similar enhanced HLA-unrestricted cytotoxic activity was seen when unfractionated cells from both seronegative and seropositive individuals were cultured in the presence of IL-2.* Recent studies have demon-

* Rook A, Koenig S: Unpublished observation.

strated that circulating cells in seropositive patients could mediate HLA-unrestricted cytolytic activity by cells that expressed CD16.[193] The activity of these cells correlated with the patient's clinical status in that the healthier individuals had more substantial activity. Since cells that bear CD16 can participate in either NK-mediated lysis or ADCC, a portion of these activated cells may be armed with low amounts of cytophilic antibody to gp120 and may effect lysis through ADCC. It would be of interest if seropositive individuals without evidence of anti-gp120 in their sera by radioimmunoprecipitation had similar cytotoxic activity in their peripheral blood mononuclear cells.

Cytotoxic T Cells

T cells with cytotoxic activities against cell-associated HIV proteins and virus have been demonstrated in the circulation and lungs of infected individuals in different assay systems. One group reported the presence of CTL to HIV envelope and gag proteins in the peripheral blood using target cells infected with a recombinant vaccinia virus expressing the proteins of HIV.[194] Cytolytic activity was seen in all seropositive patients examined, including those with ARC and AIDS, and some features of HLA restriction were found. Others have reported similar activity in the majority of healthy seropositive individuals, some patients with ARC, and rare AIDS patients with Kaposi's sarcoma, but not in those with opportunistic infections.[195] This activity did not appear to be HLA Class I restricted. A third group examining anti-envelope responses after *in vitro* priming, found very low but statistically significant HLA Class

I-restricted CTL in some seropositive individuals.[196] CD8+CTL against HIV-infected alveolar macrophages were recovered from patients with interstitial pneumonitis in an 18 hour ^{51}Cr-release assay.[197] This response appeared to be restricted to HLA-A2 in the individuals tested. In an animal model of immunity to HIV,[198] peripheral blood cells from chimpanzees immunized with recombinant vaccinia expressing HIV envelope were capable of proliferating to purified whole HIV and envelope proteins. Cloned cells from these immunized chimpanzees were cytotoxic for target cells infected with vaccinia virus expressing the recombinant envelope protein. These cytotoxic cells, however, were CD4+. It remains to be seen if both Class I and Class II HIV-specific CTLs are generated during natural infection and with immunization with different recombinant proteins and if CTL can confer any protection to the uninfected and immunized host.

CONCLUDING COMMENTS

The development of AIDS and its associated clinical disorders has resulted in a greater appreciation of the impact of immunologic impairment on human health and survival. Except for the infrequent primary immunodeficiencies, and immunologic dysfunction iatragenically induced by radiation and chemotherapy, the devastation of the immune system by HIV is unprecedented. A wealth of information has been generated on the immune responses to viruses and the effect of the entire family of retroviruses on immune function.

There are still major gaps in our understanding of the immunopathogenesis of this disorder. While the hallmark of this disease is the depletion and functional impairment of the T4-lymphocytes with the consequential loss of pivotal helper and inducer function for B cells, T cells, and monocytes in patients with AIDS, we are still at loss to explain many of the functional changes that occur early in the course of HIV function, especially at times when significant losses of T4 cells are not seen. The mechanism(s) by which T4-lymphocytes are killed *in vivo* remains a mystery and may include virally induced cytotoxic and fusogenic processes and autoimmune responses. Although many of the cell types that can support the replication of the virus are identified, precise knowledge of the important niches and reservoirs *in vivo* is lacking. Clearly, this information is critical for devising therapeutic strategies. There is a major effort to discern the molecular events that are important for viral expression. Of special interest to immunologists is the effects of cell products, namely lymphokines and monokines, on viral replication and the pathways by which this modulation of viral expression can occur.

There is currently an active endeavor to develop a vaccine against HIV that could prevent infection or clinical progression. The first candidate vaccines are being tested in humans in the United States and Africa. Unfortunately, our understanding of what type of immunity will provide a protective response to HIV is limited and therefore, the design of such a vaccine may be difficult. Given the long latency for the development of AIDS in seropositive individuals, judgments regarding efficacy of a vaccine may be difficult. Hopefully, our ignorance in this area will be short-lived.

REFERENCES

1. Gottlieb MS, Schroff R, Schanker HM et al: *Pneumocystis carinii* pneumonia and mucosal candidiasis in previously healthy homosexual men: Evidence of a new acquired cellular immunodeficiency. N Engl J Med 305:1425, 1981
2. Masur H, Michelis MA, Greene JB et al: An outbreak of community-acquired *Pneumocystis carinii* pneumonia: Initial manifestation of cellular immune dysfunction. N Engl J Med 305:1431, 1981
3. Siegel FP, Lopez C, Hammer GS et al: Severe acquired immunodeficiency in male homosexuals, manifested by chronic perianal ulcerative herpes simplex lesions. N Engl J Med 305:1439, 1981
4. Centers for Disease Control: Acquired immunodeficiency syndrome weekly surveillance report. October 19, 1987, Atlanta, GA, Centers for Disease Control.
5. Barré-Sinoussi F, Chermann JC, Rey F et al: Isolation of a T lymphotropic retrovirus from a patient at risk for acquired immune deficiency syndrome (AIDS). Science 220:868, 1983
6. Popovic M, Sarngadharan MG, Read E et al: Detection, isolation, and continuous production of cytopathic retroviruses (HTLV-III) from patients with AIDS and pre-AIDS. Science 224:497, 1984
7. Levy JA, Hoffman AD, Kramer SM et al: Isolation of lymphocytopathic retroviruses from San Francisco patients with AIDS. Science 225:840, 1984
8. Coffin J, Haase A, Levy JA et al: Human immunodeficiency viruses. Science 232:697, 1986
9. Brun–Vezinet F, Rey MA, Katlama C et al: Lymphadenopathy-associated virus type 2 in AIDS and AIDS-related complex. Lancet 1:128, 1987
10. Clavel F, Guyader M, Guetard D et al: Molecular cloning and polymorphism of the human immune deficiency virus type 2. Nature 324:691, 1986
11. Benn S, Rutledge R, Folks T et al: Genomic heterogeneity of AIDS retroviral isolates from North America and Zaire. Science 230:949, 1985
12. Asjì B, Morfeldt–Manson L, Albert J et al: Replicative capacity of human immunodeficiency virus from patients with varying severity of HIV infection. Lancet 2:660, 1986
13. Clavel F, Mansinho K, Chamaret S et al: Human immunodeficiency virus type 2 infection associated with AIDS in West Africa. N Engl J Med 316:1180, 1987
14. Poon M–C, Landay A, Prasthofer EF et al: Acquired immunodeficiency syndrome with *Pneumocystis carinii* pneumonia and *Mycobacterium avium-intracellulare* infection in a previously healthy patient with classic hemophilia. Ann Intern Med 98:287, 1983
15. Elliott JL, Hoppess WL, Platt MS et al: The acquired immunodeficiency syndrome and *Mycobacterium avium-*

intracellulare bacteremia in a patient with hemophilia. Ann Intern Med 98:290, 1983

16. Fauci AS, Masur H, Gelmann EP et al: The acquired immunodeficiency syndrome: An update. Ann Intern Med 102:800, 1985

17. Hymesk, Cheung T, Greene JB et al: Kaposi's sarcoma in homosexual men: A report of eight cases. Lancet 2: 598, 1981

18. Polsky B, Gold JWM, Whimbey E et al: Bacterial pneumonia in patients with the acquired immunodeficiency syndrome. Ann Intern Med 104:38, 1986

19. Chaisson RE, Volberding P, Sande MA: Acquired Immunodeficiency syndrome. In Parillo JE, Masur H (eds): *The Critically Ill Immunosuppressed Patient,* p. 321. Rockville, MD, Apsen, 1987

20. Reinherz E, O'Brien C, Rosenthal P et al: The cellular basis for viral-induced immunodeficiency: Analysis by monoclonal antibodies. J Immunol 125:1264, 1980

21. Gendelman HE, Phelps W, Feigenbaum L et al: Transactivation of the human immunodeficiency virus long terminal repeat sequence by DNA viruses. Proc Natl Acad Sci USA 83:9759, 1986

22. Mosca JD, Bednarik DP, Raj NBK et al: Herpes simplex virus type-1 can reactivate transcription of latent human immunodeficiency virus. Nature 325:67, 1987

23. Kornfeld H, Van de Stouwe RA, Lange M et al: T-lymphocyte subpopulations in homosexual men. N Engl J Med 307:729, 1982

24. Goldsmith JC, Moseley PL, Monick M et al: T-lymphocyte subpopulation abnormalities in apparently healthy patients with hemophilia. Ann Intern Med 98:294, 1983

25. Pinching AJ, Jeffries DJ, Donaghy M et al: Studies of cellular immunity in male homosexuals in London. Lancet 2:126, 1983

26. Detels R, Schwartz K, Visscher BR et al: Relation between sexual practices and T-cell subsets in homosexually active men. Lancet 1:609, 1983

27. Ammann AJ, Abrams D, Conant M et al: Acquired immune dysfunction in homosexual men: immunologic profiles. Clin Immunol Immunopathol 27:315, 1983

28. Rubinstein A, Sicklick M, Gupta A et al: Acquired immunodeficiency with reverse T4/T8 ratios in infants born to promiscuous and drug-addicted mothers. JAMA 249: 2350, 1983

29. Fahey JL, Prince H, Weaver M et al: Quantitative changes in T helper or T suppressor/cytotoxic lymphocyte subsets that distinguish acquired immune deficiency syndrome from other immune subset disorders. Am J Med 76:95, 1984

30. Cavaille–Coll M, Messiah A, Klatzmann D et al: Critical analysis of T cell subset and function evaluation in patients with persistent generalized lymphadenopathy in groups at risk for AIDS. Clin Exp Immunol 57:511, 1984

31. Biggar RJ, Melbye M, Ebbesen P et al: Low T-lymphocyte ratios in homosexual men. JAMA 251:1441, 1984

32. Lane HC, Masur H, Gelmann EP et al: Correlation between immunologic function and clinical subpopulations of patients with the acquired immune deficiency syndrome. Am J Med 78:417, 1985

33. Mittelman A, Wong G, Safai B et al: Analysis of T cell subsets in different clinical subgroups of patients with the acquired immune deficiency syndrome. Am J Med 78:951, 1985

34. Polk BF, Fox R, Bookmeyer R et al: Predictors of the acquired immunodeficiency syndrome developing in a cohort of seropositive homosexual men. N Engl J Med 316:61, 1987

35. Goedert JJ, Biggar RJ, Melbye M et al: Effect of T4 count and cofactors on the incidence of AIDS in homosexual men infected with human immunodeficiency virus. JAMA 257:331, 1987

36. Kaplan JA, Spira TJ, Fishbein DB et al: Lymphadenopathy syndrome in homosexual men: Evidence for continuing risk of developing the acquired immunodeficiency syndrome. JAMA 257:335, 1987

37. Fahey JL, Giorgi J, Martinez–Maza O et al: Immune pathogenesis of AIDS and related syndromes. Ann Inst Pasteur Immunol 138:245, 1987

38. Giorgi JV, Nishanian PG, Schmid I et al: Selective alterations in immunoregulatory lymphocyte subsets in early (Human T-lymphocytotropic virus Type III/lymphadenopathy associated virus) infection. J Clin Immunol 7: 140, 1987

39. Nicholson JKA, McDougal JS, Spira TJ et al: Immunoregulatory subsets of the T helper and T suppressor cell populations in homosexual men with chronic unexplained lymphadenopathy. J Clin Invest 73:191, 1984

40. Nicholson JKA, McDougal JS, Spira TJ: Alterations of functional subsets of T helper and T suppressor cell populations in acquired immunodeficiency syndrome (AIDS) and chronic unexplained lymphadenopathy. J Clin Immunol 5:269, 1985

41. Gupta S: Abnormality of Leu2$^+$7$^+$ cells in acquired immune deficiency syndrome (AIDS), AIDS-related complex, and asymptomatic homosexuals. J Clin Immunol 6:502, 1986

42. Walker CM, Moody DJ, Stites DP et al: CD8$^+$ lymphocytes can control HIV infection in vitro by suppressing virus replication. Virology 234:1563, 1986

43. McDougal JS, Mawle A, Cort SP et al: Cellular tropism of the human retrovirus HTLV-III/LAV. J Immunol 135:3151, 1985

44. Popovic M, Read–Connole E, Gallo RC: T4 positive human neoplastic cell lines susceptible to and permissive for HTLV-III. Lancet 1:79, 1984

45. Klatzmann D, Barré–Sinoussi F, Nugeyre MT et al: Selective tropism of lymphadenopathy associated virus (LAV) for helper-inducer T lymphocytes. Science 225: 59, 1984

46. Folks TM, Benn S, Rabson A et al: Characterization of a continuous T-cell line susceptible to the cytopathic effects of the acquired immunodeficiency syndrome (AIDS)-associated retrovirus. Proc Natl Acad Sci USA 82:4539, 1985

47. Klatzmann D, Champagne E, Charmaret S et al: T-lymphocyte T4 molecule behaves as the receptor for human retrovirus LAV. Nature 312:767, 1984

48. Dalgleish AG, Beverly CL, Clapham PR et al: The CD4 (T4) antigen is an essential component of the receptor for the AIDS retrovirus. Nature 312:763, 1984

49. Sattentau QJ, Dalgleish AG, Weiss RA et al: Epitopes of the CD4 antigen and HIV infection. Science 234:1120, 1986

50. McDougal JS, Kennedy MS, Sligh JM et al: Binding of HTLV-III/LAV to T4$^+$ T cells by a complex of the 110 K viral protein and the T4 molecule. Science 231:382, 1985

51. Hoxie JA, Flaherty LE, Haggarty BS et al: Infection of T4 lymphocytes by HTLV-III does not require expression of the OKT4 epitope. J Immunol 136:361, 1986

52. Folks T, Justement S, Mitchell SR et al: The T4 epitope is not required for a normal replicative cycle of human immunodeficiency virus. J Infect Dis 155:592, 1987

53. Maddon PJ, Dalgleish AG, McDougal JS et al: The T4 gene encodes the AIDS virus receptor and is expressed in the immune system and the brain. Cell 47:333, 1986

54. Mann DL, Lesane F, Blattner WA et al: HLA-DR is involved in the HIV receptor [Abstr]. In *III International Conference on Acquired Immunodeficiency Syndrome (AIDS)*, p. 209. Washington, DC, U.S. Department of Health and Human Services, 1987

55. Hoxie JA, Alpers JD, Rackowski JL et al: Alterations in T4 (CD4) protein and mRNA synthesis in cells infected with HIV. Science 234:1123, 1986

56. Asjì B, Ivhed I, Gidlund M et al: Susceptibility to infection by the human immunodeficiency virus (HIV) correlates with T4 expression in a parental monocytoid cell line and its subclones. Virology 157:359, 1987

57. Lifson JD, Feinberg MB, Reyes GR et al: Induction of CD4-dependent cell fusion by the HTLV-III/LAV envelope glycoprotein. Nature 323:725, 1986

58. Sodroski J, Goh WC, Rosen C et al: Role of the HTLV-III/LAV envelope in syncytium formation and cytopathicity. Nature 322:470, 1986

59. Epstein LG, Sharer LR, Joshi VV et al: Progressive encephalopathy in children with acquired immune deficiency syndrome. Ann Neurol 17:488, 1985

60. Ewing EP, Chandler FW, Spira TJ et al: Primary lymph node pathology in AIDS and AIDS-related lymphadenopathy. Arch Path Lab Med 109:977, 1985

61. Shaw GM, Hahn BH, Arya SK et al: Molecular characterization of human T cell leukemia (lymphotropic) virus type III in AIDS. Science 226:1165, 1984

62. Klatzmann D, Montagnier L: Approaches to AIDS therapy. Nature 319:1011, 1986

63. Ziegler JL, Stites DP: Hypothesis: AIDS is an autoimmune disease directed at the immune system and triggered by a lymphotropic retrovirus. Clin Immunol Immunopathol 41:305, 1986

64. Harper E, Marselle LM, Gallo RC et al: Detection of lymphocytes expressing human T-lymphotropic virus type III in lymph nodes and peripheral blood from infected individuals by in situ hybridization. Proc Natl Acad Sci USA 83:772, 1986

65. Winkelstein A, Klein RS, Evans TL et al: Defective in vitro T cell colony formation in the acquired immunodeficiency syndrome. J Immunol 134:151, 1985

66. Donahue RE, Johnson MM, Zon LI et al: Suppression of in vitro haematopoiesis following human immunodeficiency virus infection. Nature 326:200, 1987

67. Pollack MS, Callaway C, LeBlanc D et al: Lymphocytotoxic antibodies to non-HLA antigens in the sera of patients with acquired immunodeficiency syndrome (AIDS). In Non-HLA Antigens in Health, Aging, and Malignancy, p 209, New York, Alan R Liss, 1983

68. Kloster BE, Tomar RH, Spira TJ: Lymphocytotoxic antibodies in the acquired immune deficiency syndrome (AIDS). Clin Immunol Immunopathol 30:330, 1984

69. Williams RC, Jr, Masur H, Spira TJ: Lymphocyte-reactive antibodies in acquired immune deficiency syndrome. J Clin Immunol 4:118, 1984

70. Dorsett B, Cronin W, Chuma V et al: Anti-lymphocyte antibodies in patients with the acquired immune deficiency syndrome. Am J Med 78:621, 1985

71. Tomar RH, John PA, Hennig AK et al: Cellular targets of antilymphocyte antibodies in AIDS and LAS. Clin Immunol Immunopathol 37:37, 1985

72. Stricker RB, McHugh TM, Moody D et al: An AIDS-related cytotoxic autoantibody reacts with a specific antigen on stimulated CD4+ T cells. Nature 327:170, 1987

73. Golding H, Robey FA, Gates FT III et al: Homologous peptides from HIV P41 and HLA class II bind CD4 on human T cells [Abstr]. In *III International Conference on Acquired Immunodeficiency Syndrome (AIDS)*, p 209. Washington, DC, U.S. Department of Health and Human Services, 1987

74. Kowalski M, Potz J, Basiripour L et al: Functional regions of the envelope glycoprotein of human immunodeficiency virus type 1. Science 237:1351, 1987

75. Lasky LA, Nakamura G, Smith DH et al: Delineation of a region of the human immunodeficiency virus type 1 gp120 glycoprotein critical for interaction with the CD4 receptor. Cell 50:975, 1987

76. Belsito DV, Sanchez MR, Baer RL et al: Reduced Langerhan's cell Ia antigen and ATPase activity in patients with the acquired immunodeficiency syndrome. N Engl J Med 310:1279, 1984

77. Tischler E, Groh V, Popovic M et al: Epidermal Langerhans cells: A target for HTLV-III/LAV infection. J Invest Dermatol 88:233, 1987

78. Armstrong GA, Horne R. Follicular dendritic cells and virus-like particles in AIDS-related lymphadenopathy. Lancet 2:370, 1984

79. Patterson S, Knight SC: Susceptibility of human peripheral blood dendritic cells to infection by human immunodeficiency virus. J Gen Virol 68:1177, 1987

80. Levy JA, Shimabukuro J, McHugh T et al: AIDS-associated retrovirus (ARV) can productively infect other cells besides human T helper cells. Virology 147:441, 1985

81. Ho DD, Rota TR, Hirsch MS: Infection of monocyte/macrophage by human T lymphotropic virus type II. J Clin Invest 77:1712, 1986

82. Nicholson JKA, Cross GD, Callaway CS et al: In vitro infection of human monocytes with human T-lymphotropic virus type III/lymphadenopathy-associated virus (HTLV-III/LAV). J Immunol 137:323, 1986

83. Salahuddin SZ, Rose RM, Groopman JE et al: Human T lymphotropic virus type II infection by human alveolar macrophages. Blood 68:281, 1986

84. Gartner S, Markovits P, Markovits DM et al: The role of mononuclear phagocytes in HTLV-III/ALV infection. Science 233:215, 1986

85. Koenig S, Gendelman HE, Orenstein JM et al: Detection of AIDS virus in macrophages in brain tissue from AIDS patients with encephalopathy. Science 233:1089, 1986

86. Wiley CA, Schrier RD, Nelson JA et al: Cellular localization of human immunodeficiency virus infection within the brains of acquired immunodeficiency syndrome patients. Proc Natl Acad Sci USA 83:7089, 1986

87. Gartner S, Markovits P, Markovitz DM et al: Virus isolation from and identification of HTLV-III/LAV-producing cells in brain tissue from a patient with AIDS. JAMA 256:2365, 1986

88. Stoler MH, Eskin TA, Benn S et al: Human T-cell lymphotropic virus type III infection of the central nervous system. JAMA 256:2360, 1986

89. Vazeux R, Brousse N, Jarry A et al: AIDS subacute en-

cephalitis: Identification of HIV-infected cells. Am J Pathol 126:403, 1987

90. Rieber P, Riethmüller G: Loss of circulating T4⁺ monocytes in patients infected with HTLV-III. Lancet 1:270, 1986

91. Lee MR, Ho DD, Gurney ME: Functional interaction and partial homology between human immunodeficiency virus and neuroleukin. Science 237:1047, 1987

92. Dewhurst S, Bresser J, Stevenson M et al: Susceptibility of human glial cells to infection with human immunodeficiency virus (HIV). FEBS Letters 213:138, 1987

93. Chiodi F, Fuerstenberg S, Gidlund M et al: Infection of brain-derived cells with the human immunodeficiency virus. J Virol 93:1244, 1987

94. Koyanagi Y, Miles S, Mitsuyasu RT et al: Dual infection of the central nervous system by AIDS viruses with distinct cellular tropisms. Science 236:819, 1987

95. Montagnier L, Gruest J, Chamaret S et al: Adaption of lymphadenopathy associated virus (LAV) to replication in EBV-transformed B lymphoblastoid cells lines. Science 225:63, 1984

96. Adachi A, Koenig S, Gendelman HE et al: Productive, persistent infection of human colorectal cell lines with human immunodeficiency virus. J Virol 61:209, 1987

97. Fouchard M, Reveil B, Mbayo K et al: Evidence for HTLV-III/LAV expression by primary cultures of T8 cells. Int J Cancer 38:657, 1986

98. Lane HC, Depper JM, Greene WC et al: Qualitative analysis of immune function in patients with the acquired immunodeficiency syndrome. N Engl J Med 313:79, 1985

99. Smolen JS, Bettelheim P, Köller U et al: Deficiency of the autologous mixed lymphocyte reaction in patients with classic hemophilia treated with commercial factor VIII concentrate. J Clin Invest 75:1828, 1985

100. Gupta S, Gillis S, Thornton M et al: Autologous mixed lymphocyte reaction in man. XIV. Deficiency of the autologous mixed lymphocyte reaction in acquired immune deficiency syndrome (AIDS) and AIDS related complex (ARC). In vitro effect of purified interleukin-1 and interleukin-2. Clin Exp Immunol 58:395, 1984

101. Mann DL, Lasane F, Popovic M et al: HTLV-III large envelope protein (gp 120) suppresses PHA-induced lymphocyte blastogenesis. J Immunol 138:2640, 1987

102. Zagury D, Bernard J, Leonard R et al: Long-term cultures of HTLV-III-infected T cells: A model of cytopathology of T-cell depletion in AIDS. Science 2:850, 1985

103. Margolick JB, Volkman DJ, Folks TM et al: Amplification of HTLV-III/LAV infection by antigen-induced activation of T cells and direct suppression by virus of lymphocyte blastogenic responses.

104. Shearer GM, Payne SM, Joseph LJ et al: Functional T lymphocyte immune deficiency in a population of homosexual men who do not exhibit symptoms of acquired immune deficiency syndrome. J Clin Invest 74:496, 1984

105. Shearer GM, Salahuddin SZ, Markham PD et al: Prospective study of cytotoxic T lymphocyte responses to influenza and antibodies to human T lymphotropic virus-III in homosexual men. J Clin Invest 76:1699, 1985

106. Sheridan JF, Aurelian L, Donnenberg AD et al: Cell-mediated immunity of cytomegalovirus (CMV) and herpes simplex virus (HSV) antigens in the acquired immune deficiency syndrome: Interleukin-1 and interleukin-2 modify in vitro responses. J Clin Immunol 4:304, 1984

107. Rook AH, Manischewitz JD, Frederick WR et al: Deficient, HLA-restricted, cytomegalovirus-specific cytotoxic T cells

108. Rook AH, Masur H, Lane HC et al: Interleukin-2 enhances the depressed natural killer and cytomegalovirus-specific cytotoxic activities of lymphocytes from patients with the acquired immune deficiency syndrome. J Clin Invest 72:398, 1983

109. Mizuochi T, Goldberg H, Rosenberg AS et al: Both L3T4⁺ and Lyt-2⁺ helper cells initiate cytotoxic T lymphocyte responses against allogeneic major histocompatibility antigens but not against trinitrophenyl-modified self. J Exp Med 162:427, 1985

110. Greene WC, Depper JM, Krìnke M et al: The human interleukin-2 receptor: Analysis of structure and function. Immunol Rev 92:29, 1986

111. Tsuchiya S, Imaizumi M, Minegishi M et al: Lack of interleukin-2 production in a patient with OKT4⁺ T-cell deficiency. N Engl J Med 308:1294, 1983

112. Hauser GJ, Bino T, Rosenberg H et al: Interleukin-2 production and response to exogenous interleukin-2 in a patient with the acquired immune deficiency syndrome (AIDS). Clin Exp Immunol 56:14, 1984

113. Alcocer–Varela J, Alarcon–Segovia D, Abud–Mendoza C: Immunoregulatory circuits in the acquired immune deficiency syndrome and related complex. Production of and response to interleukins 1 and 2, NK function and its enhancement by interleukin-2 and kinetics of the autologous mixed lymphocyte reaction. Clin Exp Immunol 60:31, 1985

114. Ebert EC, Stoll DB, Cassens BJ et al: Diminished interleukin production and receptor generation characterize the acquired immunodeficiency syndrome. Clin Immunol Immunopathol 37:283, 1985

115. Murray HW, Welte K, Jacobs JL et al: Production of and in vitro response to interleukin 2 in the acquired immunodeficiency syndrome. J Clin Invest 76:1959, 1985

116. Gupta S: Study of activated T cells in man. Clin Immunol Immunopathol 38:93, 1986

117. Arya SK, Gallo RC: Human T-cell growth factor (interleukin 2) and γ-interferon genes: Expression in human T-lymphotropic virus type III- and type I-infected cells. Proc Natl Acad Sci USA 82:8691, 1985

118. Prince HE, Kermani–Arab V, Fahey JL: Depressed interleukin 2 receptor expression in acquired immune deficiency and lymphadenopathy syndromes. J Immunol 133:1313, 1984

119. Cavaille–Coll M, Brisson E, Klatzmann D et al: Exogenous interleukin-2 and mitogen responses in AIDS patients. Lancet 1:1245, 1984

120. Tsang KY, Fudenberg HH, Galbraith GMP: In vitro augmentation of interleukin-2 production and lymphocytes with the Tac antigen marker in patients with AIDS. N Engl J Med 310:987, 1984

121. Murray JL, Hersh EM, Reuben JM et al: Abnormal lymphocyte response to exogenous interleukin-2 in homosexuals with acquired immune deficiency syndrome (AIDS) and AIDS related complex (ARC). Clin Exp Immunol 60:25, 1985

122. Fauci AS, Rosenberg SA, Sherwin SA et al: Immunomodulators in clinical medicine. Ann Intern Med 106:421, 1987

123. Cunningham–Rundles S, Michelis MA, Masur H: Serum suppression of lymphocyte activation in vitro in acquired immunodeficiency disease. J Clin Immunol 3:156, 1983

124. Farmer JL, Gottlieb AA, Nishihara T: Inhibition of inter-

leukin 2 production and expression of the interleukin 2 receptor by plasma from acquired immune deficiency syndrome patients. Clin Immunol Immunopathol 38:235, 1986

125. Siegel JP, Djeu JY, Stocks NI et al: Sera from patients with the acquired immunodeficiency syndrome inhibit production of interleukin-2 by normal lymphocytes. J Clin Invest 75:1957, 1985

126. Laurence J, Gottlieb AB, Kunkel HG: Soluble suppressor factors in patients with acquired immune deficiency syndrome and its prodrome. J Clin Invest 72:2072, 1983

127. Laurence J, Mayer L: Immunoregulatory lymphokines of T hybridomas from AIDS patients: Constitutive and inducible suppressor factors. Science 225:66, 1984

128. Hersh EM, Mansell PWA, Reuben JM et al: Leukocyte subset analysis and related immunological findings in acquired immunodeficiency syndrome (AIDS) and malignancies. Diag Immunol 1:168, 1983

129. Benveniste E, Schroff R, Stevens RH et al: Immunoregulatory T cells in men with a new acquired immunodeficiency syndrome. J Clin Immunol 3:359, 1983

130. Lane HC, Masur H, Edgar LC et al: Abnormalities of B-cell activation and immunoregulation in patients with the acquired immunodeficiency syndrome. N Engl J Med 309:453, 1983

131. Smith PD, Ohura K, Masur H et al: Monocyte function in the acquired immune deficiency syndrome. J Clin Invest 74:2121, 1984

132. Poli G, Bottazzi B, Acero R et al: Monocyte function in intravenous drug abusers with lymphadenopathy syndrome and in patients with acquired immunodeficiency syndrome: Selective impairment with acquired immunodeficiency syndrome: Selective impairment of chemotaxis. Clin Exp Immunol 62:136, 1985

133. Washburn RG, Tuazon CU, Bennett JE: Phagocytic and fungicidal activity of monocytes from patients with acquired immunodeficiency syndrome. J Infect Dis 151:565, 1985

134. Murray HW, Gellene RA, Libby DM et al: Activation of tissue macrophages from AIDS patients: In vitro response of AIDS alveolar macrophages to lymphokines and interferon-γ. J Immunol 135:1501, 1985

135. Braun DP, Harris JE: Abnormal monocyte function in patients with Kaposi's sarcoma. Cancer 57:1501, 1986

136. Hofmann B, Odum N, Jakobsen BK: Immunological studies in the acquired immunodeficiency syndrome. Scand J Immunol 23:669, 1986

137. Estevez ME, Ballart IJ, Diez RA et al: Early defect of phagocytic cell function in subjects at risk for acquired immunodeficiency syndrome. Scand J Immunol 24:215, 1986

138. Kleinerman ES, Ceccorulli LM, Zwelling LA et al: Activation of monocyte-mediated tumoricidal activity in patients with acquired immunodeficiency syndrome. J Clin Oncol 3:1005, 1985

139. Enk C, Gerstoft J, Moller S et al: Interleukin 1 activity in the acquired immunodeficiency syndrome. Scand J Immunol 23:491, 1986

140. Pennington JE, Groopman JE, Small GJ et al: J Infect Dis 153:609, 1986

141. Heagy W, Kelley VE, Strom TB et al: Decreased expression of human class II antigens on monocytes from patients with acquired immune deficiency syndrome. J Clin Invest 74:2089, 1984

142. Prince HE, Moody DJ, Shubin BJ et al: Defective mono-

cyte function in acquired immune deficiency syndrome (AIDS): Evidence from a monocyte-dependent T-cell proliferative system. J Clin Immunol 5:21, 1985

143. Chess Q, Daniels J, North E et al: Serum immunoglobulin elevations in the acquired immunodeficiency syndrome (AIDS): IgG, IgA, IgM, and IgD. Diag Immunol 2:148, 1984

144. Papadopoulos NM, Frieri M: The presence of immunoglobulin D in endocrine disorders and diseases of immunoregulation, including the acquired immunodeficiency syndrome. Clin Immunol Immunopathol 32:248, 1984

145. Anderson KC, Boyd AW, Fisher DC et al: Isolation and functional analysis of human B cell populations. J Immunol 134:820, 1985

146. Pahwa SG, Quilop MTJ, Lange M et al: Defective B-lymphocyte function in homosexual men in relation to the acquired immunodeficiency syndrome. Ann Intern Med 101:757, 1984

147. Ammann AJ, Schiffman G, Abrams D et al: B-cell immunodeficiency in acquired immune deficiency syndrome. JAMA 251:1447, 1984

148. Birx DL, Redfield RR, Tosato G: Defective regulation of Epstein–Barr virus infection in patients with acquired immunodeficiency syndrome (AIDS) or AIDS-related disorders. N Engl J Med 314:874, 1986

149. Pahwa S, Pahwa R, Saxinger C et al: Influence of the human T-lymphotropic virus/lymphadenopathy-associated virus on functions of human lymphocytes: Evidence for immunosuppressive effects and polyclonal B-cell activation by banded viral preparations. Proc Natl Acad Sci USA 82:8198, 1985

150. Yarchoan R, Redfield RR, Broder S: Mechanisms of JB cell activation in patients with acquired immunodeficiency syndrome and related disorders. J Clin Invest 78:439, 1985

151. Schnittman SM, Lane HC, Higgins SE et al: Direct polyclonal activation of human B lymphocytes by the acquired immune deficiency syndrome virus. Science 233:1084, 1986

152. Pahwa S, Pahwa R, Good RA et al: Stimulatory and inhibitory influences of human immunodeficiency virus on normal B lymphocytes. Proc Natl Acad Sci USA 83:9124, 1986

153. Borst J, van de Griend RJ, van Oostveen JW et al: A T-cell receptor γ/CD3 complex found on cloned functional lymphocytes. Nature 325:683, 1987

154. Rook AH, Hooks JJ, Quinnan GV et al: Interleukin 2 enhances the natural killer cell activity of acquired immunodeficiency syndrome patients through a γ-interferon–independent mechanism. J Immunol 134:1503, 1985

155. Reddy MM, Chinoy P, Grieco MH: Differential effects of interferon-α_2a and interleukin-2 on natural killer cell activity in patients with acquired immune deficiency syndrome. J Biol Res Mod 3:379, 1984

156. Lew F, Tsang P, Solomon S et al: Natural killer cell function and modulation of α-IFN and IL-2 in AIDS patients and prodromal subjects. Clin Lab Immunol 14:115, 1984

157. Creemers PC, Stark DF, Boyko WJ: Evaluation of natural killer cell activity in patients with persistent generalized lymphadenopathy and acquired immunodeficiency syndrome. Clin Immunol Immunopathol 36:141, 1985

158. Hersh EM, Gutterman JU, Spector S et al: Impaired in vitro interferon, blastogenic, and natural killer cell re-

sponses to viral stimulation in acquired immune deficiency syndrome. Cancer Res 45:406, 1985

159. Katzman M, Lederman MM: Defective postbinding lysis underlies the impaired natural killer activity in factor VIII-treated, human T lymphotropic virus type III seropositive hemophiliacs. J Clin Invest 77:1057, 1986

160. Bonavida B, Katz J, Gottlieb M: Mechanism of defective NK cell activity in patients with acquired immunodeficiency syndrome (AIDS) and AIDS-related complex. J Immunol 137:1157, 1986

161. DeStefano E, Friedman RM, Friedman–Kien AE et al: Acid-labile human leukocyte interferon in homosexual men with Kaposi's sarcoma and lymphadenopathy. J Infect Dis 146:451, 1982

162. Buimovici–Klein E, Lange M, Klein RJ et al: Long-term follow-up of serum-interferon and its acid-stability in a group of homosexual men. AIDS Research 2:99, 1985

163. Hersh EM, Reuben JM, Rios A et al: Elevated serum thymosin alpha$_1$ levels associated with evidence of immune dysregulation in male homosexuals with a history of infectious diseases or Kaposi's sarcoma. N Engl J Med 308:45, 1983

164. Bhalla RB: Abnormally high concentrations of beta 2 microglobulin in acquired immunodeficiency syndrome (AIDS) patients. Clin Chem 29:1560, 1983

165. Sarin PS, Sun DK, Thornton AH et al: Neutralization of HTLV-III/LAV replication by anti-serum to thymosin α_1. Science 232:1135, 1986

166. McDougal JS, Hubbard M, Nicholson JKA: Immune complexes in the acquired immunodeficiency syndrome (AIDS). J Clin Immunol 5:130, 1985

167. Gupta S, Licorish K: Circulating immune complexes in AIDS. N Engl J Med 310:1530, 1984

168. Eales LJ, Ke N, Parkin JM et al: Genetic factors in susceptibility to HIV infection and to HIV related diseases: Variation in Gc subtypes. Lancet 1:999, 1987

169. Gilles K, Louie L, Newman B et al: Genetic susceptibility to AIDS: Absence of an association with group-specific component. N Engl J Med 317:630, 1987

170. Daiger SP, Brewton GW, Rios AA et al: Letter. N Engl J Med 317:631, 1987

171. Coolfont report: A PHS plan for prevention and control of AIDS and the AIDS virus. Public Health Rep 101:341, 1986

172. Robert–Guroff M, Brown M, Gallo RC: HTLV-III-neutralizing antibodies in patients with AIDS and AIDS-related complex. Nature 316:72, 1985

173. Weiss RA, Clapham PR, Cheingsong–Popov R et al: Neutralization of human T-lymphotropic virus type III by sera of AIDS and AIDS-risk patients. Nature 316:69, 1985

174. Weiss RA, Clapham PR, Weber JN et al: Variable and conerved neutralization antigens of human immunodeficiency virus. Nature 324:572, 1986

175. Matthews TJ, Langlois AJ, Robey WG et al: Restricted neutralization of divergent human T-lymphotropic virus type III isolates by antibodies to the major envelope glycoprotein. Proc Natl Acad Sci USA 83:9709, 1986

176. Ranki A, Antonen J, Valle S et al: Characterization of the latent period and the development of neutralizing antibodies in early sexually transmitted HIV infection [Abstr]. In *III International Conference on Acquired Immunodeficiency Syndrome (AIDS)*. Washington, DC, U.S. Department of Health and Human Services, 1987

177. Lasky LA, Groopman JE, Fennie CW et al: Neutralization of the AIDS retrovirus by antibodies to a recombinant envelope glycoprotein. Science 233:209, 1986

178. Putney SD, Matthews TJ, Robey WG et al: HTLV-III/LAV-neutralizing antibodies to an *E. coli*-produced fragment of the virus envelope. Science 234:1392, 1986

179. Krohn K, Robey WG, Putney S et al: Specific cellular immune response and neutralizing antibodies in goats immunized with native or recombinant envelope proteins derived from human T-lymphotropic virus type III$_B$ and in human immunodeficiency virus-infected men. Proc Natl Acad Sci USA 84:4994, 1987

180. Smith G, Cochran GL, Ericson BL et al: Full-length and truncated HIV envelope polypeptides produced in an insect cell expression system elicit high titer neutralizing antibodies in animals [Abstr]. In *III International Conference on Acquired Immunodeficiency Syndrome (AIDS)*, p. 107. Washington, DC, U.S. Department of Health and Human Services, 1987

181. Matsushita S, Koito A, Sutoh H et al: A neutralizing monoclonal antibody reactive against an external envelope glycoprotein of HTLV-III/LAV (human immunodeficiency virus) [Abstr]. In *III International Conference on Acquired Immunodeficiency Syndrome (AIDS)*, p. 106. Washington, DC, U.S. Department of Health and Human Services, 1987

182. Zagury D, Lurhuma Z, Mbayo K et al: Experimental immune activation against AIDS virus in human [Abstr]. In *III International Conference on Acquired Immunodeficiency Syndrome (AIDS)*, p 62. Washington, DC, U.S. Department of Health and Human Services, 1987

183. Ahearne PM, Weinhold KJ, Matthews TJ et al: Cellular immune response to viral peptides in patients exposed to HIV [Abstr]. In *III International Conference on Acquired Immunodeficiency Syndrome (AIDS)*, p 8. Washington, DC, U.S. Department of Health and Human Services, 1987

184. Cease KB, Margalit H, Cornette JL et al: Helper T-cell antigenic site identification in the acquired immunodeficiency syndrome virus gp120 envelope protein and induction of immunity in mice to the native protein using a 16-residue synthetic peptide. Proc Natl Acad Sci USA. 84:249, 1987

185. Robert–Guroff M, Reitz MS, Robey WG et al: In vitro generation of an HTLV-III variant by neutralizing antibody. J Immunol 137:3306, 1986

186. Montelaro RC, Parakh B, Orrego A et al: Antigenic variation during persistent infection by equine infectious anemia virus, a retrovirus. J Bio Chem 259:10539, 1984

187. Earl P, Moss B, Morrison RP et al: T-lymphocyte primary and protection against Friend leukemia by vaccinia-retrovirus env gene recombinant. Science 234:728, 1986

188. Rook AH, Lane HC, Folks T et al: Sera from HTLV-III/LAV antibody-positive individuals mediate antibody-dependent cellular cytotoxicity against HTLV-III/LAV-infected T cells. J Immunol 138:1064, 1987

189. Ojo-Amaize EA, Nishanian P, Keith DE et al: Antibodies to human immunodeficiency virus in human sera induce cell-mediated lysis of human immunodeficiency virus-infected cells. J Immunol 139:2458, 1987

190. Ljunggren K, Bittiger B, Biberfeld G et al: Antibody-dependent cellular cytotoxicity-inducing antibodies against human immunodeficiency virus. J Immunol 139:2263, 1987

191. Weber JN, Clapham, Weiss RA et al: Human immunodeficiency virus infection in two cohorts of homosexual men: Neutralizing sera and association of anti-gag antibody with prognosis. Lancet 1:119, 1987

192. Ruscetti FW, Mikovits JA, Kalyanaraman VS et al: Analysis of effector mechanism against HTLV-1 and HTLV-III/LAV infected lymphoid cells. J Immunol 136:3619, 1986

193. Weinhold KJ, Lyerly HK, Matthews TJ et al: Gp120-specific cell-mediated cytotoxicity in patients exposed to HIV. In *III International Conference on Acquired Immunodeficiency Syndrome (AIDS),* p 59. Washington, DC, U.S. Department of Health and Human Services, 1987

194. Walker BD, Chakrabarti S, Moss B et al: HIV-specific cytotoxic T lymphocytes in seropositive individuals. Nature 328:345, 1987

195. Koenig S, Earl P, Powell D et al: Cytotoxic T cells directed against target cells expressing HIV-1 proteins [Abstr]. In *III International Conference on Acquired Immunodeficiency Syndrome (AIDS),* p 59. Washington, DC, U.S. Department of Health and Human Services, 1987

196. Quinnan GV: Detection of HLA restricted human immunodeficiency virus (HIV) envelope antigen-specific cytotoxic lymphocytes (CTL) [Abstr]. In *III International Conference on Acquired Immunodeficiency Syndrome (AIDS),* p 59. Washington, DC, U.S. Department of Health and Human Services, 1987

197. Plata F, Autran B, Pedroza Martins L et al: AIDS virus-specific cytotoxic T lymphocytes in lung disorders. Nature 328:348, 1987

198. Zarling JM, Eichberg JW, Moran PA et al: Proliferative and cytotoxic T cells to AIDS virus glycoproteins in chimpanzees immunized with a recombinant vaccinia virus expressing AIDS virus envelope glycoproteins. J Immunol 139:988, 1987

The Life-Cycle of Human Immunodeficiency Virus as a Guide to the Design of New Therapies for AIDS

Samuel Broder

5

The purpose of this chapter is to summarize possible therapeutic interventions that are based on the emerging knowledge of the life-cycle of the retrovirus that causes AIDS and its related disorders. A great deal of our knowledge regarding pathogenic human retroviruses in general and therapeutic strategies for attacking such agents in particular is dependent on the long-standing commitment of the National Cancer Institute to the problem of oncogenic viruses, including retroviruses. The viral cancer and developmental therapeutic programs of the Institute laid the foundation for much of our current understanding of AIDS and its therapy.

Acquired immunodeficiency syndrome (AIDS) was initially defined as the development of either an opportunistic infection or Kaposi's sarcoma (an unusual neoplasm that had previously been associated with certain immunosuppressed states) in a person without a known cause for immunodeficiency.[1,2] Shortly thereafter it became apparent that these patients had a cellular immunodeficiency characterized by an inexorable depletion of helper/inducer (T4[+] or CD-4[+]) T cells, and within 3 years it had been proven that a retrovirus that has the capacity to replicate within cells of the immune system (and in turn cause the destruction of CD-4[+] T cells) is the cause of AIDS.[3,4] The retrovirus is the third known human T-lymphotropic virus (HTLV-III), and a great deal is now known about this new pathogen.[4–12] The virus has also been called lymphadenopathy virus; however, the most generally accepted name at this time is human immunodeficiency virus (HIV). While this virus is T-cell tropic, it is important to note that it can infect other cell types, especially macrophages. Moreover, the virus has the capacity to enter the brain and bring about significant neurologic damage in certain patients. The neurologic sequelae of HIV infection may be particularly prominent in children with AIDS, and sometimes dementia can dominate the clinical picture. While it is still not known for sure how the virus enters the brain and how it brings about neurologic damage, it is a virtual certainty that successful therapeutic strategies must address the consequences of and probably prevent, viral replication within the central nervous system. Fortunately, the prevailing assumption that AIDS-virus dementias were uniformly irreversible is clearly not valid with the advent of antiretroviral chemotherapy.

As with any virus, the different stages in the life cycle of HIV present a variety of distinct potential targets for antiviral agents (Table 5-1). Reverse transcriptase is one of the most attractive targets and there have been successes at a clinical level using this as a target for new therapies, notably with 3'-azido-2',3'-dideoxythymidine (AZT).[13,14] The testing of new antiretroviral agents has been facilitated by the availability of rapid and sensitive *in vitro* screening systems that determine whether a putative drug can inhibit the replication and T-cell killing activity of HIV.[15] At the outset, it is worth stressing that effective therapy of HIV infections may well depend on a combination of strategies that attack multiple steps in viral replication and cytopathogenicity, in part because the emergence of drug-resistant strains might be less likely.

HIV AS A RETROVIRUS

In the era before the etiology of AIDS was recognized, one of the most notable features of retroviruses was the capacity to induce neoplastic transformation in infected target cells; hence the expression *RNA tumor virus* or *leukemia virus* appeared in the literature to denote this category of virus.[16] But the virus that causes AIDS has not been shown to have a transforming capacity. By definition, retroviruses replicate through a DNA intermediate (i.e., at one step of their cycle of replication, genetic information flows from RNA to DNA, a reverse or "retro" direction).[17,18] Before the recognition of human

79

Table 5-1
Stages of HIV Replication That May Be Targets for Therapeutic Intervention

Stage	Possible Intervention
Binding to target cell	Antibodies to virus or cellular receptor; genetically engineered, soluble CD-4 receptors; dextran-sulfate?
Entry into target cell and uncoating of RNA	Drugs (by analogy with calmodulin antagonists for Epstein–Barr infection or amantadine for type A influenza virus infection)
Transcription of RNA to DNA by reverse transcriptase	Reverse transcriptase inhibitors (AZT and other dideoxy or didehydronucleoside congeners)
Degradation of RNA by RNase activity (encoded by viral pol gene)	RNase H inhibitors
Integration of DNA into host genome	Agents that inhibit pol-encoded integrase function may be found
Transcriptional efficiency/ translation of viral RNA	Inhibitors of tat-III or art-trs; "anti-sense" constructs
Ribosomal frameshifting	Possibly specific "frameshift inhibitors" can be found
Viral component production	Myristylation, glycosylation, or protease inhibitors (e.g., aspartyl proteinase-specific inhibitors)
Viral budding	Interferons; antibodies to a viral antigen

retroviruses, all retroviruses were known to contain *gag, pol,* and *env* genes as basic components of a replicating genome. Reverse transcriptase (the viral DNA polymerase) that catalyzes this step is encoded by the *pol* gene of the virus, a gene that is conserved to a considerable extent in its amino acid and nucleotide sequences among retroviruses.[19] The reverse transcriptase gene is one component of the *pol* region, and in general this region is expressed as a polyprotein that includes a protease, reverse transcriptase and an endonuclease (integrase). Post-translational cleavage is thought to yield the protease, reverse transcriptase, and so on as functioning molecules.

HIV, in common with previously known animal retroviruses, has as its major structural components a core of genomic RNA; group-specific antigen (*gag*) proteins, which play a role both in the structure of the core and assembly of the virion; a lipid bilayer; and an outside envelope glycoprotein. A retroviral fusion protein (*gag-pol*) can undergo post-translational cleavage events from active *gag* and *pol* products; retroviruses (including HIV) use a ribosomal frame shift phenomenon to produce *gag* and *pol* proteins, and we will return to this point later.

HIV is the most complex retrovirus yet characterized[20] in that it contains at least eight genes, with several never previously known to exist in retroviruses. The functions of several of these novel genes are still not known or are poorly understood. One such gene (designated *sor*) has very recently been linked to the ability to replicate by a pathway of cell-free virion infection.[21,22] The *sor* gene encodes a 23-kilodalton protein that plays a crucial role in the efficient generation of infectious virus. HIV with proviral genomes that contain mutant *sor* genes were quite limited in their capacity to establish stable infection *in vitro.* Therefore, in the future, it is conceivable that drugs or biologics could be developed to interfere with *sor* and thereby attenuate the pathogenicity of HIV infection either in individuals who are already infected or as part of an adjunct to an immunization program for individuals who are at risk of acquiring HIV infection. The functions of two other genes, *tat-III*[23] and *art*[24] or *trs,*[25] will be discussed later.

Cell Binding and Entry

The first step in the infection of a cell by HIV is its binding to the target cell receptor. In the case of helper/inducer T cells, this receptor seems to be linked to the cell-surface protein that is recognized by T4 or CD-4 antibodies.[26,27] The process of specific binding between the T4 antigen and parts of the viral envelope glycoprotein may be vulnerable to attack by antibodies either to the virus or to the receptor, and theoretically certain chemicals or small peptides[28] could be designed to occupy the receptor and serve the same purpose.

It might be worthwhile deviating from the chronology of the retroviral life cycle briefly to address the cytopathogenicity of the virus that causes AIDS. There is as yet no consensus on how the virus kills T cells. From one perspective, the T4 molecule and the envelope glycoprotein of the virus determine events both at the beginning and end of the life cycle of HIV within susceptible T cells. In addition to a role in the receptor-mediated entry of the virus into target T cells, the T4 receptor plays a part in the susceptibility of a target T cell, once it begins to produce virus, to be killed by that virus. Precisely how HIV destroys T cells *in vivo* is not known. The cytopathic effect is thought to be mediated in part by an interaction between the T4 molecule and the HIV envelope protein that brings about lethal cell-to-cell fusions (syncytia) or a surface autofusion phenomenon that destroys the integrity of the cell membrane.[29,30] But other factors are also thought to play a role in the cytopathic effects of the virus. Recent results raise the possibility that the carboxyl terminus of the envelope protein, a region different from the portion that directly binds to the T4 molecule, is important in the destruction of T cells by the virus.[31]

Conceivably, therapeutic agents could be designed to alter the certain properties (for example, the lipid composition) of the viral surface or target cell surface to reduce viral infectivity or cytopathic effects. An alternative target is the envelope protein itself. Although there can be considerable variation in the protein from one viral isolate to another, the range of alterations in the binding site is most likely constrained by the need to bind to T4, which is relatively constant in structure. An antibody directed against this site might bind to (and neutralize) most strains of HIV and perhaps kill infected cells as they begin to express envelope antigens so that spread of virus to uninfected cells can be reduced.

Thus, monoclonal antibodies to the envelope protein could have a therapeutic role in patients with AIDS or related diseases. We have recently been able to produce a complement-fixing human IgG$_k$ monoclonal antibody against the major envelope glycoprotein of the first known pathogenic human T-lymphotropic retrovirus (HTLV-I),[32] and similar approaches could be used to develop human monoclonal antibodies against HIV. A potential difficulty of this approach, however, is that virally infected cells could make infectious cell-to-cell contacts. (It is interesting to note that even viral mutants which are defective in *sor*, and are thereby poorly transmitted by cell-free virion infection, may still be transmitted by a process of cell-to-cell spread *in vitro*.) Antibodies might not gain access to relevant epitopes and the envelope protein under certain circumstances. Also, it has been shown that AIDS can occur in the face of what *in vitro* appear to be neutralizing antibodies to HIV. Whether this occurs because the titers of such antibodies are low or because such antibodies do not block epitopes that mediate *in vivo* cytopathogenicity is under investigation. One must at least consider that humoral immunity *per se* does not protect the host, and what protection is possible is mediated by cellular immunity.

After binding to a cell, HIV enters the target cell by an incompletely defined mechanism, most likely by a fusion process. It is conceivable that drugs could be developed to block this step just as calmodulin antagonists block the entry of Epstein–Barr virus into B cells. Another theoretical target is the stage of "uncoating" of the virus after it enters a target cell. In this stage, the virus loses its envelope-coat and RNA is released into the cytoplasm (each virion is thought to convey a dimer of two identical genomic RNA subunits into the cell). Pharmacologic agents that block viral uncoating might eventually be developed in the treatment of AIDS.

Uncoated viral RNA is used as a template for the production of DNA by reverse transcriptase. As already mentioned, this enzyme has become a prime target for antiretroviral agents both because it should be possible to find inhibitors that will discriminate between this en-

zyme and the DNA polymerases of the host cell, thus lessening side effects, and because a great deal is already known about *pol* and reverse transcriptase.[17,18,33,34] (It is likely that the reverse transcriptase gene will yield important information when studied by site-directed mutagenesis.) HIV reverse transcriptase uses a lysine transfer RNA primer to make a minus-strand DNA copy of the viral RNA as an RNA–DNA hybrid. Retroviral DNA polymerase (reverse transcriptase) possesses an inherent RNase H activity that specifically degrades the RNA of the RNA–DNA hybrid. The C-terminal region of the reverse transcription protein is a domain with RNase H activity. Theoretically, inhibition of this process would suppress viral replication. The reverse transcriptase then catalyzes the production of a positive-strand DNA, and eventually, a double-stranded viral DNA is formed. In some cells, the double-stranded viral DNA can migrate to the nucleus by an as yet poorly understood mechanism.

The reverse transcriptase of HIV has been purified and seems to exist as a p51 and a p66 molecule. Large quantities of the HIV reverse transcriptase should become readily available because the enzyme has been expressed in bacteria and yeast using recombinant DNA technology. This should aid the testing of potential reverse transcriptase inhibitors. The use of such agents in patients with AIDS is predicated on the assumption that there is continuing viral replication in the disease and that its inhibition will permit some regeneration, or at least prevent further deterioration, of the immune system. Two drugs (suramin and HPA-23), that were chosen early for clinical trials because they inhibit reverse transcriptase (and were already being given to humans for other purposes), have not appeared to confer clinical benefits to AIDS patients.[35-37]* Nevertheless, agents that inhibit reverse transcriptase have the greatest likelihood of achieving an immediate clinical impact on the virus. Several potent agents that inhibit this enzyme are either already available, having been developed for the therapy of conventional viral diseases (e.g., phosphonoformate[38]), or are being developed specifically for AIDS on the basis of *in vitro* screening systems for activity against HIV.[13,15] We will return to one class of such inhibitors, the dideoxynucleosides, later. One member of this class of nucleosides (AZT), has already been shown to prolong survival in patients with AIDS and to confer certain other clinical benefits as well.

Integration, Latency, and Reactivation

The DNA copy of HIV may be circularized during or soon after its formation, and apparently can either remain in an unintegrated form or can become integrated into the genome of the host cell. The capacity of ret-

---

* Suramin has the capacity to interfere with the binding of certain growth factors to tumor cell-membrane receptors, and the drug has antitumor effects in patients. These properties are being investigated by C. Stein, C. Myers, and others at the NCI

roviruses to integrate into the genome of host target cells was initially thought to render retroviral diseases inherently untreatable. In the future, it is possible that chemicals could be developed to interfere with the viral endonuclease or "integrase" (thought to be a function of one of the *pol* gene products) that mediates this integration step.

Later in the viral life cycle, perhaps after activation of the infected cell by a physiological signal such as antigen or a regulatory interleukin, the viral DNA is transcribed to mRNA and viral genomic RNA using host-cell RNA polymerases, and this RNA is then translated to form viral proteins, again using the biochemical apparatus of the host cell.

Retroviruses use a novel mechanism for the translation of certain genes. For example, they can synthesize a single *gag–pol* polyprotein from two separate reading frames on an RNA template. The coupling of these reading frames requires that the ribosome correctly shifts from one reading frame to another,[33,34] which mammalian cells are not thought to do as part of a physiologic genetic translation process. It is theoretically possible that specific chemicals or antibiotic-like agents could interrupt this process of ribosomal frame shifting, leading to impaired viral expression and thereby improved clinical status in infected patients.

It has recently been shown that HIV has a gene (*tat*-III) coding for a diffusible protein that markedly enhances the expression of other viral genes and viral replication. The *tat*-III gene, like the *tat* genes of the other two known human pathogenic retroviruses, is so called because it was originally thought to mediate a *trans*-activation of transcription, that is, it worked through a mechanism that affected the transcription of genes not in direct proximity to itself.[23,24] But ideas about the *tat*-III gene are still evolving.[39,40] The *tat*-III protein seems to cause an increase of viral products at a transcriptional level. However, the protein may also increase viral expression by acting beyond transcription of DNA to RNA by enhancing either mRNA stability or translational efficiency, or both. Whatever the mechanisms are, the *tat*-III protein is thought to provide the virus with a positive feedback loop by which a viral product can amplify the production of new virions. The protein is small (86 amino acids) with a cluster of positively charged amino acids, and is thought to affect the synthesis of other proteins by binding to critical regulatory sequences at the 5' end of viral mRNA. It may be possible to find drugs that inhibit the *tat*-III product itself, a crucial nucleic-acid binding site for this protein, or both. Employing the same mRNA that codes for *tat*-III, but using a different reading frame, the *art* or *trs* gene of HIV produces a different small (116-amino-acid) positively charged protein, which is thought to function as a second essential *trans*-acting factor in viral replication.[24,25] Again, drugs that bind or deactivate this protein would be expected to inhibit viral replication. In the absence of this second regulatory factor, *gag*- and *env*-encoded protein synthesis is severely diminished. Al-

though there is no doubt about the existence of this new regulatory gene, its mechanism of action is still a matter for study. The suggested mechanism of action of the gene was first described as an abrogation of negative regulatory effects on translation of viral mRNA-encoding HIV structural proteins (hence the name *art* for antirepression *trans*-activator).[24] It is possible that *tat*-III controls *art,* which in turn regulates the activity of *gag–pol* and *env.* A more recent report by Feinberg and colleagues suggests that the gene product balances the amount of spliced and unspliced viral RNA to permit the preservation of *gag–pol* and *env* mRNA (hence the alternative name, *trs* for *trans*-acting regulator of splicing).[25]

Thus, although the precise mechanisms are matters of future study, it is clear that this retrovirus has evolved an astonishingly complex system of genetic regulation. Perhaps this is because of the race between viral replication within a cell and the destruction of the cell that the virus has commandeered, leaving no tolerance for inefficiency or improper timing in the synthesis of viral components. We can expect that the very complexity of the virus will contribute to its defeat.

Protein Production and Assembly

It is conceivable that drugs that interfere with the structure and function of retroviral mRNA transcribed from integrated DNA in infected cells could be of therapeutic value in AIDS. One drug, ribavirin, is believed to act as a guanosine analog that interferes with the 5'-capping of viral mRNA in other viral systems, and perhaps could be useful in retrovirally induced disorders.[41] However, the clinical data to date have not yet demonstrated a clinical role for ribavirin in the therapy of HIV infections.

Another approach would be the use of "anti-sense" oligodeoxynucleotides, already tested *in vitro.*[42] Basically, this approach employs short sequences of DNA (sometimes chemically modified to enable better cell penetration and resistance to enzymatic degradation) whose base-pairs are complementary to a vital segment of the viral genome. In theory, such anti-sense oligodeoxynucleotides could block expression of the viral genome through a kind of hybridization arrest of translation or possibly interfere with the binding of a regulatory protein such as *tat*-III. Indeed, it is possible that one anti-sense oligodeoxynucleotide could interrupt two functions that are vital for HTLV-III replication. Matsakura and others discuss the *in vitro* use of phosphorothioate analogs of various oligodeoxynucleotides; some of these analogs are exceedingly potent inhibitors of the AIDS virus (and other lentiviruses) *in vitro.*[43] However, there may be an unexpected level of nonspecificity in terms of the oligonucleotide sequence, and the precise anti-viral mechanism is not known. Whether these phosphorothioate analogs work through a process of hybridization arrest or affect earlier stages of viral replication such as template/primer binding to reverse transcriptase is now under study.

The final stages in the replicative cycle of HIV involve crucial secondary processing of certain viral proteins by a protease (a function of one of the *pol* gene products) and myristylating and glycosylating enzymes (provided by the host) as a prelude to assembly of infectious virions. Therefore, additional strategies for the treatment of AIDS might conceivably involve certain kinds of protease inhibitors or drugs that dampen or alter myristylation and glycosylation steps in the synthesis of viral components.[44] Finally, retroviruses are released by a process of viral budding, which may be inhibited by interferons.[45]

Although the discussion has focused on how to suppress HIV replication *per se,* it might be worth noting that the virus could set off a chain of secondary events *in vivo* (autoimmune reaction, toxic lymphokine production, etc.) necessary for the expression of clinical disease. It is also intriguing to speculate that a combination of antiretroviral therapy coupled with bone marrow transplantation, lymphocyte replacement, or stimulation of bone marrow precursor cells by colony-stimulating factors might be successful in certain subsets of patients with HIV infections.

DIDEOXYNUCLEOSIDES

We will now turn to a discussion of a broad family of 2′,3′-dideoxynucleoside analogs (including certain didehydro congeners) that can be metabolized to become potent chain-terminating inhibitors of HIV reverse transcriptase. Even at large viral doses, these analogs can completely inhibit *in vitro* HIV replication and its capacity to destroy T-cell cultures at concentrations that are 10 to 20 times lower than those that impair the proliferation and survival of target cells.[46] In several cases studies of these compounds have been done over the past 20 years or so,[47–53] and in triphosphate form they are familiar to every molecular biologist as reagents for the Sanger DNA-sequencing procedure.[53] But their application to human antiretroviral therapy demands a new perspective. The dideoxynucleoside analogs are of special interest because they prove that a simple chemical modification of the sugar moiety can predictably convert a normal substrate for nucleic acid synthesis into a compound with a potent capacity to inhibit the replication and cytopathic effect of HIV, at least *in vitro.*[46]

We are currently developing 2′,3′-dideoxycytidine and dideoxyadenosine as possible agents for treating patients infected with HIV. On a molar basis, dideoxycytidine is the most potent antiviral nucleoside we have tested, but, of course, *in vitro* potency need not necessarily be linked to a therapeutic effect. Under certain conditions *in vitro,* the drug can suppress HIV at concentrations ≤ 10 nanomolar. This dideoxynucleoside analog was selected for clinical development because of its *in vitro* potency against HIV,[46] relative resistance to cytidine deaminase (a major catabolic enzyme for cytidine analogues),[54] good oral bioavailability,

straightforward pharmacokinetic clearance by the kidney, failure to reduce normal intracellular pyrimidine pools, and comparative lack of toxicity when administered to animals. We have recently begun to administer this drug to patients. The preliminary results will be addressed in Chapter 16. In brief, this drug has the capacity to suppress HIV replication *in vivo* as measured by p24 antigenemia. The dose-limiting toxicity is a painful peripheral neuropathy. At present, it is not possible to conclude whether the peripheral neuropathy can be circumvented; however, several regimens for avoiding this toxicity are being explored and look promising. In the near future, it is expected that dideoxyadenosine will be administered in large-scale tests. The adenosine analog is interesting in terms of its low relative toxicity for human bone marrow cells *in vitro.*

Although many issues related to the antiretroviral effects of 2′,3′-dideoxynucleosides are not yet resolved, as they are successively phosphorylated in the cytoplasm of a target cell to yield 2′,3′-dideoxynucleoside-5′-triphosphates, they become analogs of the 2′-deoxynucleoside-5′-triphosphates that are the natural substrates for cellular DNA polymerases and reverse transcriptase. (It is generally thought that nucleoside-5′-triphosphates do not cross cell membranes and are not active as drugs because of their ionic character and comparatively low lipophilicity.) Such analogs could compete with the binding of normal nucleotides to DNA polymerases (with high relative affinity for reverse transcriptase), or could be incorporated into DNA and bring about DNA chain termination because normal 5′–>3 phosphodiester linkages cannot be completed. We know that, at concentrations achievable in human cells, dideoxynucleotide analogs can serve as substrates for the HIV reverse transcriptase to elongate a DNA chain by one residue, after which the chain is terminated.[55]

Pyrimidine and purine dideoxynucleoside analogs can inhibit the *in vitro* replication and pathogenic effects of a range of animal and human retroviruses, even when the pathogenic effect being monitored (transformation) requires only a single round of replication; moreover, with certain lentiviruses (a family of animal retroviruses related to HIV[56]), these drugs can reduce the *in vitro* viral infectivity by more than five orders of magnitude.[57] We have found that two dideoxynucleosides, 2′,3′-dideoxycytidine and 3′-azido-2′,3′-dideoxythymidine (see below) can block the infectivity of another human retrovirus, HTLV-I, against helper/inducer T-cells *in vitro.* Indeed, we have not yet observed any type or strain of retrovirus that is resistant to 2′,3′-dideoxynucleoside analogs in appropriate target cells; however, the emergence of drug-resistant mutants must always be considered possible. One might speculate by analogy to herpes simplex that *pol* mutations might lead to attenuation in pathogenicity of the mutant virus. It is important to stress that the phosphorylation reactions crucial to the activation of the nucleoside analogs are catalyzed by host-cell kinases, and therefore, extreme caution must be used in extrapolating from cells of one type (or species) to another.

Cell lines derived from different species show striking differences in their sensitivity to the cytostatic and antiretroviral activity, as well as the intracellular metabolism, of AZT and dideoxycytidine (ddC)*. AZT and ddC are considerably more cytostatic to human cells than murine cells. In human lymphoid cells (ATH8, Molt/4F) and caprine ovary (Tahr) cells, AZT accumulates as its 5′-monophosphate (AZT-MP), whereas in murine leukemia (L1210) cells it is readily metabolized to the 5′-triphosphate (AZT-TP). The rapid conversion of AZT to AZT-TP in murine cells may explain why AZT has a pronounced activity against Moloney murine sarcoma virus (MSV)-induced transformation of murine C3H cells *in vitro* and MSV-induced tumor development in certain newborn mice *in vivo*. By contrast, ddC has comparatively little activity in these murine assay systems, and this may seem related to the poor conversion of ddC to its 5′-triphosphate in murine cells. In human cells, however, ddC is more extensively phosphorylated to its 5′-triphosphate than in murine cells. When radiolabeled AZT and ddC were compared for their metabolism in human ATH8 and Molt/4F cells, under the same conditions substantial levels of ddCTP built up gradually. Thus, levels of ddCTP much higher than those of AZT-TP were achieved in human lymphoid cells, an observation that may be particularly relevant from a therapeutic point of view.

If the relevant kinases are lacking in the host cell, the retrovirus will appear resistant to the nucleoside analogs, but if the retrovirus is permitted to replicate in a different target cell that has the appropriate enzymes for anabolic phosphorylation, it will appear sensitive again. Similarly, we have observed that one dideoxynucleoside (2′,3′-dideoxythymidine) behaves as a relatively poor substrate inhibitor for human thymidine kinase. The substitution of an azido group at the 3′-carbon of this analog, yielding 3′-azido-2′,3′-dideoxythymidine (AZT), produces a compound that is an excellent substrate for thymidine kinase (Km = 3 μM) and is a very potent inhibitor of HIV replication. On the other hand, the substitution of a cyano moiety at the 3′-carbon does not yield a good antiretroviral agent. (Some methods of synthesizing this compound yielded significant quantities of the didehydro analog of thymidine, leading to an initial error of interpreting and assigning antiretroviral effects.)

There are data to suggest that the HIV reverse transcriptase is much more susceptible to the inhibitory effects of these drugs as triphosphates than is mammalian DNA polymerase alpha, an enzyme that has key DNA synthetic and repair functions in the life of a cell. Indeed, the reverse transcriptase has a higher affinity for dideoxynucleotides than normal substrates. This parallels what had been learned in animal retroviral systems.[46,58] Although most 2′,3′-dideoxynucleoside-5′-tri-

phosphates can inhibit mammalian DNA polymerase beta (a repair enzyme) and DNA polymerase gamma (a mitochondrial enzyme),[58] we have observed that dideoxynucleosides can suppress HIV replication and protect sensitive helper/inducer T-cell target cells *in vitro* for long periods without interfering with the function and survival of target T cells.[55] It is interesting to note that AZT as a triphosphate is a comparatively poor inhibitor of DNA polymerase alpha *and* beta, compared to its inhibitory capacity for reverse transcriptase. As discussed above, our working explanation for the activity of these drugs against pathogenic retroviruses is that, following anabolism to nucleoside-5′-triphosphates, they bind to the viral DNA polymerase and/or bring about a selective chain termination as the RNA form of the virus attempts to make DNA copies of itself.

AZT (RETROVIR)

Several clinical features of AZT will be discussed in Chapter 16. Synthesized over 20 years ago by Horwitz and co-workers under a grant from the National Cancer Institute[48] and shown to inhibit C-type murine retrovirus replication *in vitro* by Ostertag and colleagues more than 12 years ago,[59] no medical application of 3′-azido-2′,3′-deoxythymidine (AZT) had emerged prior to our studies. We found that AZT is a very potent inhibitor *in vitro* of HIV replication and its cytopathic effect in susceptible target T cells, and that it has an antiretroviral effect against widely divergent strains of HIV.[13] As discussed above, the drug undergoes anabolic phosphorylation in human T cells to a nucleoside-5′-triphosphate,[60] which can compete with thymidine-5′-triphosphate (TTP) and serve as a chain-terminating inhibitor of HIV reverse transcriptase. In that sense, AZT parallels the other dideoxynucleosides. But it can also bring about severe alterations of nucleoside metabolism within some host cells, which may be of clinical significance. For example, thymidine kinase catalyzes the formation of a monophosphate derivative of AZT, which then serves as a competitive inhibitor, with very low V_{max}, of thymidylate kinase (an enzyme that catalyzes the second phosphorylation step to thymidine diphosphate), leading to the reduced formation of the third phosphorylation product, TTP.[60] How this reduction of normal pyrimidine pools might affect the balance between antiretroviral activity and drug-induced cytotoxicity remains unknown. Nevertheless, a form of partial pyrimidine depletion is likely to contribute to bone marrow suppression, one of the key side effects of AZT. This feature of the drug might lend itself to regimens that combine AZT with an agent that does not appear to deplete normal intracellular pyrimidine pools, such as ddC. Within the intramural program, a pilot protocol involving a weekly regimen of AZT alternating with ddC has been initiated to see if the non-overlapping toxicities of these drugs could be put to clinical advantage. In the case of AZT, the key toxicity one would seek to obviate

---

* Balzarini J, Broder S, unpublished

would be bone marrow suppression; in the case of ddC, it would be peripheral neuropathy.

What can be said is that AZT, a drug chosen on the basis of its selective *in vitro* antiviral effect against HIV, has been shown as a single agent to confer a clinical benefit in patients with advanced disease.[14,61] Although the drug does have prominent side effects in some patients, it has a noteworthy lack of cardiac, renal, and hepatic toxicity. AZT represents a first step in developing practical chemotherapy against pathogenic human retroviruses. Moreover, the development of AZT is a validation of the key assumptions underlying antiviral strategies for intervening against established AIDS: HIV replication can be suppressed *in vivo* and such suppression can lead to prolonged survival and improved quality of life for patients with HIV infections. I am optimistic that other therapies based on a knowledge of the HIV life-cycle will emerge in the near future.

REFERENCES

1. Gottlieb MS, Schroff R, Schanker HM et al: *Pneumocystis carinii* pneumonia and mucosal candidiasis in previously healthy homosexual men: Evidence of a new acquired cellular immunodeficiency. N Engl J Med 305:1425, 1981

2. Broder S, Gallo RC: A pathogenic retrovirus (HTLV-III) linked to AIDS. N Engl J Med 311:1292, 1984

3. Gallo RC, Salahuddin MG, Popovic M et al: Frequent detection and isolation of cytopathic retroviruses (HTLV-III) from patients with AIDS and at risk for AIDS. Science 224:500, 1984

4. Popovic M, Sarngadharan MG, Read E et al: Detection, isolation, and continuous production of cytopathic retroviruses. Science 224:497, 1984

5. Barré-Sinoussi F, Chermann JC, Rey F et al: Isolation of a T cell lymphotropic virus from a patient at risk for acquired immunodeficiency syndrome (AIDS). Science 220:868, 1983

6. Levi JA, Hoffmann AD, Kramer SM et al: Isolation of lymphocytopathic retroviruses from San Francisco patients with AIDS. Science 225:840, 1984

7. Coffin J, Haase A, Levy J et al: What to call the AIDS virus? Nature 321:10, 1986

8. Shaw GM, Harper ME, Hahn BH et al: HTLV-III infection in brains of children and adults with AIDS encephalopathy. Science 227:177, 1985

9. Ho DD, Rota TR, Schooley RT et al: Isolation of HTLV-III from cerebrospinal fluid and neural tissue of patients with neurologic syndromes related to the acquired immunodeficiency syndrome. N Engl J Med 313:1493, 1985

10. Resnick L, diMarzo-Veronese F, Schüpbach J et al: Intrablood-brain-barrier synthesis of HTLV-III specific IgG in patients with neurologic symptoms associated with AIDS or AIDS-related complex. N Engl J Med 313:1498, 1985

11. Gartner S, Markovits P, Markovitz DM et al: The role of mononuclear phagocytes in HTLV-III/LAV infection. Science 233:215, 1986

12. Koenig S, Gendelman HE, Orenstein JM et al: Detection of AIDS virus in macrophages in brain tissue from AIDS patients with encephalopathy. Science 233:1089, 1986

13. Mitsuya H, Weinhold KJ, Furman PA et al: 3'-azido-3'-deoxythymidine (BW A509U): An antiviral agent that inhibits the infectivity and cytopathic effect of human T-lymphotropic virus type III/lymphadenopathy-associated virus in vitro. Proc Natl Acad Sci USA 82:7096, 1985

14. Yarchoan R, Klecker RW, Weinhold KJ et al: Administration of 3'azido-3'-deoxythymidine: An inhibitor of HTLV-III/LAV replication, to patients with AIDS or AIDS-related complex. Lancet i:575, 1986

15. Mitsuya H, Matsukura M, Broder S: Rapid in vitro systems for assessing activity against HTLV-III/LAV. In Broder S (ed): AIDS: Modern Concepts and Therapeutic Challenges p. 303. New York, Marcel Dekker, 1987

16. Gross L: Oncogenic Viruses, 3rd ed. Oxford, Pergammon Press, 1983

17. Baltimore D: Viral RNA dependent DNA polymerase. Nature 226:1209, 1970

18. Temin H, Mizutani S: RNA dependent DNA polymerase in virions of rous sarcoma virus. Nature 226:1211, 1970

19. Toh H, Hayashida H, Miyata T et al: Sequence homology between retroviral reverse transcriptase and putative polymerases of hepatitis and cauliflower mosaic virus. Nature 305:827, 1983

20. Ratner L, Haseltine W, Patarca R et al: Complete nucleotide sequence of the AIDS virus, HTLV-III. Nature 313:277, 1985

21. Fisher AG, Ensoli B, Ivanoff L et al: The sor gene of HIV-1 is required for efficient virus transmission in vitro. Science 237:888, 1987

22. Strebel K, Daugherty D, Clouse K et al: The HIV 'A' (sor) gene product is essential for virus infectivity. Nature 328:728, 1987

23. Sodroski J, Rosen C, Wong-Staal F et al: Trans-acting transcriptional regulation of human T-cell leukemia virus type III long terminal repeat. Science 312:171, 1985

24. Sodroski J, Goh WC, Rosen C et al: A second post-transcriptional *trans*-activator gene required for HTLV-III replication. Nature 412, 1986

25. Feinberg MB, Jarrett RF, Aldovini A et al: HTLV-III expression and production involve complex regulation at the level of splicing and translation of viral RNA. Cell 46:807, 1986

26. Dalgleish AG, Beverley PCL, Clapham PR et al: The CD4 (T4) antigen is an essential component of the receptor for the AIDS retrovirus. Nature 312:763, 1984

27. Klatzman D, Champagne E, Chamaret S et al: T lymphocyte T4 molecule behaves as the receptor for human retrovirus LAV. Nature 312:767, 1984

28. Pert CB, Hill JM, Ruff MR et al: Octapeptides deduced from the neuropeptide receptor-like pattern of antigen T4 in brain potently inhibit human immunodeficiency virus receptor binding and T cell infectivity. Proc Natl Acad Sci USA 83:2672, 1986

29. Sodroski J, Goh WC, Rosen C et al: Role of HTLV-III/LAV envelope in syncytium formation and cytopathicity. Nature 322:470, 1986

30. Lifson JD, Feinberg MB, Reyes GR et al: Induction of CD4-dependent cell fusion by the HTLV-III/LAV envelope glycoprotein. Nature 323:725, 1986

31. Fisher AG, Ratner L, Mitsuya H et al: Infectious mutants of HTLV-III with changes in the 3' region and markedly reduced cytopathic effects. Science 233:655, 1986

32. Matsushita S, Robert-Guroff M, Trepel J et al: Human monoclonal antibody directed against an envelope glycoprotein of human T cell leukemia virus type I. Proc Natl Acad Sci USA 83:2672, 1986

33. Jacks T, Varmus H: Expression of the Rous sarcoma virus *pol* gene by ribosomal frameshifting. Science 230:1237, 1985

34. Craigen WJ, Caskey CT: Translational frameshifting: Where will it stop? *Cell* 50:1, 1987

35. Mitsuya H, Popovic M, Yarchoan R et al: Suramin protection of T cells in vitro against infectivity and cytopathic effect of HTLV-III. Science 226:172, 1984

36. Broder S, Yarchoan R, Collins JM et al: Effects of suramin on HTLV-III/LAV infection presenting as Kaposi's sarcoma or AIDS-related complex. Lancet 2:627, 1985

37. Rosenbaum W, Dormont D, Spire B et al: Antimoniotungstate (HPA23) treatment of three patients with AIDS and one with prodrome. Lancet 1:450, 1985

38. Sandstrom EG, Kaplan JC, Byington RE et al: Inhibition of human T-cell lymphotropic virus type III in vitro by phosphonoformate. Lancet 1:1480, 1985

39. Cullen BR: Trans-activation of human immunodeficiency virus occurs via a biomodal mechanism. Cell 46:973, 1986

40. Okamoto T, Wong–Staal F: Demonstration of virus-specific transcriptional activator(s) in cells infected with HTLV-III by an in vitro cell-free system. Cell 47:29, 1986

41. McCormick JB, Getchell JP, Mitchell SW et al: Ribavirin suppresses lymphadenopathy-associated virus in culture of human adult lymphocytes. Lancet 2:1367, 1984

42. Zamecnik PC, Goodchild J, Taguchi Y et al: Inhibition of replication and expression of human T-cell lymphotropic virus type III in cultured cells by exogenous synthetic oligodeoxynucleotides complementary to viral RNA. Proc Natl Acad Sci USA 83:4143, 1986

43. Matsukura M, Shinozuka K, Zon G et al: Phosphorothioate analogs of oligodeoxynucleotides: Inhibitors of replication and cytopathic effects of human immunodeficiency virus (HIV). Proc Natl Acad Sci USA 84:7706, 1987

44. Schultz AM, Oroszlan S.: In vivo modification of retroviral *gag* gene-encoded polyproteins by myristic acid. J Virol 46:355, 1983

45. Ho DD, Hartshorn KL, Rota TR et al: Recombinant human interferon alpha- suppresses HTLV-III replication in vitro. Lancet 1:602, 1985

46. Mitsuya H, Broder S: Inhibition of the in vitro infectivity and cytopathic effect of human T-lymphotropic virus type III/lymphadenopathy-associated virus (HTLV-III/LAV) by 2',3'-dideoxynucleosides. Proc Natl Acad Sci USA 83:1911, 1986

47. Robins MJ, Robins RK: The synthesis of 2',3'-dideoxyaden-osine from 2'-deoxyadenosine. J Am Chem Soc 86:3585, 1964

48. Horwitz JP, Chua J, Noel M: The monomesylates of 1-(2'-deoxy-b-D-lyxofuranosyl) thymine. J Org Chem 29:2076, 1964

49. Doering AM, Janse M, Cohen SS et al: Polymer synthesis in killed bacteria: Lethality of 2',3'-dideoxyadenosine. J Bact 92:565, 1966

50. Horwitz JP, Chua J, Noel M et al: Nucleosides. XI. 2',3'-dideoxycytidine. J Org Chem 32:817, 1967

51. Atkinson MR, Deutscher MP, Kornberg A et al: Enzymatic synthesis of deoxyribonucleic acid. XXXIV. Biochemistry 8:4897, 1969

52. Toji L, Cohen SS: Termination of deoxyribonucleic acid in *Escherichia coli* by 2',3'-dideoxyadenosine. J Bact 103:323, 1970

53. Sanger F, Nicklen S, Coulsen AR: DNA sequencing with chain terminating inhibitors. Proc Natl Acad Sci USA 74:5463, 1977

54. Cooney DA, Dalal M, Mitsuya H et al: Initial studies on the cellular pharmacology of 2',3'-dideoxycytidine, an inhibitor of HTLV-III infectivity. Biochem Pharmacol 35:2065, 1986

55. Mitsuya H, Jarrett RF, Matsukura M et al: Long-term inhibition of HTLV-III/LAV DNA synthesis and RNA expression in T-cells protected by 2',3'-dideoxynucleosides. Proc Natl Acad Sci USA 84:2033, 1987

56. Chiu I–M, Yaniv A, Dahlberg JE et al: Nucleotide sequence evidence for relationship of AIDS retrovirus to lentivirus. Nature 317:366, 1985

57. Dahlberg JE, Mitsuya H, Broder S et al: Broad spectrum antiretroviral activity of 2',3'-dideoxynucleosides. Proc Natl Acad Sci USA 84:2469, 1987

58. Waqar MA, Evans MJ, Manly KF et al: Effects of 2',3'-dideoxynucleosides in mammalian cells and viruses. J Cell Physiol 121:402, 1984

59. Ostertag W, Roesler G, Krief CJ et al: Induction of endogenous virus and of thymidine kinase by bromodeoxyuridine in cell cultures transformed by Friend virus. Proc Natl Acad Sci USA 71:4980, 1974

60. Furman PA, Fyfe JA, St. Clair MH et al: Proc Natl Acad Sci USA 83:8333, 1986

61. Yarchoan R, Brouwers P, Spitzer AR et al: Preliminary observation of the response of HTLV-III/LAV-associated neurological diseases to the administration of 3'-azido-3'-deoxythymidine. Lancet 1:132, 1987

Strategies for the Development of Vaccines to Prevent AIDS

Peter J. Fischinger

6

Human acquired immunodeficiency syndrome (AIDS) is an expanding pandemic involving over 57,000 cases in the United States alone. As currently defined, clinical AIDS is generally lethal. Infection with the causative agent, now generically named human immunodeficiency virus (HIV), is apparently irreversible. Descriptions of cohorts of infected individuals describe a long-term progressive depletion of T4-helper lymphocytes, which eventually results in an immune status of such debility that opportunistic infections or rare tumors occur. Intermediate levels of symptoms and signs such as those defined by the AIDS-related complex (ARC) and by serious neurologic involvement are common and often prodromal to AIDS. Most if not all HIV antibody-positive individuals carry HIV, which as a retrovirus is integrated into the DNA of the cell. Current strategies of intervention are based on a few drugs of the chain-terminating family that lessen the probability of progression to further serious events in patients who already have AIDS. Because there do not appear to be any clearly defined individuals who have been initially infected but have either eliminated or adequately controlled the HIV infection, preventive approaches that involve vaccine strategies appear to be critically important. Although AIDS in the developed world is still generally confined to defined high-risk populations with an estimated infected population of 1 to 2 million, the greatest proportional new increases have occurred in the previously not-at-risk heterosexual group. A major objective is to prevent HIV from becoming just another sexually transmitted disease, because if numbers of HIV-infected individuals were to become comparable to the high numbers of individuals infected with herpes or chlamydia, it would be an even more severe health problem. It is widely recognized that although AIDS in the developed countries is confined to high-risk groups, in several parts of the world, especially in equatorial Africa, AIDS already appears to be a serious threat as a heterosexually trans-mitted disease. It is estimated that several million individuals may be infected with HIV in those countries. Prevention of further spread by an AIDS vaccine in these populations is acutely needed.

Although a number of approaches to develop a vaccine against AIDS are being followed concurrently, recent results from several animal challenge experiments, outlined below, indicate that the simple conventional approaches may not be enough. Nonetheless, these failures do point out the more correct direction to be pursued to develop a broadly effective vaccine against AIDS. This chapter provides an overview of the current experiments most likely to succeed and outlines alternative efforts being deferred because others take priority or because needed resources are unavailable.

PRIORITIZING VACCINE STRATEGIES

Many possible approaches exist for an anti-HIV vaccine and these have been reviewed in detail.[1-3] A basic tenet is that especially in this disease the vaccine has to be safe and broadly effective. Several approaches are immediately practical, whereas others are still theoretical. The first objective is to narrow down the number of approaches. The baseline logic of what could work was defined by partial successes of active and passive immunization in the field of classical animal retroviruses.[4-11] Table 6-1 outlines and assesses a priority system of the current approaches and reflects the initial attempts being carried out by a number of academic and industrial laboratories.

Historically efficacious approaches for many human viruses such as the generation of nonpathogenic infectious agents or the use of killed virus are considered somewhat less likely for the AIDS retrovirus. Nonpathogenic variants can today be genetically engineered in the sense that critical genes could be modified or de-

Table 6-1
Priority of Current Approaches to Development of Anti-HIV Vaccines

	Feasibility	Safety	Probable Efficacy	Priority
Nonpathogenic, infectious	++	?	+	4
Killed HIV	++	?	±	3
ISCOMS (parts of killed HIV)	++	+	+	
Subunits				
Native	+	+	++	
Genetically engineered	++	+	++	1
Peptides	++	+	+	2
Infectious recombinants				
Vacc, APC, VZV	++	+?	++	1
Anti-idiotypes	±	+	+	5

leted without affecting the expression of antigens involved in the generation of protective responses.[12] However, in the area of retroviruses, killed virus is notoriously a poor inducer of protective immunity; in fact, kittens immunized with killed feline leukemia virus (FeLV) fared worse after live virus challenge than controls.[13] Even purified HIV is significantly contaminated by cellular proteins such as DR antigens while virion proteins considered important such as envelope (*env*) glycoproteins (gp) are lost.[14] Recently it has been reported that a noncytopathogenic variant could revert to pathogenicity on culture.[15] However, the most salient objection against these two approaches is that they contain viral nucleic acids. Even a very small part of long-terminal repeats (LTRs) of retroviruses contain promoters and enhancers that, if integrated next to an oncogene, could eventually result in a tumor.[16] The HIV in particular has in addition to LTRs several "rheostat" type genes, for example, *tat,* which have powerful transactivating effects in experimental systems.[17-23]

The use of subunits in various formats, demonstrably as pure proteins/glycoproteins, is attractive because advances in biotechnology now allow for an unlimited supply of safely produced individual products from a wide choice of vectors grown in bacteria, yeast, insect, or mammalian cells. A system can be selected for epitope selection, glycosylation, superinducibility, transport, and whatever translational and posttranslational modifications thought to be useful. In the last year a significant number of such products has become available that are currently being tested.

A shortcut approach to a subunit HIV vaccine may involve the use of ISCOMS, which are artificial matrices composed of amphipathic viral proteins sticking in saponin-like micelles. In several systems, including the FeLV retrovirus, this approach promises to be highly feasible.[10,24,25] ISCOMS have already been made with HIV; however, the incorporation of pure unmodified major envelope glycoprotein (gp120) into the micelle is limited. On the other hand, some HIV proteins such as the most abundant protein (p24) of the viral core are

completely excluded. A major problem is that ISCOMS prepared from the purified HIV also incorporate significant amounts of cellular membrane type proteins.[14] Figure 6-1 shows such a preparation of ISCOMS made with the HTLV-IIIb isolate of HIV.

A special subset of virion proteins is defined by totally synthetic peptides defining epitopes that could stimulate protective cellular or humoral responses. This is being done by a sequential reduction in size of larger immunogenic proteins to smaller pieces that induce a parameter of immunity analogous to the larger molecule. Alternatively, special computer programs can search for continuous amphipathic helices, which are known to represent T-cell–specific epitopes in a variety of immunogenic vaccine proteins. Both of these approaches have recently been successful in part.[26-29] Peptides may be directly sufficient for a vaccine; alternatively they may be important for primary or recall functions and may be especially critical in inducing a strong cellular immunity.

The infectious recombinant virus approach remains of the highest priority. Although a number of virus vehicles such as adenovirus, varicella-zoster, and herpes simplex can be used, most emphasis has been put on vaccinia as the vector of choice.[30-32] Various animal vaccines have been designed with this agent, which has the advantage of replicating with an estimable safety record, and which could readily be used worldwide under field conditions. Essentially any HIV gene(s) can be incorporated, and positive humoral and cellular responses to HIV envelope glycoproteins have been elicited by several groups using closely related HIV variants, LAV-1 and HTLV-IIIb.[33,34]

Research on anti-idiotypes, which are theoretically of great interest, has been hampered by the lack of good monoclonal antibodies to various HIV proteins, for example, those that would be neutralizing for HIV. Antibodies to such monoclonals could serve as antigens because they represent an internal image of the protein. For a number of viral test systems such antibody "three" is not only active against the virus but generally could

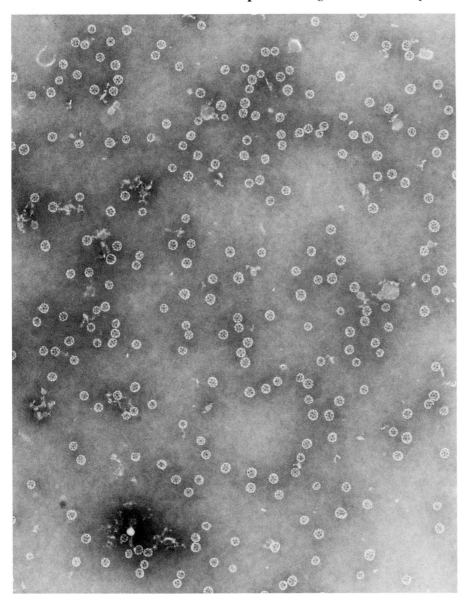

FIG. 6-1. A preparation of IS-COMS derived from partially purified HTLV-IIIb isolate of HIV. Each structure is about 35 nm in size (×90,000).

elicit a broader response than the isolated antigen. This feature would be particularly relevant because of the wide heterogeneity of HIV isolates.[35] Recently, monoclonals to HIV core and especially envelope glycoproteins are being described that do have specific biologic functions of interest.

CHOICE OF VIRAL TARGET

Besides its normal contingent of structural genes, HIV has a series of extra functional genes. Several of these genes, which are generally not found in classical oncornaviruses, function to increase/decrease virus production and may play a role in latency.[19,20,23] These are depicted in Figure 6-2. Considerable complexity has been observed for these genes, such as the use of all three reading frames and of multiple spliced genes. Based on other retroviruses, the viral gene product most likely to induce a protective humoral immune response would be the major external viral glycoprotein of the 5′ end of the envelope (*env*) gene, gp120 in the case of HIV.[36] At the 3′ end of *env* is the transmembrane protein (tmp) gp41 that anchors the gp120. The interaction of these two proteins with the virion envelope is fragile because even on gentle purification they generally fall off the virus. Glycoprotein 120 has been reported to induce not only reactive antibodies but also type-specific neutralizing antibodies (NAs), antibodies that inhibit viral-mediated fusion, as well as antibodies causing

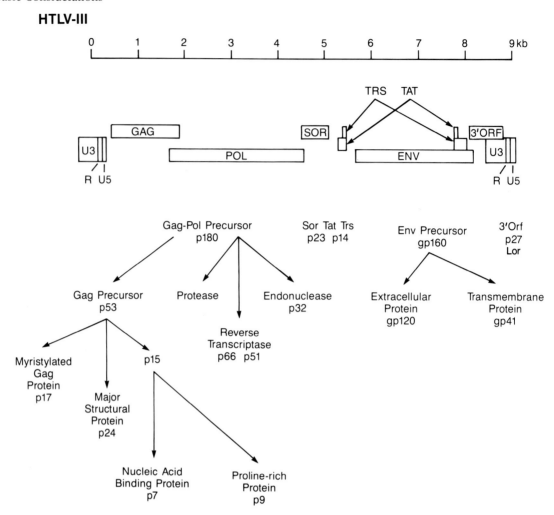

FIG. 6-2. A simplified gene map of HIV. Different lines represent various possible reading frames. Some gene products derive from spliced messengers indicated by discontinuities. The long-terminal repeats have the usual U_3, R, U_5 structures as found in all retroviruses. The relative size is expressed in kilobases of nucleotides.

both complement-mediated (ACC), and cell-mediated (ADCC) cytotoxicity phenomena.[37–40] Glycoprotein 41 induces highly reactive antibodies but with some exceptions has not induced NAs.[26,27] Table 6-2 briefly describes the function of each known viral gene and currently recognized immune responses.

Core and viral proteins coded by group-specific antigen (*gag*) gene, reverse transcriptase or polymerase (*pol*) gene, and perhaps other genes have been shown in some viral systems to be able to elicit a protective antibody.[41,42] At times in some retroviral systems *gag* proteins could appear at the infected cell surface.[43] Also an individual *gag* protein may be specifically recognizable and cytotoxic antibodies could be induced, for example, the p12 in the murine leukemia virus (MuLV) system.[44,45] In HIV p17 may play such a role based on the description of HIV-neutralizing antibodies induced

by a synthetic peptide derived from the p17 sequence.[46] Although no specific positive data have been obtained from studies of responses to other internal HIV proteins, a thorough analysis of each of these would be useful.

A very important subset of immune responses is represented by the cellular arm known to be important for recovery from many viral diseases. A specific subset of these are mediated by T-cell–specific epitopes that are different from B-cell epitopes. The former are generally defined by short, contiguous, conserved amino acid sequences with an amphipathic profile. They are also important in specific antibody recall phenomena as well as T-helper and cytotoxic cell functions. Recently, several such T-cell immunoreactive sequences have been identified in the gp120 of HIV.[29] Specific processing of the viral protein also takes place for the recognition of these peptides. In this case particularly, the

Table 6-2
Viral Targets for Vaccine Considerations

Gene	Product	Imm. Reactive	Function	Needed for Growth
env	gp41	Pathognomonic	Transmembrane protein	Yes
	gp160	Strong	Attachment	Induce cytopathic effect
	gp120 (Small peptides T_1, T_2, etc.)	Yes	B&T cell epitopes	
gag	p24	Good	Core	Yes
	p17	Good		Yes
	p6–p7	Good		Yes
pol	p60	Good	Reverse transcriptase	Yes
sor	p23–p25	Yes	Nonstructural	No
lor	p22–p28	Yes	Nonstructural	No
tat	p14	Yes	+ Rheostat	Yes
trs		Yes	− Rheostat	No
R		Yes		?

localization of these peptides may well be within any number of the internal HIV proteins.

The isolated "native" protein products of HIV may be of particular importance because of extensive glycosylation of gp120 (~50% by weight) and to a lesser degree of gp41.[36,37] Figure 6-3 shows a full-sized gp120 purified from H9 cells infected with the HTLV-IIIb variant. The carbohydrate moiety may be itself immunogenic or may affect the configuration of the molecule and possibly its specific epitopes, as is known for MuLVs.[47-49] Although a number of synthetic products have been made of the HIV gp120, only those produced in mammalian or insect cells appear to be extensively or even fully glycosylated.[50-52] Whether glycosylation of HIV *env* gene proteins synthesized in insect or yeast cells may differ enough in the type of sugar linkages to be important in the production of protective immunity has to be determined. At present, however, at least some of the apparently significant responses such as the induction of the type-specific NA has been localized to the nonglycosylated protein backbone of gp120 and can be further defined to be on a short, apparently continuous amino acid sequence.[50] A key element may be the presentation of an antigen to function as a good immunogen. This not only involves a choice of adjuvants, but also the configuration or the combination of the antigens. For example, in FeLV, gp70 by itself does not induce a protective antibody, but in association with its transmembrane protein (tmp), p15E, or as part of an infected cell membrane complex did result in protective responses.[8,9] The formation of "rosettes" that have hydrophobic portions on the inside and the hydrophilic moieties on the outside is known to result in a highly favorable response defined by a much smaller amount of antigen, which induces a good antibody response.[5,53,54] The ISCOMS mentioned above may be particularly advantageous in this regard.

INTRINSIC DIFFICULTIES

The major acknowledged problem appears to be the extensive heterogeneity of HIV isolates. Of the more than 100 separate isolates only a few closely matched pairs were observed, and some of these were isolated contemporaneously. Different geographic regions yielded viruses with significantly different sequences. The degree of dissimilarity could be profound and is manifest especially in the envelope gene product. It is not unusual to find an approximate 20% amino acid difference in the gp120s of a pair of isolates. What is more troubling is that yet another variant would also have a 20% divergence from each member of first pair of isolates.[55,56] Even within a single individual, a number of variants could be isolated sequentially. It is of interest, however, that the isolates from a single infected person will tend to show rather fine differences from each other rather than dramatic changes.[57] So far, most of the change has been reminiscent of rapid mutation as opposed to recombinational events, in which whole sections of sequences from a gene of a much less related variant are incorporated *en bloc* into the variant, as has been described for murine leukemia recombinant viruses.[58]

The localization of variations predominantly within the major external viral glycoprotein is indicative of functional change presumably as a maneuver designed to evade host defenses. HIV is more closely related to animal lentiviruses than to any other known family of retroviruses. Lentiviruses present a number of interesting models that demonstrate how disease progression could occur in the presence of an active immune response.[59] A significant feature of some lentiviruses is progressive change in the envelope sequences, which allows the new variants not to be neutralized by the pre-existing neutralizing serum effective against the previous variants. This progressive change has best been defined in the equine infectious anemia virus system as nucleotide changes in the envelope gene coding for the major viral glycoprotein, gp90. Successive episodes of disease were associated with the generation of new gp90 variants in each cycle of the disease within a single pony.[60] It is assumed that HIV could also undergo similar changes over the years of infection prior to clinical AIDS development, although the states of disease and wellness are much less distinct. One of the possible outcomes would be that any field isolate could be composed of multiple genomes even if the predominant envelope is of a single phenotype. This would be analogous to the MuLV system, in which often xenotropic or recombinant viruses adopt the envelope of the ecotropic variant, which can exist freely in the face of host responses, whereas the others cannot. The result is a predominant genotype in a single envelope type with the existence of scarcer genotypes masked by that tolerated envelope.[61]

The protracted pathogenic process by which AIDS occurs many years after infection is not well understood. The major and obvious event is the progressive destruction of the T4 population. The HIV itself is fully capable of killing T4 cells by inducing a fusion response with a subsequent cytopathogenic effect. Possible phenomena that may be involved are the presence and induction of cytotoxic molecules and the generation of a specific immune cytotoxic response against the HIV-infected cell. One of the critical questions is whether any single viral protein designated to be a vaccine could by itself have an adverse effect on the immune system. For example, the gp120 that normally attaches itself to the CD4a receptor on T4-helper cells could interfere with normal immune cellular instructive and interactive networking. More recently, gp120 was clearly identified as a superior target for ADCC in the absence of infection. Free native gp120 bound to an uninfected T4 cell would render that cell susceptible to killing by anti-gp120 antibody and effector cells.[40] This scenario might occur under the unknown dynamics of the *in vivo* situation, where booster immunizations with gp120 would render T4 cells susceptible to killing by the recently induced antibody. This possibility was carefully examined in vaccinated chimpanzees by sequential T4 and T4:T8 ratio analysis by fluorescence-activated cell sorting. No adverse effects were seen on the chimpanzee T4-helper cell status.[62] Additionally, the responses in the only analyzed human inoculated with the vaccine infectious recombinant virus containing the IIIb envelope gene were shown not to be significantly detrimental to his T4 population.*

Other viral molecules should also be examined for specific effect on the immune system. For example, in the FeLV retrovirus system, the tmp, p15E (analogous

to the gp41 of HIV), by itself has a depressive effect on the immune system.[4,9] However, when complexed to the major external viral glycoprotein, gp70, the "rosette" is highly protective and is not detrimental to the immune response.[8] So far, the highly immunogenic tmp gp41 of HIV has never been isolated in amounts significant enough for such a study, although nonglycosylated fragments such as peptide-121 did not show any adverse effect in several species, including rhesus monkeys.[27] Glycoprotein 41 does have sequences homologous to fusion proteins found in other viruses and may partake in the fusion process mediated by the gp120 of HIV.[63] The potential detrimental role of other viral proteins, especially those of the functional "rheostat" genes, are unknown.

Immune Responses to Native or Engineered Viral Proteins or Peptides

Immune responses subsequent to HIV infection in man are generally broad and are manifest in both the humoral and the cellular arms of the immune system. All known viral proteins are immunoreactive in infected species. These are manifest as broadly reactive precipitating antibodies that recognize widely divergent HIV variants as determined in a number of tests. Although ACC was not demonstrated in infected humans, it was shown to exist in chimpanzees chronically infected with HIV.[39] ADCC was shown to exist in both infected humans and chimpanzees.[40,64] The latter was a useful prognostic indicator in that worsening status was correlated with a reduced ADCC, primarily due to reduced effectiveness of the effector cells.[64] Classical cell-mediated immunity is difficult to measure in this infection; however, a number of different tests indicated that such immunity may either be scarce or exist at times during infection.[65–68]

A large number of HIV-exposed individuals were tested to determine whether persons could be identified who have been initially infected with HIV but have subsequently either eliminated the virus or so well controlled it that they remain and will be expected to remain asymptomatic. Antibody-positive, well patients were examined to determine whether there are specific patterns of humoral or cellular immunity that would indicate an immune and protected status. Major attention was paid to virus NA status at various stages of the disease. Although a broadly responsive NA was generally observed, it did not predict protection well, because at times progressive disease was accompanied with high titers of NA.[36,69] However, this does not mean, *a priori,* that pre-existing antibody or cellular immunity could not protect a person from the initial infection. Nonetheless, any attempt at inducing a state of protection in man with a vaccine preparation has to be considered without a pre-existing model of an immune state indicative of protection.

The HIV subunit material of greatest initial interest was the major envelope glycoprotein, gp120.[36,37] Most investigators dealt with the two very similar early isolates

* Zagury D: Personal communication.

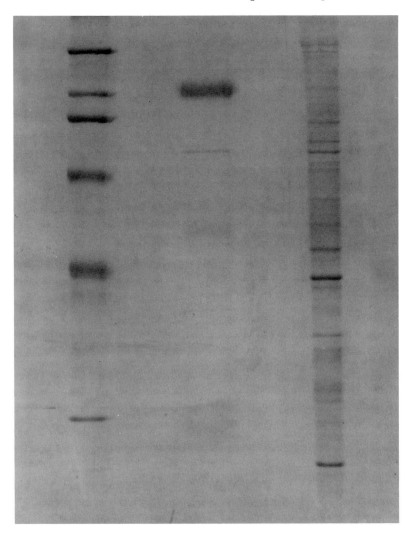

FIG. 6-3. A purified preparation of the HIV native gp120 from the IIIb isolate. The left lane represents molecular weight markers. The right lane shows the relative impurity of HIV after several cycles of density gradient centrifugation. The gp120 band is almost invisible in that virus preparation. The strong gp120 band seen in the intermediate lane can be highly purified after considerable effort.

of HIV, HTLV-IIIb and LAV-1, especially because these were molecularly cloned before most other isolates. Native gp120 was isolated from the IIIb virus supernates and infected cell membranes and was initially tested for safety and immunogenicity in a number of lower species with various adjuvants.[37] A purified native gp120 preparation used for vaccination is shown in Figure 6-3. A fairly rapid initial response as well as normal anamnestic responses were seen in mice, guinea pigs, rabbits, goats and horses which consisted of broadly reactive precipitating antibody and a highly type-specific NA.[30] Similar responses were seen with the gp120 in rhesus monkeys and in chimpanzees that were immunized with alum and muramyl dipeptide as adjuvants. In the higher primate the gp120 bound readily to the CD4a molecule of the lymphocyte, but no effect was observed relative to the T4 helper population.[62] In all species, the precipitating and the type-specific NA decayed with time even after more than eight consecutive immunizations. At no time was a group-specific NA observed.[38,62] In the chimpanzee the ts NA titers were generally lower perhaps because of the limiting amounts of immunogen. Similar responses were seen with the deglycosylated IIIb gp120, which approximated a p59 in size.[50] Although again only type-specific NA was observed, it suggested that the epitopes on the gp120 eliciting NA were on the protein backbone. The second native gp120 used in multiple species was that derived from the RFII, the Haitian isolate of HIV. Although the latter gp120 differed by about 20% in amino acid sequence, the responses in multiple species were analogous to the IIIb gp120 in that similar levels of antibody were seen, which was again highly specific in neutralization only for the homologous type.*

Expression of the gp120, initially the IIIb molecular clone BH10, was attempted in bacterial and mammalian cells using various vectors. Of a larger number of products made in bacteria, a polypeptide termed PB-1, in the 5′ third of the *env* gene appeared to be highly active in inducing NA.[50] It was curious that other larger con-

* Nara P, Arthur L, Fischinger P: Unpublished data.

structs from the *env* gene, including one that encompassed the entire PB-1 sequence, were not able to elicit substantial NA. The PB-1 inoculation into a number of species including chimpanzees again stimulated only a type-specific NA. Other PB-1 variant molecules from five different HIV isolates are now available for comparison. Because PB-1 is not glycosylated, it is implicit that the type-specific NA–inducing epitope is represented by a sequence of amino acids. Further subdivision of the PB-1 polypeptide into smaller pieces, and alternative approaches using overlapping *env* gene peptides both showed that the dominant epitope is represented by a contiguous amino acid sequence in positions 307 to 330.* Of interest is that, although PB-1 induces NA, theoretically it would not have a negative effect on T-helper cell populations.[50]

Alternative synthesis of the gp120 molecule of HIVs were feasible in a mammalian vector system. There the entire, presumably fully glycosylated, gp120 structure which was quite immunoreactive and also induced a type-specific NA, was synthesized. A slight broadening of neutralizing response to one other, less related HIV was reported.[51]

An alternative approach to the generation of fully glycosylated HIV *env* gene products was to express the gene in an insect cell system. An insect baculovirus has intrinsic molecular promoters that control the expression of a protein called polyhedrin to extremely high levels. It was possible to use this promoter system to construct and drive various other genes to high expression levels. The entire *env* gene of several HIV variants was also introduced and resulted in high levels of expression of the entire uncleaved precursor, gp160.[52] The uncleaved precursor may have advantages in generating higher levels of antibody because in other retrovirus systems an artificial reassociation of the major glycoprotein and the transmembrane protein was much more effective than the glycoprotein alone in inducing protective immunity.[7,8] Experimentally, the baculovirus-derived gp160 did induce higher amounts of antibody; however, as in the case of other purified gp120s, the NA was still quite type specific. The role of binding of gp160 to the CD4a receptor is under study, as are the cellular immune responses that might have been induced.[52] One commercial group has shown relative safety and a lack of toxicity of the gp160 in higher primates and has applied for permission from the U.S. Food and Drug Administration to initiate human Phase I trials. This has recently been granted, the first HIV vaccine material to reach this stage although there is no current evidence of efficacy. Human volunteer studies using seronegative, healthy members of a high-risk group are being initiated.

The other end of the spectrum of viral proteins as vaccines deals with minimalist approaches. Because at least one major epitope that induced type-specific NA is contiguous and can be configured as a small 15- to 25-amino-acid peptide, such peptides can be synthesized chemically without using molecular engineering.

Several such peptides have been described.[26,28] An added advantage is that the entire gene can be readily scanned with a series of overlapping peptides. The supposition is that glycosylation may be less important because these small polypeptides could assume varying shapes. If the epitope of interest were noncontinuous, that is, composed of two stretches far apart in sequence but brought together three-dimensionally by folding, one could still rather simply construct such an artificial epitope. Various molecular folding possibilities are being worked on with advanced computing programs because the sequence of various divergent HIVs are currently known.

A second subset of peptides may be critical to the induction of adequate immunity to peptides that induce antibodies. This second set is represented by amino acid sequences in a larger molecule that are used as recognition signals for T-helper cells to generate B-cell responses. For example, a B-cell epitope that can induce the right type of antibody may not by itself serve to give a booster response on reinoculation because different sequences are required for T-cell–mediated recall functions.[29] These T-cell epitopes are generally short, contiguous stretches of amino acids that are generally well conserved. A second identifying feature is that they are amphipathic, that is, that each peptide in itself has short hydrophobic and hydrophilic stretches. This biophysical configuration has been used to generate computer programs that could search for such stretches in a larger protein. Recently, several such peptide groups have been identified in the HIV gp120. Two of these, named T_1 and T_2, were synthesized and examined for immunologic reactivity. Initial studies demonstrated that these two peptides were involved in the generation of appropriate initial and recall T-cell responses.[29] As such, they can serve as adjuncts to boost immune responses and may of themselves be important in the stimulation of cellular immunity. Another feature is that artificial constructs may be made of multiple T-cell epitopes that can be joined to B-cell epitopes to result in artificial but theoretically compelling composites that could induce levels of immunity superior to those obtained by standard means.

Yet another variation was to use the infectious recombinant vaccinia virus vector containing the entire *env* gene of either IIIb or LAV-1. Expression in cell culture systems was adequate, and both gp160, gp120, and gp41 were observed. Antibodies to the precursor and both of the cleavage products were induced in a number of species, including lower and higher primates.[33,65] The construct composed of the HIV IIIb *env* gene in infectious vaccinia virus was also experimentally inoculated into man and did not engender any toxicity. However, a low level of type-specific NA response was observed as well as some indications of possible cellular immunity.*

Other HIV proteins have been examined to a lesser extent. For example, the native gp41, the transmembrane protein that serves as the anchor for gp120, is very

---

* Putney S, Haynes B: Personal communication.

* Zagury D: Personal communication.

immunogenic but most difficult to purify. On repeated attempts, small amounts of gp41 have been obtained from the HTLV-IIIb isolate and inoculated into mice and rabbits. Expected broadly precipitating antibodies, including several monoclonal ones, have been obtained.* No neutralization of several HIVs tested has been observed with the resulting sera; however, two reports of an immunogenic synthetic peptide and a genetically engineered peptide state that some broadly neutralizing antibody was detected.[26,68] Apparently, some cell fusion function may be inherent in the HIV tmp based on sequence prediction and sequence substitution studies.[63] One of the first genetically engineered HIV peptides was derived from the IIIb tmp sequence and was termed *peptide-121*.[27] This nonglycosylated peptide-121 contained the immunodominant region of the tmp and was highly reactive in many tests. When inoculated into several lower species and rhesus monkeys with or without adjuvants, the resulting antibodies did not neutralize either homologous or heterologous HIVs. It is not clear whether peptide-121 or the larger native product induce any cellular immunity. Because in some retrovirus systems antibodies to tmp could be neutralizing, at least an adjunct role for this molecule in the induction of immunity has to be maintained.[70]

Many of the remaining HIV proteins deserve serious consideration in the potential construction of a vaccine. One of these is the p17 core protein, which is quite immunogenic. In type C retroviruses there are situations, as in the murine leukemia virus, in which group-specific antigen core region precursors appear at the cell surface, are glycosylated, and serve as targets for an immune attack, for example through the ACC system. A significant target then is the murine p12 molecule, a core protein that engenders an active cytotoxic antibody *in vivo*.[45] Sequences in the p17 of HIV have also been found to share homology with the α-1-thymosin growth factor molecule. When a peptide was made from such a common region of the two molecules, it was found to be immunoreactive in rabbits and to induce some apparently broadly neutralizing antibody.[46] Further confirmatory studies are anticipated.

Other core proteins such as the major structural conserved element, p24, induce good antibodies, but neither NA nor cellular immune responses have been reported. With the advent of the capability of synthesizing and expressing all structural and functional components of HIV, including reverse transcriptase, each of these can be considered and tested for the ability to induce humoral and cellular immunity. An overview and status of all known HIV vaccine preparations using envelope gene glycoproteins and peptides is presented in Table 6-3. The extent of progress of each preparation is presented as a lateral line. Of note is the significant number of bacterial-vector–expressed, immunogenic peptides from several HIV isolates. These at times span natural *env* cleavage points. In addition, the important

epitopes can now be pared down to very much reduced stretches of the PB-1 immunogen. Because a number of these studies that are also occurring within the private sector are therefore not as yet known, an overview of the status in this area cannot be complete. Other than the above mentioned synthetic peptide of the p17 *gag* protein product mentioned above, no significant attempts are known to be currently pursued.

Because progression to AIDS can occur in the presence of significant humoral response, special attention may have to be paid to particular aspects of cellular immunity.

Cytotoxic responses to HIV-infected cells may be important in preventing infection or progression to AIDS after infection. One set of these are mediated by antibody and can be mediated by complement, that is, antibody- and complement-mediated cytotoxicity (ACC). The second is antibody-dependent cell-mediated cytotoxicity (ADCC). Cytotoxic responses may be especially important in HIV infection because transmission is suspected to occur through intact cells. HIV-infected cells additionally appear to have the capability of maintaining the provirus in a latent form. As such, the presence of a cytotoxic system would be critical to eliminating the cell beginning to express HIV antigens. Just the NA may not be enough. For example, AKR mouse cells expressing MuLV simply down-regulate virus production in the presence of NA and complement and resume virus production when the antibody is withdrawn.[71] In man, absence of ACC is one criterion of difference from the infected chimpanzee and several gp120-immunized species, and as such may play a role in AIDS.[39] ADCC is also present in HIV-infected individuals, and recent data indicate that it may be related to disease progression in that more severely affected individuals have lower ADCC levels because of a diminution of effector cells.[40,64] Forms of classical cell-mediated immunity have been described in HIV-infected individuals, after immunization with vaccinia-HIV-*env*-infections recombinant virus and more recently after gp120 immunization.[65–68] The presence of a T8-specific cytotoxic population capable of killing HIV infection cell may be related to state of disease. Studies with peptides may be relevant to induction of an enhanced cellular immune response arm. Amphipathic, conserved amino acid regions could stimulate a cellular response and may also be important to enhancing the entire panoply of immune responses to HIV.[29,68]

STRATEGIES FOR BROADENING THE IMMUNE RESPONSE

Up to now all the various vaccine preparations using native or engineered gp120 moieties have resulted in a weak to relatively strong NA that was type specific. Whatever responses were seen in ACC or ADCC after immunization with viral subunits, these were again exquisitely type specific. The specificity is based on tissue culture experiments that show that serum from a vac-

---

* Zweig M: Unpublished data.

Table 6-3
Synoptic View of AIDS Vaccine Development

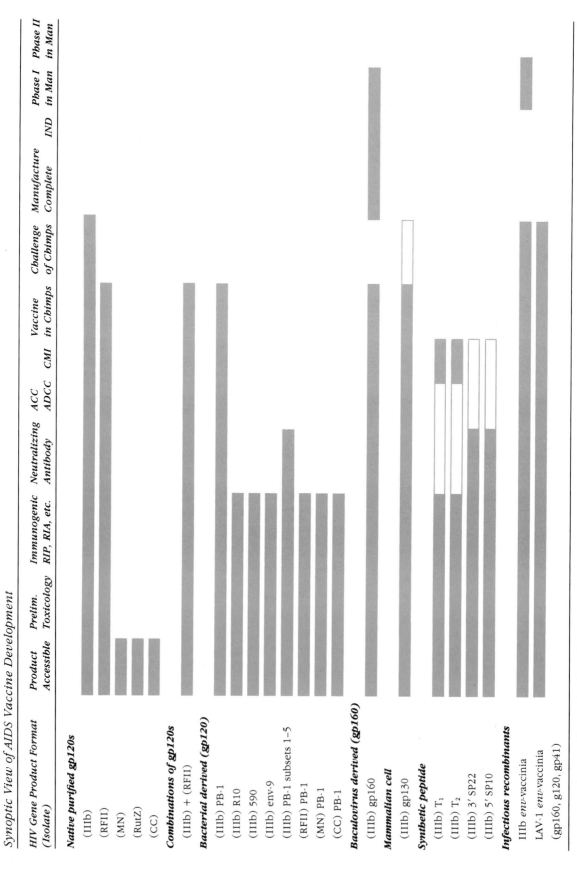

Various HIV isolates are abbreviated and set off in parentheses. RIP, radioimmunoprecipitation; RIA, radioimmunoassay. ACC, antibody- and complement-mediated cytotoxicity; ADCC, antibody-dependent cell-mediated cytotoxicity; CMI, cell-mediated immunity; IND, investigational new drug status approved by the Food and Drug Administration. Solid horizontal bars indicate that the stage was traversed. Empty bars indicate that experiments were attempted. A gap denotes that a stage(s) was skipped for various reasons.

cinee could kill the homologous type virus, but not a much less related virus.[37,38,62] Most experiments have used various native or synthetic envelope gp120s of HIV from the IIIb isolate as the immunogen and the RFII Haitian isolate as the virus to be inactivated because each represents a thoroughly characterized virus type. Recently, the reverse was also found to be successful. Using the RFII gp120, a good type-specific NA was obtained, but this antibody could not neutralize IIIb or several other unrelated HIV variants.* Thus, there does not seem to be any intrinsic special features of IIIb gp120 that do not allow for engendering a broad immune NA. However, more variants may have to be examined because it appears that some isolates such as ARV appear to be acutely susceptible to neutralization with many human sera, some of which will neutralize only select HIV variants.[72] It may be that some variants may readily present antigens that elicit a group-specific NA and other broad immune responses.

A basic question is whether a single HIV variant could induce a broad NA. Because infected individuals in high-risk groups are potentially exposed to many variants in sequence, the resulting NA may represent a series of type-specific NAs, or subgroup-specific antibodies. It is clear that sera from HIV-infected humans could have high-titer broadly neutralizing antibodies. However, the responses are quite variable both in strength of NA found, which ranges from almost undetectable to very high titers, and in specificity. In terms of the latter, not readily explainable patterns of response are found. At times a human neutralizing serum would neutralize some HIV variants strongly, but not others. A special situation was found in at least one such serum, which could neutralize a number of divergent HIV types, but not the virus reisolated from the same individual.[72] The above observations could be potentially defined by the series of exposures in the individuals tested and by the evasive action of the infecting virus by subtly mutating away from the current NA, as has been described above for lentiviruses such as the infectious equine anemia virus.[59,60]

Accordingly, experiments were recently performed in the chimpanzee that were designed to answer the question whether a single defined HIV variant could induce group-specific NA. Two approaches were used: immunization with subunits from several divergent isolates, and infection with a single defined variant HIV type. Again, the IIIb and the RFII native gp120s were used for sequential immunization of several species including the chimpanzee. The results were clear: the IIIb gp120 alone induced a type-specific NA for the IIIb, and the RFII gp120 induced a type-specific NA only for itself. An RFII gp120 immunization of a IIIb-gp120–immunized goat or chimpanzee resulted in a second type-specific NA response for the RFII variant. Thus, the outcome was two type-specific NA responses, one for each immunogen. When these dual type-specific NA sera

* Nara P et al: Unpublished data.

Table 6-4
Approaches Using HIV Subunits That Elicit Immunologic Responses Potentially Capable of Protecting Against a Variety of Distantly Related HIV Types

Combination of subunits, e.g., gp120, gp41
Multiple gp120s from divergent variants
Preparations of subunits from special serotypes
Targeting against the common cell receptor specific site
Use of HIV-infected cell membrane fractions
Special adjuvants and presentations of antigens
Search for the group-specific neutralizing antibody site by overlapping peptides
Use of multiple conserved epitopes that elicit cellular responses

were tested against three other HIV variants unrelated to either immunogen gp120, the MN, Rut Z, CC variants, none of these were neutralized even after four RFII gp120 superimmunizations, indicating that no detectable true group-specific NA was obtained.*

The alternative approach for examining the NA response in the infected chimpanzee proved more successful in defining that a single HIV variant could give rise to group-specific NA. Several chimpanzees were infected with low levels of the tissue-culture–derived IIIb variant stock. The resulting antibodies were group specific in precipitation and diagnostic tests. Initially, however, type-specific NA was observed as the predominant response. With time, a strong group-specific NA became detectable that even improved in titer between 1 and 2 years after infection. The serum from these animals readily neutralized five of the divergent prototypes used.[73] Additionally, the ACC pattern in all infected chimpanzees was also group specific. To determine whether this might have been due to the evolution of significantly altered variants with time, the virus was reisolated from the chronically infected chimpanzees over 2 years after infection. Using highly specific two-dimensional chymotryptic maps, it was shown that the reisolated virus was the IIIb variant and that only very minor changes were observed in the gp120 protein structure.[73] These findings imply that induction of a group-specific response may be feasible by using materials from a single HIV variant in man as well.

The determinants that induce this strong group-specific NA are currently being identified. A number of possibilities could be considered (Table 6-4). A major possibility is that the presentation of the antigen, for example, on an infected cell, may be critical. Tactics such as using HIV-infected cell membrane fractions may be useful. (A reasonably functional veterinary vaccine in current use employs the retroviral FeLV-infected cell membrane fraction, which does give a broadly protective response in the field.[9]) The variety of feasible adjuvants should be explored to determine whether some of these may be more conducive in eliciting a broad response. The search for the group-specific NA-inducing epitope could take many tacks; among the more obvious is the induction of antibody specific for the common CD4a cellular attachment site of the gp120 of the virus. A more thorough analysis could involve a sequential search of peptides defined by overlaps to determine which induce a broader antibody response. Whether such specific epitopes exist as single entities or are defined by a saturation of multiple contiguous three-dimensional sites will become more clear with time.

ANIMAL MODELS USEFUL TO DETERMINE PROTECTIVE CAPACITY OF HIV VACCINES

Chimpanzee is the only species that can readily be infected with several of the HIV strains tested.[74,75] Dozens of animals have been readily infected by various routes. Only several hundred animals may be available for vaccine purposes worldwide. Recently a species of gibbon (*Hylobates lar*) has also been infected, but that species is also as scarce as or even scarcer than the chimpanzee.* It is clear from the foregoing that, first, challenge experiments with HIV *in vivo* in chimpanzees will have to be carefully selected and second, the chimpanzee is not a perfect model for human AIDS. No chimpanzee, including those followed for about 3 years, has come down with clinical AIDS. At most, lymphadenopathy was observed in a rare animal, but this regressed spontaneously.[74] Currently, examination of chimpanzee T4 cells and T4/T8 ratios in several of the animals infected for several years are within normal (i.e., uninfected) animal range.[62]

On the other hand, one of the most significant features is that this species is acutely sensitive to primary infection with HIV. An assessment of an HIV-IIIb stock designated as a "pool" for *in vivo* challenge studies was performed to compare tissue culture infectious units by various assays using human cells and the *in vivo* dose capable of infecting 50% of the animals (ID_{50}). Although only a small number of animals could be used, it was remarkable that only about four tissue culture infectious doses equaled an ID_{50} in the chimpanzee. Furthermore, in all animals destined to become infected, the longest it took to detect seroconversion or to isolate virus was 6 weeks; the majority of animals scored positive by 4 weeks.† Thus, by determining the outcome as primary infection or no infection, the relatively shorter hiatus would be very advantageous in that long multi-year terms necessary to evaluate human AIDS in a vaccine trial could be avoided if an analogous endpoint could be considered in humans (see below).

* Gallo R: Personal communication.
† Arthur L: Unpublished data.

A comparable analysis of infected humans and chimpanzees shows many similarities and a few salient differences. Initially, after infection reactive antibodies can generally be observed against all the HIV proteins in both species. There is considerable variability in man as to the strength of response to some HIV antigens.[36,37,39] A notable and unfavorable sign in man is the loss of the anti-p24 protein antibody that is associated with resurgent p24 antigenemia.[76] This has not been observed in the infected chimpanzee. A second comparable response in the two species is the induction of neutralizing antibodies. In all the chimpanzees so tested, a strong group-specific NA has been observed.[73] In man the group-specific response does exist, but there is variability in that better neutralization of some virus strains occurs preferentially.[72] HIV can be readily isolated from both species despite the presence of neutralizing antibody.[69,73] It may be notable that virus isolation is easily achieved by co-cultivation of infected cells of both species. Cell free virus in man was initially documented by infectivity of Factor VIII preparations. Limited attempts in the chimpanzee have not yielded evidence for the isolation of cell-free HIV from sera or plasma in animals from which virus was isolated by cell co-cultivation.[73]

In several other retrovirus systems as well, much of the virus is so cell associated that only allogeneic stimulation induces the retrovirus to express viral messenger RNA and its proteins, presumably the targets the immune system could attack.[77] Because it has been speculated that HIV infection can occur by transmucosal membrane passage of infected cells, it was considered important to determine whether specific mechanisms designed for the induction of infected cell killing occur in HIV-infected chimpanzees. As described above, both ACC and ADCC acting in a group-specific fashion are found in infected chimpanzees.[39,64] Because ACC was not found in infected humans, the ACC response represents the only significant currently known difference in infected but clinically asymptomatic individuals of the two species. The major similarities and differences between infected humans and chimpanzees are listed in Table 6-5.

With the advent of indigenous viruses in African green monkeys and sooty mangabey termed *simian T-cell lymphotrophic virus (STLV-III)* or *simian immune deficiency virus (SIV)*, which resemble HIV closely in genomic organization and partially by sequence analysis, a search ensued for an animal model in which both infection and disease are observable. Neither of the two species in which this virus was found in nature appear to suffer any ill effects.[78,79] STLV-III or SIV was actually first described as occurring spontaneously in macaques that suffered lymphomas and immune deficiencies.[80] However, one has to differentiate further from a very analogous simian AIDS-like disease in rhesus monkeys held in several primate centers that appears to be caused by a D type retrovirus, which is quite different from the HIV-SIV large familial grouping that more closely resemble the lentiviruses in genomic information and organization.[11] Conventional wisdom has it that the disease

Table 6-5
Similarities and Differences of Immunologic Responses in HIV-Infected Humans and Chimpanzees

Test	Humans	Chimpanzees
Precipitating antibodies	Respond to all HIV antigens	Respond to all HIV antigens
Neutralizing antibodies	Mostly group specific, variable strength	Group specific, high titer
Antibody- and complement-mediated cytotoxicity	Never observed regardless of clinical status	Found regularly
Antibody-mediated, cell-dependent cytotoxicity	Found in man, related to disease state	Found regularly
Cell-mediated responses	Found in man, depends on test procedures	Found uniformly

in laboratory rhesus monkeys was obtained via a direct transmission in the laboratory setting from the African species to the Asian species.

The disease in the rhesus appears to spread only by animal to animal direct contact which may be analogous to HIV in man. Assessed by laboratory transmission criteria, SIV can cause clinical disease in several months in rhesus monkeys, which has been described in detail.[80] Because this species is not scarce, a model system parallel to HIV could be developed, in which the nature of the vaccine, its preparation and efficacy could all be reasonably predicted if protection could be achieved in SIV-challenged rhesus monkeys. Recently, the sooty mangabey transmission has been achieved via rhesus to the pig-tailed macaque (*M. nemestrina*). Early attempts at further transmission in this species resulted in a fulminant pansystemic disease in the recipients in which death occurred within 2 weeks. Although many pathologic signs are compatible and virus could be recovered by passage, biologic limiting dilution isolation must be performed to establish clear and direct causality in the absence of adventitious agents responsible for a contribution to this very rapid disease.* Needless to say, should the *M. nemestrina* model prove to be caused directly by SIV, this could be viewed as an almost ideal parallel model to human HIV infection, which results in AIDS. In this species, a rapid prevention of clinical disease could be considered a measure of efficacy for a vaccine preparation.

CHALLENGE EXPERIMENTS WITH INFECTIOUS HIV

The scarcity of the chimpanzee as a research resource would dictate that only critical experiments be carried out in this species. The animals currently the first to be used are those that have been previously infected with human hepatitis A, B, and non-A, non-B (NANB) viruses.

* McClure H et al: Unpublished data.

Because of the uncertain infectious status for man of NANB-infected animals, these already have to be contained. In the case of AIDS experimentation, preinfection with these human viruses could not be a detriment, since in the current largest risk group in the United States, homosexual males, there is a high percentage of individuals exposed to human hepatitis viruses, unlike the rest of the U.S. population.

With the existence of a chimpanzee-titered pool of the HIV challenge virus one could estimate the dose that infects 100% of the animals and any additional multiples of that dose. The level of response to immunization by native or genetically engineered products of the HIV envelope gene as measured by NA has been either undetectable or moderate in this species and in all cases highly type specific.[62,81] ACC or ADCC levels have been very low to undetectable, but some cell-mediated responses have been observed.[62,81] The levels of response were presumably low because of the suboptimal levels of the immunogen gp120, which was not available in greater amounts. Which of these responses is more or less indicative of protection is at present unknown because there is no known state of immunity in the human that could be predictive. Several elements would appear to be of initial importance in challenge experiments: (1) The type of challenge virus should be the one exactly homologous to the type of proteins derived from the immunizing strain because tissue culture assays indicate that a heterologous strain would not be inactivated. Should the challenge with homologous HIV be withstood, then a subsequent challenge with heterologous virus would be indicated. (2) The titer of challenge virus can be adjusted to compensate for the presently observed low level of immune responses. One of the criteria for quantification would be to assess the homologous virus surviving fraction *in vitro* in the presence of the animals' serum and then adjust the minimum challenge dose so that there is still a 100% infection if the vaccine is not protective. This is now possible to assess with at least one challenge HIV, the IIIb, which is being assessed for *in vivo* infectivity. (3) The infectious inoculum would initially be cell-free virus injected intravenously, but later alternative routes of infection and use of human or chimpanzee infected cells would also be relevant.

Several groups have now reported on the outcome of HIV challenge experiments in the vaccinated chimpanzees. One of them made use of the animals inoculated with the infectious vaccinia recombinant virus vector containing the entire LAV-1 envelope gene.[81] Neutralizing antibody responses were essentially unobservable, although evidence of cellular immunity was present. The animals were challenged with high titers of LAV-1, the infectious potential of which was high for this species but never quantitated precisely. The challenge virus readily infected both vaccinated animals. Evidence of priming by the vaccinia-vector–derived HIV *env* gene products was clear because after infection there was a rapid rise of broadly specific neutralizing antibody.[81]

The second set of challenge experiments was performed in two chimpanzees immunized four times with native IIIb gp120. The challenge dose was the 100% infectious dose in one animal and ten times that dose in the other. Based on HIV surviving fraction analysis it appeared that about 99% of the homologous incoming challenge virus would be neutralized. The first response in both animals was an anamnestic response of the NA to high levels and a much broadened group specificity, unlike the type specificity observed prior to challenge. Virus was isolated from both animals by 6 weeks. Initially, a small delay was seen in the lower-dose–infected animal, but reverse transcriptase activity was found readily thereafter. Additional isolations of HIV confirmed the infection. At that time, group-specific ADCC also occurred in both animals. It appeared initially that the level of immune response was inadequate for protection even with the homologous virus type. However, when the type-specific neutralization spectrum of the recovered virus was analyzed in more detail, the early virus recovered from the two vaccinated animals appeared much less susceptible to neutralization by standard anti-HIV-IIIb typing serum. Thus, it appears likely that infection with the predominant HIV type in the stock was prevented, but that either preexisting variants or rapidly appearing mutants were able to overcome the initial levels of defense.* Retrospectively, this is not surprising because the IIIb stock of HIV is a composite of viral genome and recently even the otherwise closely related HXB2 and HXB3 infectious proviral DNA clones derived from the IIIb stock were found to be much less susceptible to standard neutralizing sera prepared against the IIIb stock, whose main species of glycoprotein appears to be from the BH-10 clone.†

Thus, several important guidelines derive from these experiments. HIV stocks may be admixtures of mutants and variants some of which may be genomically

* Fischinger PJ et al: Unpublished data.
† Wong–Staal F et al: Personal communication.

masked and some of which may have variant envelopes. The quest for inducing a true group-specific response seems to be all the more important. The ability of a single species of HIV to induce a true group-specific NA and the existence of broadly specific cell-mediated response all augur well for the generation of such responses prior to subsequent challenge experiments.[65,68,73]

MULTIPLE PERMUTATIONS IN VACCINE PROTOCOLS ARE NECESSARY

The initial problems lie in the numbers of choices that have to be considered. A series of permutations can be considered as matrices defined as products of multiple choices. For example, after selecting an antigen and its configuration one has to think of the routes of immunization, antigen dosage, and the times of inoculation for initial as well as booster immunizations. So far, the levels of response have been low, suggesting the need for adjuvants other than alum that could be more potent and could elicit a spectrum of responses broader than those observed.

After immunization a series of immune responses can be assessed. The accentuation of one or more of these may be relevant to the perception of what responses would best reflect protective immunity. Usually initial experiments are performed in lower species to test for safety and immunoreactivity. In terms of response assessment, immunizations can proceed until a significant level of humoral and/or cellular immunity are observed. However, responses in lower species may or may not be relevant to the outcome of challenge in higher species such as chimpanzees or man.

The challenge matrix can be considered only in terms of the chimpanzee to determine whether prevention of primary infection could be achieved. Whether immunization in man could protect against disease but not against infection, at whatever portal of entry, cannot be determined in the chimpanzee. The rapid jump in titer and the broadening of the specificity of neutralizing antibody may suggest that primary inoculation by a gp120 vaccine could be of benefit in man. However, an alternate animal model using SIV may be helpful. HIV and SIV clearly belong to the same larger retroviral subgroup, and the existence of an intermediately related human pathogen, HIV-2 suggests that vaccine studies in monkeys may be useful. Although SIV is not pathogenic in the species of origin such as the African green monkey, SIV infection in macaques does lead to full blown AIDS-like disease.[80] Accordingly, parallel studies are being initiated to ascertain whether a preparation of SIV for any of the proposed vaccine formats could actually protect from disease.

In the chimpanzee model, the number of animals worldwide is extremely limited, so that particular care has to be taken that nothing is tested but the preparations that proved most promising had been pretested in lower primates. The difficulty is all the more acute because the many HIV types that can be considered to challenge should be previously titered in the same species to establish doses of challenge virus commensurate with the level of immunity. Besides the variability of timing and the routes of challenge, (e.g., intravenous, oral, anal, vaginal), one also has to consider the possibility that under field conditions virus-carrying human cells rather than free virus may represent the actual source of infection. Accordingly, challenges could be considered with various acutely or chronically infected cells again using at least several HIV variants. This enumeration of possibilities suggests that the number of permutations may be in the order of thousands and may thus easily exceed by a factor of several times all the chimpanzees available worldwide for research.

DECISION SWITCH POINTS

Table 6-6 presents a tentative schema of what could be attempted if there is a failure to protect a species from primary HIV infection. If humoral or cellular levels of immunity were relatively low, then a higher antigen dose with better adjuvants could be attempted. The presentation format could be critical and alternatives of the same antigen in micelles, "rosettes," and membrane fractions could be more efficacious. Different inoculation routes and schedules may be useful. Peptides containing T-cell epitopes could be added with the standard immunogen to boost immunity; alternatively, the use of artificial constructs linking B-cell epitopes together with multiple T-cell epitopes could make for a more potent preparation, with higher recall and more long-lasting immunity. One possibility may be that some HIV variants might be intrinsically more prone to expose the group-specific neutralizing epitopes and might accordingly induce a broader state immunity.[32] Many others alternate ways of improving a given product of choice such as

gp120. Protection versus homologous, but not heterologous, variants would present an additional challenge. However, should a given preparation again fail to protect from minimal challenge dose, even with homologous HIV type, then one should consider switching to the next most promising preparation.

DIRECTIONS

As our understanding of the virology of HIV and of the pathogenesis of its infection increases, more significant approaches can be launched in the area of AIDS vaccines. The most salient contribution of modern science has been the ability to engineer and express literally every protein and peptide of HIV. As cloning is completed for any new variant, its regions of disparity can be analyzed and the products compared. Although the number of choices are currently large, the availability of reagents is not expected to be a limiting feature. Based on present conventional wisdom, the most promising proteins and glycoproteins of HIV are being tested, and at least several of these are now at the level of trials in man.

There are two possible levels of outcome if a given vaccine proves efficacious. If primary infection with HIV could be unequivocally prevented in man by a vaccine, then further steps to larger-scale efficacy testing would be rapid. If prevention of infection is not feasible but prevention of disease would occur, the time plan for the development of a vaccine would have to span a number of years because of the length of time between exposure and disease. In the latter case multiple trials might be initiated to produce a better preparation that could prevent the primary HIV infection. This biphasic approach may run concurrently.

Many technical and ethical considerations are relevant but fall outside the scope of this discussion. One major feature that can complicate all AIDS vaccine trials is that both the vaccinees and their controls have to be instructed not to practice high-risk behavior because the efficacy of any preparation will be unknown. However, in this disease it will be easy for the vaccinees to distinguish themselves from controls by various forms of tests available now and in the future. This may modify the behavior in each group as to the propensity of practices that lead to infection. If a vaccine is imperfect, even long-term results could be very ambiguous. Despite these caveats, the panoply of available testing materials, and the astoundingly rapid pace of new information argue well for the rapid development of a safe and effective vaccine against AIDS.

Table 6-6
Preparation "Switch Points"

Failure of Protection
  Prep: Priority n

Intermediate Modes
1. Increase titer
2. Increase CMI
3. Alter presentation
4. Change adjuvants
5. Add T cell epitopes, etc.
6. Alternative HIVs

Retest for Protection
  Minimal homologous type HIV
  Failure: Switch n + 1   Success: IND
                           Human Phase I Trials

REFERENCES

1. Fischinger PJ, Robey WG, Koprowski H et al: Current status and strategies for vaccines against diseases induced by human T-cell lymphotropic retroviruses (HTLV I, II and III). Cancer Res [Suppl]45:4694s, 1985

2. Gallo RC, Fischinger PJ, Bolognesi DP: Vaccine strategies against the human retroviruses associated with AIDS. In Goldman JM, Jarrett JO (eds): Mechanisms of Viral Leukaemogenesis, Chap 6, p 89. London, Churchill Livingston, 1985

3. Fischinger PJ, Gallo RC, Bolognesi DP: Towards a vaccine against AIDS: Rationale and current progress. Mt Sinai J Med (NY) 53:639, 1986

4. Jarrett WFH: The development of vaccines against feline leukemia. In Origins of Human Cancer, p 1215. New York, Cold Spring Harbor Laboratory, 1977

5. Schafer W, Bolognesi DP: Mammalian C-type oncornaviruses: Relationships between viral structural and cell surface antigens and their possible significance in immunological defense mechanisms. Contemp Top Immunol 6: 127, 1977

6. Hunsmann G, Moennig V, Schafer W: Properties of mouse leukemia viruses. IX. Active and passive immunization of mice against Friend leukemia with isolated viral GP71 glycoprotein and its corresponding antiserum. Virology 66: 327, 1975

7. Hunsmann G, Schneider J, Schulz A: Immunoprevention of Friend virus-induced erythroleukemia by vaccination with viral envelope glycoprotein complexes. Virology 113: 602, 1981

8. Hunsmann G, Pedersen NC, Theilen GH et al: Active immunization with feline leukemia virus envelope glycoprotein suppresses growth of virus-induced feline sarcoma. Immunology 171:233, 1983

9. Lewis MG, Mates LE, Olson RG: Protection against feline leukaemia by vaccination with a subunit vaccine. Infect Immun 34:888, 1981

10. Osterhaus A, Weijer K, Uytdehaag F et al: Induction of protective immune response in cats by vaccination with feline leukemia virus iscom. J Immunol 135:591, 1985

11. Marx PA, Pedersen N, Lerche N et al: Prevention of simian acquired immune deficiency syndrome with a formalin inactivated type D virus vaccine. J Virol 60:431, 1986

12. Fisher AG, Ratner L, Mitsuya H et al: Infectious mutants of HTLV-III with changes in the 3′ region and markedly reduced cytopathic effects. Science 233:655, 1986

13. Olsen RG, Hoover EA, Schaller VP et al: Abrogation of resistance to feline oncornavirus disease by immunization with killed feline leukemia virus. Cancer Res 37:2082, 1977

14. Henderson LE, Sowder R, Copeland TD et al: Direct identification of class II histocompatibility DR proteins in preparations of human T-cell lymphotropic virus type III. J Virol 61:629, 1987

15. Willey RL, Smith DH, Laskey LA et al: In vitro mutagenesis identifies a region within the envelope gene of the human immunodeficiency virus that is critical for infectivity. J Virol (Submitted), 1987

16. Hayward W, Neel B, Astrin S: Avian leukosis viruses activation of cellular "oncogenes." In Klein G (ed): Advances in viral oncology, p 297. New York, Raven Press, 1982

17. Arya SK, Guo C, Josephs SF et al: Trans-activator gene of human T-lymphotropic virus type III (HTLV-III). Science 229:69, 1985

18. Rosen CA, Sodroski JG, Haseltine WA: The location of cisacting regulatory sequences in the human T-cell lymphotropic virus type III (HTLV-III/LAV) long terminal repeat. Cell 41:813, 1985

19. Dayton AI, Sodroski JG, Rosen CA et al: The trans-activator gene of the human T-cell lymphotropic virus type III is required for replication. Cell 44:941, 1986

20. Fisher AG, Feinberg HB, Josephs SF et al: The trans-activator gene of HTLV-III is essential for virus replication. Nature 320:367, 1986

21. Kan NC, Franchini G, Wong–Staal F et al: Identification of HTLV-III/LAV sor gene product and detection of antibodies in human sera. Science 231:1553, 1986

22. Rosen C, Sodroski JG, Goh WC et al: Post-transcriptional regulation accounts for the trans-activation of the human T-lymphotropic virus type III. Nature 319:555, 1986

23. Sodroski J, Goh WC, Rosen C et al: Replicative and cytopathic potential of HTLV-III/LAV with sor gene deletions. Science 231:1549, 1986

24. Morein B, Helenius A, Simons K et al: Effective subunit vaccines against an enveloped animal virus. Nature (London) 276:715, 1978

25. Morein B, Sundquist B, Hoglund S et al: ISCOM: a novel structure for antigenic presentation of membrane proteins from envelope viruses. Nature 308:457, 1984

26. Kennedy RC, Henkel RD, Pauletti D et al: Antiserum to a synthetic peptide recognizes the HTLV-III envelope glycoprotein. Science 231:1556, 1986

27. Chang TW, Kato I, McKinney S et al: Detection of antibodies to human T-cell lymphotropic virus III (HTLV-III) with immunoassay employing a recombinant Escherichia coli derived viral antigenic peptide. Biotechnology 3:905, 1985

28. Palker TJ, Matthews TJ, Clark ME et al: A conserved region at the COOH terminus of the human immune deficiency virus gp120 envelope protein contains an immunodominant epitope. Proc Natl Acad Sci USA 84:2479, 1987

29. Cease KB, Margalit H, Cornette JL et al: Helper T-cell antigenic site identification in the acquired immunodeficiency syndrome virus gp120 envelope protein and induction of immunity in mice to the native protein using a 16-residue synthetic peptide. Proc Natl Acad Sci USA 84: 4249, 1987

30. Paoletti E, Lipinskas BR, Samsonoff C et al: Construction of live vaccines using genetically engineered poxviruses. Biological activity of vaccinia virus recombinants expressing the hepatitis B virus surface antigen and the herpes simplex virus glycoprotein D. Proc Natl Acad Sci USA 81: 193, 1984

31. Mackett M, Smith GL, Moss B: Vaccinia virus: A selectable eukaryotic cloning and expression vector. Proc Natl Acad Sci USA 79:7415, 1982

32. Perkus ME, Piccini A, Lipinskas BR et al: Recombinant vaccinia virus: immunization against multiple pathogens. Science 229:981, 1985

33. Chakrabarti S, Robert–Guroff M, Wong–Staal F et al: Expression of the HTLV-III envelope gene by a recombinant vaccinia virus. Nature (London) 320:535, 1986

34. Hu S–L, Kosowski SG, Dalrymple JM: Expression of AIDS virus envelope gene in recombinant vaccinia viruses. Nature (London) 320:537, 1986

35. Koprowski H: Unconventional vaccines: Immunization with anti-idiotype antibody against viral disease. Cancer Res [Suppl] 45:4689s, 1985

36. Robey WG, Safai B, Oroszlan S et al: Characterization of envelope and core structural gene products of HTLV-III with sera from AIDS patients. Science 228:593, 1985

37. Robey WG, Arthur LO, Matthews TJ et al: Prospects for prevention of human immunodeficiency virus infection: Purified 120-KDA envelope glycoprotein induces neutralizing antibodies. Proc Natl Acad Sci USA 83:7023, 1986

38. Matthews TJ, Langlois AJ, Robey WG et al: Restricted neu-

tralization of divergent HTLV-III/LAV isolates by antibodies to the major envelope glycoprotein. Proc Natl Acad Sci USA 83:9709, 1986

39. Nara PL, Robey WG, Gonda MA et al: Absence of cytotoxic antibody to HTLV-III-infected cells in man and its induction in animals after infection or immunization with purified gp120. Proc Natl Acad Sci USA 84:3797, 1987

40. Lyerly HK, Matthews TJ, Langlois AJ et al: Human T-cell lymphotropic virus IIIB glycoprotein (gp120) bound to CD determinants on normal lymphocytes and expressed by infected cells serves as a target for immune attack. Proc Natl Acad Sci USA 84:4601, 1987

41. Yewdell JW, Bennink JR, Smith GL et al: Influenza A virus nucleoprotein is a major target antigen for cross-reactive anti-influenza A virus cytotoxic T lymphocytes. Proc Natl Acad Sci USA 82:1780, 1985

42. Townsend ARM, Gotch FM, Davey J. Cytotoxic T cells recognize fragments of the influenza nucleoprotein. Cell 42:457, 1985

43. Schwarz H, Hunsmann G, Moennig V et al: Properties of mouse leukemia viruses. XII. Immunoelectron microscopic studies on viral structural antigens on the cell surface. Virology 69:169, 1976.

44. Grant JP, Bigner DD, Fischinger PJ et al: Expression of murine leukemia-virus structural antigens on surface of chemically-induced murine sarcomas. Proc Natl Acad Sci USA 71:5037, 1974

45. Ihle JN, Lee JC, Hanna MG Jr: Characterization of natural antibodies in mice to endogenous leukaemia virus. In Yuhan JM, Tennant RW, Regan JD (eds): The biology of radiation carcinogenesis, p 261. New York, Raven Press, 1976

46. Sarin PS, Sun DK, Thornton AH et al: Neutralization of HTLV-III/LAV replication by antiserum to thymosin α_1. Science 232:1135, 1986

47. Elder JH, McGee JS, Alexander S: Carbohydrate side chains of Rauscher leukaemia virus envelope glycoproteins are not required to elicit a neutralizing antibody response. J Virol 57:340, 1985

48. Schafer W, Fischinger PJ, Collins JJ et al: Role of carbohydrate in biological functions of Friend murine leukaemia virus gp71. J Virol 22:35, 1977

49. Pierotti M, Deleo AB, Pinter A et al: The GIX antigen of murine leukemia virus: An analysis with monoclonal antibodies. Virology 112:450, 1981

50. Putney SD, Matthews TJ, Robey WG et al: HTLV-III/LAV-neutralizing antibodies to an E. coli-produced fragment of the virus envelope. Science 234:1392, 1986

51. Laskey LA, Groopman JE, Fennie CW et al: Neutralization of the AIDS retrovirus by antibodies to a recombinant envelope glycoprotein. Science 233:209, 1986

52. Rusche JR, Lynn DL, Robert-Guroff M et al: Humoral immune response to the entire human immunodeficiency virus envelope glycoprotein made in insect cells. Proc Natl Acad Sci USA (in press), 1987

53. Bolognesi DP, Bauer H, Gelderblom H et al: Polypeptides of avian RNA tumor viruses. IV. Components of the viral envelope. Virology 47:551, 1972

54. Bolognesi DP, Montelaro RC, Frank H: Assembly of type C oncornaviruses: A model. Science 199:183, 1978

55. Hahn BH, Gonda MA, Shaw GM et al: Genomic diversity of acquired immune deficiency syndrome virus HTLV-III: Different viruses exhibit greatest divergence in their envelope genes. Proc Natl Acad Sci USA 82:4813, 1985

56. Starich BR, Hahn BH, Shaw GM et al: Identification and characterization of conserved and variable regions in the envelope gene of HTLV-III/LAV, the retrovirus of AIDS. Cell 45:637, 1986

57. Hahn BH, Shaw GM, Taylor ME et al: Genetic variation in HTLV-III/LAV over time in patients with AIDS or at risk for AIDS. Science 232:1548, 1986

58. Fischinger PJ: Molecular mechanisms of leukemogenesis by murine leukemia viruses. In Goldman JM, Jarrett O (eds): Leukemia and Lymphoma Research, Vol 1, p 89. London, 1984

59. Gonda MA, Wong-Staal F, Gallo RC et al: Sequence of homologous and morphologic similarity of HTLV-III and visna virus, a pathogenic lentivirus. Science 227:173, 1985

60. Payne S, Fang FD, Liu CP et al: Antigenic variation and lentivirus persistence: Variation in envelope gene sequences during EIAV infection resemble changes reported for sequential isolates of HIV. Virology (in press), 1987

61. Fischinger PJ, Blevins CS, Dunlop NM: Genomic masking of nondefective recombinant murine leukemia virus in Moloney virus stocks. Science 201:457, 1975

62. Arthur LO, Pyle SW, Nara PL et al: Serological responses in chimpanzees inoculated with a potential human immunodeficiency virus subunit vaccine. Proc Natl Acad Sci USA (in press), 1987

63. Kowalski M, Potz J, Basirpour L et al: Functional regions of the envelope glycoprotein of human immunodeficiency virus type I. Science 236:1351, 1987

64. Weinhold KJ, Lyerly HK, Matthews TJ et al: Cellular anti-gp120 cytolytic reactivities in HIV seropositive individuals. Nature (Submitted), 1987

65. Zarling JM, Morton W, Moran PA et al: T-cell responses to human AIDS virus in macaques immunized with recombinant vaccinia virus. Nature 323:344, 1986

66. Walker BD, Chakrabarti S, Moss B et al: HIV-specific cytotoxic T lymphocytes in seropositive individuals. Nature 328:345, 1987

67. Plata F, Autran B, Martins LP et al: AIDS virus-specific cytotoxic T lymphocytes in lung disorders. Nature 328:348, 1987

68. Krohn K, Robey WG, Putney S et al: HIV specific cellular immune response and neutralizing antibodies in goats immunized with native or recombinant envelope proteins derived from HTLV-IIIB, and in HIV infected men. Proc Natl Acad Sci USA 84:4994, 1987

69. Robert-Guroff M, Brown M, Gallo RC: HTLV-III-neutralizing antibodies in patients with AIDS and AIDS-related complex. Nature 316:72, 1985

70. Fischinger PG, Schafer W, Bolognesi DP: Neutralization of homologous and heterologous oncornaviruses by antisera against the p15(E) and gp71 polypeptides of Friend murine leukemia virus. Virology 71:169, 1976

71. Fischinger PJ, Dunlop NM, Schwarz H et al: Properties in mouse leukemia viruses. XVIII. Effective treatment of AKR leukemia with antibody to gp71 eliminates the neonatal burst of ecotropic AKR virus producing cells. Virology 119:68, 1982

72. Weiss RA, Clapham PR, Weber JN et al: Variable and conserved neutralization antigens of human immunodeficiency virus. Nature 324:572, 1986

73. Nara PL, Robey WG, Arthur LO et al: Persistent infection of chimpanzees with human immunodeficiency virus (HIV): Serological responses and properties of reisolated viruses. J Virol 61:3173, 1987

74. Alter HJ, Eichberg JW, Masur H et al: Transmission of HTLVIII infection from human plasma to chimpanzees, an animal model for AIDS. Science 226:549, 1984

75. Fultz PN, McClure HM, Swenson CR et al: Persistent infection of chimpanzees with human T-lymphotropic virus type III/lymphadenopathy associated virus: A potential model for acquired immunodeficiency syndrome. J Virol 58:116, 1986

76. Pedersen C, Nielsen CM, Vestergaard BF et al: Temporal relationship of antigenemia and loss of antibodies to core antigens to development of clinical disease in HIV infection. Br Med J 316:567, 1987

77. Burny A, Bruck C, Chantrenne H et al: Bovine leukemia virus: Molecular biology and epidemiology. In Klein G (ed): Viral oncology, p 231. New York, Raven Press, 1980

78. Kanki PJ, Alroy J, Essex M. Isolation of T-lymphotropic retrovirus related to HTLV-III/LAV from wild-caught African green monkeys. Science 230:951, 1985

79. Murphey–Corb M, Martin LN, Rangan SRS et al: Isolation of an HTLV-III-related retrovirus from macaques with simian AIDS and its possible origin in asymptomatic mangabeys. Nature 321:435, 1986

80. Letvin NL, Daniel MD, Sehgal PK et al: Induction of AIDS-like disease in macaque monkeys with T-cell tropic retrovirus STLV-III. Science 230:71, 1985

81. Hu SL, Fultz PN, McClure HM et al: Effect of immunization with a vaccinia-HIV *env* recombinant on HIV infection of chimpanzees. Nature (in press), 1987

PART II

Clinical Aspects

Clinical Aspects of Infection with AIDS Retrovirus: Acute HIV Infection, Persistent Generalized Lymphadenopathy, and AIDS-Related Complex

Robert Yarchoan
James M. Pluda

7

In 1981, a number of young adults in coastal cities of the United States were observed to have developed either unusual opportunistic infections or a hitherto rare skin cancer, Kaposi's sarcoma.[1-4] The infections in these young adults had previously been found only in immunosuppressed patients, and indeed, these individuals were observed to have severe depression of their cellular immunity.[1-3] Also, nearly all the patients in whom these disease manifestations were initially found were noted either to have used intravenous drugs or to have had homosexual contacts. The patients with these disease manifestations generally fared poorly, and many died within months. These developments could not be easily explained by any known disease, and the clinical, epidemiologic, and immunologic information available suggested that this represented a new disorder now known as acquired immunodeficiency syndrome (AIDS).[1-4]

This term was initially used to denote patients with any of a number of characteristic opportunistic infections or with Kaposi's sarcoma (as long as other causes of immunodeficiency were excluded and, in the case of Kaposi's sarcoma, the patient was under 60 years of age).[5] This definition, which was established by the Centers for Disease Control and underwent several minor modifications over the next several years,[6] was especially useful from an epidemiologic point of view as patients meeting the criteria formed a rather distinct group. It was soon recognized, however, that a number of individuals in the same risk groups (i.e., homosexuals or intravenous drug users) had generalized lymphadenopathy, fevers, night sweats, or malaise and that many had a decrease in their ratio of helper/suppressor ($CD4^+/CD8^+$) T cells.[7,8] There was initially some un-

certainty as to whether these findings represented an earlier manifestation of the same disease process or were rather the result of other infections resulting from these same high-risk behaviors. It gradually became apparent, however, that some of these patients went on to develop AIDS and that generalized lymphadenopathy or AIDS-related complex, terms used to describe these less severe syndromes, were manifestations of the same disease process as AIDS. It was also observed that some patients in the same risk groups developed other disorders with increased frequency such as high-grade B-cell lymphomas, other malignancies, and less characteristic opportunistic infections.[7,9,10]

In 1983, a novel T-cell tropic retrovirus, now termed human immunodeficiency virus (HIV), was isolated from a patient with lymphadenopathy syndrome by Barré–Sinoussi and co-workers.[11] Several months later, Gallo and colleagues reported the isolation and propagation of similar viruses from a number of patients with AIDS or AIDS-related complex (ARC) and the finding that nearly every patient with AIDS or AIDS-related complex had detectable antibodies to this virus.[12-14] The ability to identify persons infected with HIV proved useful in appreciating the clinical spectrum of infection with this agent. It is now recognized that HIV can (either directly or indirectly) affect nearly every organ system in the body and that a wide range of clinical manifestations can result from infection with this agent. Some of these appear to result directly from infection with the virus while others may result from the altered immune function in infected patients and the resulting opportunistic infections or change in normal flora. In this chapter, we will provide an overview of the clinical presentations of HIV infection. In particular, we will detail some of the early and less severe disease manifestations, including acute HIV infection, persistent generalized lymphadenopathy, and ARC. This chapter will also serve as an introduction to subsequent chapters in this section which will cover certain manifestations of HIV infection in greater detail.

CLASSIFICATION OF HIV-ASSOCIATED DISEASE

As noted above, it has become clear over the past several years that HIV can cause a wide spectrum of clinical disease, ranging from acute infection to an asymptomatic state to severe immunodeficiency with chronic infections and wasting. The term *AIDS* has been used to describe the more severe manifestations of this disorder, particularly opportunistic infections and unusual tumors associated with the immunodeficiency (for the most recent surveillance definition of AIDS as proposed by the Centers for Disease Control, see reference 15). However, study of the less advanced forms of HIV infection has been somewhat impeded by the lack of similar uniform definitions. In general, the term *persistent generalized lymphadenopathy* (*PGL*) has been used to denote a relatively healthy group of patients with lymphadenopathy (lymph nodes greater than 1 cm) found at two or more extrainguinal sites for 3 or more months, while the term *AIDS-related complex* (ARC) has generally been applied to patients who have constitutional signs such as weight loss, fevers, night sweats, or infections that did not define the patient as having AIDS. However, these terms have been used differently by different authors, causing a certain amount of confusion in the literature.

In the past couple of years, two classification schemes have been developed for patients with HIV infection that have attempted to encompass both patients with AIDS and those with less severe HIV infection. One of these, proposed by the Centers for Disease Control, divides patients into four main groups and a number of subgroups (Table 7-1).[16] A patient in this system is viewed as being in only one group, and the four major groups are viewed as being temporally hierarchial; that is, if a patient is classified in a group, he would not move into a lower numbered group if the symptoms resolved. However, within group IV, a patient may be classified in one or more subgroups. Some physicians have been bothered because the groups do not correlate with generally used designations of AIDS or ARC; patients with AIDS, for example, may be included in several of the subgroups of group IV, while only category C-1 in subgroup C will be composed exclusively of AIDS patients. However, it has been useful as a general clinical classification scheme.

Another classification scheme for patients with HIV infection has been proposed by researchers at the Walter Reed Army Institute of Research (Table 7-2).[17] In this scheme, HIV-infected patients are divided into one of six stages that define increasingly compromised laboratory or clinical immune function. In addition, certain other clinical parameters are designated by the addition of letters after the stage (fevers, weight loss, or diarrhea by the letter *B;* Kaposi's sarcoma by the letter *K;* HIV-induced neurologic disease by the letters *CNS;* and neoplasms other than Kaposi's sarcoma by the letter *N*). Thus, a patient with thrush, no AIDS-defining oppor-

Table 7-1
Centers for Disease Control Classification Schema for HIV Infection

Group I.   Acute HIV infection
Group II. Asymptomatic HIV infection
Group III. Persistent generalized lymphadenopathy (PGL). Lymphadenopathy (>1 cm diameter) at 2 or more extra-inguinal sites lasting more than 3 months without another condition to explain the findings.
Group IV. Other HIV Disease
  Subgroup A: Constitutional disease. One or more of the following: Fever for >1 month, 10% weight loss, diarrhea lasting <1 month, and no other condition to explain the findings.
  Subgroup B: Neurologic disease. One or more of the following: Dementia, myelopathy, or peripheral neuropathy, and no other condition to explain the findings.
  Subgroup C: Secondary infectious diseases
    C-1: One of the 12 specified symptomatic or invasive diseases which define AIDS: *Pneumocystis carinii* pneumonia, chronic cryptosporidiosis, toxoplasmosis, extra-intestinal strongyloidiasis, isoporiasis, candidiasis (esophageal, bronchial, or pulmonary), cryptococcosis, histoplasmosis, *Mycobacterium avium* complex or *M. kansasii*, cytomegalovirus, chronic mucocutaneous or disseminated herpes simplex infection, or progressive multifocal leukoencephalopathy.
    C-2: Symptomatic or invasive disease with one of the following: Oral hairy leukoplakia, multidermatomal herpes zoster, recurrent *Salmonella* bacteremia, nocardiosis, tuberculosis, or oral candidiasis
  Subgroup D: Secondary cancers. Diagnosis of one of the following known to be associated with HIV infection: Kaposi's sarcoma, non-Hodgkin's lymphoma (small, non-cleaved lymphoma or immunoblastic sarcoma), or primary lymphoma of the brain
  Subgroup E: Other conditions in HIV infection. Includes a variety of clinical findings which may be attributable to HIV disease, including chronic lymphoid interstitial pneumonitis, constitutional symptoms not meeting subgroup IV-A, patients with infectious diseases not meeting subgroup IV-C, and patients with neoplasms not meeting subgroup IV-D.

(Adapted from Centers for Disease Control: Classification system for human T-lymphotropic virus type III/lymphadenopathy-associated virus infections. MMWR 35:334, 1986)

Table 7-2
The Walter Reed Staging Classification for HIV Infection

Stage	HIV Ab or Virus Isolation	Chronic Lymphadenopathy	CD4+ T Cells (/mm³)	DTH*	Thrush	OI
WR0	−	−	>400	NL*	−	−
WR1	+†	−	>400	NL	−	−
				NL		
WR2	+	+	>400		−	−
WR3	+	+ or −	**<400**	NL	−	−
WR4	+	+ or −	**<400**	**Partial***	−	−
WR5	+	+ or −	**<400**	**Anergy and/or**	+	−
WR6	+	+ or −	**<400**	Partial or anergy	+ or −	+

* DTH, delayed type hypersensitivity; NL, normal; partial, partial anergy (defined as induration of 5 mm or greater to only one of the test antigens tetanus, trichophyton, mumps, and candida).
† The essential criteria for each stage are denoted by bold type.
(Adapted from Redfield RR, Wright CD, Tramont EC: The Walter Reed Staging Classification for HTLV-III/LAV infection. N Engl J Med 314: 131, 1986)

tunistic infections, and Kaposi's sarcoma would be labeled WR5K. Advantages of this classification system are that it can be used to follow the declining immune function that occurs in many patients with HIV infection (in the absence of therapy)[17] and that it can be used to select relatively uniform groups of patients for clinical trials.

ACUTE ILLNESS ASSOCIATED WITH HIV SEROCONVERSION

With this background, we can turn our attention to some of the clinical syndromes associated with HIV infection. During the last several years, it has been recognized that a number of individuals develop a mononucleosis-like illness at the time of their initial infection with HIV. Interestingly, the first reports of an such an acute illness did not appear until 3 years after the initial description of AIDS. In 1984, a patient was reported to develop a transient mononucleosis-like illness after being transfused with blood from a patient who subsequently developed AIDS.[18] Later that year a nurse was reported to develop a transient flu-like illness with lymphadenopathy and a rash 13 days after a needlestick injury from an AIDS patient; 49 days after the needlestick, she developed antibodies to HIV.[19] In 1985, Cooper and others reported a series of 12 patients with a symptom complex that was ascribed to acute infection with HIV.[20] The symptom complex was generally of sudden onset, lasted from 3 to 14 days, and typically consisted of fevers, cutaneous eruptions, myalgias, arthralgias, malaise, lymphadenopathy, sore throat, gastrointestinal symptoms, headache and photophobia. In addition, some patients had weight loss, neurologic symptoms, or elevated serum transaminase levels. Development of antibodies to HIV occurred anywhere from 19 to 56 days after the onset of the illness. There was sometimes se-

vere lymphopenia associated with the acute illness without an inversion in the T-cell helper:suppressor ratio. After resolution of the acute illness, an atypical lymphocytosis developed in some patients in conjunction with a decrease in the helper:suppressor ratio. Interestingly, this ratio changed mostly because of an increase in the number of circulating CD8+ (T8+) lymphocytes, rather than a decrease in CD4+ (T4+) T-cells. This increase in CD8+ lymphocytes is similar to that found in Epstein–Barr virus- or cytomegalovirus-induced mononucleosis.[8]

Later that same year, Ho and colleagues reported a similar illness in several patients.[21] They estimated that symptoms first developed 3 to 6 weeks after the probable exposure to HIV, and that seroconversion occurred at 8 to 12 weeks from exposure. Two of their patients had a lymphocytic meningitis with HIV isolated from the cerebrospinal fluid. Not all patients, however, appear to develop a clinically significant illness at the time of their initial infection; this group and others documented seroconversion in a number of patients who denied having symptoms over the previous 3 months.[21,22] Thus, seroconversion may or may not be associated with a discernable illness.

The rash that occurs during the acute illness is perhaps the most recognizable sign and has been described by a number of authors.[20,21,23–25] It generally consists of a roseola-like rash, occurring mainly on the trunk and limbs. However, it can involve the face, hands, and feet. The rash generally resolves within 2 weeks of onset.[23,24] The erythematous macular eruption can also be associated with a diffuse enanthema of the oral cavity with angular stomatitis.[25] Recently, a distinctive vesiculopapular exanthematous rash has been reported to develop.[26]

As noted above, various neurologic symptoms can be found in conjunction with the acute illness associated with seroconversion. An acute, reversible encephalopathy manifested by altered mentation, personality changes, and even grand mal seizures has been reported.[27] Also, a self-limited aseptic meningitis can be seen with seroconversion that is thought to be a direct effect of HIV infection in the central nervous system.[21,28] One can speculate that the spontaneous remission of such symptoms after several weeks may be related to the development of humoral and/or cellular immunity against HIV in these patients; indeed, several authors have documented a decline in the viral load at the time that antibodies develop.[21,29,30] This finding that the immune response to HIV indeed can reduce the replication of the virus may have implications in the development of a vaccine against HIV and is an area worthy of further research.

Seroconversion can also be associated with peripheral neurologic symptoms including an acute neuropathy or a Guillain–Barré–like syndrome, either during or up to 20 weeks following the acute illness.[31-33] An acute myelopathy with paraparesis and hyperreflexia of the arms, with isolation of HIV from both blood and cerebrospinal fluid, has been reported.[34] Most recently, a case of acute brachial neuritis has been documented.[26]

As additional cases of acute HIV infection have been reported, several other disease manifestations have been identified, including an intensely erythematous pharyngitis, transient leukopenia, and thrombocytopenia.[35] Also, while immunosuppression is not generally felt to be characteristic of acute HIV infection, several researchers have documented transient cutaneous anergy and decreased response to phytohemagglutinin in some patients.[36]

In some patients, antibodies to HIV can be found within 2 weeks after the onset of acute infection; in nearly all cases, they can be detected by two months.[37,38] The first antibody to appear is directed at the *gp160* envelope glycoprotein as measured by radioimmunoprecipitation (RIPA).[38] This technique is, however, quite labor intensive and is not generally used in clinical laboratories. Soon after anti-*gp160* antibody is detectable, antibodies to *p24* can be measured by Western blot; antibodies to *gp120, p15, p55,* and *gp41* appear slightly later.[39,40] Antibodies to HIV as measured by enzyme-linked immunosorbent assay (ELISA) generally do not appear as early as that detected by these more specific assays, and this technique is less useful for making a definitive diagnosis of acute infection.[38]

As noted above, the recognition of a syndrome associated with acute infection with HIV lagged by several years behind the recognition of AIDS as a new illness. In part, the identification of the illness required the ability to measure antibodies against HIV.[14,20] Also, acute HIV infection, if associated with symptoms at all, appears in most instances to be relatively nonspecific in its manifestations. Indeed, this lack of specificity can pose diagnostic problems for physicians confronted with such a patient. Acute HIV infection should be considered in patients who present with an acute febrile mononucle-

osis-like illness, particularly if they are in high-risk groups or have a rash or neurologic symptoms. In regard to making a definitive diagnosis, such patients often do not develop antibodies to HIV for several weeks, and culture of HIV from blood or cerebrospinal fluid is expensive and technically difficult, and is not always successful. Recently, it has been shown that HIV antigen can be detected in serum of patients with acute HIV infection using a capture ELISA before seroconversion occurs.[29,30] Such assays will be invaluable in diagnosing patients with acute HIV infection, and several commercial kits are presently being evaluated by the U.S. Food and Drug Administration for this purpose. It is likely that such assays will be available for clinical use in the near future.

ASYMPTOMATIC HIV INFECTION AND PERSISTENT GENERALIZED LYMPHADENOPATHY

As noted above, there is a wide spectrum of clinical manifestations in patients infected with HIV. In a "prototype" patient, there is a progression from acute illness through an asymptomatic state, through persistent generalized lymphadenopathy, through more symptomatic AIDS-related complex (ARC), and finally to frank AIDS; these changes are associated with a progressive decline in the number of CD4$^+$ T cells. It should be stressed that the time that it takes to progress to frank AIDS may vary considerably, and that at this point, it is not clear that all patients infected with HIV will develop AIDS.[41] Also, in some patients clearly defined intermediate stages can be identified, whereas in others the initial clinical manifestation of HIV infection may be the development of Kaposi's sarcoma or *Pneumocystis carinii* pneumonia.

As noted above, it was recognized even in the early 1980s that a number of persons in risk groups for acquiring AIDS appeared to have generalized lymphadenopathy, and that a number of these persons had a decreased ratio of helper/suppressor T cells.[7,8] It was also appreciated that a certain percentage of these patients went on to develop AIDS,[41-43] and the suggestion was made that this might represent a prodrome of AIDS or a less severe form of the illness. It has since clearly been shown that generalized lymphadenopathy in such patients is associated with HIV infection;[13,14] it is perhaps worth noting that the first reported isolation of HIV was made from a patient with lymphadenopathy.[11]

Persistent generalized lymphadenopathy (PGL) (defined as lymph nodes greater than 1 cm in diameter at two extrainguinal sites persisting for 3 months or longer, not attributable to other causes, and not associated with other substantial constitutional symptoms) is commonly found in patients with early HIV infection.[44,45] The term *lymphadenopathy syndrome* is sometimes used to describe this disorder, and such patients are now classified as being in group III in the

CDC classification (see Table 7-1). In some cases, the lymphadenopathy is first noticed by the patient, whereas in other cases it is first identified during a physical examination.[45,46] It should be stressed that a high percentage of patients with HIV infection have generalized lymphadenopathy; in one large study, for example, 70.9% of HIV-seropositive homosexual or bisexual men without AIDS had lymphadenopathy when examined, and 29% had marked lymphadenopathy (greater than 9 cm total diameter of all lymph nodes).[45] While lymphadenopathy is sometimes found in seronegative men from the same risk groups, the incidence is considerably lower (only 2% had marked lymphadenopathy in the same study[45]), and lymphadenopathy can be considered as being a sign suggestive of HIV infection in this population.

Although lymphadenopathy is very common in patients with HIV infection, it is clear that some patients may be infected without having any signs or symptoms attributable to HIV (group II in the CDC classification). It is perhaps obvious that the incidence of such a clinical state is dependent on how carefully the patient is questioned and examined; for example, in one recent study, over 80% of patients who initially denied symptoms on an initial questionnaire were found to have signs or symptoms of HIV infection after careful study.[46]

Returning to those patients who have evidence of lymphadenopathy, a number of researchers have attempted to elucidate the pathology and pathogenesis of the enlarged nodes.[47-51] In general, the pathology of lymph nodes from such patients are nonspecific, with the most common finding being hyperplastic lymphadenopathy with follicular hyperplasia.[47-51] Patients with more severe disease or frank AIDS generally have follicular depletion (or lymphoid atrophy).[47-51] One group has delineated a spectrum of changes in patients with HIV infection ranging from follicular hyperplasia, to involution with follicular fragmentation, to involution with follicular atrophy;[50] these were viewed as stages progressing to follicular depletion.

Several groups have investigated the subclasses of lymphocytes in nodes from such patients in an attempt to better understand the changes observed on light microscopy.[49,50,52] The most consistent finding is an overall reduction in the number of CD4[+] (helper) lymphocytes in the nodes of such patients, accompanied by an increase in the number of CD8[+] (suppressor-cytotoxic) lymphocytes.[49,50,52] In general, the 4:8 ratio (CD4[+]:CD8[+] ratio) is greater in the lymph nodes than in the peripheral blood, but it is still substantially less than in normal nodes. There has also been observed an increased number of OKT-10[+] plasma cells and aggregates of Leu-6[+] dendritic cells in the nodes of HIV-infected patients. Finally, although there were increased HLA-DR[+] paracortical cells (suggestive of T-cell activation), the number of interleukin-2 receptor positive (TAC[+]) T cells was reduced.[49,50,52] Thus, overall, there appears to be a proliferation of CD8[+] T cells in the nodes of the patients (particularly early in the disease), while later on there is a progressive depletion of all lymphoid elements, particularly CD4[+] (helper) T cells.

Although lymphadenopathy is an early and prominent feature in patients with HIV infection, little HIV can actually be detected in the lymph nodes using available techniques. For example, Shaw and colleagues were able to find HIV using Southern blot hybridization in only 7 of 34 lymph nodes from patients with AIDS or ARC.[53] Using a more sensitive technique, *in situ* hybridization, Biberfeld and co-workers found cells expressing HIV RNA in each of 14 nodes (from HIV-seropositive patients) studied; however, HIV-positive cells were very rare, with only 1 to 10 such cells detected per section.[54] Most of the HIV-expressing cells were found in the follicular regions, which interestingly have relatively few T cells. Finally, Le Tourneau and associates reported the finding of rare HIV-like particles in the nodes from patients with PGL using electron microscopy.[55] Interestingly, such particles were generally found in the extracellular space near the dendritic reticular cells. Taken together, these studies indicate that the lymphadenopathy in patients with HIV infection is a reactive process and is not the result of the majority of cells being infected with HIV. In addition, they provide suggestive evidence that many of the HIV-infected cells in lymph nodes are dendritic cells. This latter finding is consistent with the recent observation by Gartner and others that certain isolates of HIV preferentially replicate in monocyte/macrophages and the suggestion that macrophages may be the initial target cell in patients with HIV infection.[56]

A question posed by many clinicians taking care of AIDS patients is how to define the role of lymph node biopsies in assessing patients with PGL. Several early reports suggested that such biopsies might have value in making the diagnosis of PGL.[51] However, as noted above, the pathologic findings in PGL are nonspecific, and the development of serologic and antigenic assays for the detection of HIV infection has reduced the value of such biopsies.[13,30,48] In the opinion of many clinicians dealing with AIDS patients, such biopsies are most useful for diagnosing lymphoma, Kaposi's sarcoma, or other secondary disorders affecting the lymph node in patients with HIV infection.

AIDS-RELATED COMPLEX

A number of reports in the literature over the past 5 years have detailed a variety of clinical and laboratory abnormalities that accompany patients with HIV-associated lymphadenopathy.[44-46,57] Some of the frequently occurring symptoms in such patients are fatigue, painful lymphadenopathy, skin rash, fevers, diarrhea, muscle pain, night sweats, and weight loss.[44-46,57,58] Also, some patients with HIV infection (but without frank AIDS) develop oral candidiasis, herpes zoster, or other infections suggestive of an impaired immune system but not necessarily life-threatening.[44-46,57,58]

Some patients are minimally affected by these disease manifestations, whereas others are nearly incapacitated, and a number of authors have used the terms *AIDS-related complex (ARC), lesser-AIDS,* or *pre-AIDS* to describe such patients with constitutional symptoms. As noted above, different authors have used these terms differently, causing a certain amount of confusion in the literature. In the recent CDC classification, such patients are included in subgroups A, C-2, or E of Group IV (see Table 7-1). Those with fever persisting more than 1 month, involuntary weight loss of greater than 10% of baseline, or diarrhea lasting more than 1 month and no other condition to explain the findings are assigned to subgroup A. Patients with other secondary infectious diseases are now listed in subgroup C-2, while other patients with other constitutional symptoms are now listed in subgroup E. It is clear from this that the boundary between group III (PGL) and group IV, subgroup E remains somewhat arbitrary, and authors writing clinical descriptions of such patients are encouraged to specify the criteria used to distinguish between these two groups. Also, as an editorial comment, it is perhaps best to avoid the term pre-AIDS for such patients, as it conveys a perhaps unnecessarily pessimistic prognosis.

Patients with asymptomatic HIV infection, PGL, and ARC present with a spectrum of immunologic abnormalities ranging from minimal alterations in the immune system to severe cellular immunodeficiency comparable to those of patients with AIDS and opportunistic infections.[7,8,10,59] Many of the patients who clinically fall into the category of PGL or ARC are anergic.[45] As will be detailed in another chapter in this book, they may also manifest abnormalities of other aspects of their immune systems such as hypergammaglobulinemia, hypersplenism, and sometimes (but not always) a diminution in primary antibody responses.[10,44,60,61] In addition, as will be discussed below, many of these patients have mild anemia, leukopenia, or thrombocytopenia. There is a rough association between the presence of constitutional symptoms and the depression of the immune system in these patients;[44,45] however, some patients with constitutional symptoms have relatively high numbers of CD4[+] T cells,[44] whereas we have seen occasional asymptomatic patients with fewer than 30 CD4[+] cells/mm[3].*

There was initially some uncertainty as to whether PGL (or ARC) was a disease endpoint in itself or could progress to AIDS;[58] however, it has become clear over the past several years that many of the patients who have these disorders will progress to frank AIDS over a 5-year period.[41,43,57] Several research groups have conducted prospective studies of groups of patients with PGL or ARC to determine the incidence of progression to AIDS and the features that were prognostic of disease progression. Although there is not perfect consensus on this point,[62] most authors have found that the absolute number of CD4[+] T cells/mm[3] was highly predictive of

the probability of developing AIDS over the next 2 to 4 years.[41,43,57,63] For example, in a study by Goedert and colleagues, 43% of patients with fewer than 300 CD4[+] T cells/mm[3] developed AIDS over a 3-year follow-up, compared to only 5% of patients with over 550 CD4[+] T cells/mm[3].[63] Also, the progression from ARC to AIDS is frequently associated with a progressive decline in the absolute number of CD4[+] T cells. Once the number of CD4[+] T cells drops below 150, there appears to be a substantial increase in the incidence of opportunistic infections and development of AIDS.[63]

Oral candidiasis appears to portend a particularly poor prognosis in patients with ARC; in a study by Klein and co-workers, for example, 59% of patients with oral candidiasis developed AIDS over a follow-up period of 1 to 23 months (median time to AIDS was 3 months).[64] Other features that appear to predict a higher likelihood for developing AIDS include fevers, weight loss, anergy as measured by cutaneous delayed-type sensitivity, and (to a lesser extent) herpes zoster.[41,43,57,63,65,66] In contrast, the presence of lymphadenopathy does not appear to have predictive value for the development of AIDS.[63]

Although the rate of progression to AIDS varied somewhat in these longitudinal studies, in general, about 12% to 35% of patients with PGL developed AIDS over a 3-year period.[41,57,63,66] The variation probably reflects differences in the patient populations at the time of their entry into the studies. A common observation, however, in these studies was that the risk of developing AIDS does not decrease with time but instead may increase; if this trend continues, then all patients with PGL or ARC may eventually develop AIDS.[41,43,63,66] It should be stressed, however, that this is an extrapolation and that it is not known whether a subset of patients with HIV infection (or even with ARC) will be able to avoid progressing to AIDS. Additional studies are presently underway to address this point and to further determine the incubation period for the development of AIDS from the time of initial infection with HIV.

As noted in the section on acute HIV infection, ELISA technology has recently been developed to measure HIV p24 *gag* antigen in the serum of patients with HIV infection.[30] This antigen is frequently detectable at the time of acute infection but then disappears when the patients develop antibody to HIV.[30] Additional studies have shown that serum p24 antigen subsequently becomes detectable at the time that patients begin to develop constitutional symptoms; this late resurgence of p24 antigen is associated with a selective loss of anti-p24 antibody[67,68] and is predictive of a high incidence of AIDS developing over the subsequent year (even when corrected for the CD4[+] count in such patients).[68] Anti-p24 antibody will compete with the ability to measure p24 antigen in patients' serum, and the question has been raised whether the recurrence of p24 antigen in such patients represents an increase in the viral load or simply a decrease in the competing anti-p24 antibody. It has been pointed out, however, that the increase in p24 antigen is associated with a selective loss of anti-

---

* Yarchoan R: Unpublished observation

p24 antibody (while antibodies to other viral antigens do not decline), suggesting that there is truly an increase in viral replication, which then forms immune complexes with the antibody.[68] This suggests that the progression from ARC to AIDS may be associated with a burst of HIV replication, possibly as a result of the immune system failing to control the infection.

HEMATOLOGIC MANIFESTATIONS OF HIV INFECTION

In addition to the hallmark depression of their immune system, many persons with HIV infection have hematologic abnormalities. These are in general most pronounced in persons with frank AIDS, but they are also observed in persons with PGL or ARC.[44,46] The most commonly observed abnormalities are a mild depression of one or more blood elements, and these are frequently observed in patients even with relatively mild symptoms. For example, in one large study, 10.1% of patients with PGL were found to have a depressed hematocrit of <40%, 7.8% had a platelet count of <150,000/mm³, 7.8% had a neutrophil count of <1800/mm³, and 7.6% had a total lymphocyte count of <1000/mm³.[44] In general, these mild abnormalities do not in themselves cause clinical problems and do not require specific therapy; however, as will be discussed below, such patients appear to be at greater risk for developing toxicity when administered 3′-azido-2′,3′-dideoxythymidine (AZT).[69,70]

In addition to these relatively mild depressions of hematologic elements, a certain subset of patients with PGL or ARC develop more substantial depressions of their formed blood elements. Perhaps the most common of these is thrombocytopenia. As early as 1982, Morris and co-workers described a group of homosexual men without AIDS who had thrombocytopenic purpura with platelet counts ranging down to 3000/mm³.[71] It has subsequently become clear that this thrombocytopenic purpura is found with increased incidence in patients with HIV infection and that this can be a manifestation of ARC.[72-76] These patients almost always have increased numbers of megakaryocytes in the bone marrow, suggesting that the thrombocytopenia results from a destructive process.[71] Like patients with classic idiopathic thrombocytopic purpura, these patients generally have no palpable spleen.[72-74]

The mechanism of the thrombocytopenia associated with HIV infection is still unclear. Circulating immune complexes are found in the serum of HIV-positive persons and have also been shown to be bound to the surface of platelets.[74] One current hypothesis is that the thrombocytopenia may be related to the deposition of immune complexes on platelets with subsequent ingestion by the macrophages.[74] Some researchers have suggested that specific autoantibodies, either to a platelet membrane antigen[75] or to the F(ab′)$_2$ portion of immunoglobulin[77] can be identified in the serum of patients with HIV-associated thrombocytopenic purpura

and may contribute to this condition. The relative contribution of these laboratory abnormalities to the depressed platelet counts in these patients is still unclear and will require further research.

As with classic autoimmune thrombocytopenic purpura, a variety of approaches may be used in the management of patients with thrombocytopenia from HIV infection. As many as 50% of patients will not require treatment and are clinically asymptomatic.[72] In addition, up to a fifth of patients may have a spontaneous recovery of normal platelet counts.[78] Prednisone has been tried in many of these patients, and response rates are roughly similar to what may be found with classic autoimmune thrombocytopenic purpura, with most patients having a substantial rise in their platelet counts.[72-74] However, many patients either do not achieve normal platelet counts with this therapy or relapse after the steroids are withdrawn, and only about 10% will achieve a sustained complete response.[74] Perhaps of greater concern in the use of steroids, however, is that they will further depress the cellular immune system in patients where this is already a major problem. Thus, steroids perhaps would be best reserved for patients who are at substantial risk for significant bleeding.[74]

Another approach that has been used in a number of patients with substantial depressions of their platelet counts has been splenectomy; even in patients who have failed steroid therapy, normalization of the platelet count has been observed in more than 90% of patients and a prolonged complete response was observed in over half of the patients studied.[73,74,78] Additional approaches have included administration of vincristine,[79] α-interferon,[80] and intravenous gammaglobulin.[76] It is perhaps ironic that the latter should be effective, since patients with HIV-associated thrombocytopenia generally have hypergammaglobulinemia. However, substantial responses are frequently observed, and because of the low incidence of side-effects associated with its use, intravenous gammaglobulin administration should probably be considered the initial treatment of choice when therapy is clinically indicated.

Finally, mention should be made that some patients with AIDS or ARC have been reported to have substantial rises in their platelet counts upon being given AZT,[81,82] including the first patient ever to have received this drug.[81] The mechanism of action of this response is unclear at present, but may be somehow related to a diminution of the viral load of HIV in treated patients. (As will be discussed in Chapter 16, thrombocytopenia may also be a side-effect of AZT administration, although this is predominantly found in patients who have received prolonged therapy with the drug and have other evidence of bone marrow toxicity.[69,70] AZT should be considered in patients with HIV-associated thrombocytopenia who meet the other criteria for AZT administration, and clinical studies are warranted to further explore the role of AZT in this disorder.

As noted above, in addition to thrombocytopenia,

depression of the erythroid and myeloid blood elements can be observed in HIV-infected patients, even those with minimal immunosuppression.[83,84] Bone marrow evaluation in patients with such cytopenias has revealed a variety of abnormalities. The marrow is generally normocellular to hypercellular, and plasmacytosis, aggregates of atypical lymphocytes, histiocytic hemophagocytosis, and increased reticulin are frequently observed.[83-86] For reasons that are unclear, stainable iron may be decreased in the marrow of up to 50% of patients.[83] In patients with severe HIV infection, myelodysplastic changes associated with abnormalities in maturation of all cell lines may be found; these changes are most pronounced in the granulocyte series, and are similar to those seen in preleukemia or myelodysplastic syndromes.[87]

The pathogenesis of these hematologic abnormalities is not clear at present, and it is likely that they are multifactorial. Several investigators have studied this using *in vitro* culture techniques of bone marrow elements. Using such an approach, Donahue and associates found that the marrow progenitors from patients with AIDS or ARC grew normally in the presence of erythropoietin or granulocyte–monocyte colony stimulating factor (GM-CSF).[88] However, in the presence of antibodies to HIV envelope glycoprotein (gp 120), the growth of these progenitor cells was suppressed. Thus, it appears that antibodies to HIV gp120 may bind to HIV-infected bone marrow progenitors and inhibit their growth. Furthermore, this group found that, unlike that from normals, sera from AIDS patients lacked bone-marrow growth stimulating activity when tested on normal marrow progenitors, and they further hypothesized that a lack of growth-factor production may contribute to the cytopenias in these patients.[88] Other groups have found evidence for different potential mechanisms, including suppression of the hematopoietic progenitor cells by the excess CD8[+] cells in AIDS patients[89] and antineutrophil antibodies in the circulation of AIDS patients.[90]

In addition to these mechanisms, which may be directly related to HIV infection in these patients or the associated immunologic disorders, several secondary mechanisms may contribute to marrow suppression in certain patients. We have observed that as many of 10% of patients with AIDS may have low serum vitamin B_{12} levels; vitamin B_{12} absorbtion was abnormal in patients in whom this was studied, and it did not correct with intrinsic factor.* Also, it has been our experience that patients with *Mycobacterium avium* complex or with symptomatic cytomegalovirus infections frequently have substantial anemia and neutropenia.† Whether these organisms contribute to the bone marrow suppression or whether both the infections and marrow abnormalities

* Yarchoan R, Lassam NJ, Broder S: Unpublished data

† Yarchoan R, Pluda JM, Broder S: Unpublished data

are manifestions of profound HIV infection is unclear at this time.

Finally, it should be stressed that bone marrow suppression in patients with HIV infection is particularly problematic in patients who are given AZT.[69,70,82] As will be discussed in Chapter 16, marrow suppression, particularly of the erythroid blood elements, is the dose-limiting toxicity with this drug. Patients with frank AIDS, with pretreatment anemia or neutropenia, or with vitamin B_{12} or folic acid deficiencies appear to be particularly sensitive to this, and physicians prescribing AZT are encouraged to measure serum vitamin B_{12} and folic acid levels and to initiate replacement therapy if low or even low-normal levels are found.[69,70,82]

Because bone-marrow suppression frequently limits AZT therapy in patients with AIDS or ARC, a number of approaches are now being explored to address this problem. As noted above, there is suggestive evidence that patients with AIDS may have reduced levels of bone marrow growth stimulating factors; thus, it is possible that administering such factors may reduce this toxicity. In this regard, one of these factors, GM-CSF, has been shown to increase the neutrophil and monocyte counts in patients with AIDS,[91] and a study is now underway at the National Cancer Institute to test a regimen of GM-CSF alternating with AZT. Other groups are investigating the possible use of erythropoietin in this setting.

In addition to depression of formed-blood elements, a lupus-like anticoagulant has been found to be present in the sera of some patients with HIV infection.[92,93] Patients with this anticoagulant have prolongation of several tests of coagulation, including the thromboplastin time, the dilute thromboplastin inhibition assay, and the Russell viper venom clotting time. The anticoagulant appears to be associated with the occurence of opportunistic infections and in most cases is not clinically significant. However, hemorrhagic complications may occur in the presence of thrombocytopenia or hypoprothrombinemia,[92,93] and it is particularly important that appropriate clotting studies be obtained in HIV-positive patients undergoing invasive procedures. Also, it should be noted that thromboembolic events can paradoxically be seen with lupus anticoagulant, and this possibility should be considered when evaluating HIV-infected patients with such problems.[92]

OTHER DISEASE MANIFESTATIONS OF ARC AND AIDS

As noted above, patients with HIV infection frequently develop lymphadenopathy, and many develop a variety of constitutional symptoms including fevers, night sweats, diarrhea, malaise, and fatigue. In addition to these, HIV infection, either as a primary disease manifestation or as a secondary process, can affect virtually every organ system in the body, including the joints, heart, muscles, kidneys, and endocrine systems.[94-96] Some of the individual organ systems involved will be discussed in the following chapters. At this point, however, it may be worthwhile to briefly discuss several other frequent specific disease manifestations that may occur in patients with HIV infection.

Cutaneous and Oral Manifestations of HIV Infection

Patients with HIV infection frequently develop any of a wide variety of cutaneous and oral abnormalities. Indeed the sudden appearance of Kaposi's sarcoma in a number of young patients was one of the factors that led to the recognition of AIDS as a new syndrome.[4] In addition to Kaposi's sarcoma, however, patients with HIV infection frequently develop a wide variety of skin abnormalities; in one large study, 13.7% of HIV seropositive patients reported the development of a new skin rash within the previous 6 months.[45] In addition to the rash associated with primary infection (described above), a variety of nonspecific skin manifestations may develop in patients with PGL, ARC, or AIDS; these include acneiform folliculitis, seborrheic dermatitis, cutaneous vasculitis, acquired ichthyosis, xerosis, and psoriasis.[97,98] In addition to these, an entity called the "yellow nail syndrome," an unusual symptom complex of yellow nails, lymphedema, pulmonary symptoms, and sinusitis, appears to be associated with *Pneumocystis carinii* infections in patients with AIDS.[97]

For reasons that are not understood, HIV-infected individuals develop drug eruptions to a number of agents more frequently than do other patients. This is especially true of sulfonamides (including trimethoprim–sulfamethoxazole). Up to 60% of AIDS patients may develop drug eruptions following administration of these drugs, which substantially affect the treatment of opportunistic infections like *Pneumocystis carinii* and toxoplasmosis.[99]

Other cutaneous manifestations in patients with HIV infection can be more directly linked to their immunodeficiency, and such patients are prone to develop a variety of cutaneous infections. Candidiasis is particularly common in these patients, with the mouth or intertriginous regions being frequently involved;[97] as noted above, the development of oral candidiasis in a patient with ARC is a poor prognostic sign for the development of AIDS.[64] Other fungal infections that are frequently seen include dermatophytosis, especially *Trichophytum rubrum,* tinea pedis, onychiomycosis, and skin lesions associated with disseminated histoplasmosis or cryptococcosis.[98] A variety of viruses can also involve the skin in such patients. Herpes simplex virus (type I and II) infections frequently occur, and indeed, an increased incidence of such infections in homosexual men was historically an early sign that a new disorder of acquired immunodeficiency was occurring in this patient population.[3] Herpesviruses can

cause a chronic mucocutaneous infection in such patients as well as severe gingivostomatitis;[99,100] these infections can usually be controlled with the antiherpes drug acyclovir. Varicella–zoster infections are also found in increased incidence in patients with AIDS or ARC, and although in many patients it is restricted to a single dermatome, in others it may become disseminated. Finally, molluscum contagiosum is common in this population, and in addition, the patients sometimes develop warty lesions that may be caused by papillomaviruses; in particular, condyloma accuminatum can be troublesome and may occur at both genital and extragenital sites.[99]

Skin infections with protozoal or bacterial organisms are also more common in patients with HIV infection than in the general population.[98,99] Skin infections with *Acanthamoeba castellani* have been seen, although this condition is somewhat uncommon. A more common problem is the development of multiple skin abscesses or furunculosis; staphylococcus is the most commonly cultured organism, and extensive impetigo may develop if the infection is severe. Lesions associated with disseminated mycobacterial infections can be seen, generally in association with *Mycobacterium avium-intracellulare* or tuberculosis.[99] Finally, it should be noted that persons caring for patients with HIV infection should be particularly alert for the occurrence of syphilis, and that a secondary syphilitic rash has been observed in an HIV-infected patient who had a negative syphilis serology.[101] Such patients, who may be particularly challenging from a diagnostic point of view, may be identified by the observance of treponemal organisms in a skin biopsy.[101]

Although this will be the subject of another chapter, mention should be made that a variety of malignant processes, including Kaposi's sarcoma, lymphoma, and squamous cell carcinoma may involve the mouth and skin of patients with HIV infection.[4,9,10,99,100] Certain types of lymphomas, particularly high-grade B-cell lymphomas, appear to be occurring at high frequencies in patients with HIV infection,[9] and cutaneous lesions may be the first evidence of this complication.

Patients with HIV infection are also susceptible to a number of clinical manifestations that involve the mouth, and alert dentists may be the first to diagnose HIV infection disease in some patients. As noted above, such patients may develop oral herpes infections, thrush, or Kaposi's sarcoma.[100] In addition, they are sometimes troubled by severe periodontal disease with gingival recession and loss of alveolar bone.[102] Apthous ulcerations have been observed in the setting of acute HIV infection,[29] and it has been our impression that they affect patients with AIDS or ARC more than the general population.* HIV-infected patients who are moderately to severely immunosuppressed sometimes develop what is called *oral hairy leukoplakia;* this appears as white,

---

* Yarchoan R, Broder S: Unpublished observations

corrugated, poorly demarcated lesions that do not wipe away, usually occurring on the lateral aspect of the tongue, but occasionally involving the floor of the mouth or buccal mucosa.[103] Replicating Epstein–Barr virus (EBV) has been demonstrated in the epithelial cells of such lesions, as has papilloma virus.[104] Supporting a role for replicating EBV (or another herpesvirus) in the pathogenesis of this lesion, several patients have recently been reported to have resolution of oral hairy leukoplakia upon being administered ganciclovir or acyclovir.[105,106] Such therapy is not generally recommended for this disorder, however, as the lesions are asymptomatic.

Ocular Complications of HIV Infection

Ocular disease has been found to be a common feature of AIDS and severe HIV infections. Cotton-wool spots are the most common finding,[107–109] occurring in from 50% to 100% of patients who are carefully examined. They are thought to be caused by local ischemia that occurs as the result of a retinal microvasculopathy caused by immune complex deposition.[108] More recently, HIV has been reported to be present in endothelial cells within the retina of infected individuals, and the possibility of vascular alterations resulting directly from HIV infection has been suggested.[110] Other noninfectious abnormalities seen include conjunctival Kaposi's sarcoma, conjunctivitis, keratitis, retinal phlebitis, retinal microaneurysms, ischemic maculopathy, retinal hemorrhages, and Roth's spots.[107,108]

Various infections found in HIV-infected individuals can also involve the eye. Cytomegalovirus retinitis is a common and devastating complication of AIDS.[107–109] Several open trials have shown that this can resolve with ganciclovir therapy.[111] Maintenance therapy with ganciclovir is usually recommended as the retinitis may return in its absence. Even with this therapy, however, such patients often die within several months; the patients who develop cytomegalovirus retinitis are usually quite immunocompromised, and ganciclovir causes bone marrow suppression (which can limit therapy and/or contribute to the immune suppression).

The retina is normally protected by a blood–ocular barrier, and the development of retinal infections in HIV-infected patients suggests that there might be breaks in this barrier. Such breaks may occur as the result of the deposition of immune complexes and ischemia.[108]

Other infections that may occur in patients with HIV infection include cryptococcal chorioretinitis, *Mycobacteria avium-intracellulare* granulomas in the retina and choroid, herpes simplex retinitis, herpes zoster opthalmicus, and toxoplasma or candidal chorioretinitis.[107–109] *Pneumocystis carinii* has been reported to be found in the retina of a patient with cotton-wool spots and *P. carinii* pneumonia;[112] however, this must be viewed as a rare occurrence.[113,114]

INFECTIONS WITH OTHER PATHOGENIC HUMAN RETROVIRUSES

So far in this chapter, we have discussed the manifestations of HIV infection in humans. Although a detailed discussion of other retroviral infections is beyond the scope of this chapter, it is perhaps worth noting briefly that at least five retroviruses are now known to infect humans: HTLV-I, HTLV-II, HIV, LAV-2, and HTLV-V.[11,13,115–119] Two of these, human T-cell lymphotropic viruses, types I and V (HTLV-I and HTLV-V) are predominantly associated with T-cell proliferative disorders;[115,119] HTLV-I can also cause tropical spastic paraparesis[120] and may be associated with immunodeficiency.[121] A virus related to HIV, called lymphadenopathy-associated virus type II (LAV-II) has been noted to cause a disorder similar to AIDS.[118] Human T-cell lymphotropic virus type II (HTLV-II) has been isolated from occasional patients with hairy-cell leukemia; however, the association with that disease is still unclear.[116] Finally, it should be noted that an increasing number of persons, particularly intravenous drug users, have recently been reported to be simultaneously infected with more than one retrovirus, and at least one such patient has been reported to have an unusual CD8+-proliferative sarcoid-like disorder.[122] Clinicians should be on the alert for other such unusual manifestations of retroviral infections as these viruses continue to spread through segments of the population.

SUMMARY

As we have seen, HIV infection may have many clinical manifestions, ranging from an asymptomatic state to devastating multisystem illness, and as the incidence of this disease increases, it is likely that clinicians will continue to observe new disease manifestations that may be attributable to HIV. Most of the attention in disease has been focused on the patients who fulfill the criteria for AIDS; the number of AIDS cases are tracked by the Centers for Disease Control on a weekly basis and in the eyes of many, it is this number that defines the extent of the pandemic. However, this accounting provides a gross underestimation of the extent of the disease in this country; it is estimated that 1 to 2 million Americans are infected with HIV and many more persons are infected throughout the world. It is clear that many of these individuals will have some symptoms attributable to their infection, and many others who still do not meet the criteria for AIDS will have substantial symptomatology that may interfere with their daily life and even prevent them from working. It is thus imperative that we develop effective strategies for treating HIV infection, not only for persons with frank AIDS, but also for those with less advanced disease. In such patients, therapy should be evaluated not only for its ability to prevent the development of AIDS, but also for its ability to reduce the existing symptomatology. As will be discussed in Chapter 16, at least one antiretroviral drug, AZT, has been shown to accomplish both of these goals,[69,82,123] and it is hoped that more effective therapies will be developed in the near future.

REFERENCES

1. Gottlieb MS, Schroff R, Schanker HM et al: *Pneumocystis carinii* pneumonia and mucosal candidiasis in previously healthy homosexual men: Evidence of a new acquired immunodeficiency. N Engl J Med 305:1425, 1981
2. Masur H, Michelis MA, Greene JB et al: An outbreak of community acquired *Pneumocystis carinii* pneumonia: Initial manifestations of cellular dysfunction. N Engl J Med 305:1431, 1981
3. Siegal FP, Lopez C, Hammer GS et al: Severe acquired immunodeficiency in male homosexuals, manifested by chronic perianal ulcerative ulcerative herpes simplex lesions. N Engl J Med 305:1439, 1981
4. Hymes KB, Cheung T, Greene JB et al: Kaposi's sarcoma in homosexual men: A report of eight cases. Lancet 2: 598, 1981
5. Centers for Disease Control: Update on acquired immunodeficiency syndrome (AIDS)—United States. Morbid Mortal Week Rept 31:507, 1982
6. Centers for Disease Control: Revision of the case definition of acquired immunodeficiency syndrome for national reporting—United States. Morbid Mortal Week Rept 34:373, 1985
7. Gottlieb MS, Groopman JE, Weinstein WM et al: The acquired immunodeficiency syndrome. Ann Intern Med 99: 208, 1983
8. Fahey JL, Prince H, Weaver M et al: Quantitative changes in the T helper or T suppressor/cytotoxic lymphocyte subsets that distinguish acquired immune deficiency syndrome from other immune subset disorders. Am J Med 76:95, 1984
9. Ziegler JL, Becjstead JA, Volberding PA et al: Non-Hodgkin's lymphoma in 90 homosexual men. Relation to generalized lymphadenopathy and the acquired immunodeficiency syndrome. N Engl J Med 311:565, 1984
10. Fauci AS, Macher AM, Longo DL et al: Acquired immunodeficiency syndrome: Epidemiologic, clinical, immunologic, and therapeutic considerations. Ann Intern Med 100:92, 1984
11. Barré–Sinoussi F, Chermann JC, Rey F et al: Isolation of a T cell lymphotropic virus from a patient at risk for acquired immunodeficiency syndrome (AIDS). Science 220:868, 1983
12. Popovic M, Sarngadharan MG, Reed E and Gallo RC: Detection, isolation, and continuous production of cytopathic retroviruses (HTLV-III) from patients with AIDS and pre-AIDS. Science 224:497, 1984
13. Gallo RC, Salahuddin SZ, Popovic M et al: Frequent detection and isolation of cytopathic retroviruses (HTLV-III) from patients with AIDS and at risk for AIDS. Science 224:500, 1984
14. Sarngadharan MG, Popovic M, Bruch L et al: Antibodies reactive with human T-lymphotropic viruses (HTLV-III) in the serum of patients with AIDS. Science 224:506, 1984
15. Centers for Disease Control: Revision of the CDC surveillance case definition for acquired immunodeficiency syndrome. Morbid Mortal Week Rept [Suppl] 36:1S, 1987
16. Centers for Disease Control: Classification system for human T-lymphotropic virus type III/lymphadenopathy-associated virus infections. Morbid Mortal Week Rept 35: 334, 1986
17. Redfield RR, Wright DC, Tramont EC: The Walter Reed Staging Classification for HTLV-III LAV infection. N Engl J Med 314:131, 1986
18. Feorino PM, Kalyanaraman VS, Haverkos HW et al: Lymphadenopathy associated with virus infection of a blood donor-recipient pair with acquired immunodeficiency syndrome. Science 225:69, 1984
19. Anonymous: Needlestick transmission of HTLV-III from a patient infected in Africa. Lancet 2:1376, 1984
20. Cooper DA, Maclean P, Finlayson R et al: Acute AIDS retrovirus infection. Lancet 1:537, 1985
21. Ho DD, Sarngadharan MG, Resnick L et al: Primary human T-lymphotrophic virus type III infection. Ann Intern Med 103:880, 1985
22. Weber JN, Rogers LA, Scott K et al: Three year prospective study of HTLV-III infection in homosexual men. Lancet 1:1179, 1986
23. Lindskov R, Orskov Lindhardt B et al: Acute HTLV-III infection with roseola-like rash. Lancet 1:447, 1986
24. Wantzin GRL, Orskov Lindhardt B, Weismann K et al: Acute HTLV-III infection associated with exanthema, diagnosed by seroconversion. Br J Dermatol 115:601, 1986
25. Rustin MHA, Ridley CM, Smith MD et al: The acute exanthem associated with seroconversion to human T-cell lymphotropic virus in a homosexual man. J Infect Dis 12:161, 1986
26. Calabrese LH, Proffitt MR, Levin KH et al: Acute infection with the human immunodeficiency virus (HIV) associated with acute brachial neutitis and exanthematous rash. Ann Intern Med 107:849, 1987
27. Carne CA, Smith A, Elkington SG et al: Acute encephalopathy coincident with seroconversion for anti-HTLV-III. Lancet 2:1206, 1985
28. Ho DD, Rota TR, Schooley RT et al: Isolation of HTLV-III from cerebrospinal fluid and neural tissues of patients with neurologic syndromes related to the acquired immunodeficiency syndrome. N Engl J Med 313:1493, 1985
29. Kessler HA, Blaauw B, Spear J et al: Diagnosis of human immunodeficiency virus infection in seronegative homosexuals presenting with an acute viral syndrome. JAMA 258:1196, 1987
30. Goudsmit J, Paul DA, Lange JMA et al: Expression of human immunodeficiency virus antigen (HIV-Ag) in serum and cerebrospinal fluid during acute and chronic infection. Lancet 2:177, 1986
31. Piette AM, Tusseau F, Vignon D et al: Acute neuropathy coincident with seroconversion for anti-LAV/HTLV-III. Lancet 1:852, 1986
32. Hagberg L, Malmvall BE, Svennerholm L et al: Guillain-Barré syndrome as an early manifestation of HIV central nervous system infection. Scand J Infect Dis 18:591, 1986
33. Vendrell J, Hcrcdia C, Pujol M et al: Guillain-Barré syndrome associated with seroconversion for anti-HTLV-III. Neurology 37:544, 1987
34. Denning DW, Anderson J, Rudge P et al: Acute myelopathy associated with primary infection with human immunodeficiency virus. Br Med J 294:143, 1987

35. Valle SL: Febrile pharyngitis as the primary sign of HIV infection in a cluster of cases linked by sexual contact. Scand J Infect Dis 19:13, 1987

36. Buchanan JG, Goldwater PN, Somerfield SD et al: Mononucleosis-like syndrome associated with acute AIDS retrovirus infection. N Zealand Med J 99:405, 1986

37. Allain JP, Paul DA, Laurian Y et al: Serological markers in early stages of human immunodeficiency virus infection in haemophiliacs. Lancet 2:1233, 1986

38. Gaines H, Sonnerborg A, Czajkowski J et al: Antibody response in primary human immunodeficiency virus infection. Lancet 1:1249, 1987

39. Cooper DA, Imrie AI, Penny R: Antibody response to human immunodeficiency virus after primary infection. J Infect Dis 155:1113, 1987

40. Ulstrup JC, Skaug K, Figenschau KJ et al: Sensitivity of Western blotting (compared with ELISA and immunofluorescence) during seroconversion after HTLV-III infection. Lancet 2:1151, 1986

41. Goedert JJ, Biggar RJ, Weiss SH et al: Three-year incidence of AIDS in five cohorts of HTLV-III-infected risk group members. Science 231:992, 1986

42. Metroka CE, Cunningham-Rundles S, Pollack MS et al: Generalized lymphadenopathy in homosexual men. Ann Intern Med 99:585, 1983

43. Eyster ME, Gail MH, Ballard JO et al: Natural history of human immunodeficiency virus infections in hemophiliacs: Effects of T-cell subsets, platelet counts, and age. Ann Intern Med 107:1, 1987

44. Kaslow RA, Phair JP, Friedman HB et al: Infection with the human immunodeficiency virus: Clinical manifestations and their relationship to immune deficiency. Ann Intern Med 107:474, 1987

45. Lang W, Anderson RE, Perkins H et al: Clinical, immunologic, and serologic findings in men at risk for acquired immunodeficiency syndrome. JAMA 257:326, 1987

46. Howard J, Sattler F, Mahon R et al: Clinical features of 100 human immunodeficiency virus antibody-positive individuals from an alternate test site. Arch Intern Med 147:2131, 1987

47. Jaffe ES, Clark J, Steis R et al: Lymph node pathology of HTLV and HTLV-associated neoplasms. Cancer Res 45[Suppl]:4662s, 1985

48. O'Murchadha MT, Wolf BC, Neiman RS: The histologic features of hyperplastic lymphadenopathy in AIDS-related complex are nonspecific. Am J Surg Pathol 11:94, 1987

49. Garcia CF, Lifson JD, Engleman EG et al: The immunohistology of persistent generalized lymphadenopathy syndrome (PGL). Am J Clin Pathol 86:706, 1986

50. Biberfeld P, Porwit-Ksiazek A, Böttiger B et al: Immunohistology of lymph nodes in HTLV-III infected homosexuals with persistent adenopathy or AIDS. Cancer Res 45[Suppl]:4665s, 1985

51. Brynes RK, Chan WC, Spira TJ et al: Value of lymph node biopsy in unexplained lymphadenopathy in homosexual men. JAMA 250:1313, 1983

52. Modlin RL, Meyer PR, Hofman FM et al: T-lymphocyte subsets in lymph nodes from homosexual men. JAMA 250:1302, 1983

53. Shaw GM, Harper ME, Hahn BH et al: Molecular characterization of human T-cell leukemia (lymphotropic) virus type III in the acquired immune deficiency syndrome. Science 227:177, 1985

54. Biberfeld P, Chayt KJ, Marselle LM et al: HTLV-III expression in infected lymph nodes and relevance to the pathogenesis of lymphadenopathy. Am J Pathol 123:436, 1986

55. Le Tourneau A, Audouin J, Diebold J et al: LAV-like viral particles in lymph node germinal centers in patients with the persistent lymphadenopathy syndrome and the acquired immunodeficiency syndrome-related complex: An ultrastructural study of 30 cases. Hum Pathol 17:1047, 1986

56. Gartner S, Markovitz P, Markovitz DM et al: The role of mononuclear phagocytes in HTLV-III/LAV infection. Science 233:215, 1986

57. Mathur-Wagh U, Enlow RW, Spigland I et al: Longitudinal study of persistent generalized lymphadenopathy in homosexual men: Relation to acquired immunodeficiency syndrome. Lancet 1:1033, 1984

58. Abrams DI, Lewis BJ, Beckstead JH et al: Persistent diffuse lymphadenopathy in homosexual men: Endpoint or prodrome? Ann Intern Med 100:801, 1984

59. Shearer GM, Payne SM, Joseph LJ et al: Functional T lymphocyte immune deficiency in a population of homosexual men who do not exhibit symptoms of acquired immune deficiency syndrome. J Clin Invest 74:496, 1984

60. Yarchoan R, Redfield RR, Broder S: B cell activation in patients with HTLV-III/LAV infection: Contribution of B cells producing antibody to HTLV-III/LAV, of Epstein-Barr virus-infected B cells, and of HTLV-III/LAV-induced immunoglobulin production. J Clin Invest 78:439, 1986

61. Huang K-L, Ruben FL, Rinaldo CR et al: Antibody responses after influenza and pneumococcal immunization in HIV-infected homosexual men. JAMA 257:2047, 1987

62. Weber JN, Wadsworth J, Rogers LA et al: Three-year prospective study of HTLV-III/LAV infection in homosexual men. Lancet 1:1179, 1986

63. Goedert JJ, Biggar RJ, Melbye M et al: Effect of T4 counts and cofactors on the incidence of AIDS in homosexual men infected with human immunodeficiency virus. JAMA 257:331, 1987

64. Klein RS, Harris CA, Small CB et al: Oral candidiasis in high-risk patients as the initial manifestation of the acquired immunodeficiency syndrome. N Engl J Med 311:354, 1984

65. Friedman-Kien AE, Lafleur FL, Gendler E et al: Herpes zoster: A possible early clinical sign for development of acquired immunodeficiency syndrome in high-risk individuals. J Am Acad Derm 14:1023, 1986

66. Kaplan JE, Spira TJ, Fishbein DB et al: Lymphadenopathy syndrome in homosexual men. Evidence for continuing risk of developing the acquired immunodeficiency syndrome. JAMA 257:335, 1987

67. Lange JMA, Paul DA, Huisman HG et al: Persistent HIV antigenaemia and decline of HIV core antibodies associated with the transition to AIDS. Br Med J 293:1459, 1986

68. Allain J-P, Laurian Y, Paul DA et al: Long-term evaluation of HIV antigen and antibodies to p24 and gp41 in patients with hemophilia. N Engl J Med 317:1114, 1987

69. Yarchoan R, Broder S: Development of antiretroviral therapy for the acquired immunodeficiency syndrome and related disorders: A progress report. N Engl J Med 316:557, 1987

70. Richman DD, Fischl MA, Grieco MH et al: The toxicity of azidothymidine (AZT) in the treatment of patients with

AIDS and AIDS-related complex. N Engl J Med 317:192, 1987

71. Morris L, Distenfeld A, Amorosi E et al: Autoimmune thrombocytopenic purpura in homosexual men. Ann Intern Med 96:714, 1982

72. Walsh C, Krigel R, Lennette E et al: Thrombocytopenia in homosexual men. Ann Intern Med 103:542, 1985

73. Abrams DI, Kiprov DD, Goedert JJ et al: Antibodies to human T-lymphotropic virus type III and development of the acquired immunodeficiency syndrome in homosexual men presenting with immune thrombocytopenia. Ann Intern Med 104:47, 1986

74. Walsh CM, Nardi NA, Karpatkin S: On the mechanism of thrombocytopenic purpura in sexually active homosexual men. N Engl J Med 311:635, 1984

75. Stricker RB, Abrams DI, Corash L et al: Target platelet antigen in homosexual men with immune thrombocytopenia. N Engl J Med 313:1375, 1985

76. Delfraissy JF, Tertian G, Dreyfus M et al: Intravenous gamma-globulin, thrombocytopenia, and the acquired immunodeficiency syndrome. Ann Intern Med 103:478, 1985

77. Yu J–R, Lennette ET, Karpatkin S: Anti-F(ab')$_2$ antibodies in thrombocytopenic patients at risk for acquired immunodeficiency syndrome. J Clin Invest 77:1756, 1986

78. Schneider PA, Abrams DI, Rayner AA et al: Immunodeficiency-associated thrombocytopenic purpura (IDTP): Response to splenectomy. Arch Surg 122:1175, 1987

79. Mintzer DM, Real FX, Jovino L et al: Treatment of Kaposi's sarcoma and thrombocytopenia with vincristine in patients with the acquired immunodeficiency syndrome. Ann Intern Med 102:200, 1985

80. Ellis ME, Neal KR, Leen CLS, et al: Alpha-2a recombinant interferon in HIV associated thrombocytopenia. Br Med J 295:1519, 1987

81. Gottlieb MS, Wolfe PR, Chafey S: Case report: Response of AIDS-related thrombocytopenia to intravenous and oral azidothymidine (3'-azido-3'-deoxythymidine). AIDS Research Human Retroviruses 3:109, 1987

82. Yarchoan R, Weinhold KJ, Lyerly HK et al: Administration of 3'-azido-3'-deoxythymidine, an inhibitor of HTLV-III/LAV replication, to patients with AIDS or AIDS-related complex. Lancet 1:575, 1986

83. Abrams DI, Chinn EK, Lewis BJ, et al: Hematologic manifestations in homosexual men with Kaposi's sarcoma. Am J Clin Pathol 81:13, 1984

84. Spivak JL, Bender BS, Quinn TC: Hematologic abnormalities in the acquired immunodeficiency syndrome. Am J Med 77:224, 1984

85. Osborne BM, Guarda LA, Butler JJ: Bone marrow biopsies in patients with the acquired immunodeficiency syndrome. Hum Pathol 15:1048, 1984

86. Zon LI, Arkin C, Groopman JE: Haematologic manifestations of the human immunodeficiency virus (HIV). Br J Haematol 66:251, 1987

87. Schneider GR, Picker LJ: Myelodysplasia in the acquired immunodeficiency syndrome. Am J Clin Pathol 84:144, 1985

88. Donahue RE, Johnson MM, Zon LI et al: Suppression of in vitro haematopoiesis following human immunodeficiency virus infection. Nature 326:200, 1987

89. Stella CC, Ganser A, Hoelzer D: Defective in vitro growth of the hemopoietic progenitor cells in the acquired immunodeficiency syndrome. J Clin Invest 80:286, 1987

90. Murphy MF, Metcalfe P, Waters AH et al: Incidence and mechanism of neutropenia and thrombocytopenia in patients with human immunodeficiency virus infection. Br J Haematol 66:337, 1987

91. Groopman JE, Mitsuyasu RT, DeLeo MJ et al: Effect of recombinant human granulocyte-macrophage colony-stimulating factor on myelopoesis in the acquired immunodeficiency syndrome. N Engl J Med 317:593, 1987

92. Bloom EJ, Abrams DI, Rodgers G: Lupus anticoagulant in the acquired immunodeficiency syndrome. JAMA 256:491, 1986

93. Cohen AJ, Philips TM, Kessler CM: Circulating coagulation inhibitors in the acquired immunodeficiency syndrome. Ann Intern Med 104:175, 1986

94. Cohen IS, Anderson DW, Virmani R et al: Congestive cardiomyopathy in association with the acquired immunodeficiency syndrome. N Engl J Med 315:628, 1986

95. Winchester R, Bernstein DH, Fischer HD et al: The co-occurrence of Reiter's syndrome and acquired immunodeficiency. Ann Intern Med 106:19, 1987

96. Rao TK, Friedman EA, Nicastri AD: The types of renal disease in the acquired immunodeficiency syndrome. N Engl J Med 316:1062, 1987

97. Goodman DS, Teplitz ED, Wishner A et al: Prevalence of cutaneous disease in patients with acquired immunodeficiency syndrome (AIDS) or AIDS-related complex. J Am Acad Dermatol 17:210, 1987

98. Sindrup JH, Lisby G, Weismann K et al: Skin manifestations in AIDS, HIV infection, and AIDS-related complex. Int J Dermatol 2:267, 1987

99. Resnik L, Herbst JS: Dermatological (non-Kaposi's sarcoma) manifestations associated with HTLV-III/LAV infection. In Broder S (ed): AIDS: Modern Concepts and Therapeutic Challenges, p 285. New York, Marcel Dekker, 1987

100. Andriolo M, Wolf JW, Rosenberg JS: AIDS and AIDS-related complex: Oral manifestations and treatment. JADA 113:586, 1986

101. Hicks CB, Benson PM, Lupton GP et al: Seronegative secondary syphilis in a patient infected with the human immunodeficiency virus (HIV) with Kaposi's sarcoma. Ann Intern Med 107:492, 1987

102. Silverman S, Migliorati CA, Lozada–Nur F et al: Oral findings in people with or at high risk for AIDS: A study of 375 homosexual males. JADA 112:187, 1986

103. Greenspan D, Conant M, Silverman S et al: Oral "hairy" leucoplakia in male homosexuals: Evidence of association with both papilloma virus and a Herpes-group virus. Lancet 2:831, 1984

104. Greenspan JS, Greenspan D, Lennette ET et al: Replication of Epstein–Barr virus within the epithelial cells of oral "hairy" leukoplakia, an AIDS-associated lesion. New Engl J Med 313:1564, 1985

105. Newman C, Polk BF: Resolution of oral hairy leukoplakia during therapy with 9-(1,3-dihydroxy-2-propoxymethyl) guanine (DHPG). Ann Intern Med 107:348, 1987

106. Resnick L, Herbst JS, Ablashi D et al: Regression of oral hairy leukoplakia after orally administered acyclovir therapy. JAMA 259:384, 1988

107. Holland GN, Pepose JS, Pettit TH et al: Acquired immunodeficiency syndrome: Ocular manifestations. Am Acad Opthalmol 90:859, 1983

108. Pepose JS, Holland GN, Nestor MS et al: Acquired im-

munodeficiency syndrome: Pathogenic mechanisms of ocular disease. Opthalmology 92:472, 1985

109. Schuman JS, Friedman AH: Retinal manifestations of the acquired immunodeficiency syndrome (AIDS): Cytomegalovirus, *Candida albicans,* cryptococcus, toxoplasmosis and *Pneumocystis carinii.* Trans Opthalmol Soc UK 103:177, 1983

110. Pomerantz RJ, Kuritzkes DR, de la Monte SM et al: Infection of the retina by human immunodeficiency virus type 1. N Engl J Med 317:1643, 1987

111. Felsenstein D, D'Amico DJ, Hirsch MS et al: Treatment of cytomegalovirus retinitis with 9-[2-hydroxy-1(hydroxymethyl) ethoxymethyl] guanine. Ann Intern Med 103:377, 1985

112. Kwok S, O'Donnell JJ, Wood IS: Retinal cotton-wool spots in a patient with *Pneumocystis carinii* infection. N Engl J Med 307:184, 1982

113. Holland GN, Gottlieb MS, Foos RY: Retinal cotton-wool patches in acquired immunodeficiency syndrome. N Engl J Med 307:1704, 1982

114. Sobel HJ: Retinal cotton-wool patches in acquired immunodeficiency syndrome. N Engl J Med 307:1704, 1982

115. Poiesz BJ, Ruscutti FW, Gazdar AF et al: Detection and isolation of type C retrovirus particles from fresh and cultured lymphocytes of a patient with cutaneous T-cell lymphoma. Proc Natl Acad Sci USA 77:7415, 1980

116. Kalyanaraman VS, Sarngadharan MG, Robert–Guroff M et al: A new sub-type of human T cell leukemia virus (HTLV-II) associated with a T-cell variant of hairy cell leukemia. Science 218:571, 1982

117. Kanki PJ, Barin F, M'Boup S et al: New human T-lymphotropic retrovirus related to simian T-lymphotropic virus type III (STLV-III$_{AGM}$). Science 232:238, 1986

118. Clavel F, Guetarad D, Brun–Vezinet F et al: Isolation of a new human retrovirus from west African patients with AIDS. Science 233:343, 1986

119. Manzari V, Gismondi A, Birillari G et al: HTLV-V: A new human retrovirus isolated in a Tac-negative T cell lymphoma/leukemia. Science 238:1581, 1987

120. Gessain A, Barin F, Vernant JC et al: Antibodies to human T-lymphotropic virus type I in patients with tropical spastic papaparesis. Lancet 2:407, 1985

121. Essex M, McLane MF, Kanki P et al: Retroviruses associated with leukemia and ablative syndromes in animals and human beings. Cancer Res 45[Suppl]:4534s, 1985

122. Harper ME, Kaplan MH, Marselle LM et al: Concomitant infection with HTLV-I and HTLV-III in a patient with T8 lymphoproliferative disease. N Engl J Med 315:1073, 1986

123. Fischl MA, Richman DD, Grieco MH et al: The efficacy of azidothymidine (AZT) in the treatment of patients with AIDS and AIDS-related complex. A double-blind placebo-controlled trial. N Engl J Med 317:185, 1987

Diagnostic Tests for HIV Infection: Serology

S. Gerald Sandler
Roger Y. Dodd
Chyang T. Fang

8

Current serologic tests for HIV infection are based on the observation that most persons infected by the human immunodeficiency virus (HIV) develop specific antibodies within a few weeks, and nearly all persons develop antibodies within a few months. These HIV-specific antibodies persist during the course of latent infection and, to varying degrees, during subsequent progression to overt disease, that is, acquired immunodeficiency syndrome (AIDS).[1-7] Although antibodies have been detected to nearly all HIV gene products,[8-10] those antibodies usually evaluated for the serologic diagnosis of HIV infection correspond to *gag*-encoded core proteins (p55, p24, p17), *env*-encoded glycoproteins (gp160, gp120, gp41), or *pol*-encoded reverse transcriptase (p66, p51) or endonuclease (p31). This chapter provides information on the serologic tests that are currently used for clinical laboratory diagnosis of HIV infection and outlines their relative advantages and limitations.

ENZYME IMMUNOASSAYS

Test Kits

Early studies of HIV infection established the effectiveness of enzyme immunoassays (EIAs), or enzyme-linked immunosorbent assays (ELISAs), for detecting virus-specific serologic responses.[1,2,11,12] The formats of these prototype enzyme immunoassays were adapted promptly by commercial manufacturers. By March 1985 the Food and Drug Administration (FDA) issued the first license for an enzyme immunoassay to detect HIV antibodies, and by September 1985, three FDA-licensed test kits were available in the United States.[13,14] By October 1987, eight manufacturers had received FDA licenses to market enzyme immunoassay test kits for HIV antibodies in the United States (Table 8–1).

All FDA-licensed test systems used in the United States are indirect solid-phase immunoassays using partially purified, disrupted and inactivated HIV as the reagent antigen. Six of these FDA-licensed EIAs are manufactured from an HIV isolate originally described as human T-lymphotropic virus type III (HTLV-III) and propagated in the National Cancer Institute's T-lymphocyte cell line H9/HTLV-III$_B$.[8] The Cellular Products test kit uses an HIV isolate cultured in lymphocytes from the same donor as the H9 cell line and identified as HUT-78. The Genetic Systems LAV EIA uses an HIV isolate originally described as lymphadenopathy-associated virus (LAV) by the Institute Pasteur and propagated in the CEM cell line.[15] Since the HIV preparations used for EIAs may also contain detectable host-cell components, differences in cell culture lines, such as their expression of histocompatibility locus antigens (HLAs) may contribute to different performance characteristics for certain EIAs. The Wellcozyme anti-HTLV III (Wellcome Diagnostics, Dartford), is a solid-phase competitive enzyme linked immunosorbent assay using microplate strips.[16,17] Wellcome kits are widely used in the United Kingdom and Europe, but they are not licensed by the FDA for use in the United States.

Test Kit Formats

Of the eight FDA-licensed EIA test kits for HIV antibodies, two use HIV-coated beads and six use HIV-coated microtiter wells as the solid phase (see Table 8-1). The methodologic principles, however, are identical for bead-coated and microtiter well-coated solid-phase test systems (Fig. 8-1).[18] Samples of serum or plasma to be tested for the presence of HIV antibodies are added to the HIV-antigen solid-phase and incubated. If HIV antibodies are present in the sample, they will bind to the HIV-antigen during incubation and be detected by

Table 8-1
Specifications of Enzyme Immunoassays for HIV Antibodies Licensed by the Food and Drug Administration*

Manufacturer	HIV Viral Isolate/ Cell Line	Reagent Antihuman Globulin	Format	Total Incubation Time (hr)	Number Controls Neg/Pos
Abbott Laboratories	HTLV-III H9	Polyclonal	Bead/Tray	$3\frac{1}{2}$	2/3
Cellular Products†	In-House HUT-78	Polyclonal	Microplate	$2\frac{1}{2}$	2/4
Du Pont/Biotech‡	HTLV-III H9	Polyclonal	Microplate	2	2/4
Electron-Nucleonics	HTLV-III H9	Polyclonal	Microplate	$1\frac{1}{2}$	2/3
Genetic Systems	LAV/CEM	Polyclonal	Microplate	$2\frac{1}{2}$	3/2
Organon Teknika	HTLV-III H9	Polyclonal	Bead/Microplate	$2\frac{1}{4}$	3/1
Ortho Diagnostics	HTLV-III H9	Monoclonal	Microplate	$2\frac{1}{2}$	3/2
Travenol-Genetech	HTLV-III H9	Monoclonal	Microplate	$3\frac{1}{2}$	4/2

* As of October 1987.
† Distributed by Eastman Kodak.
‡ Distributed by E. I. Du Pont De Nemours and Company, Inc.

an antiglobulin-enzyme conjugate followed by an enzyme-substrate reaction. A chromogen produces a spectrophotometrically detectable color reaction that, within certain technical limitations, is proportional to the amount of HIV antibodies bound to HIV antigens.

Sensitivity

The sensitivity of a clinical laboratory screening test is conventionally defined as the proportion of positive test results obtained when a population of true positives is tested.[19] The sensitivity of a test also defines the expected frequency of false negatives which is equal to the value of 1 minus sensitivity.[19] In the absence of standardized reference antisera for determining sensitivity, the FDA established an operational definition based on the ability of test kits to generate positive test results in populations of patients with AIDS (presumed to represent 100% positive tests).[13] To provide measurements of sensitivity, manufacturers conducted clinical trials in high-risk populations, and the results are reproduced in each manufacturer's package insert. However, because manufacturers tested different populations, there is minimal commonality. Claims by manufacturers pertaining to sensitivity that are based on data in their product inserts cannot be compared meaningfully. Studies directly comparing the ability of test kits to detect known positive and negative samples on a panel provide more useful information.[17,20-25]

Specificity

The specificity of a clinical laboratory test is conventionally defined as the frequency of negative results obtained when a population of true negatives is tested.[19] The frequency of false positives is equal to the value of 1 minus specificity. Manufacturers of EIA test kits obtained data by testing at least 1,000 blood donors prescreened for AIDS or other low-risk populations presumed on the basis of health history and other nonserologic information to have absence of HIV antibodies. This definition was a practical and efficient approach to providing a basis for FDA-licensure of the first generation of EIA test kits, which were urgently needed by blood donor services. However, there are limitations to the validity of these measurements since the results indicate that these low-risk populations did, in fact, include some HIV-infected individuals.

False-Negative Test Results

An important limitation of current EIAs for HIV antibodies is the potential for false-negative serologic test results, particularly during the early incubation period and acute viral syndrome.[26-30] To understand why false-negative EIA tests occur it is important to distinguish between (1) a negative EIA test result occurring when HIV antibodies are truly present and detectable by another serologic test; (2) a negative EIA test result oc-

Partially purified, inactivated human immunodeficiency virus (HIV) (antigen, △) is absorbed on microplate wells or polystyrene beads (solid phase, ⧄⧄).

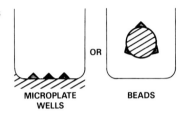

Samples to be tested are added, incubated with the HIV antigen, and washed. HIV-specific antibodies (⋏), if present, bind to absorbed antigens and are not removed by washing.

Enzyme-conjugated anti-human immunoglobulin (anti-Ig) (⏚) binds to anti-HIV.

Chromogen (⊟) develops color in proportion to quantity of enzyme-conjugated Ig.

Chromogen reaction is stopped. Optical absorbance is read by spectrophotometer, and test results are interpreted by relating optical density to cut-off value established by controls.

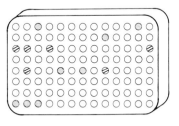

FIG. 8-1. General principles of the indirect enzyme immunoassay for HIV antibodies using antigen-coated beads or microplate wells as the solid phase. Valid test results require strict adherence to each test kit manufacturer's instructions as specified in the package insert.

curring in the absence of any detectable HIV antibodies in an individual proven to be infected by a nonserologic method, for example, viral isolation; and (3) operational errors.

False-negative EIA test results have been reported during the period immediately following a primary infection and prior to seroconversion. These false-negative test results have been attributed to lack of sensitivity for low-titer antibodies to *env*-encoded glycoproteins,[5,31,32] *gag*-encoded core proteins,[4,33,34] and isolated IgM anti-

bodies.[6] There is no consensus on which HIV-antibodies appear first and, therefore, which antibodies are most critical for the detection of an early serologic response. The identification of an acute viral syndrome following HIV infection[6,7,35–40] provides a clinical indicator of acute HIV infection and an important opportunity to focus studies on the early serologic response to HIV infection. Immunofluorescence assays (IFAs) may detect IgM HIV antibodies as early as 5 days after onset of symptoms of the acute viral illness, whereas current EIAs may not detect HIV antibodies until 31 to 58 days after the onset of symptoms, depending on the test kit used.[6] Free HIV antigen and/or low-titer antibodies to recombinant HIV proteins may be detected 6 to 14 months before HIV antibodies are detectable.[41] Attempts to narrow the vulnerable seronegative "window period" between the time of a primary HIV infection and the earliest detectable antibody response include the development of more sensitive EIAs using highly specific recombinant antigens.[42–45] Nevertheless, intrinsic limitations to the approach of testing for HIV antibodies will always remain. Another approach to narrowing of the seronegative "window period" is direct detection of HIV, DNA, or circulating viral proteins,[41,46–48] but the effectiveness of these tests has yet to be ascertained. This subject is discussed in further detail in Chapter 9.

Rarely, a second seronegative "window period" may occur in the terminal stages of AIDS, particularly in patients with Kaposi's sarcoma or *Pneumocystis carinii* pneumonia.[49] This finding represents the ultimate expression of humoral immunodeficiency and may be manifested by declining titers of antibodies to certain *gag*-encoded proteins (p24, p55), as well as the detection of circulating p24 protein.

False-Positive (Falsely Reactive) Test Results

Falsely reactive test results may be observed with any of the currently available EIAs for HIV antibodies, although the cause and frequency of these reactions vary for individual test kits. General principles that may be applied to interpreting reactive and falsely reactive EIA test results are outlined in Figure 8-2 and are described below. Readers are cautioned that valid interpretation of any EIA test result requires strict adherence to instructions in each manufacturer's package insert.

Falsely Reactive Test Results: EIA Not Repeatedly Reactive

A sample that tests "reactive" by an initial EIA ("initially reactive"), but nonreactive when the sample is retested by two additional EIAs may be considered "negative for HIV antibodies" (see Fig. 8-2). Such nonrepeatedly reactive EIA test results are usually attributable to technical errors or high negative test signals, for the following reasons:

TECHNICAL ERRORS. An erroneous reactive EIA test result may be due to a wide range of technical factors, including improper washing of microplate wells, cross-contamination of nonreactive samples by strongly reactive samples, contamination of chromogen reagents, or excessive color development. When automated washing devices are used, it is not uncommon for nonrepeatedly reactive test results to occur when enzyme conjugate is incompletely removed during the final wash.[19]

HIGH NEGATIVE SIGNAL. EIAs for HIV antibodies have been designed with priority for high sensitivity. Among other reasons, this priority was established because the first application of FDA-licensed test kits was detection of HIV-infected blood donors.[50] To achieve this objective, the optical density (OD) for cutoff values for nonreactive test results were, by design, selected to classify all equivocal test signals as reactive. The outcome is a certain number of nonrepeatedly reactive results in each test run which must be retested to obtain a valid serologic result. As a consequence of this design, minor variations in handling may cause samples with borderline high nonreactive signals to migrate over the cutoff and appear to be weak nonrepeatable reactives. Some clinical laboratories report increased sensitivity using commercial EIAs by intentionally redefining criteria for initially reactive test results, and retesting all samples with high nonreactive or otherwise equivocal signals.[51]

Falsely Reactive Test Results: EIA Is Repeatedly Reactive

If a sample tests "reactive" by the initial EIA and by at least one of two additional EIAs on repeat testing, the test result is reported to be "EIA repeatedly reactive for HIV antibodies, additional testing required" (see Fig. 8-2).[52] These samples should be tested by additional, more specific procedures, for example, immunoblot (Western blot) or indirect immunofluorescence antibody assay (IFA). If HIV antibodies are not confirmed by additional testing, the EIA test result is most probably falsely reactive. There are several possible causes of a repeatedly reactive, falsely positive reaction:

SEROLOGIC CROSS-REACTIVITY WITH LYMPHOCYTE ANTIGENS. HIV preparations used as antigen for EIAs may express HLA reactivity of the lymphocytes in cell cultures. The H9/HTLV III_B cell line used for most FDA-licensed EIAs has the HLA phenotype A1, Bw62, Bw6, Cw3, DR4, DQw3.[53] The HUT-78 cell line has the identical HLA phenotype.[54] Although prototype EIAs prepared from H9-derived HIV exhibited only minor reactivity when tested by HLA typing sera,[53] large-scale testing using commercial EIAs revealed that some falsely positive, repeatedly reactive EIA test results do occur and are the consequence of cross-reactions with class II HLA antigens.[54] These cross-reactions are usually specific for HLA-DR4,[55] but may involve other lymphocyte components as well.[55–58] Cross-reactions due to HLA antibodies in test samples are not a common problem with the Genetic Systems LAV EIA since the CEM cell line used in for manufacture of this kit does not express class II HLA antigens.

OTHER CAUSES OF FALSELY POSITIVE EIAS. Among other causes of falsely positive EIA test results are factors that might result in nonspecific adherence of immunoglobulin to the solid phase, such as repeated freezing

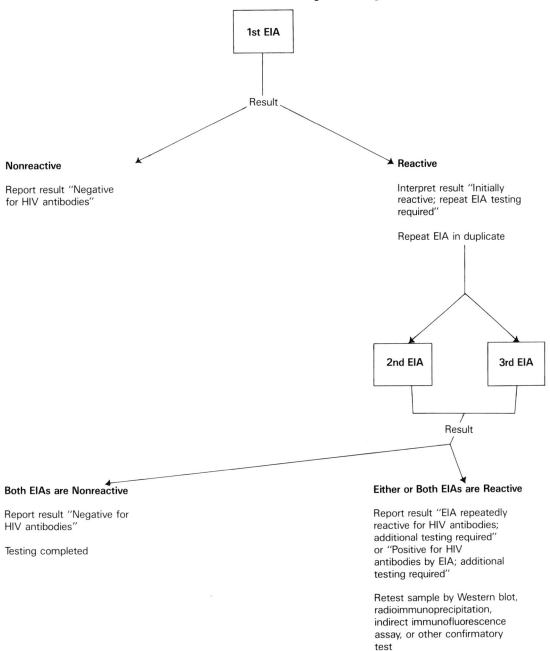

FIG. 8-2. Outline for interpreting test results of enzyme immunoassay for HIV antibodies. Usually, the likelihood of a truly positive result (positive predictive value) for an EIA test increases with the strength of the test signal (optical density). However, an occasional false-positive EIA reaction may be associated with a strong signal. For that reason, additional testing, such as immunoblot or indirect immunofluorescence antibody assay, is recommended for a valid serologic diagnosis.

and thawing of specimens,[25] "stickiness" of stored sera from malarial regions of Africa,[59,60] unexplained factors in samples from parenteral drug abusers,[61,62] and persons with alcoholic liver disease.[63] Cross-reactions with other retroviruses may also occur. For example, 15 of 20 sera from asymptomatic persons infected by lymphadenopathy-associated virus type 2 (LAV-2/HIV-2) reacted with an HIV EIA.[64] Such cross-reactivity with retroviral core proteins is not unexpected, since the name *gag* was given to these proteins because the prototype retroviral core protein (p30) was found to bear major antigenic determinants for *group-specific antigenicity* in early studies. Interestingly, sera containing HTLV-1 antibodies failed to cross-react when tested by an EIA for HIV antibodies, although 10% to 18% of samples containing HIV antibodies did cross-react in an EIA for HTLV-1 antibodies.[65]

Finally, variations in the performance (lot-to-lot consistency) of the test kits has been identified to be a factor contributing to false-positive, repeatedly reactive EIA test results. Between March 1985 and February 1986, for example, the rate of repeatedly reactive EIA test results for the Abbott Laboratories HTLV-III EIA varied by a factor of more than three times, from an initial rate of 14 per 10,000 samples to a high of 48 per 10,000 samples. During this same period, there was a stepwise decrease in the rate of true, confirmed positives (immunoblot) for HIV antibodies (Fig. 8-3).[66] This observation has been interpreted to reflect a high rate of false-positive, repeatedly reactive EIA test results based on follow-up studies of the implicated individuals who, in nearly all cases, had no history of high risk behavior and were found to be EIA nonreactive and immunoblot negative when subsequent samples were tested.

False-positive reactions are less of a problem in high-risk populations, such as promiscuous male homosexuals, than in low-risk populations, such as blood donors. An EIA that has a specificity of 99.8% will generate 20 false-positive results per 10,000 samples (0.2%) in any population. In a population with a true positive rate of 90%, the impact of 20 false positives among 9,000 true positives is not readily apparent. However, in low-risk blood donor populations where the true positive rate is approximately 1.5 per 10,000, 20 false positive results per 10,000 tests present a significant problem.

PASSIVELY TRANSFERRED HIV ANTIBODIES. Concern has been raised that passively transferred HIV antibodies might result in an erroneous interpretation of a truly positive EIA test result performed on a sample from a recent recipient of immune globulin (IG), hepatitis B immune globulin (HBIG) or intravenous immune

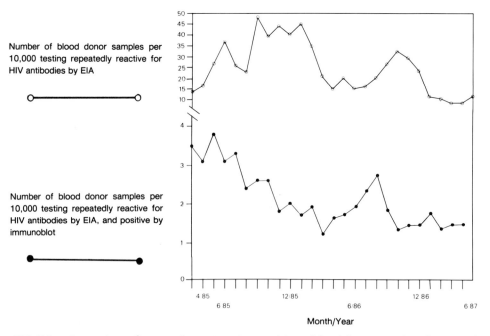

Number of blood donor samples per 10,000 testing repeatedly reactive for HIV antibodies by EIA

○——————○

Number of blood donor samples per 10,000 testing repeatedly reactive for HIV antibodies by EIA, and positive by immunoblot

●——————●

Month/Year

FIG. 8-3. Comparison of test results on American Red Cross blood donor samples when tested by EIA (only) and subsequently by immunoblot (Western blot). During the initial 11 months of testing, there was a gradual decrease in true positive results, reflected by immunoblot test results. In contrast, there was a threefold increase in the number of repeatedly reactive EIA test results during the same period. The discrepancy has been attributed to changes in the specificity of the manufacturer's test kits, since nearly all donors whose samples tested repeatedly reactive by EIA and negative by immunoblot had negative EIA test results on subsequent testing. Each month's results reflect approximately 500,000 tests.

globulin (IVIG).[67] This concern is based, in part, on the fact that some immune globulin products available in 1986–87 were manufactured from plasma collected prior to the introduction of donor testing for HIV antibodies and, therefore, may contain HIV antibodies.[68] Tests conducted at the FDA and Centers for Disease Control (CDC) have shown that as many as two-thirds of production lots of HBIG, as well as some lots of IG and IVIG, manufactured between 1982–85 may have detectable HIV antibodies.[68] Although the risk that a recipient of a standard dose of IG (0.06 mL/kg) will have a false positive EIA has been calculated to be more theoretical than real,[69] HIV antibodies were transiently detectable in the serum of some recipients of 1 to 5 ampules of HBIG that tested strongly reactive for HIV antibodies.[70]

IMMUNOBLOT (WESTERN BLOT)

Early studies of AIDS patients and asymptomatic HIV carriers demonstrated the importance of the immunoblot (enzyme linked immunoelectrotransfer; Western blot technique)[71,72] for detecting and identifying HIV antibodies.[1,73] The principal advantage of this test for serologic diagnosis is the separation and identification of individual HIV antibodies occurring naturally in complex mixtures, according to the molecular weights of corresponding HIV antigens.

Methodology

Variations of the immunoblot technique may be used by different laboratories, but the basic principles are similar (see Fig. 8-3). Partially purified, disrupted HIV is fractionated according to molecular weight by electrophoresis on polyacrylamide gel. HIV-specific proteins are transferred from the polyacrylamide gel to a nitrocellulose membrane by electroblotting. Individual nitrocellulose strips, now bearing HIV-specific proteins (reagent antigens), are incubated with test samples to detect the presence of HIV antibodies in an enzyme-linked anti–human-immunoglobulin reaction analogous to that of an EIA (compare Figs. 8-1 and 8-4). If HIV antibodies are present in a test sample, they will bind to HIV antigens on the nitrocellulose strip. After washing to remove any excess unbound immunoglobulin, HIV-specific antibodies are visualized by the enzyme anti–human-immunoglobulin chromogen reaction that stains the nitrocellulose strips in characteristic bands.

Diagnostic Criteria

Between 1985 and 1987, immunoblot tests were performed using a wide range of techniques and diagnostic criteria, and interlaboratory standardization was minimal. The American Red Cross Blood Services collabo-

rated with Abbott Laboratories to standardize immunoblot testing and required the presence of p24, gp41 and at least one other HIV-specific band (i.e., p51, p55, p66, gp120/160) as a criterion for a positive immunoblot test result. Since 1987, the American Red Cross national headquarters laboratory has required at least one band corresponding to *gag, env* and *pol* proteins to establish a serologic diagnosis of HIV infection. In 1985, the CDC issued guidelines recommending that the Western blot test result should be considered positive if band p24 or gp41 is present either alone or in combination with other bands.[52] These guidelines have been widely accepted for general clinical applications. In March 1987, the Second Consensus Conference of the Association of State and Territorial Public Health Laboratory Directors adopted criteria for a positive Western blot as the presence of at least two of the three major bands: p24, gp41, or gp120/160.[74] In April 1987, the FDA issued the first license for an HIV immunoblot test kit (Biotech/Du Pont HIV Western Blot Kit; E. I. Du Pont De Nemours and Company, Inc., Wilmington, DE).[75] This immunoblot test kit may identify as many as nine HIV-specific antibodies in strongly reactive samples (p17, p24, p31, gp41, p51, p55, p66, gp120, gp160) (Table 8-2).[76,77] Preliminary experience suggests that the Biotech/Du Pont Western Blot Kit has equivalent sensitivity to most FDA-licensed EIAs for detecting HIV antibodies. Diagnostic criteria for positive, indeterminate, and negative immunoblot test results using this test kit have been proposed (Table 8-3).

Indeterminate Immunoblot Results

Occasionally, a sample that tests repeatedly reactive for HIV antibodies by EIA may give an indeterminate result by immunoblot, i.e., bands are present but they do not fulfill diagnostic criteria for a positive test (Fig. 8-5). The frequency of these reactions depends on the population tested, the EIA test kit used to select the samples for immunoblot testing, and the immunoblot method itself. The clinical diagnosis of an individual whose sample tests indeterminate by immunoblot may be clarified by additional information obtained by personal interview, additional laboratory testing of the sample (i.e., IFA, radioimmunoprecipitation), or testing serial samples over a period of several weeks to months. Indeterminate or "atypical" immunoblot results may be the result of several different circumstances:

EVOLVING, EARLY ANTIBODY RESPONSE DURING SEROCONVERSION. The humoral response following primary HIV infection typically involves multiple HIV-specific antibodies. A sample obtained during this early response before the full complement of antibodies is detectable may yield an indeterminate immunoblot band pattern. There are some reports that immunoblot patterns limited to antibodies to p24 and other core proteins may represent early seroconversion,[33] whereas others indicate that antibodies to gp120 and gp160 are

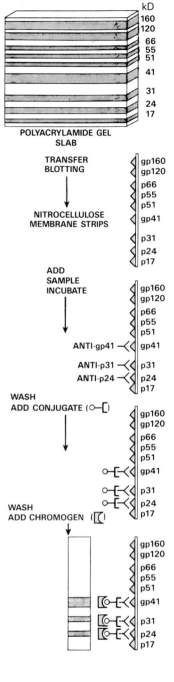

Disrupted, partially purified human immunodeficiency virus (HIV) is fractionated by polyacrylamide gel electrophoresis, distributing viral components according to molecular weight expressed in kilodaltons (kD).

HIV proteins (p) and glycoproteins (gp) are transferred to nitrocellulose membranes, which are cut into individual strips. HIV proteins and glycoproteins function as specific antigens (◁).

Nitrocellulose strips are incubated with serum or plasma, binding HIV-specific antibodies (─◁), if present, to corresponding antigens.

Enzyme-conjugated anti-human immunoglobulin binds to strips in areas that correspond to antibody-antigen reactions.

FIG. 8-4. General principles of the immunoblot (Western blot) technique for HIV antibodies. In this example, three HIV-specific antibodies (anti-gp41, -p31, and -p24) are presumed present in the test sample. Bands appear on the nitrocellulose strip in positions determined by the molecular weights of the corresponding HIV proteins.

Added chromogen develops color and stains strips in bands that correspond to distribution of antibody-antigen reactions.

more typical of early seroconversion.[31] Since these reports are based on screening with different EIA test kits as well as using different immunoblot methods, it is not possible to address the apparent discrepancy and distinguish between true biologic patterns and artificial differences due to variations in laboratory methods. When samples from seroconverting individuals are tested by the Biotech/Du Pont Western blot, antibodies to both *env*-and *gag*-encoded proteins are detectable (Fig. 8-6). The increased sensitivity of this immunoblot test for

detecting antibodies to gp120 and gp160 is attributed to a modification in the heating step before electrophoresis and blotting.[78] In a study conducted by the Netherlands Red Cross, 12 stored serum samples from known seroconverting male homosexuals were retested using the new Biotech/Du Pont Western blot, and all 12 samples had detectable antibodies to gp120, gp160, and p24. The original Western blot tests on these samples conducted during the period 1980–1982 prior to technical upgrading of the test kits revealed only anti-p24.[78]

Table 8-2

HIV-Specific Antibodies Detected by Immunoblot in Samples From AIDS Patients and Asymptomatic Carriers[76,77]

| | | Samples With Detectable Immunoblot Bands (%) | | |
| | | | Asymptomatic Carriers | |
Bands	HIV Gene Product	AIDS Patients (n = 127)	Positive (n = 914)	Indeterminate (n = 969)
gp160	Precursor of *env* glycoproteins	100	100	0
gp120	Outer *env* glycoprotein	100	99	0
p66	Reverse transcriptase component of *pol* translate	99	99	1.8
p55	Precursor of *gag* proteins	99	99	79.4
p51	Reverse transcriptase component of *pol* translate	99	98	1.8
gp41	Transmembrane *env* glycoprotein	100	100	0
p31	Endonuclease component of *pol* translate	94	95	0
p24	Core *gag* protein	98	99	18.2
p17	Core *gag* protein	84	89	38.7
	Samples reacting with all nine bands	76	85	0

* Biotech/Du Pont Western Blot Kit (Du Pont Company, Wilmington, DE)

Table 8-3

Criteria for Establishing a Serologic Diagnosis of HIV Infection Using FDA-Licensed Immunoblot Test Kit[76]

Immunoblot Bands Pattern	Interpretation
No bands present	Negative
A band is present at p24, p31, *and* either gp41 or gp160	Positive†
Band(s) present but pattern does not meet criteria for positive	Indeterminate

* Biotech/Du Pont HIV Western Blot Kit (Du Pont Company, Wilmington, DE)

† These criteria are proposed to apply to the interpretation of test results on samples from blood donors and other individuals without a corroborating history of risk for HIV infection. Less stringent criteria, for example only bands at gp41 and p24, may be applied for situations where the serologic diagnosis is corroborated by clinical information. A negative test in an individual with a high likelihood of HIV infection may indicate that the sample was obtained prior to seroconversion and testing of a second sample obtained 2 to 6 weeks later should be seriously considered.

Because of the many uncertainties in resolving indeterminate immunoblot test results, it is prudent to assume that all indeterminate immunoblot test results are potentially indicative of early seroconversion. If the implicated sample has not been tested using an FDA-licensed immunoblot kit, such retesting may be useful. Also, testing serial samples at 2- to 4-week intervals, depending on the urgency of the situation, may clarify whether the atypical band pattern is stable or evolving.

NONEVOLVING ANTIBODY RESPONSES LIMITED TO ANTI-p24 AND/OR OTHER GAG-ENCODED PROTEINS. More commonly, indeterminate immunoblot results are limited to anti-p24 and/or antibodies to other core proteins.[56,77–82] Usually, if the sample has been obtained from an individual without risk behavior for HIV infection, subsequent samples obtained over months and even years will reveal no additional antibodies to *env-, pol-,* or other gene products. In a recent study, 969 "indeterminate" blood donor samples were retested using the Biotech/Du Pont Western blot. The most frequently occurring antibodies were *gag*-related anti-p55, p17, and p24 (see Table 8-2).[77] Typically, individuals with nonevolving atypical immunoblot results do not have risk behavior for HIV infection, and limited studies in such individuals have failed to grow HIV in culture[80,83] or to demonstrate other signs of HIV infection. Sera that contain nonevolving antibodies to HIV core proteins may also react with HTLV-IV and HTLV-1 core proteins.[79] The etiology of these atypical serologic reactions, which appear to be limited to retroviral core proteins, is not known. Blood donors with such test results should be deferred and their blood excluded for transfusion purposes. Individuals with a history of risk behavior for HIV infection and such atypical immunoblot test results should be retested, perhaps in some instances for as long as 14 months after the initial sample was obtained.[41]

LOSS OF ANTIBODIES TO CORE PROTEINS DURING AIDS. As many as 50% of AIDS patients may lack detectable antibodies to *gag*-encoded proteins p24, p55, and p17, although they maintain antibodies to *env*-encoded membrane glycoproteins.[31] Immunoblots for such patients may not fulfill diagnostic criteria for a positive test result for HIV antibodies, but the clinical diagnosis in such cases is rarely equivocal (Fig. 8-7). In some instances, loss of HIV antibody reactivity has been

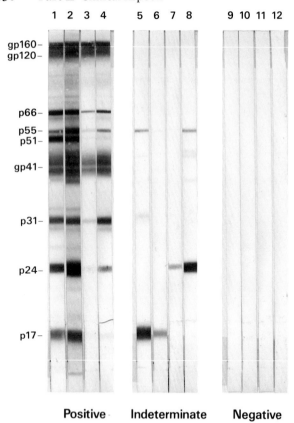

FIG. 8-5. Immunoblots demonstrating positive (lanes 1–4), indeterminate (lanes 5–8) and negative (lanes 9–12) results. *Establishing a serologic diagnosis* requires bands indicative of *env-*, *pol-*, and *gag*-encoded products. An indeterminate result indicates detection of at least one band, but constitutes insufficient criteria for a positive interpretation. A negative result indicates absence of all bands, but requires simultaneous positive controls to ensure valid test procedure. If there is a high clinical suspicion of HIV infection, most clinicians would regard bands at p24 and gp41 to be adequate for *confirming a clinical diagnosis.*

attributed to concomitant treatment with high-dose glucocorticoids or other immunosuppressive drugs for cancer or organ transplantation.

OTHER RETROVIRAL INFECTIONS. Atypical HIV immunoblot patterns may occur when samples are tested from individuals who are infected by another retrovirus. Sera from patients infected by HIV-2, HTLV-IV, and HTLV-1 may be reactive when tested by HIV EIAs, but immunoblot bands are limited to *gag*-encoded proteins.

ERRORS IN TECHNIQUE OR INTERPRETATION. The immunoblot test has not been well standardized and technical proficiency varies widely from one laboratory to another. In a quality assurance program conducted

by the United States Army, identical panels of samples were distributed to five large commercial laboratories performing HIV immunoblot tests on a fee-for-service basis.[84] Each panel consisted of 15 samples known to be nonreactive for HIV antibodies and 5 samples obtained from HIV-infected patients with clearly positive immunoblot test results for HIV antibodies. Four of the five laboratories reported at least one false-positive immunoblot test result. The single most common result was erroneous reporting of a band at p24 when testing normal samples. The FDA-licensed Biotech/Du Pont Western blot kit includes a strongly reactive control as a guide to the relative positioning of HIV bands. Also, this kit includes a weakly reactive control that exhibits bands at p24 and gp160 as a measure of sensitivity to ensure valid test results. These quality control measures should eliminate most cases of erroneous interpretation.

Errors of overinterpretation of immunoblots may also contribute to the reporting of erroneous results.[57] Because the viral antigen preparation used for immunoblots contain nonviral cellular proteins, not all bands appearing on an immunoblot are necessarily HIV spe-

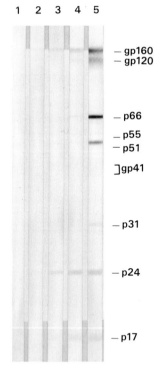

FIG. 8-6. Immunoblot results illustrating HIV seroconversion, demonstrated on serial samples from an individual following primary HIV infection. Lane 1, negative. Lane 2, weak p24 and weak gp160 (Day 1). Lane 3, p24, gp160, weak p17, trace gp120 (Day 14). Lane 4, p24, p17, gp160, weak gp120, weak p66, trace p55, p51 (no gp41) (Day 35). Lane 5, all bands (a few weeks later). (Courtesy of Dr. Steve Alexander, Biotech Research Laboratories)

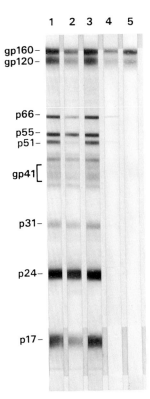

FIG. 8-7. Immunoblot results from five AIDS patients, demonstrating loss of serologic reactivity to core proteins. Lanes 1–3, samples from AIDS patients demonstrating a full complement of HIV-specific antibodies. Lanes 4 and 5, samples from two AIDS patients with far advanced immunodeficiency, demonstrating reactivity to *env*-encoded gp120 and gp160, but absence of reactivity to all *gag*-encoded proteins.

cific.[57,85] Laboratory staff reporting immunoblot results must be expert in recognizing non-HIV band patterns to avoid overinterpretation as a cause of false-positive immunoblot test results.

Retesting after False-Positive EIA Results: "Reentry Protocol"

The availability of an FDA-licensed immunoblot test kit has made it possible to reevaluate the HIV antibody status of blood donors and other individuals without risk behavior who were previously found to have a repeatedly reactive EIA test result, but whose immunoblot tests were clearly negative.[86] Evidence supporting this protocol included studies of more than 1,000 blood donors with repeatedly reactive EIAs, but negative immunoblots, who had negative viral cultures for HIV and/or showed no signs or symptoms of HIV infection.[87,81,83] The protocol was based on the assumption that if the discrepant EIA and immunoblot test results were due to early seroconversion, repeat testing after 6 months

would demonstrate HIV antibodies by immunoblots, as well by EIA.

The principal application of this protocol has been to clarify the serologic status of blood donors whose repeatedly reactive ("positive") EIA for HIV antibodies required permanent deferral in accordance with FDA directives and Public Health Service recommendations for testing blood donors for HIV antibodies.[52] An outline of the protocol for retesting these donors was distributed by the FDA in April 1987. The protocol provides for the reentry of such donors if retesting of a frozen aliquot of the original sample and a sample obtained 6 months later gives negative results by two different EIA tests, and if the second sample also tests negative by an FDA-licensed immunoblot test (Fig. 8-8).[87]

INDIRECT IMMUNOFLUORESCENCE (IFA)

Although IFA is a very useful serologic test for detecting or confirming the presence of HIV antibodies,[88–96] it has not been as widely used as the immunoblot test procedure.[95]

Methodology

IFA is used by clinical laboratories for serologic diagnosis of infection by a wide range of viruses, including influenza virus, mumps virus, measles virus, rabies virus, herpes viruses, and adenoviruses.[97–99] The IFA procedure for detecting viral antibodies consists of incubating test samples with virus-infected cells that have been spread and fixed on glass slides. Virus-specific antibodies, if present, bind to antigens expressed on the infected cells and are detected by fluorescein-conjugated anti–human-immunoglobulin. Reactions are read by fluorescence microscopy. The principles of this procedure have been adapted for detection of HIV antibodies using the HUT-78,[49] or H9 cell lines.[90] Reliable IFA test results have been achieved following incubations as short as 20 minutes.[88] Positive IFA reactions are defined as diffuse cytoplasmic fluorescence, but positive staining patterns may be focal, capping, or limited to membrane staining.[96] A negative reaction is defined as the absence of fluorescence staining. A dull nondiscriminatory staining pattern, which may include nuclear staining, suggests "nonspecific" serologic reactivity, such as antinuclear, anti-HLA,[90] anti-*Mycoplasma*[57] or other non-HIV antibodies. Recognition of nonspecific reactivity may be facilitated by preparing slides with a mixture of HIV-infected and uninfected culture cells in a known ratio (i.e., 1:3). Fluorescence on more than 25% of the cells on the smear indicates presence of "nonspecific" or cross-reacting antibodies. Nonspecific reactivity may be eliminated by absorption of sera with uninfected cells,[88,91] but this procedure may interfere with the detection of weak, low-titer HIV antibodies if they are present also.[90]

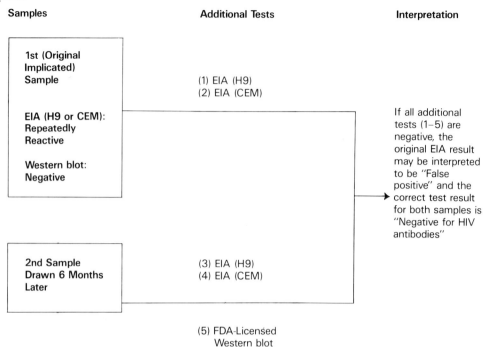

FIG. 8-8. Recommended protocol for retesting a blood donor with a repeatedly reactive EIA test result that is presumed to be falsely positive because of a negative immunoblot and the individual's denial of risk for HIV infection. According to FDA guidelines, donor samples are retested by the EIA from the same kit manufacturer as the original test, and by an EIA manufactured using a different cell culture line (H-9 or CEM). If all EIAs are negative (i.e., on the 6-month sample and on a frozen aliquot of the original sample) and if an FDA-licensed additional test (i.e., Western blot) on the 6-month sample is also negative, the donor may be re-entered as a prospective donor.

As experience with this protocol accumulates, it may be possible to simplify the retest procedures. In clinical situations, it should be possible to expand the application of this protocol, or simplified adaptations, to other categories of individuals with discrepant EIA (repeatedly reactive) and immunoblot (negative) test results, and without risk of HIV infection. Additional data will be needed, however, before the results of such variations in the retest protocol can be ensured valid.

Advantages and Disadvantages

IFA is easier to perform than immunoblot procedures, and may be equally sensitive and specific.[88,95] However, the availability of marketed FDA-licensed immunoblot (Western blot) kits, including standardized reagent test strips, puts expert immunoblot testing within the reach of most clinical laboratories. The principal advantage of IFA is that test results may be available in 30 minutes,[95] whereas current immunoblot procedures usually require an overnight incubation. Another advantage of IFA is the convenience of a one-step procedure compared to the two-step detection/confirmation protocol for EIA/ immunoblot. For this reason, IFA is advantageous for low-volume reference laboratories that test samples from high-risk populations.[96]

The principal advantage of immunoblot over IFA is its capacity to identify individual HIV-specific antibodies, which may confirm the clinical diagnosis (see Figs.

8-5, 8-6, 8-7). For blood donor services, the additional confidence that is added by visualization of nine or more virus-specific bands is substantial. In contrast to testing in hospital laboratories where samples are referred to *confirm* clinical suspicions of HIV infection, blood donor services test samples from persons who *deny* risk behavior for HIV infection. Thus, visualization of several characteristic antigen–antibody bands on a positive immunoblot adds confidence to a serologic diagnosis of HIV infection when the laboratory test result is a contradiction, not a confirmation, of the available clinical history.

RADIOIMMUNOPRECIPITATION ASSAY (RIPA)

Radioimmunoprecipitation is a research method that may have application for resolving selected, complex serologic diagnostic problems. Because RIPAs are ex-

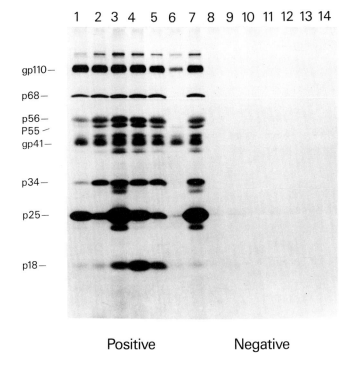

1 2 3 4 5 6 7 8 9 10 11 12 13 14

gp110—
p68—
p56—
P55—
gp41—
p34—
p25—
p18—

Positive   Negative

FIG. 8-9. Radioimmunoprecipitation of human sera reactive and nonreactive with specific HIV viral proteins. HIV virus was radiolabeled with ^{35}S-methionine and a radioimmunoprecipitation performed according to methods described previously.[103] Lanes 1–7 show reactivity of human sera to specific HIV viral proteins. Lanes 8–14 show human sera nonreactive to HIV. Human sera positive for HIV show reaction to a spectrum of viral proteins representing envelope proteins (gp110, gp41), core proteins (p55, p25, p18), and polymerase proteins (p68, p56, p34). (Courtesy of Genetic Systems)

pensive and labor intensive and require containment facilities for handling live HIV, they are not used routinely in clinical laboratories.[57,100]

Methodology

In radioimmunoprecipitation assays, HIV antibodies are detected by using radiolabeled lysates of purified virus or HIV-infected cells. Test samples are incubated with the cell lysate. If HIV-specific antibodies are present, they will bind to the corresponding radiolabeled viral antigens. All antibody molecules are then precipitated from the reaction mixture, including bound, but not unbound, radiolabeled viral antigens. The antibody–antigen complexes are separated by polyacrylamide gel electrophoresis of the precipitates, and the labeled antigens are identified by autoradiography.[57,100–103] HIV antibodies detected by RIP assays include viral proteins encoded by *env-* (gp110/120, gp41), *gag-* (p55, p24/25, p17/18) and *pol-* genes (p66/68, p51/56, p31/34) (Fig. 8-9).[103]

Advantages and Disadvantages

The radioimmunoprecipitation assay is particuary useful for detecting antibodies to the *env-*encoded HIV glycoproteins gp120 and gp41, which may not be consistently detected by immunoblot. Radioimmunoprecipitation assays are also useful for distinguishing HIV from closely related viral strains.[64,102,104] The principal disadvantages of radioimmunoprecipitation assays are high

cost and the need for highly specialized virus handling facilities. As immunoblot methods are improved and standardized, radioimmunoprecipitation assays may be needed less frequently to confirm the presence of weakly reactive antibodies to HIV glycoproteins.

REFERENCES

1. Sarngadharan MG, Popovic M, Bruch L et al: Antibodies reactive with human T-lymphotropic retroviruses (HTLV-III) in the serum of patients with AIDS. Science 224:506, 1984
2. Brun–Vezinet F, Barre–Sinoussi F, Saimot AG et al: Detection of IgG antibodies to lymphadenopathy-associated virus in patients with AIDS or lymphadenopathy syndrome. Lancet 1:1252, 1984
3. Pan L–Z, Cheng–Mayer C, Levy JA: Patterns of antibody response in individuals infected with the human immunodeficiency virus. J Infect Dis 155:626, 1987
4. Groopman JE, Chen FW, Hope JA et al: Serological characterization of HTLV-III infection in AIDS and related disorders. J Infect Dis 153:736, 1986
5. Allain J–P, Paul DA, Laurian Y et al: Serological markers in early stages of human immunodeficiency virus infection in haemophiliacs. Lancet 2:1233, 1986
6. Cooper DA, Imrie AA, Penny R: Antibody response to human immunodeficiency virus after primary infection. J Infect Dis 155:1113, 1987
7. Ho DD, Sarngadharan MG, Resnick L et al: Primary human T-lymphotropic virus type III infection. Ann Intern Med 103:880, 1985
8. Gallo RC, Salahuddin SZ, Popovic M et al: Frequent detection and isolation of cytopathic retroviruses (HTLV-

III) from patients with AIDS and at risk for AIDS. Science 224:500, 1984

9. Franchini G, Robert–Guroff M, Aldovini A et al: Spectrum of natural antibodies against five HTLV-III antigens in infected individuals: Correlation of antibody prevalence with clinical status. Blood 69:437, 1987

10. Kalyanaraman VS, Cabradilla CD, Getchell JP et al: Antibodies to the core protein of lymphadenopathy-associated virus (LAV) in patients with AIDS. Science 225:321, 1984

11. Saxinger C, Gallo RC: Application of the indirect enzyme-linked immunosorbent assay microtest to the detection and surveillance of human T cell leukemia-lymphoma virus. Lab Invest 49:371, 1983

12. Spira TJ, DesJarlis DC, Marmor M et al: Prevalence of antibody to lymphadenopathy-associated virus among drug-detoxification patients in New York. N Eng J Med 311:467, 1984

13. Petricciani JC: Licensed test for antibody to human T-lymphotropic virus type III: Sensitivity and specificity. Ann Intern Med 103:726, 1985

14. Marwick C: Blood banks give HTLV-III test positive appraisal at five months. JAMA 254:1681, 1985

15. Barre–Sinoussi F, Chermann JC, Rey F et al: Isolation of T-lymphotropic retrovirus from a patient at risk for acquired immune deficiency syndrome (AIDS). Science 220:868, 1983

16. Taylor H–L, Moulsdale HJ, Mortimer PP: Blood donor screening by Wellcome anti-HIV kits. Lancet 1:631, 1987

17. Evans RP, Shanson DC, Mortimer PP: Clinical evaluation of Abbott and Wellcome enzyme linked immunosorbent assays for detection of serum antibodies to human immunodeficiency virus (HIV). J Clin Pathol 40:552, 1987

18. Kurstak E: Enzyme Immunodiagnosis, p 25. Orlando, FL, Academic Press, 1986

19. Dodd RY: Testing for HTLV-III/LAV. In Menitove JE, Kolins J (eds): AIDS, p 55. Arlington, VA, American Association of Blood Banks, 1986

20. Reesink HW, Huisman JG, Lelie PN et al: Evaluation of six enzyme immunoassays for antibody against human immunodeficiency virus. Lancet 2:483, 1986

21. Nishanian P, Taylor JMG, Korns E et al: Significance of quantitative enzyme-linked immunosorbent assay (ELISA) results in evaluation of three ELISAs and Western blot tests for detection of antibodies to human immunodeficiency virus in high-risk population. J Clin Microbiol 25:395, 1987

22. Fang CT, Williams KW, Wilkinson JS et al: Comparative study on pre-licensure screening kits for HTLV-III antibodies. Transfusion [abstr] 25:480, 1985

23. Fang CT, Darr F, Kleinman SP: Relative specificity of enzyme-linked immunosorbent assays to human T-lymphotropic virus type-III: Relationship to Western blot. Transfusion 26:208, 1986

24. Carlson JR, Hinrichs SH, Levy NB: Evaluation of commercial AIDS screening test kits. Lancet 1:1388, 1985

25. Vercauteren G, van der Groen G, Piot P: Comparison of enzyme immunoassays and an immunofluorescence test for detection of antibody to human immunodeficiency virus in African sera. Eur J Clin Microbiol 6:132, 1987

26. Marlink RG, Allan JS, McLane MF et al: Low sensitivity of ELISA testing in early HIV infection. N Eng J Med 315:1549, 1986

27. Zuck TF: Greetings—with comments on lessons learned this past year from HIV antibody testing and from counseling blood donors. Transfusion 26:493, 1986

28. McFadden T, Jason JM, Feorino P: HTLV-III/LAV-seronegative, virus-negative sexual partners and household contacts of hemophiliacs. JAMA 255:1702, 1986

29. Goedert JJ, Eyster ME, Bodner AJ et al: A search for HTLV-III and its antibodies in hemophilia families. [abstr] p 48, First International Conference on AIDS, Atlanta, GA, 1985

30. Jason JM, McDougal JS, Dixon G et al: HTLV-III/LAV antibody and immune status of household contacts and sexual partners of persons with hemophilia. JAMA 255:212, 1986

31. Barin F, McLane MF, Allan JS et al: Virus envelope protein of HTLV-III represents major target antigen for antibodies in AIDS patients. Science 228:1094, 1985

32. Ulstrup JC, Skaug K, Figenschaun KJ et al: Sensitivity of Western blotting (compared with ELISA and immunofluorescence) during seroconversion after HTLV-III infection. Lancet 1:1151, 1986

33. Esteban JI, Shih JWK, Tai CC et al: Importance of Western blot analysis in predicting infectivity of anti-HTLV/III/LAV positive blood. Lancet 2:1083, 1985

34. Lange JMA, Coutinho RA, Kronc WJA et al: Distinct IgG recognition patterns during progression of subclinical and clinical infection with lymphadenopathy-associated virus/human T-lymphotropic virus. Br Med J 292:228, 1986

35. Cooper DA, Gold J, Maclean P et al: Acute AIDS retrovirus infection: Definition of a clinical illness associated with seroconversion. Lancet 1:537, 1985

36. Tindall B, Barber S, Donovan B et al: Characterization of the acute clinical illness associated with human immunodeficiency virus infection. Arch Intern Med (in preparation), 1987

37. Lindskov R, Lindhardt BO, Weismann K et al: Acute HTLV-III infection with roseola-like rash. Lancet [letter] 1:447, 1986

38. Boiteux F, Vilmer E, Girot R et al: Lymphadenopathy syndrome in two thalassemic patients after LAV contamination by blood transfusion. N Eng J Med 312:648, 1985

39. Tucker J, Ludlam CA, Craig A: HTLV-III infection associated with glandular-fever-like illness in a haemophiliac. Lancet 1:585, 1985

40. L'Age–Stehr J, Schwarz A, Offermann G: HTLV-III infection in kidney transplantation recipients. Lancet [letter] 2:1361, 1985

41. Ranki A, Krohn M, Allain J–P: Long latency precedes overt seroconversion in sexually transmitted human-immunodeficiency-virus infection. Lancet 2:589, 1987

42. Burke DS, Brandt BL, Redfield RR et al: Diagnosis of human immunodeficiency virus infection by immunoassay using a molecularly-cloned and expressed virus envelope polypeptide. Ann Intern Med 106:671, 1987

43. Kenealy W, Reed D, Cybulski R: Analysis of human serum antibodies to human immunodeficiency virus (HIV) using recombinant ENV and GAG antigens. AIDS Res Hum Retrovir 3:95, 1987

44. Schulz TF, Aschauer JM, Hengster P et al: Envelope gene-derived recombinant peptide in the serodiagnosis of human immunodeficiency virus infection. Lancet 2:111, 1986

45. Chang TW, Kato I, McKinney S et al: Detection of antibodies to human T-cell lymphotropic virus III (HTLV-III) with an immunoassay employing a recombinant *Escherichia coli* derived viral antigenic peptide. Biotechnol 3:905, 1985

46. Paul DA, Falk LA: Detection of HTLV-III antigens in serum. J Cell Biochem [Suppl] 10A:224, 1986

47. Goudsmit J, Paul DA, Lange JMA et al: Expression of hu-

man immunodeficiency virus antigen (HIV-Ag) in serum and cerobrospinal fluid during acute and chronic infection. Lancet 2:177, 1986

48. Kessler HA, Blaauw B, Spear J et al: Diagnosis of human immunodeficiency virus infection in seronegative homosexuals presenting with an acute viral syndrome. JAMA 258:1196, 1987

49. Pan L–Z, Cheng–Mayer C, Levy JA: Patterns of antibody response in individuals infected with the human immunodeficiency virus. J Infect Dis 155:626, 1987

50. Allen JR: Scientific and public health rationales for screening donated blood and plasma for antibody to LAV/HTLV-III. In Petricciani JC, Gust ID, Hoppe PA et al (eds): AIDS: The safety of blood and blood products, p 141. New York, John Wiley & Sons, 1987

51. Barr A, Muir W, Dow BC et al: Detection of anti-HTLV-III: Modification of a commercial enzyme immunoassay. Med Lab Sci 44:97, 1987

52. Centers for Disease Control: Provision Public Health Service inter-agency recommendations for screening donated blood and plasma for antibody to the virus causing acquired immunodeficiency syndrome. Morbid Mortal Week Rep 34:1, 1985

53. Weiss SH, Mann DL, Murray C et al: HLA-DR antibodies and HTLV-III antibody ELISA testing. Lancet 2:157, 1985

54. Sayers MH, Beatty PG, Hensen JA: HLA antibodies as a cause of false-positive reactions in screening enzyme immunoassays for antibodies to human T-lymphotropic virus type III. Transfusion 26:113, 1986

55. Kuhnl P, Seidl S, Holzberger G: HLA DR4 antibodies cause positive HTLV-III antibody ELISA results. Lancet 1:1222, 1985

56. Bieberfeld G, Bredberg–Raden U, Bottiger B et al: Blood donor sera with false-positive Western blot reactions to human immunodeficiency virus. Lancet 2:289, 1986

57. O'Shaughnessy MV: LAV/HTLV-III antibody confirmatory testing. In Petricciani JC, Gust ID, Hoppe PA et al (eds): AIDS: The safety of blood and blood products, p 171, New York, John Wiley & Sons, 1987

58. Rucheton M, Graafland H, Fanton H et al: Presence of circulating antibodies against gag-gene MuLV proteins in patients with autoimmune connective tissue disorder. Virology 144:468, 1985

59. Biggar RJ, Gigase PL, Melbeye M et al: Elisa HTLV retrovirus antibody reactivity associated with malaria and immunocomplexes in healthy Africans. Lancet 2:520, 1985

60. Schupbach J, Tanner M: Specificity of human immunodeficiency virus (LAV/HTLV-III)-reactive antibodies in African sera from southeastern Tanzania. Acta Tropica 43: 195, 1986

61. Moore JD, Cone EJ: HTLV-III seropositivity in 1971–1972 parenteral drug abusers: A case of false positives or evidence of viral exposure. N Eng J Med 314:1387, 1986

62. D'Aquila R, Williams AB, Kleber HD et al: Prevalence of HTLV-III infection among New Haven, Connecticut parenteral drug abusers in 1982–1983. N Eng J Med 314:117, 1986

63. Mendenhall CL, Roselle GA, Grossman CJ et al: False positive tests for HTLV-III antibodies in alcoholic patients with hepatitis. N Eng J Med 314:921, 1986

64. Brun–Vezinet F, Katlama C, Roulot D et al: Lymphadenopathy-associated virus type 2 in AIDS and AIDS-related complex. Lancet 1:128, 1987

65. Porter L, Le P, Akins R et al: Serological crossreactions between HIV and HTLV-I. Transfusion [Abstr], (in preparation) 1987

66. Schorr JB, Berkowitz A, Cumming PD et al: Prevalence of HTLV-III antibody in American blood donors. N Eng J Med [letter] 313:384, 1985

67. Steele DR: HTLV-III antibodies in human immune gamma globulin. JAMA [letter] 255:609, 1986

68. Centers for Disease Control: Safety of therapeutic immune globulin preparations with respect to transmission of human T-lymphotropic virus type III/lymphadenopathy-associated virus infection. Morbid Mortal Week Rep 35: 231, 1986

69. Wolfe WH, Miner JC, Armstrong FP et al: More on HTLV-III antibodies in immune globulin. JAMA 256:2200, 1986

70. Tedder RS, Uttley A, Cheingsong–Popov R: Safety of immunoglobulin preparation containing anti-HTLV-III. Lancet [letter] 1:815, 1985

71. Towbin H, Staehelin T, Gordon J: Electrophoretic transfer of proteins from polyacrylamide gels to introcellulose sheets: Procedures and some applications. Proc Natl Acad Sci USA 76:4350, 1979

72. Tsang VCW, Peralta JM, Simons AR: Enzyme-linked immunoelectrotransfer blot techniques (EITB) for studying the specificities of antigens and antibodies separated by gel electrophoresis. Meth Enzymol 92:377, 1983

73. Popovic M, Sarangadharan MG, Read E et al: Detection, isolation, and continuous production of cytopathic retroviruses (HTLV-III) from patients with AIDS and pre-AIDS. Science 224:497, 1984

74. Association of State and Territorial Public Health Laboratory Directors: Second Consensus Conference on HIV Testing: Report and Recommendations. March 16–18, 1987, Atlanta, GA.

75. Nightingale SL: HIV Western blot kit approved. JAMA 257:3030, 1987

76. Human immunodeficiency virus (HIV) Biotech/Du Pont HIV Western blot kit: For detection of antibodies to HIV [package insert]. Wilmington, DE. Specialty Diagnostics/E.I. duPont De Nemours and Company, Inc., 1987

77. Fang C, Le P, Mallory D et al: Western blot patterns of antibodies to human immunodeficiency virus (HIV). Transfusion [Abstract], 27:539, 1987

78. Lelie PN, van der Poel CL, Reesink HW: Interpretation of isolated HIV anti-p24 reactivity in Western blot analysis. Lancet 1:632, 1987

79. Dock NL, Lamberson HV, O'Brien TA et al: Evaluation of HIV antibody reactivity in blood donors with atypical Western blot patterns [Abstr WP 226] p 148, Abstracts Volume III International Conference on AIDS, Washington, DC, 1987

80. van der Poel CL, Reesink HW, Tersmette TH: Blood donations reactive for HIV in Western blot, but non-infective in culture and recipients of blood. Lancet 2:752, 1986

81. McClure J, Dykers T, Shriver K et al: Analysis of sera exhibiting atypical reactions with LAV/HTLV. Transfusion 26:577, 1986

82. Courouce A–M, Muller J–Y, Richard D: False-positive Western blot reactions to human immunodeficiency virus in blood donors. Lancet 2:921, 1986

83. Ward JW, Grindon AJ, Feorino PM et al: Laboratory and epidemiologic evaluation of an enzyme immunoassay for antibodies to HTLV-III. JAMA 256:357, 1986

84. Burke DS, Redfield RR: False-positive Western blot tests for antibodies to HTLV-III. JAMA 256, 1986

85. Roy S, Portnoy J, Wainberg MA: Need for caution in in-

terpretation of Western blot tests for HIV. JAMA 257:1047, 1987

86. Sandler SG: Retesting category 8 donors by FDA-licensed Western blot test kits. American Red Cross Blood Services Letter No. 87-32 (May 1, 1987), National Headquarters, Washington, D.C.

87. Esber EC: Recommended testing protocol to clarify status of donors with a reactive anti-HIV screening test [Memorandum]. U.S. Food and Drug Administration, Bethesda, MD, April 29, 1987

88. Gallo D, Diggs JL, Shell GR et al: Comparison of detection of antibody to the acquired immune deficiency syndrome virus by enzyme immunoassay, immunofluorescence, and Western blot methods. J Clin Microbiol 23:1049, 1986

89. Sanstrom EG, Schooley RT, Ha DD et al: Detection of human anti-HTLV-III antibodies by indirect immunofluorescence using fixed cells. Transfusion 25:308, 1985

90. Carlson JR, Yee J, Hinrichs SH et al: Comparison of indirect immunofluorescence and Western blot for detection of anti-human immunodeficiency virus antibodies. J Clin Microbiol 25:494, 1987

91. Kaminsky LS, McHugh T, Stites D et al: High prevalence of antibodies to acquired immune deficiency syndrome (AIDS): associated retrovirus (ARV) in AIDS and related conditions but not in other disease states. Proc Natl Acad Sci USA: 82:5535, 1985

92. Blumberg RS, Sandstrom EG, Paradis TJ: Detection of human T-cell lymphotropic virus type III-related antigens and anti-human T-cell lymphotropic virus type III antibodies by anticomplementary immunofluorescence. J Clin Microbiol 23:1072, 1986

93. Hedenskog M, Dewhurst T, Ludwigsen C et al: Testing for antibodies to AIDS-associated retrovirus (HTLV-III/LAV) by indirected fixed cell immunofluorescence: Specificity, sensitivity and application. J Med Virol 19:325, 1986

94. McHugh TM, Stites DP, Casavant CH et al: Evaluation of the indirect immunofluorescent assay as a confirmatory test for detecting antibodies to the human immunodeficiency virus. Diag Immunol 4:233, 1986

95. Levy JA: Indirect immunofluorescence assays can readily detect antibodies to the human immunodeficiency virus. JAMA 257:1176, 1987

96. Lennette ET, Karpatkin S, Levy JA: Indirect immunofluorescence assay for antibodies to human immunodeficiency virus. J Clin Microbiol 25:199, 1987

97. Menegus MA, Douglas G Jr: Viruses, rickettsiae, chlamydiae, and mycoplasmas. In Mandell GL, Douglas RG Jr, Bennett JE (eds): Principles and Practices of Infectious Diseases, 2nd ed, p 138, New York, John Wiley & Sons, 1985

98. Gardner PS, McQuillin J: Rapid virus diagnosis. London, Butterworths, 1974

99. White DO, Fenner FJ: Medical Virology, 3rd ed, p 325, Academic Press, Inc. NY, 1986

100. Saah AJ: Serologic tests for human immunodeficiency virus (HIV). In AIDS: Information on AIDS for the practicing physician, Vol 2, p 11. Chicago, American Medical Association, 1987

101. Huisman HG, Winkel IN, Lelie PN et al: Future of confirmatory testing: Sensitivity of immunoblot analysis and radio-immunoprecipitation assay for the detection of antibodies to LAV/HTLV-III. In Petricciani JC, Gust ID, Hoppe PA et al (eds): AIDS: The safety of blood and blood products, p 199, New York, John Wiley & Sons, 1987

102. Chiodi F, Bredberg–Raden U, Biberfeld G et al: Radioimmunoprecipitation and Western blotting with sera of human immunodeficiency virus infected patients: A comparative study. AIDS Res Hum Retrovir 3:165, 1987

103. Gosting LH, McClure J, Dickinson ES et al: Monoclonal antibodies to gp110 and gp41 of human immunodeficiency virus. J Clin Microbiol 25:845, 1987

104. Kanki PJ, Barin F, Souleyman M et al: New human T-lymphotropic retrovirus related to simian T-lymphotropic virus type III (STLV-III$_{AGM}$). Science 232:238, 1986

Detection of Human Retroviruses

Bernard J. Poiesz
Garth D. Ehrlich
Lawrence D. Papsidero
John J. Sninsky

9

There are four known human retroviruses: Human T-cell lymphoma/leukemia viruses (HTLV) types I and II[1,2] and human immunodeficiency viruses (HIV) types I and II.[3,4,5] HTLV-I and -II are oncornaviruses and are associated with CD4[+] T-lymphocytic malignancies.[6,7] HTLV-I has been recently linked to a chronic progressive neurologic disorder termed tropical spastic paraparesis or HTLV-I–associated myelopathy (HAM).[8,9] HTLV-I is endemic in southern Japan, central Africa, and the Caribbean, while HTLV-II has been identified only in sporadic cases in the United States. HIV-I and II are lentiviruses[10,11] and are the etiologic agents of acquired immunodeficiency syndrome (AIDS) and its prodromal forms.[12,13] As with HTLV-I, HIV-I has also been associated with a neuropathic syndrome.[14,15] While HIV-I has been responsible for the worldwide pandemic of AIDS, HIV-II infection appears to be primarily confined to western Africa and Europe.[16–18] All of these viruses except HIV-II have been isolated from American patients and represent a serious public health problem in the United States.

The genomic structures of two of these viruses and their principle encoded structural and functional proteins are illustrated in Figure 9-1. In this chapter, discussion will be confined to the viral core and envelope structural proteins and to the retroviral DNA polymerase protein, reverse transcriptase (RT). As can be seen, these viruses contain other functional genes that encode for proteins (*TAT, ART, SOR*, etc.) which affect trans-activation of viral and cellular RNA transcription and translation; viral messenger RNA splicing and stability; and viral infectivity, respectively.[19–21] These functional genes are discussed in detail in Chapter 2.

Strategies employing a variety of serologic assays (e.g., ELISA, Western blot, RIPA) to detect natural antibodies to the viral structural proteins are currently used to identify patients who have been exposed to human retroviruses and to exclude potentially infected blood products from being transfused.[22] These assays are described in Chapter 8. When used together, they have sensitivities and specificities of greater than 99%. Although some of these techniques are suitable for mass screening for viral exposure, it is clear for several reasons that they provide insufficient information for complete analyses of these retroviral infections. First, it is now apparent that until patients mount an immune response they can be infected with a retrovirus and be seronegative for several months to more than a year after exposure to these viruses.[23–24] In addition, for unexplained reasons, a finite number of infected patients with clinical disease remain seronegative for prolonged periods of time.[25] Second, although seropositivity to a particular human retrovirus and a set of clinical symptoms has been used to establish diagnoses (e.g., adult T-cell leukemia [ATL], AIDS, or AIDS related complex [ARC]), it would seem probable that staging patients by establishing their "viral load" and sites of involvement would provide additional important prognostic information. Indeed, it seems possible that certain seropositive individuals are not infected at all and, hence, would have excellent clinical courses and lower biohazard potential. Furthermore, given the high mutation rate of HIV-I,[26–27] the variable number of HIV-I proviral DNA copies[28] (either integrated and/or non-integrated) and the apparent randomness of proviral integration in general,[29–30] it will continue to be important to actually detect, quantitate, isolate, and characterize the particular retroviral isolate infecting a given cell type, individual, and/or population. Finally, the ability to perform such viral analyses will be necessary to understand the epidemiology and pathogenesis of these retroviral infections and to monitor the efficacy of vaccines and antiviral therapies.

This chapter, then, will deal with the methodologies suitable for retroviral detection, quantitation, isolation, and characterization. The discussion will focus primarily on HTLV-I and HIV-I because they are currently the

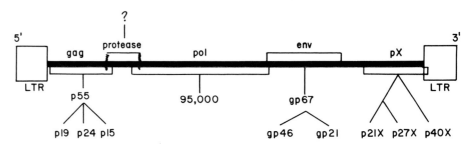

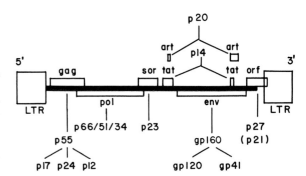

FIG. 9-1. Proviral genomic DNAs of HTLV-I (*top*) and HIV-I (*bottom*). The *LTR* (long terminal repeats) contains sequences for regulating RNA transcription from the viral genome. The *gag* (group antigen specific) gene encodes for the core proteins. The *pol* gene encodes for the reverse transcriptase and endonuclease proteins. The *env* gene encodes for two outer-envelope proteins. The other genes, *tat, art,* etc., encode for highly specialized functional viral proteins, which are discussed in depth elsewhere in this text.

most clinically relevant isolates. However, the methodologies discussed will apply to any of the human retroviruses now known or yet to be discovered.

RETROVIRAL LIFE CYCLE

In order to understand the techniques used to detect, isolate, and characterize a retrovirus, it is important to understand how they are physically packaged and how they replicate. As shown in Figure 9-2, a mature virus contains two single strands of 35S, full length, genomic RNA contained in a protein core or capsid. The *gag* gene protein products (p19, p24, p15 for HTLV-I; p17, p24, p12 for HIV-I) comprise the structural elements of the core. The virus's unique DNA polymerase, reverse transcriptase, is also packaged in the core and is intimately associated with the viral RNA.[31] The core is surrounded by an outer envelope comprised of the two *env* gene protein products embedded in a lipid membrane. One or both of these proteins are usually glycosylated with the exact nature of the carbohydrate moiety dependent upon the type of host cell in which the virus was grown. One of these proteins exists solely on the outer surface of the envelope and is termed the *spike protein,* while the other traverses the envelope and is termed the *transmembrane protein.* Historically it has been felt that the most 5' *gag* gene product (p19 for HTLV-I and p17 for HIV-I) (see Fig. 9-1) was associated with the core only. However, both HTLV-I p19 and HIV p17 are

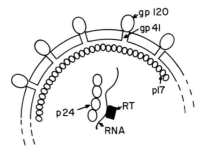

FIG. 9-2. Schematic of the assembled viral proteins in a mature HIV-I virion.

myristylated[32,33] and this may explain why both of these proteins are also found embedded in the inner surface of the viral envelope and host cell membranes (see Fig. 9-2). Since the viral particle ultimately is formed by budding of the virion from the host cell surface, the viral envelope also contains host cellular membrane components (lipids, sugars, and proteins) that can obfuscate results of antibody or antigen detection (Fig. 9-3) (see Chap. 8). Another source of confusion in interpreting antiretroviral antibody or retroviral antigen analyses is that the structural protein products of each of the retroviral genes are initially translated as large polyproteins which are ultimately cleaved into mature functional peptides by a virally encoded protease (usually located within the 3' *gag* gene and/or 5' *pol* gene

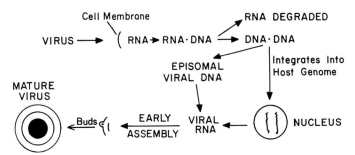

FIG. 9-3. Life cycle of the human retroviruses. Mature virions bind to specific cell surface receptors then enter the cell and undergo uncoating. Within minutes, the RNA is copied into double-stranded viral DNA by the reverse transcriptase and ribonuclease H activity of one of the *pol* gene products. In HTLV-I and HTLV-II the proviral DNA integrates into the host chromosomal DNA at a site affected by the endonuclease activity of the 3′ *pol* gene product. In HIV-I infections, however, the proviral DNA can also be present in a nonintegrated form. The proviral DNA can remain latent for years but ultimately will be transcribed into RNA, which will subsequently be translated into viral polyproteins, which are cleaved into their individual components. The proteins and viral genomic RNA assemble at the cell surface, and virions bud out and mature extracellularly. In this budding process the virions retain cellular membrane moieties. Further, glycosylation of their envelope proteins will be determined by metabolic processes within the cell. Hence, the ultimate protein, carbohydrate, and lipid content of the virions produced is very dependent on the particular host cell expressing the virus.

(Fig. 9-4; see also Figs. 9-1 and 9-3).[34] Since this process of protease cleavage is not always completed as virions mature, the virus often contains a mixture of individual lower molecular-weight (MW) proteins and higher MW polyproteins.[35,36]

Retroviruses have a unique life cycle, as shown in Figure 9-3. In order to infect a cell, mature virions must first bind by means of their outer envelope proteins (Fig. 9-2) to specific cell surface receptors. The presence of these receptors is a major factor in determining the cellular and species specific tropism of a given retrovirus. The lack of appropriate receptors prevents infection and therefore disease. Once bound, the virus enters the cell either by direct fusion with the cellular membrane or by endocytosis. While the primary receptor for HIV-I has been demonstrated to be the CD4 antigen present on some T-lymphocytes, B-lymphocytes, and macrophages,[37,38] the receptors for the other human retroviruses are unknown. Assays exist, however, for measuring retroviral binding to the cell surface.[39] These should allow for further characterization of these receptors and for *in vitro* and *in vivo* studies on agents (particularly vaccines and monoclonal antibodies) that could interfere with this interaction.

After the virus enters the cell it loses its outer envelope. The viral nucleocapsid, which contains two 35S genomic RNA molecules, each associated with an RT protein,[31] is then activated in the cytoplasm to commence synthesis of a double-stranded cDNA from the virion-associated RNA. The synthesis of full-length cDNA is probably dependent on the intact structure of the viral core.* The genomic RNA molecules each have a transfer

RNA (tRNA) binding site, positioned 3′ to the U5 region, to which a cellular tRNA is bound in the virion.[40,41] This RNA duplex serves as a template primer system that is recognized by the viral RT, which then synthesizes a DNA (cDNA) strand complementary to the 5′ end of the genomic RNA.[31] This is termed *strong stop DNA.* An integrally associated ribonuclease H activity of the RT then degrades the RNA strand of the heteroduplex, and the second DNA strand is synthesized. Following several polymerization and degradation steps, a double-stranded DNA provirus is produced with two complete LTRs (see Fig. 9-1).[42] The unintegrated provirus can exist in either a linear or circular form, but recent studies suggest that it is the linear molecule that integrates into the host's genome.[43] This newly formed DNA can either remain as an episomal element, as is sometimes the case with HIV,[44] or be integrated into the host's genome, as is the requirement for HTLV-I and II and also occurs with HIV. This integration event depends upon the endonuclease activity of a *pol* gene product,[45,46] on sequences present in the viral LTRs,[42,47] and probably on chromatin structure or the presence of active DNA synthesis in the host target DNA.[29,30,48]

Whether present as an integrated and/or nonintegrated form, the proviral DNA can do one of two things: it can remain latent without substantial expression of the structural genes or, using cellular RNA polymerases and substrates, it can begin to transcribe the genomic and subgenomic RNAs necessary for the production of the virus-associated genome and its structural and functional proteins, respectively. The subgenomic RNAs are translated into the viral polyproteins, which are subsequently cleaved into mature peptides (see Figs. 9-3, 9-4). Viral RNA and core proteins assemble at the cell

---

* Coffin J: Personal communication.

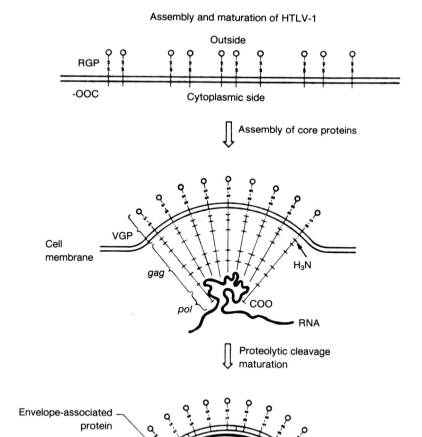

FIG. 9-4. Schematic illustrating the assembly and maturation of HTLV-I. While some protein cleavage occurs intracellularly, full maturation does not occur until after the virions bud from the cell. The degree of maturation will affect the infectivity of the virions produced.

surface, ultimately budding out as immature particles. After budding, there is further cleavage of the polyproteins and subsequent nuclear capsid condensation. Typically, only a small minority (1:1000) of the extracellular virions produced represent mature infectious particles.[49]

RETROVIRUS DETECTION AND ISOLATION

Previous studies of animal retroviruses provided many clues regarding techniques useful for their detection and isolation. These methodologies have also proven useful in the discovery of all of the human retroviruses. The first of these was that cellular transmission, proviral DNA integration and expression, and virus production all were augmented when target cells for viral transmission or infected cells for viral expression were induced to proliferate.[50,51] Pioneers in the field of human retrovirology had long espoused a belief that, like bovine leukemia virus, human retroviruses would prove to be predominantly latent *in vivo,* and infected cells would have to be cultured *in vitro* for prolonged periods before detectable levels of virus could be achieved.[52–54] Indeed, it was in part the necessity to identify hematopoietic growth factors to facilitate retroviral research that led to the discovery of T-cell growth factor or IL-2.[55] This protein enables the propagation *in vitro* of normal and malignant human T-lymphocytes[56,57], and its use has been absolutely critical in the initial discovery and isolation of all of the known human retroviruses.

Routine isolation of virus from individuals infected with HTLV-I or HTLV-II has proven relatively simple since these cells express elevated levels of the IL-2 receptor.[58] They therefore have a distinct growth advantage over uninfected cells when cultured in the presence of delectinated, partially purified IL-2. Typically, even in patients with a very low percentage of infected cells (e.g., ≤ 1:100 peripheral blood mononuclear cells [PBM]), it is possible to detect virus after a month in culture. Also, since these cells are transformed, they sometimes can be weaned off exogenous IL-2 and be easily and cheaply cultured in bulk (≥100 liters). HIV-I and HIV-II proved much harder to isolate, primarily because they are typically present in a much smaller fraction of PBM (≤1:10,000) than HTLV-I and II and, rather than being oncogenic, they are cytopathic and result in the destruction, not the immortalization, of the infected cells. French investigators were the first to overcome these HIV-I–associated phenomena when they periodically added fresh, PHA-stimulated PBMs

from normal individuals to cultures containing IL-2 and PHA-stimulated PBM from AIDS/ARC patients.[59] By allowing the newly synthesized HIV-I virions to infect the activated PBM, they were able to achieve continuous production of HIV-I *in vitro*. Although this has proved to be a reasonable technique for routine virus culture for antiviral drug studies (Table 9-1), it does not provide a facile, inexpensive method for bulk production of HIV-I. The latter was accomplished by investigators at the National Institutes of Health (NIH) when they transmitted HIV-I to resistant clones of a CD4+, uninfected, IL-2–independent, T-cell leukemic cell line.[4] This clonal cell line, H9, or its parent culture, HUT 78,[60] and other immortal cell lines now serve as excellent co-cultivation partners and long-term HIV-I producers.[61] Recently, other investigators have shown that removing the AIDS/ARC patient's CD8-positive cells from the co-culture increased HIV-I production presumably by removing cells that would be cytotoxic or suppressive for HIV-I infected cells.[62] Results in our laboratory corroborate these findings, and we have further found that the optimal way to passage an isolate is to use cell-free, conditioned media from cultures of the patients' PBMs co-cultivated with HUT-78 to infect previously uninfected HUT-78 cells (Table 9-2).

Table 9-1
Incidence of Seronegativity to Either HTLV-I or HIV-I

Diagnosis	Total No. of patients	No. seropositive *	No. seronegative, DNA positive
AIDS/ARC	1160	1158 (99.8%)	2 (0.17%)
ATL, TSP, HTLV-I carrier	500	493 (98.6%)	7 (1.4%)

* ATL, TSP, HTLV-I carriers tested against HTLV-I; AIDS/ARC tested against HIV.

Table 9-2
Different HIV-I Genotypes as Determined by Enzymatic Gene Amplification

Sample No.	Diagnosis	Primer Pairs				
		5' gag SK01, 02	3' gag SK17, 18	LTR SK29, 30	pol SK32, 33	env SK68, 69
1	AIDS	−	+	−	−	−
2	Asymptomatic male homosexual	+	+	+	−	−
3	AIDS	+	+	+	−	−
4	AIDS	−	+	−	−	+
5	AIDS	−	−	−	−	+/−
6	AIDS	+	−	+	+	+
7	AIDS	−	+	−	−	−
8	AIDS	+	+	+	+	+/−
9	AIDS	+	+	+	+	−
10	AIDS	+	+	−	−	−

Several techniques have been developed that will modestly increase virus production *in vitro,* namely the addition of polybrene to stabilize virus/receptor binding,[4] the addition of the nucleoside analog, 5'-iododeoxyuridine,[1] and the addition of dexamethasone, which binds to a steroid receptor within the retroviral LTR sequences and thereby enhances RNA transcription. However, the addition of antibodies to α-interferon to the cell cultures has had little impact in our studies. The probable reason for this is that, while the AIDS/ARC patients have an acid-labile α-interferon in their plasma[63] that inhibits retroviral transmission, *in vitro* their cell cultures produce γ-interferon, which does not affect virus replication.[64]

The standard technique for detecting a new retrovirus has been and still is to screen concentrated cell-culture–conditioned media (by polyethylene glycol precipitation or by centrifugation at $40,000 \times g$) for reverse transcriptase activity. Retroviruses and related eukaryotic transposable elements are the only life forms that contain this unique DNA polymerase, which preferentially copies RNA into DNA rather than DNA into DNA.[65] Although RTs can copy any form of RNA into DNA, they are most efficient when synthetic template primers are used (Fig. 9-5). These typically contain 12 to 18 bases of a DNA primer annealed to 300 bases of an RNA template. In the presence of the appropriate radioactively labeled nucleoside triphosphates, divalent cation (usually Mn^{++} or Mg^{++}), and potassium, the RT released when virions are disrupted by detergent (typically Triton-X 100) can efficiently incorporate the labeled nucleotide into the extended DNA strand as directed by the nucleotide sequence of the RNA strand. This results in an acid precipitable, radioactively labeled RNA:DNA hybrid. This product is then analyzed in a liquid scintillation counter; and results are expressed as picomoles of nucleoside monophosphate incorporated per hour or, if compared to a standard, as RT units. Two particular synthetic template-primers are routinely used in these assays: poly rA-oligo dT; and poly rC-oligo dG.[1] Some confusion can occur, however, when poly rA-oligo dT is used because certain DNA-dependent DNA polymerases (e.g., human DNA polymerase γ and *Mycoplasma sp.* polymerase) can also efficiently use this template primer and can potentially be present in the co-cultures. Fortunately, the template-primer, poly rC-oligo dG, is quite retrovirus specific and, although not used equally well by all animal retroviruses, it is utilized efficiently by all of the identified human retroviral RTs, particularly in the presence of Mg^{++} (see Fig. 9-5).

During the initial years of screening patients for HTLV-I or HIV-I, investigators relied largely on analyses of cell cultures for reverse transcriptase. As can be seen in Figure 9-6, this approach allows for reasonable separation between index cases and presumably normal populations when their respective T cells are placed in co-cultivation with a permissive cell line. However, the signal-to-noise ratio between many infected patients and normals is not large enough to avoid missing some infected persons if the cutoff is set too high, or calling some normals false positive if the cutoff is set too low. Part of the reason for this is that it is not possible to control the amount of cellular DNA polymerases produced and released into the culture media such that their concentrations can vary over several orders of magnitude among separate cultures. While these DNA-dependent DNA polymerases do not utilize poly rA-oligo dT or poly rC-oligo dG efficiently, they can utilize them to some degree and, if they are present in large amounts, can yield results that overlap with low levels of viral activity.

Classically, in order to prove that a new retrovirus has been isolated, it has been necessary to demonstrate particle-associated RT activity, the criteria for which are that it can be maintained in continuous culture, it can be serially passaged to uninfected target cells, and it can be purified in bulk form on sucrose gradients.[1,4] The latter task is performed by growing the infected cells in culture (anywhere from 1 to 100 liters of 10^6 cells/ml), pelleting the particles from the cell-culture–conditioned media at high speed ($40,000 \times g$), and banding the particles on sequential sucrose or glycerol gradients and demonstrating the presence of RT activity in fractions corresponding to the buoyant density of retroviral particles (Fig. 9-7).[1,4] The proteins and nucleic acids of

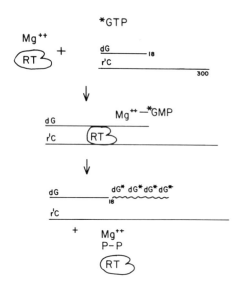

FIG. 9-5. Schematic of a reverse transcriptase assay utilizing the template-primer poly-rC oligo-dG. The 18 bases of dG DNA serve as a primer for DNA synthesis off of the 300 bases of poly-rC RNA in the presence of magnesium and radioactively labeled quanosine triphosphate. Ultimately, the results can be expressed as picomoles of quanosine monophosphate incorporated. These small synthetic template-primers are very specific for reverse transcriptase and results in much greater levels of nucleotide incorporation than an endogenous assay using viral genomic RNA as a template and cellular tRNA as a primer.

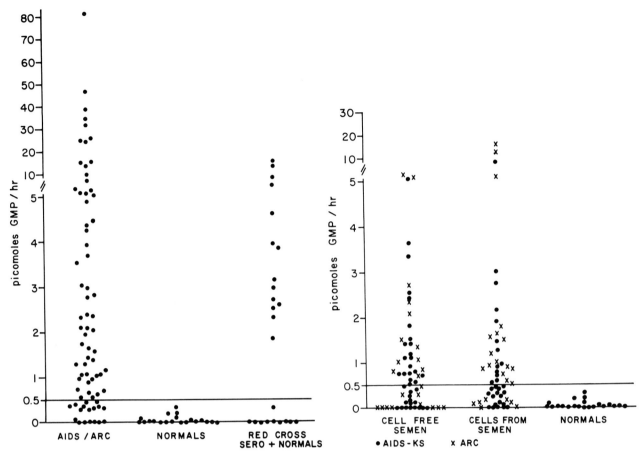

FIG. 9-6. Reverse transcriptase activity from concentrated 14-day-old cell culture conditioned media from PBM and semen cultures from AIDS/ARC patients and normals. As can be seen, there is reasonable discrimination between normals and patients (we routinely score results between 0.5 and 1.0 pM GMP incorporated as +/− and results ≥ 1.0 pM GMP as +. However, using this cutoff is still somewhat insensitive and is plagued by false negatives. Lowering the cutoff will increase the true positive rate but, as would be expected, also results in more false positives.

these purified virions can then be analyzed and used to make probes and detection systems for further studies. This is precisely what has happened with respect to HTLV-I and HIV-I.[40,44,66] Contributions from many laboratories have led to an in-depth understanding of both the HTLV-I and HIV-I genomes;[26,67] indeed, many isolates have been cloned and fully sequenced.[28,40,41,68,69] Nucleic acid probes exist for all of the human retroviruses. Furthermore, monoclonal and polyclonal antibodies to all of the major structural proteins of both HTLV-I and HIV-I have also been derived.

As these antibodies became available, it became possible to probe for the production of specific viral proteins *in vivo* and *in vitro*. As anticipated, owing to the latent nature of the human retroviruses, examination of mononuclear cells from fresh peripheral blood by indirect immunoperoxidase or immunofluorescence assays proved fruitless. The number of infected cells was too low or the viruses were not being expressed to any great degree. We and others have found, however, that protein-producing cells can be found in the lymph nodes, and in benign and malignant tissues of the patients. (Fig. 9-8).[70] These assays have facilitated the awareness that, at least in the case of HIV-I, the virus does infect non T cells *in vivo*.[71] Currently, our preferred method for detection of viral proteins is to use a triple antibody sandwich technique that works on both fresh cells and paraffin embedded fixed tissues. (Fig. 9-9).

Although analyses of fresh cells were usually unrewarding, it is possible to assay for viral proteins in T cells after they are stimulated with mitogen and cultured with IL-2. Similarly, B cells can be stimulated with anti-μ and cultured with B cell growth factor and monocytes can be stimulated with human effusion fluids or normal

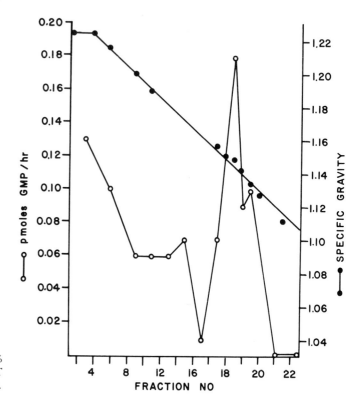

FIG. 9-7. Sedimentation profile of HIV-I virions on a 22% to 65% sucrose gradient. Fractions were analyzed for RT activity expressed as picomoles GMP incorporated per hour.

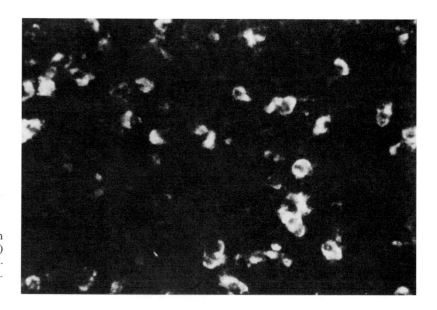

FIG. 9-8. HTLV-I positive cells in the lymph node of an ATL patient, (fluorescent cells) as detected using a double-antibody immunofluorescent assay employing an anti-HTLV-I p19 monoclonal antibody.

human sera and analyzed for virus production (Fig. 9-10). Fixed or unfixed cells can then be analyzed with indirect immunosandwich assays that tag the infected cells with either alkaline phosphatase, peroxidase, or a fluorescent dye. The cells can then be examined under routine light or fluorescent microscopes or on a fluorescent activated cell sorter (Fig. 9-11).

Although these assays are useful, they are neither sensitive enough nor efficient enough for determining the efficacy of antiviral drugs in *in vitro* and *in vivo* studies. Over time a series of ELISA formats has evolved to detect soluble viral antigens (Fig. 9-12). These include competitive ELISAs[72] and "antigen capture" assays[73-75] that are quite sensitive and produce linear

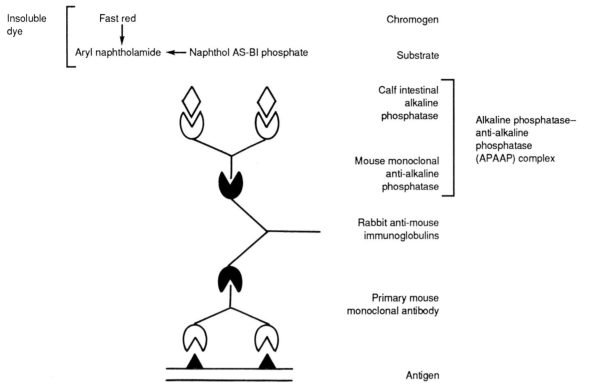

Insoluble dye [Fast red ↓ Aryl naphtholamide ◄— Naphthol AS-BI phosphate]

Chromogen

Substrate

Calf intestinal alkaline phosphatase

Mouse monoclonal anti-alkaline phosphatase

Alkaline phosphatase–anti-alkaline phosphatase (APAAP) complex

Rabbit anti-mouse immunoglobulins

Primary mouse monoclonal antibody

Antigen

FIG. 9-9. Schematic for the triple antibody sandwich technique, optimal for detecting human retroviral proteins in fixed tissue.

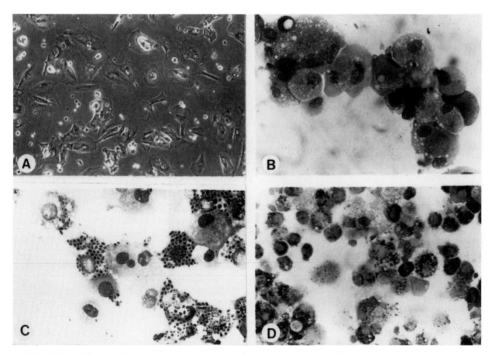

FIG. 9-10. Cultured human monocytes stimulated with human effusion fluids. Cells will proliferate until they become confluent.

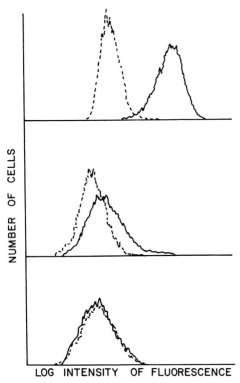

FIG. 9-11. Histograms of fluorescent activated cell sorter analyses of indirect fluorescent antibody staining of cells from three different cell cultures reacting with either an anti-HTLV-I p19 monoclonal antibody (*solid line*) or a negative control murine monoclonal antibody of the same isotype (*broken line*). Top, HTLV-I infected cell line MT-2; *middle,* HTLV-I infected cell line UMC-CTL-5B; and *bottom,* normal human T cells.

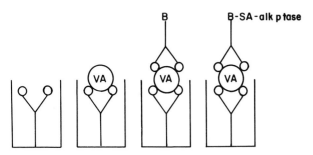

FIG. 9-12. Schematic for a typical antigen capture assay. Polyclonal or monoclonal anti-HIV-I immunoglobulin is bound to the bottom of a plastic well. Human body fluid samples or cell culture conditioned media are then added to the well. After washing, viral antigen present in the fluids will remain bound to the first antibody. It can then be detected by a biotinylated second polyclonal or monoclonal antiviral antibody. Strepavidin bound to alkaline phosphatase is then added and reacted with an appropriate substrate indicator dye. Samples are then evaluated on an automated plate reader, and optical densities are compared to a known viral antigen standard.

results. These assays can be designed to be very specific, depending upon which particular single antibody or combination of antibodies is used. They also can be designed to be epitope specific and therefore can be used to immunophenotype different viral isolates, which should prove useful for a highly mutable virus such as HIV-I. Currently, these assays are being used in our laboratory as an initial screen for the *in vitro* anti-HIV-I effect of neutralizing antibodies or antiviral drugs (Figs. 9-13, 9-14). They also have been chosen to quantitate plasma or serum viral antigenemia and cell culture viral production in most current clinical trials of anti-AIDS agents.

Measuring viral antigens in fresh plasma, fresh cell lysates, or cultured material has proved useful; but for several reasons these assays do not necessarily provide accurate data about the level of viral infection in a given patient. First, only a minority of retrovirally infected patients will test positive in their fresh plasma and cells. Second, cultures of patients' cells are not necessarily always positive, and if they are positive do not necessarily reflect "viral load." Many variables will influence the ultimate viral protein yield. These include the original proviral DNA copy number, the level of cell stimulation and virus expression, the ability of the expressed virus to infect other target cells in the culture, and the degree of the cytopathic effect on the original and newly infected cells by both the virus and the immunocytes in the culture. Additionally, culture techniques for both HTLV-I and HIV-I are both time consuming and expensive.

For all of these reasons, it would be desirable to measure viral nucleic acid directly from fresh tissues and PBM. Since standard techniques such as Southern blotting and dot blotting require at least 1 copy of virus per 100 cells, they are useful only in patients with a leukemic phase. This occurs only with HTLV-I or II when an infected T-cell clone has expanded *in vivo.* Most HIV-I infected patients and many HTLV-I infected patients have too few infected cells to be detected by these techniques. *In situ* hybridization methods can be used for the detection of a low number of infected cells,[76] but these techniques are primarily dependent on RNA expression and are tedious and laborious to perform. In order to overcome these constraints, we have successfully employed an *in vitro* enzymatic gene amplification process, the polymerase chain reaction (PCR),[77,78] to increase exponentially small regions of the genomes of all of the known human retroviruses.[70,79,80]

Figure 9-15 illustrates in schematic form the PCR method of enzymatic gene amplification. This technique is absolutely dependent upon prior knowledge of the nucleic acid sequences to be detected. Fortunately, such information is available for all of the human retroviruses. With this sequence information oligonucleotides (20–30 bases long) are synthesized to the respective 5' ends of opposite strands of the region of the retroviral genome to be amplified. These oligonucleotides will be

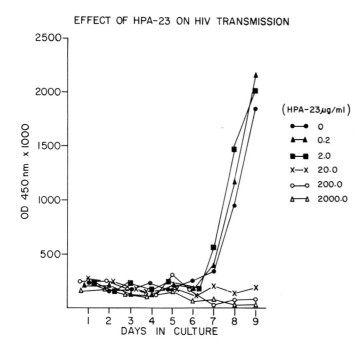

EFFECT OF HPA-23 ON HIV TRANSMISSION

(HPA-23 μg/ml)

- ●—● 0
- ▲—▲ 0.2
- ■—■ 2.0
- x—x 20.0
- ○—○ 200.0
- △—△ 2000.0

FIG. 9-13. Effect of various concentrations of the antiviral compound HPA-23 on *in vitro* transmission and/or expression of cell-free HIV-I virions added to target HUT 78 cells. Virus was added to cells that had been treated for 24 hours with the indicated drug concentrations. The cells were then placed in culture, and viral antigen in the cell culture media was analyzed 4 days later using an antigen capture assay. Inhibition was observed between 2 and 20 μg/ml of HPA-23. Although HPA-23 is believed to be a reverse transcriptase inhibitor, these results can only confirm that the drug has an effect on either transmission or expression, or both.

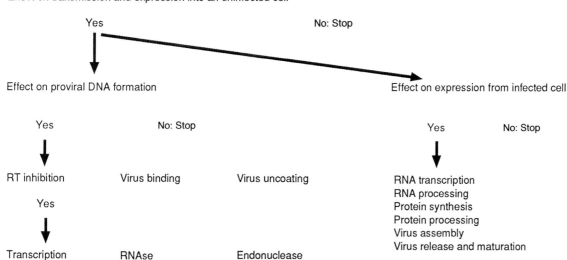

Antiviral assays

Effect on transmission and expression into an uninfected cell

Yes — No: Stop

Effect on proviral DNA formation — Effect on expression from infected cell

Yes — No: Stop — Yes — No: Stop

RT inhibition — Virus binding — Virus uncoating — RNA transcription
Yes — RNA processing
— Protein synthesis
Transcription — RNAse — Endonuclease — Protein processing
— Virus assembly
— Virus release and maturation

FIG. 9-14. Algorithm for the *in-vitro* evaluation of antiviral drugs. Agents that score positive in the screen assay described in Fig. 9-12 are evaluated in a systematic fashion for their effects on the pre- and/or post-proviral DNA stage of the virus life cycle, using enzymatic gene amplification of DNA from target T cells as the discriminating assay.

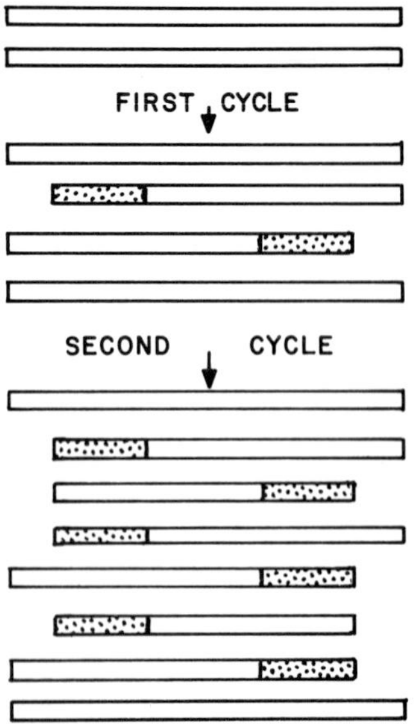

FIG. 9-15. Schematic of the polymerase chain reaction through two amplification cycles. Double-stranded human DNA, which presumably contains retroviral DNA, is denatured at 94°C to yield two single strands of DNA. Primer pairs (*stippled*) consist of small oligonucleotides to 5' regions of opposite strands of a portion of the retroviral genome. Typically, these primer pairs define a region of 100 to 300 bp in the viral genome. As the reaction is cooled, the primers will hybridize to homologous DNA sequences before the larger single strands of human DNA can reanneal; this is due to the small size and relative abundance of the primers. At the optimal temperature and in the presence of a DNA-dependent DNA polymerase and all of the nucleoside triphosphates, the single-stranded DNA template is copied 3' to the annealed primer to complete the cycle. At the end of the first cycle there are now four copies of the DNA defined by the primer pair. At the end of two cycles there are eight copies, and so forth. As can be seen, over many cycles there will be a geometric increase in the amount of the specific amplified viral DNA.

used as primers for DNA synthesis. Typically, the regions to be amplified are approximately 100 to 300 bp apart and are selected because of their relative GC nucleotide content and degree of homology with other retroviruses and human DNA (Fig. 9-16).

The DNA to be tested is added to the primer oligonucleotides in the presence of all four nucleoside triphosphates, the heat-stable DNA-dependent DNA polymerase from *Thermas aquaticus* (TAQ) and the appropriate buffer. The reaction mixture is then cycled through a three-stage amplification procedure: heat denaturation, primer annealing, and DNA extension. Each of these steps takes 1 to 2 minutes, and they are carried out sequentially at temperatures of 94°, 53°, and 65°C, respectively. The optimal time intervals and appropriate temperature may vary for a given set of primer pairs. This cycle is repeated 30 to 60 times in an automated heating/cooling block controlled by a microprocessor.

With each cycle there is a doubling of the target DNA, resulting in a geometric expansion such that within several hours, and without any further operator handling, one can easily achieve a millionfold amplification of the DNA, which is bounded by the primer pair. While most retrovirally derived primer pairs are quite specific and will only anneal to and amplify retroviral DNA, others will anneal to and amplify sequences present in normal human DNA as well. Figure 9-17 illustrates this point. We have found that selected primer pairs to the HTLV-I *tat* gene and the HIV-I *gag* genes are quite specific and result in amplified DNAs of the predicted fragment length on minigel fractionation. However, utilization of the HTLV-I *pol* gene primer pair yields bands of different sizes depending upon which target DNA is amplified. If the DNA to be analyzed actually contains HTLV-I, the predicted band pattern is observed, but if HTLV-I sequences are not present, the normal human DNA gives another specific but different pattern. This would suggest that in the presence of HTLV-I these *pol* specific primers will preferentially anneal to the target viral DNA sequences but that in its absence they will anneal to other sequences present within human DNA.

What these latter sequences represent are unknown at the moment except that they do not hybridize to specific HTLV-I *pol* gene detector oligonucleotides, which are derived from sequences located between the primer pairs. (Fig. 9-16). They may simply represent stretches of human DNA that share some homology with the HTLV-I *pol* gene, or they may represent the presence of slightly related endogenous or exogenous human retroviruses. The precise sequences of these fragments of amplified DNA are currently being determined.

As mentioned above, sometimes normal human DNA can be amplified such that one cannot be totally confident in evaluating simple incorporation assays. However, despite the occasional incorporation of nucleotides into normal DNA when the HTLV-I *pol* primer pair is used, the addition of a second step, nucleic acid hybridization, using a detector oligomer complementary to DNA located within the primer pair, imposes enough stringency to make the ultimate assay results quite specific. Hence, we now have developed a series of primer pairs and their respective detector sequences capable of specifically amplifying and identifying many regions within all of the known human retroviruses (Fig. 9-18).

Several methods exist to quantitate the amplified products. For primer pairs in which there is minimal DNA synthesis in normal samples, it is possible to use radioactively labeled nucleoside triphosphates as substrates and acid precipitate the amplified product and analyze it in a liquid scintillation counter (Fig. 9-19). If there is significant DNA synthesis occurring in normal DNA for a given primer pair, one can fractionate the product on a minigel and quantitate specific bands using a densitometer and calculate the area under the curve that corresponds to virus-specific bands (Fig. 9-20). Similarly, one could perform spot blots or Southern blots on the amplified product and quantify the amount of

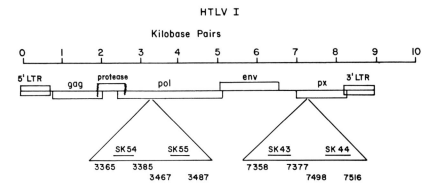

FIG. 9-16. Representative primer pairs within the HTLV-I genome located within the *pol* and *tat* genes. The detector oligonucleotides are located within the regions defined by the primer pairs. The *pol* gene primer pair shown is very specific for HTLV-I, but the *tat* gene primer pair is also homologous to a region within HTLV-II.

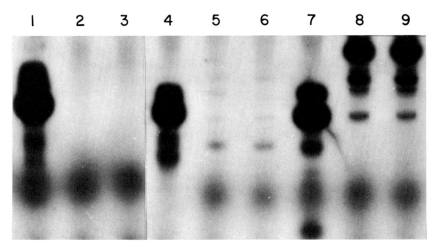

FIG. 9-17. Autoradiograph of ^{32}P-labeled radionucleotide incorporated into DNA from different sources and amplified with different viral primer pairs. Lanes 1, 5, and 7 are DNAs from HTLV-I–infected cells; lanes 2, 4, and 8 are from HIV-I–infected cells; lanes 3, 6, and 9 are from normal uninfected human cells. Lanes 1, 2, and 3 were amplified with the HTLV-I *tat* gene primer pairs SK43, 46; lanes 3, 4, and 5 were amplified with the HIV-I *gag* gene primer pairs SK38, 39; lanes 7, 8, and 9 were amplified with the HTLV-*pol* gene primer pair SK54, 55.

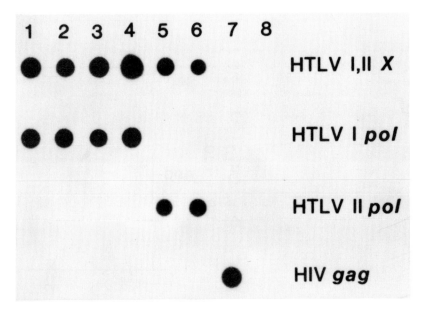

FIG. 9-18. Autoradiography of spot blots of DNA from the cells of various patients amplified with the primer pairs indicated and hybridized with the appropriate ^{32}P end-labeled detector oligonucleotide. Lanes 1–4 are HTLV-I–infected patients; lanes 5 and 6 are HTLV-II–infected patients; lane 7 is an HIV-I–infected patient; and lane 8 is a normal person.

hybridized detector. For mass screening purposes, we currently quantitate amplified virus specific bands fractionated on a minigel and stained with ethidium bromide using a densitometer. All samples that score above a certain cutoff value of viral DNA are then confirmed by hybridization studies. Hence, in many ways we have

developed a system similar to retroviral serology; studies whereby we screen with a quick, inexpensive, sensitive, quantitative but relatively nonspecific assay and confirm with a very sensitive and specific but more time-consuming and expensive second assay. It is our belief that with time technical improvements in all facets of enzymatic gene amplification will allow for its routine use in the detection of human retroviruses.

CLINICAL STUDIES USING GENE AMPLIFICATION

Employing approximately 35 cycles of amplification and one primer pair, we have been able to identify HTLV-I proviral DNA sequences in the PBMs of over 99% of patients with ATL. We have, however, found an occasional patient who has early-stage disease and the infected cells can be detected only in his tumor tissue and not in the peripheral blood or bone marrow.[70] In analyzing many DNAs obtained from samples at time of diagnosis or from autopsy specimens from these ATL patients, it has become apparent that enzymatic gene amplification is much more sensitive than light microscopic examination of these specimens by a trained hematopathologist.[82] Hence, we would advocate that gene amplification be used as a diagnostic staging tool, and also as a way to evaluate response rates in HTLV-I–associated lymphomas and leukemia.

The use of enzymatic gene amplification to detect HTLV-I sequences in HAM patients has proved to be extremely important. In a recent study[9] we were able to demonstrate that all of 12 such HTLV-I-antibody–positive patients with symptoms of noncompressive myelopathy were positive for HTLV-I DNA in their fresh PBMs via gene amplification. None of these patients were positive by Southern blot hybridization. Their viral

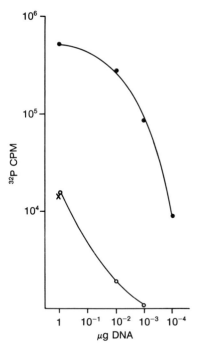

FIG. 9-19. Incorporated ^{32}P-labeled nucleotides after amplification with the HTLV-I *tat* gene primer pair SK43, 44 using varying starting concentrations of HTLV-I–infected (*solid circles*) vs uninfected (*open circles*) human DNA. The signal-to-noise ratio is optimal between 10^{-2} and 10^{-3} μg of DNA.

FIG. 9-20. Autoradiograph (*A*) and densitometer reading (*B*) of radiolabeled nucleotides incorporated into DNAs amplified with the HTLV-I *tat* gene primer pair SK43, 44. Lane 1, normal DNA; Lane 2, HTLV-I–infected patient's cells; Lanes 3–5, decreasing concentrations of standardized human DNA infected with one copy of proviral DNA per haploid genome, further diluted into human DNA such that Lane 3 equals 8×10^{-4} copies; Lane 4 equals 8×10^{-5} copies; and Lane 5 equals 8×10^{-6} copies. Densitometry analysis of lanes 3 (*solid line*), 4 (*outer broken line*), and 5 (*inner broken line*) yield areas under the curve of 61,358; 31,995; and 20,159, respectively, compared to zero for the negative control.

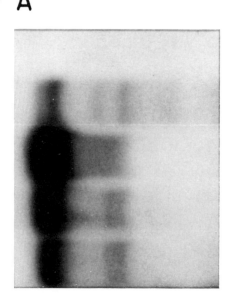

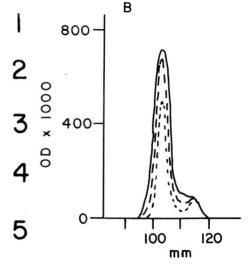

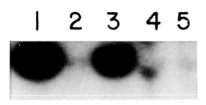

FIG. 9-21. Spot blots of DNAs from HUT 78 cells amplified for HIV-I *gag* gene sequences 6 hours after exposure to HIV-I (Lane 1) vs no virus exposure (Lane 2) or treatment with 0.2, 2 and 20 μg of HPA-23, respectively, prior to the addition of virus (Lanes 3–5).

copy number was so low that even after 3 months of continuous culture, only 3 of the 12 specimens were Southern blot positive, and 9 would have been totally missed without enzymatic gene amplification.

Genotyping the ATL and HAM patients with different primer pairs to HTLV-I has indicated that there is very little genetic variation among these isolates. The HTLV-I viruses infecting the HAM patients contain sequences homologous to the *tat-I* transactivating gene, which is believed to be in part responsible for oncogenesis. Subsequent sequencing of the amplified *pol* gene products and, ultimately, restriction endonuclease digestion and Southern blot analysis of the cultured isolates have corroborated that the ATL and HAM viruses are indistinguishable.

Although there is typically a much lower copy number of virus in HIV-I–infected individuals than in HTLV-I–infected patients, we had almost equal success in detecting HIV-I. In an analysis of DNA from fresh PBM from AIDS patients and late-stage ARC patients, we have been able to detect HIV-I in more than 90% of the patients. This has compared favorably with our detection of viral antigens produced by co-cultures containing these same PBMs. Analyses are currently underway to determine if this yield increases when DNA from the 4-week-old co-cultivated cells is similarly amplified. It is apparent from these early studies that a "quantitative" measurement of HIV-I proviral DNA can be determined by comparing the HIV signal to the signal obtained by amplification of a single copy gene, such as β globin. This should allow us to establish cutoffs for positive and negative samples and to perform large epidemiologic studies to correlate "viral load" with various clinical parameters, including survival.

Enzymatic gene amplification has also proved useful in evaluating patients with atypical or negative serologic reactions to the human retroviruses. In a prospective analysis, out of 500 ATL, HAM, and HTLV-I carrier patients tested, 493 or 98.6% were seropositive for anti-HTLV-I antibodies.[25] Seven patients (1.4%) (all ATL) were seronegative by ELISA, RIPA, and Western blot assays but positive for HTLV-I proviral DNA via enzymatic gene amplification (see Table 9-1).[25] Out of 1160 AIDS/ARC patients tested, 1158 (99.8%) were seropositive for anti-HIV-I antibodies.[25] Two patients (both ARC) were seronegative by ELISA, RIPA, and western

blot assays but positive for HIV-I proviral DNA sequences via enzymatic gene amplification. Similarly, in 20 blood donors who had "atypical" western blot patterns after scoring positive in anti-HIV-I ELISA,[83] 3 were positive for HIV-I DNA and 1 was positive for HTLV-I DNA by analysis of DNA amplified by PCR. All were negative for HTLV-II and HIV-II DNA. All of the 3 donors positive for HIV-I DNA belong to HIV-I associated risk groups and one of the 3 has ultimately developed a classic anti-HIV-I western blot pattern. Hence, enzymatic gene amplification is a useful complementary tool to serologic assays in making a diagnosis of retroviral infections. We are currently involved in large population studies to compare the relative prevalence rates of positivity for retroviral antibodies and DNA.

In addition to using PCR to quantify HIV-I, we have also been able to use this technique to compare one isolate to another. Table 9-2 illustrates results obtained when five different primer pairs, representing distinct regions of the HIV-I genome, are used to analyze different HIV-I isolates. As can be seen, it is rather easy to assign each of these isolates to a particular genotype pattern depending upon whether it is positive or negative for the sequences being amplified. We envision using 20 such primer pairs to rapidly analyze isolates from different patients, from different geographic locales over time. This should allow for correlations with clinical outcomes and for facile detection of genetic drift in the HIV-I virus. Isolates that represent substantial departure from prototype HIV-I could then be characterized further to allow for development of new antibody assays and/or vaccines to keep pace with the virus as it evolves.

Enzymatic gene amplification is also a useful tool for determining the *in vitro* and *in vivo* efficacy of antiviral drugs. The ultimate goals of such studies are to develop clinically relevant combination drug regimens utilizing agents with different mechanisms of action and no overlapping toxicities. Hence, it is imperative to establish the actual site(s) of action of a particular antiviral drug *vis-à-vis* the viral life cycle. The algorithm in Figure 9-14 illustrates our approach to this endeavor. Our screen assay measures the amount of HIV-I antigen expressed 4 days after exposure of an uninfected target cell to cell-free HIV-I virions. An inhibitory effect in such an assay (Fig. 9-13) could be due either to a decrease in transmission or to expression of the virus or both. To determine if the effect is due to transmission we measure the ultimate end product of this stage of the virus life cycle, proviral DNA, by enzymatic gene amplification of viral DNA 6 hours after exposure of the virus to the uninfected target cells. (see Fig. 9-14). A positive result can then be analyzed for inhibitory effects preceding the formation of proviral DNA (Fig. 9-21).

We have also begun to analyze HIV-I proviral DNA levels from patients *in vivo* on clinical trials. Our initial analyses have been on DNA derived from cultured cells and have suggested that enzymatic gene amplification is more specific and sensitive than RT or antigen expression analyses on these cultures. We are currently analyzing DNA from fresh PBM from these patients in addition to their cultured cells. Since various drug combinations will affect transmission and/or expressions of HIV-I we suggest that future studies measure antiviral efficacy in three ways: (1) quantitivate levels of HIV-I proviral DNA per human β-globin DNA in PBMs and/or PBM subtypes (e.g., CD4 + T cells or monocytes), cerebrospinal fluid cells, and so forth; (2) measure relative virus expression *in vivo* by analysis for viral antigens in different body fluids; and (3) assess the ability of the patients' cultured cells to produce cell-free infectious particles capable of infecting uninfected target cells.

CONCLUSION

The long held belief that retroviruses are the etiologic agents of human disease has clearly been validated. The search for new unrelated retroviruses will, of necessity, still require the laborious task of selective cell culture, virus detection by analysis for reverse transcriptase, isolation of the virus and its ultimate purification and characterization. Once the proteins and nucleic acids of these viruses are established, however, sensitive and specific techniques exist for their rapid detection and analysis. This ability should allow for the performance of important clinical studies. Given the rapid advances in human retrovirology over the past decade, one can only expect future technical improvements in this field in the near future.

REFERENCES

1. Poiesz BJ, Ruscetti FW, Gazdar AF et al: Detection and isolation of type C retrovirus particles from fresh and cultured lymphocytes of a patient with cutaneous T-cell lymphoma. Proc Natl Acad Sci (USA) 77:7415, 1980
2. Kalyanamaran VS, Sarngadharan MG, Robert–Guroff M et al: A new subtype of human T-cell leukemia virus (HTLV-II) associated with a T-cell variant of hairy cell leukemia. Science 218:571, 1982
3. Barre–Sinoussi F, Chermann JC, Rey F et al: Isolation of a T-lymphotropic retrovirus from a patient at risk for acquired immune deficiency syndrome (AIDS). Science 220:868, 1983
4. Popovic M, Sarngadharan MG, Read E et al: Detection, isolation, and continuous production of cytopathic retroviruses (HTLV-III) from patients with AIDS and pre-AIDS. Science 224:497, 1984b
5. Clavel F, Guetand D, Brun–Vezinet F et al: Isolation of a new human retrovirus from West African patients with AIDS. Science 233:343, 1986
6. Yoshida M, Miyoshi I, Hinuma Y: Isolation and characterization of retrovirus (ATLV) from cell lines of human adult T-cell leukemia and its implication in the disease. Proc Natl Acad Sci (USA) 79:2031, 1982
7. Chen ISY, McLaughlin J, Gasson JC et al: Molecular characterization of genome of a novel human T-cell leukemia virus. Nature 305:502, 1983
8. Gessain A, Barin F, Vernant JC: Antibodies to human T-lymphotropic virus type −I in patients with tropical spastic paraparesis. Lancet 2:407, 1985
9. Bhagavati S, Ehrlich GD, Kula RW et al: Detection of HTLV-I DNA and antigen in the spinal fluid and blood of cases of chronic progressive myelopathy and a clinical, radiological and electrophysiological profile of HTLV-I associated myelopathy. New Engl J Med Submitted.
10. Gonda MA, Wong–Staal F, Gallo RC et al: Sequence homology and morphologic similarity of HTLV-III and visna virus, a pathogenic lentivirus. Science 227:173, 1985
11. Stephens RM, Casey JW, Rice NR: Equine infectious anemia virus *gag* and *pol* genes: Relatedness to visna and AIDS virus. Science 231:589, 1986
12. Gallo RC, Salahuddin SZ, Popovic M et al: Frequent detection and isolation of cytopathic retroviruses (HTLV-III) from patients with AIDS and at risk for AIDS. Science 224:500, 1984
13. Centers for Disease Control: Antibodies to a retrovirus etiologically associated with acquired immunodeficiency syndrome (AIDS) in populations with increased incidences of the syndrome. Morbid Mortal Week Rep 33:377, 1984
14. Ho DD, Rota TR, Schooley RT et al: Isolation of HTLV-III from cerebrospinal fluid and neural tissues of patients with neurological syndromes related to the acquired immunodeficiency syndrome. N Engl J Med 313:1493, 1985
15. Koenig S, Gendelman HE, Orenstein JM et al: Detection of AIDS virus in macrophages in brain tissue from AIDS patients with encephalopathy. Science 233:1089, 1986
16. Courouce AM: HIV-II in blood donors and in different risk groups in France. Lancet [letter] 1:1151, 1987.
17. Ferroni P, Tagger A, Lazzanin A et al: HIV-I and HIV-II infections in Italian AIDS/HRC patients. Lancet [letter] 1:869, 1987
18. Tedde RS, O'Connor T: HIV-II in UK. Lancet [letter] 1:864, 1987
19. Sodroski J, Patarca R, Rosen C et al: Location of the trans-activating region on the genome of the human T-cell lymphotropic virus type III. Science 229:74, 1985
20. Sodroski J, Goh WC, Rosen C et al: A second post-transcriptional transactivator gene required for HTLV-III replication. Nature 321:412, 1986
21. Fisher AG, Ensoli B, Ivanoff L et al: The *sor* gene of HIV-I is required for efficient virus transmission *in vitro*. Science 237:888, 1987
22. Weiss SH, Goedert JJ, Sarngadharan MG et al: Screening test for HTLV-III (AIDS agent) antibodies, specificity, sensitivity and applications. JAMA 253:221, 1985
23. Ranki A, Krohn M, Allain J–P et al: Long latency precedes overt seroconversion in sexually transmitted human immunodeficiency virus infection. Lancet 2:584, 1987
24. Tajima K, Tominaga S, Suchi S et al: Epidemiological analysis of the distribution of antibody to adult T-cell leukemia-virus-associated antigen (ATLA): Possible horizontal transmission of adult T-cell leukemia virus. Gann 73:893, 1982
25. Poiesz BJ, Ehrlich G, Papsidero L et al: Incidence of Seronegativity to HIV and HTLV-I in individuals infected with either virus. Third International Conference on Acquired Immunodeficiency Syndrome (AIDS), June 1–5, 1987, No 23, p 114.
26. Rabson AB, Martin MA: Molecular organization of the AIDS retrovirus. Cell 40:477, 1985
27. Hahn BH, Shaw GM, Taylor ME et al: Genetic variation in HTLV-III/LAV over time in patients with AIDS or at risk for AIDS. Science 232:1548, 1986

28. Ratner L, Haseltine H, Patarca R et al: Complete nucleotide sequence of the AIDS virus, HTLV-III. Nature 313:277, 1985

29. Conklin KF, Groudine M: Varied interactions between provirus and adjacent host chromatin. Mol Cell Biol 6:3999, 1986

30. Barklis E, Mulligan RC, Jaenisch R: Chromosomal position or virus mutation permits retrovirus expression in embryonal carcinoma cells. Cell 47:391, 1986

31. Varmus H, Swanstrom R: Replication of retroviruses. In Weiss R, Teich N, Varmus H et al (eds): RNA Tumor Viruses, p 369. Cold Spring Harbor, NY, Cold Spring Harbor Laboratory, 1982

32. Kalyanamaran VS, Jarvis–Morar M, Sarngadharan MG et al: Immunological characterization of the low molecular weight *gag* gene proteins p19 and p15 of HTLV and demonstration of human natural antibodies to them. Virology 132:61, 1984

33. Otsuyama Y, Shimotohno K, Miwa M et al: Myristylation of gag protein in HTLV-I and II. Jap J Cancer Res 76:1132, 1985

34. Shimotohno K, Takahashi Y, Shimizu N et al: Complete nucleotide sequence of an infectious clone of human T-cell leukemia virus type II: An open reading frame for the protease gene. Proc Natl Acad Sci (USA) 82:3103, 1985

35. Dickson C, Eisenman R, Hung F et al: Protein biosynthesis and assembly. In Weiss R, Teich N, Varmus H et al (eds): RNA Tumor Viruses. Cold Spring Harbor, NY, Cold Spring Harbor Laboratory, p 513, 1982

36. Luftig RB, Yoshinaka Y: Rauscher leukemia virus populations enriched for "immature" virions contain increased amounts of p70, the *gag* gene product. J Virol 25:416, 1978

37. Maddon PJ, Dalgleish AG, McDougal JS et al: The T4 gene encodes the AIDS virus receptor and is expressed in the immune system and the brain. Cell 47:333, 1986

38. Stewart SJ, Fujimoto J, Levy R: Human T-lymphocytes and monocytes bear the same Leu-3 (T4) antigen. J Immunol 136:3773, 1986

39. Krichbaum–Stenger K, Poiesz BJ, Keller B et al: Specific absorption of HTLV-I to various target human and animal cells. Blood 70:1303, 1987

40. Seiki M, Hattori S, Hirayoma Y et al: Human adult T-cell leukemia virus: Complete nucleotide sequence of the provirus genome integrated in leukemia cell DNA. Proc Natl Acad Sci (USA) 80:3618, 1983

41. Wain–Hobson S, Sonigo P, Danos O et al: Nucleotide sequence of the AIDS virus, LAV. Cell 40:9, 1985

42. Panganiban AT, Temin HM: Circles with two tandem LTRs are precursors to integrated retrovirus DNA. Cell 36:673, 1984

43. Brown PO, Bowerman B, Varmus HE et al: Correct integration of retroviral DNA *in vitro*. Cell 49:347, 1987

44. Luciw PA, Potter SJ, Steimer K et al: Molecular cloning of AIDS-associated retrovirus. Nature 312:760, 1984

45. Lightfoote MM, Coligan JE, Folks TM et al: Structural characterization of reverse transcriptase and endonuclease polypeptides of the acquired immunodeficiency syndrome retrovirus. J Virol 60:771, 1986

46. Allan JS, Coligan JE, Lee TH et al: Immunogenic nature of a pol gene product of HTLV-III/LAV. Blood 69:331, 1987

47. Panganiban AT, Temin HM: The retrovirus *pol* gene encodes a product required for DNA integration: Identification of a retrovirus *int* locus. Proc Natl Acad Sci USA 81:7885, 1984

48. Rohdewohid H, Weihen H, Reik W et al: Retrovirus integration and chromatin structure: Molony murine leukemia proviral integration sites map near DNAse I hypersensitive sites. J Virol 61:336, 1987

49. Hanada S, Koyanagi Y, Yamamoto N: Infection of HTLV III/LAV in HTLV-I-carrying cells. MT-2 and MT-4 and application in a plaque assay. Science 229:563, 1985

50. Merl S, Kloster B, Moore J et al: Efficient transformation of previously activated and dividing T-lymphocytes by human T-cell leukemia/lymphoma virus. Blood 64:967, 1984

51. Duc–Dodon M, Gazzolo L: Loss of IL-2 requirement for the generation of T-cell colonies defines an early event of HTLV-I infection. Blood 69:1, 1987

52. Miller JM, Miller LD, Olson C et al: Virus-like particles in phytohemagglutinin-stimulated lymphocyte cultures with reference to bovine lymphosarcoma. J Natl Cancer Inst 43:1297, 1969

53. Klein G: Viral Oncology. New York, Raven Press, 1980

54. Gallo RC, Poiesz BJ, Ruscetti FW: Regulation of human T-cell proliferation: T-cell growth factor and isolation of a new class of type-C retroviruses from human T-cells. Haematol Blood Transfus 26:502, 1981

55. Morgan DA, Ruscetti FW, Gallo RC: Selective growth of T-lymphocytes from normal human bone marrow. Science 193:1007, 1976

56. Ruscetti FW, Morgan DA, Gallo RC: Functional and morphological characterization of human T-cells continuously grown *in vitro*. J Immunol 117:131, 1977

57. Poiesz BJ, Ruscetti FW, Mier JW et al: T-cell lines established from human T-lymphocytic neoplasias by direct response to T-cell growth factor. Proc Natl Acad Sci (USA) 77:6815, 1980

58. Kronke M, Leonard WJ, Depper JM et al: Deregulation of interleukin-2 receptor gene expression in HTLV-I-induced adult T-cell leukemia. Science 228:1215, 1985

59. Vilmer E, Barre–Sinoussi F, Rouzioux C et al: Isolation of new lymphotropic retrovirus from two siblings with hemophilia B, one with AIDS. Lancet 1:753, 1984

60. Gazdar AF, Carney DA, Russell EK et al: *In vitro* growth of cutaneous T-cell lymphomas. Cancer Treat Rep 63:587, 1979

61. Montagna RA, Poiesz BJ, Ruscetti FW et al: Use of a new HIV isolate in an ELISA test for antibodies to HIV. AIDS (Submitted)

62. Walker CM, Moody OJ, Stites DP et al: CD8+ lymphocytes can control HIV infection *in vitro* by suppressing virus replication. Science 234:1563, 1986

63. Eysler ME, Goedert JJ, Poon MC et al: Acid labile alpha interferon: A possible preclinical marker for AIDS in hemophilia. N Engl J Med 309:583, 1983

64. Moore JL, Poiesz BJ, Tomar RH et al: Gamma interferon and AIDS. New Engl J Med [letter] 312:442, 1985

65. Ehrlich GD, Poiesz BJ: Clinical and Molecular Parameters of HTLV-I infection. Clinics in Laboratory Med. 8:65, 1988

66. Hahn BH, Shaw GM, Arya SK et al: Molecular cloning and characterization of the HTLV-III virus associated with AIDS. Nature 312:166, 1984

67. Chen ISY: Regulation of AIDS virus expression. Cell 47:1, 1986

68. Sanchez–Pescador R, Power MD, Barr PJ et al: Nucleotide sequence and expression of an AIDS-associated retrovirus (ARV-2). Science 227:484, 1985

69. Myers G: AIDS virus sequence database update. Los Alamos, Los Alamos National Laboratory, 1987

70. Duggan DB, Ehrlich GD, Davey FP et al: HTLV-I induced lymphoma mimicking Hodgkin's disease diagnosis by

polymerase chain reaction amplification of specific HTLV-I sequences in tumor DNA. Blood (in press, 1988)

71. Koenig S, Gendelman HE, Orenstein JM et al: Detection of AIDS virus in macrophages in brain tissue from AIDS patients with encephalopathy. Science 233:1084, 1986

72. Limentani SA, Furie BC, Poiesz BJ et al: Separation of human plasma factor IX from HTLV-I or HIV by immunoaffinity chromatography using conformation-specific antibodies. Blood 70:1312, 1987

73. Kessler HA, Blaauw B, Spear J et al: Diagnosis of human immunodeficiency virus infection in seronegative homosexuals presenting with an acute viral syndrome. JAMA 258:1196, 1987

74. Papsidero LD, Montagna RA, Poiesz BJ: Acquired immune deficiency syndrome: Detection of viral exposure and infection. Am Clin Proc, p 17, October 1986

75. Chaisson RE, Allain J–P, Leuther M et al: Significant changes in HIV antigen level in the serum of patients treated with azidothymidine. N Engl J Med [letter] 315(25):1610, 1986

76. Harper ME, Marselle LM, Gallo RC et al: Detection of lymphocytes expressing human T-lymphotropic virus type III in lymph nodes and peripheral blood from infected individuals by *in situ* hybridization. Proc Natl Acad Sci (USA) 83:772, 1986

77. Saiki RK, Scharf S, Faloona F et al: Enzymatic amplification of beta globin genomic sequences and restriction site analysis for diagnosis of sickle cell anemia. Science 230:1350, 1985

78. Mullis KB, Faloona F: Specific synthesis of DNA *in vitro* via a polymerase catalysed chain reaction. Meth Enzymol 155:335, 1987

79. Kwok S, Mack D, Mullis KB et al: Identification of HIV viral sequences using in vitro enzymatic amplification and oligomer cleavage detection. J Virol 61:1690, 1987

80. Kwok S, Ehrlich G, Poiesz B et al: Enzymatic amplification of HTLV-I viral sequences from peripheral blood mononuclear cells and infected tissues. Blood (in press, 1988)

81. Abbott M, Poiesz BJ, Sninsky JJ et al: A comparison of methodologies to detect the products of the polymerase chain reaction. (in preparation)

82. Ehrlich GD, Davey FR, Kirshner JJ et al: A polyclonal CD4+ and CD8+ lymphocytosis in a patient doubly infected with HTLV-I and HIV-I: A clinical and molecular analysis. Am J Hematol (Submitted)

83. Dock NL, Lamberson HV, O'Brien TA et al: Evaluation of HIV antibody in blood donors with a typical western blot reactivity. Lancet (Submitted)

Pathologic Features of Patients Infected with the Human Immunodeficiency Virus

Abe M. Macher
Maria L. De Vinatea
Peter Angritt
Sylvana M. Tuur
Cheryl M. Reichert

10

The acquired immune deficiency syndrome (AIDS) is a devastating new disease caused by the human immunodeficiency virus (HIV), which renders the host profoundly immunoincompetent. The surgical and postmortem pathologic features associated with infection by HIV can be divided into four major categories: (1) morphologic manifestations of immunologic impairment; (2) secondary opportunistic infections; (3) unusual neoplasms; and (4) special problems. Infection by HIV is a dynamic process with pathologic features and patterns of involvement that vary with the chronology of the disease. Thus, hyperplastic reactive lymph nodes biopsied during the prodromal AIDS-related complex (ARC) phase of the illness bear little resemblance to the burned out, depleted lymph nodes seen terminally, and the sometimes subtle angiomatous lesions of Kaposi's sarcoma (KS) are at one end of a histologic spectrum that also encompasses lesions that may be frankly sarcomatous. An understanding of the various pathologic findings in patients infected by HIV is fundamental to an appreciation of the diverse clinical manifestations of this syndrome. Because of the multiplicity of infections and neoplastic processes encountered in patients with AIDS, and because of the potential hazards of the various therapeutic agents involved, specific pathologic diagnoses are essential for a rational approach to therapy. In this chapter we present the gross and microscopic features of both the prodromal illness caused by HIV infection and the fully developed acquired immune deficiency syndrome.[1-4]

HANDLING OF TISSUES

Strict handling precautions should be observed when handling tissues and fluids of patients infected with HIV. Many of these patients are also likely to be shedding latent (reactivated) viruses such as cytomegalovirus and Epstein–Barr virus, and are carriers of hepatitis B, as well as a variety of bacterial, fungal, protozoal, and other heretofore unidentified viral pathogens. Safety precautions recommended by our laboratory in the handling of pathologic specimens are listed in Table 10-1.[5-25]

MORPHOLOGIC MANIFESTATIONS OF IMMUNOLOGIC IMPAIRMENT

Lymph Nodes

Persistent generalized lymphadenopathy is observed in patients infected with HIV.[26] This chronic lymphadenopathy syndrome or ARC represents a prodromal phase of AIDS and occurs prior to the development of opportunistic infections, Kaposi's sarcoma, and non-Hodgkin's lymphomas. Patients may be otherwise asymptomatic, or they may suffer from a variety of constitutional symptoms, including fever, weight loss, malaise, diarrhea, and oral candidiasis. Some may also present with autoimmune phenomena including thrombocytopenic purpura[27] and hemolytic anemia.[28]

The hyperplastic lymph nodes are grossly enlarged (Fig. 10-1) up to 6 cm in greatest dimension, and are mobile, discrete, and soft. Microscopic sections of biopsied lymph nodes stained with hematoxylin and eosin reveal reactive, sometimes florid, follicular hyperplasia with prominent, irregularly shaped, mitotically active germinal centers with many tingible body macrophages (Color Plate 10-1); occasional large lymphocytes with vesicular nuclei (immunoblasts) within the interfollicular areas (Fig. 10-2); clusters of perivascular polymorphonuclear leukocytes and/or plasma cells; and rare multinucleated giant cells.[29-32] Lymphoid proliferation may also occur in other tissues, particularly lung (see Special Problems) and salivary gland. We have studied the cases of a number of HIV-seropositive patients who

Table 10-1
Guidelines for Handling of Tissues from Patients Infected with HIV

Limit access; exclude persons who are pregnant, immunosuppressed, or with open wounds.

Avoid direct contact of skin, conjunctivae, and mucous membranes with blood, other body fluids, excretions, and tissues.

Use as many disposable items as possible.

Wear goggles or wrap-around safety glasses, surgical mask, disposable gown, hair cover, shoe covers, two pairs of gloves, and a water-proof apron. Consider using full face plastic shields. These items should be removed prior to leaving the autopsy suite and placed in a plastic-lined cardboard box destined for incineration. Wash hands following completion of the procedure, after removing protective clothing, and before leaving the area.

Exercise care to avoid accidental injury from sharp instruments, aerosolization, and splattering of body fluids; minimize aerosolization of bone dust by using a vacuum attachment for the bone saw and by fitting a transparent plastic bag over the head and the saw.

Wash thoroughly all instruments, containers, and work surfaces with a soap or detergent solution before decontaminating them.

Decontaminate instruments, containers, and work surfaces with a 1:10 dilution of 5.25% sodium hypochlorite (household bleach) in water. Soak instruments in decontaminating solution for 15–30 min (longer periods of decontamination may corrode instruments). Wash again. Autoclave instruments for at least 45 min at temperatures of at least 121°C and pressures of at least 20 psi.

Place cadavers in impervious bags. Affix warning labels to the bag as well as to all identification tags.

Do not distribute organs for transplantation.

Do not distribute tissues to researchers except to those with approved HIV protocols.

Fix tissue samples thoroughly (twenty parts formalin to one part tissue) before trimming for histologic examination.

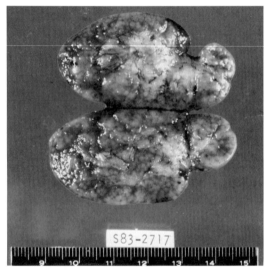

FIG. 10-1. Gross appearance of an enlarged bivalved lymph node from a patient with ARC.

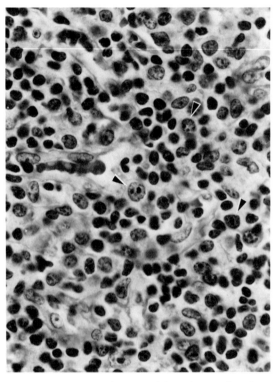

FIG. 10-2. Scattered immunoblasts (*arrows*) within interfollicular areas of a lymph node biopsy from a patient with ARC (H&E stain).

presented with unilateral or bilateral parotid enlargement; microscopic sections of salivary gland revealed marked lymphoid infiltration with florid follicular hyperplasia.

In some HIV-infected patients there is histologic progression from the pattern of follicular hyperplasia to a pattern of partial lymphoid depletion, evidenced by loss of paracortical (T-cell area) lymphocytes, poorly defined or absent follicular mantles, variable hyalinization of germinal centers, and sometimes prominent interfollicular plasmacytosis (Fig. 10-3). This pattern of partial lymphoid depletion frequently accompanies the development of opportunistic infections.

Finally, there may be further progression to a third histologic pattern, that of severe to virtually complete lymphoid depletion (burn-out) of both B-cell and T-cell areas, with only residual plasma cells and histiocytes (Color Plate 10-2). Erythrophagocytosis may also be present (Fig. 10-4). At this stage in the evolution of the syndrome, special stains for microorganisms are often

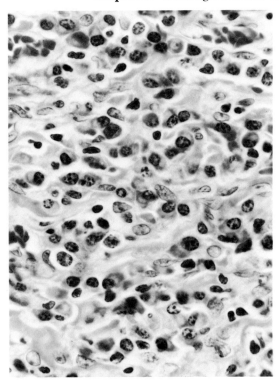

FIG. 10-3. Lymph node biopsy of a patient with AIDS reveals prominent interfollicular plasmacytosis (H&E stain).

positive in the absence of overt granulomata. We have studied patients with AIDS who have had histopathologically florid lymphadenopathic mycobacterioses,[33] mycoses,[34] isosporiasis,[35] syphilis, cat-scratch disease, and pneumocystosis.

Immunohistology of lymph nodes from HIV-infected patients demonstrates substantial abnormalities in the numbers and distribution of T-lymphocytes.[37–39] Quantitative T-cell and B-cell immunohistology of frozen sections of lymph nodes from male homosexuals with persistent generalized lymphadenopathy and with AIDS reveals fewer helper T cells and increased numbers of suppressor cytotoxic T-lymphocytes, as compared with normal controls. More cells with the suppressor T phenotype are present in follicular centers and mantle zones (B-cell areas), than are in controls. There is a decrease of cells with helper T phenotype in paracortical regions (T-cell areas) and in germinal centers. Lymph nodes with subtotal effacement of architecture demonstrate depletion of B-lymphocytes in addition to the aforementioned decreases of helper T cells and increases in suppressor-cytotoxic T-lymphocytes.

Thymus

The normal thymus varies in size and development with age. During the aging process, portions of thymus undergo involution and fatty replacement. When compared with age-matched controls, thymic specimens obtained at autopsy from pediatric and adult patients with AIDS exhibit disproportionate and premature atrophy, depletion of lymphoid elements, and focal calcification of Hassal's corpuscles (Fig. 10-5).[40]

Spleen

Splenomegaly is present to varying degrees in most patients with AIDS. We and others[41] have seen AIDS patients with massive splenomegaly (2060 g; normal average = 155 g); however, splenic enlargement is usually modest (1.5 to 3 times normal) and clinically inapparent. Histopathologically, the spleens are congested, there is a virtual absence of germinal centers, and profound depletion of lymphocytes in both T-cell and B-cell areas. Erythrophagocytosis and extramedullary hematopoiesis may be present. Patients with disseminated opportunistic infections may exhibit an acute splenitis; splenic macrophages may be engorged with acid-fast bacilli or fungal organisms. We have studied three AIDS patients with multifocal splenic necrosis caused by *Pneumocystis carinii*.[36]

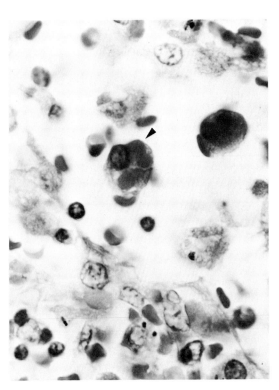

FIG. 10-4. Erythrophagocytosis (*arrow*) in a lymphocyte-depleted autopsy lymph node of patient with AIDS (H&E stain). (Reichert CM, O'Leary TJ, Levens DL et al: Autopsy pathology in the acquired immune deficiency syndrome. Am J Pathol 112:357, 1983)

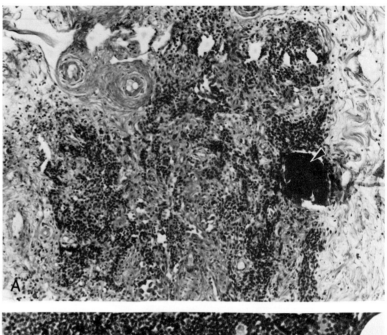

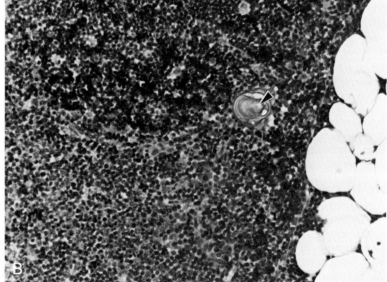

FIG. 10-5. (*A*) Lymphocyte-depleted thymus with calcified Hassall's corpuscle (*arrow*) in a patient with AIDS (H&E stain). (*B*) Thymus with normal Hassall's corpuscle (*arrow*) from a non-immunosuppressed age-matched male control (H&E stain). (Reichert CM, O'Leary TJ, Levens DL et al: Autopsy pathology in the acquired immune deficiency syndrome. Am J Pathol 112:357, 1983)

Bone Marrow

Peripheral anemia, thrombocytopenia, lymphopenia, and neutropenia occur in many of these patients. The following non-neoplastic morphologic abnormalities have been observed in the bone marrow:[42-44]

1. Moderate hypercellularity
2. Increased myeloid/erythroid ratio secondary to hyperplasia of immature myeloid elements and a decrease in erythroid precursors
3. Lymphoid hyperplasia, with focal, ill-defined lymphoid aggregates that may contain atypical lymphocytes[45]
4. Variable plasmacytosis
5. Megakaryocytic hyperplasia
6. Increased reticulin fiber deposition

Focal aggregates of histiocytes may be present secondary to disseminated mycobacterial and fungal infections. We studied one AIDS patient with multifocal bone marrow necrosis caused by *P. carinii*.[36]

Postmortem findings in bone marrow are variable. Lymphocytic hyperplasia may no longer be apparent, the overall cellularity may be normal or only moderately increased (due to hyperplasia of myeloid elements), and megakaryocytic hyperplasia is rare. Erythrophagocytosis may be prominent.

Gastrointestinal Lymphoid Tissue

During the later stages of AIDS, depletion of lymphocytes is also apparent within the Peyer's patches of the ileum, the lymphoid tissue of the appendix (Fig. 10-6), and throughout the scattered lymphoid follicles of the colon.

ULTRASTRUCTURAL FINDINGS IN TISSUES

Several unusual inclusions have been described in lymphocytes and other tissues of patients infected with HIV.

Test Tube and Ring-Shaped Forms

Sidhu and colleagues described test tube and ring-shaped forms in the lymphocytes of patients with AIDS.[46–48] These structures consist of concentrically arranged, endoplasmic reticulum cisternae with electron-dense material interposed in the cytosol between layers. Such structures have also been described in a Japanese case of HTLV-I–positive adult T-cell leukemia,[49] as well as in non-A, non-B hepatitis.[50,51]

Tubuloreticular Inclusions

Tubuloreticular inclusions are abundant in biopsied tissue specimens from patients with AIDS.[52-56] These abnormal subcellular organelles consist of nuclease- and RNase-resistant complexes of lipid-rich membranes and proteins.[57,58] They arise within the cytosecretory apparatus and are composed of fine tubular meshworks that distend the endoplasmic reticulum (Fig. 10-7).[59] Grimley and co-workers detected tubuloreticular inclusions within peripheral mononuclear cells in all of 12 patients with AIDS. Using monoclonal anti-Leu 2a antibodies, they localized tubuloreticular inclusions to suppressor/cytotoxic T-lymphocytes.[55]

Vesicular Rosettes

Ewing and colleagues found vesicular rosettes in the cytoplasm of lymphoid cells from lymph nodes in 17 of 18 patients with ARC and 3 of 6 patients with AIDS. The rosettes occurred in lymphoid cells and were composed of multiple distinct 30- to 60-nm vesicles radially clustered around an ill-defined electron-dense core. The rosettes measured 300 to 500 nm in overall diameter and were devoid of any surrounding membranes.[60]

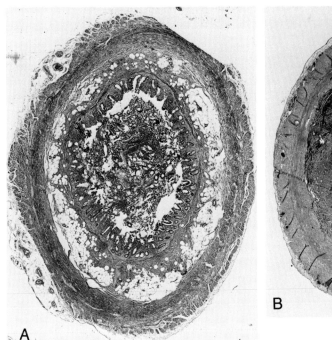
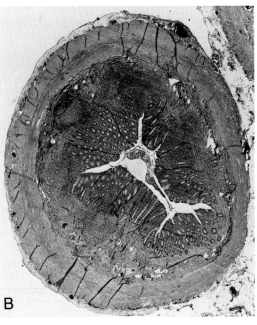

FIG. 10-6. (*A*) Cross section of an appendix from a patient with AIDS, showing virtual absence of lymphoid elements (H&E stain). (*B*) A normal appendix with abundant submucosal lymphoid tissue (H&E stain). (Reichert CM, O'Leary TJ, Levens, DL et al: Autopsy pathology in the acquired immune deficiency syndrome. Am J Pathol 112:357, 1983)

INFECTIONS

Profoundly immunodeficient, patients with AIDS are susceptible to a variety of protozoal, fungal, bacterial, viral, helminthic, and arthropodal infections, often with notably unusual opportunistic microorganisms (e.g., *Mycobacterium avium-intracellulare, Cryptosporidium*). Furthermore, infections in patients with AIDS are often severe, persistent, and/or relapsing despite appropriate therapy (e.g., *P. carinii* pneumonia, *Cryptococcus neoformans* meningitis); some infections are virtually untreatable (cryptosporidial enteritis, polyomavirus-associated progressive multifocal leukoencephalopathy).[61] Etiologic agents of infections in patients with AIDS are given in Table 10-2, and the typical gross, microscopic, and cytologic[62] findings are discussed in the accompanying text. Although not all of the infectious agents listed are considered to cause opportunistic infections that are diagnostic of the syndrome, they are included because they appear as part of the AIDS-associated spectrum of infectious complications in these patients.

Protozoa

Pneumocystis carinii

Pneumonia caused by *Pneumocystis carinii* is the most common life-threatening opportunistic infection in patients with AIDS.[63] As an extracellular protozoan, *P. carinii* exists as trophozoite and cyst forms within the pulmonary alveoli of humans and some animals. In the immunocompromised host proliferation of organisms results in consolidation of pulmonary parenchyma and progressive hypoxemia and dyspnea.

Grossly, the lungs are heavy and cut with increased resistance. Early involvement is characteristically patchy, although postmortem lungs may be diffusely consolidated. *Pneumocystis carinii* cannot be readily cultured; hence, diagnosis is dependent upon direct visualization of the protozoan. The diagnosis is usually established with centrifuged bronchial lavage specimens, touch imprints of unfixed transbronchial biopsies, and formalin-fixed, paraffin-embedded transbronchial specimens; occasionally, open lung biopsy with frozen section evaluation is required.[64] Histopathologically, in sections stained by hematoxylin and eosin, cysts of *P. carinii* are most likely to be found within eosinophilic foamy exudates that distend alveoli and terminal bronchioles (Fig. 10-8A; Color Plate 10-3). Rapid diagnosis may be accomplished with frozen sections, touch imprints, or bronchial lavage, using toluidine blue O or methenamine silver staining techniques. The cyst walls are seen as cup shaped, oval, or round structures 3 to 7 μ in diameter (Fig. 10-8B). Gram's[65] and Wright's[66] stains of lung imprints have also been successfully used for the rapid diagnosis of *P. carinii* pneumonia as up to eight internal sporozoites per cyst can be identified within

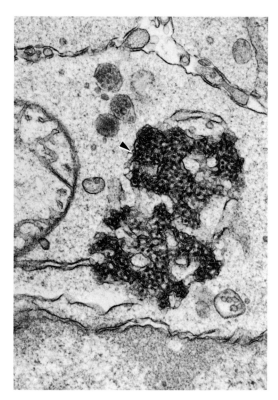

FIG. 10-7. A large tubuloreticular inclusion (*arrow*) within the cytoplasm of a peripheral blood mononuclear cell from a patient with AIDS. (Electron micrograph, ×40,000, courtesy of Dr. P. M. Grimley)

the foamy matrix background of the alveolar exudates. With these two staining procedures, the cyst wall is transparent; however, the cysts may be indirectly outlined by thin, clear, nonstaining haloes. The internal structures of *P. carinii* cysts are well seen by electron microscopy (Fig. 10-8C). In patients with AIDS the inflammatory response to pneumocystis is minimal, and when present it consists of occasional mononuclear and plasma cells within thickened alveolar septae. Because *P. carinii* pneumonia frequently presents with other concomitant opportunistic pulmonary infections, bacterial, mycobacterial, fungal, and viral cultures should be obtained, and specimens should be stained with hematoxylin and eosin, tissue Gram's stain, periodic acid-Schiff, methenamine silver, and acid-fast techniques.

Following successful treatment, the protozoa are phagocytosed over the ensuing weeks with clearing of the intra-alveolar exudates. The organisms, however, may persist for an interval in some cases despite a satisfactory response to therapy.

Finally, we have studied three patients with AIDS who had pulmonary as well as disseminated extrapulmonary infections caused by *P. carinii*. The first patient presented with left upper quadrant pain, splenomegaly, and inguinal lymphadenopathy. At splenectomy, the

Table 10-2
Infections in Patients With AIDS

Microorganism	Location	Clinical Manifestations
Protozoa		
Pneumocystis carinii	Lung, spleen, lymph node, eye, disseminated	Pneumonia, splenomegaly, lymphadenopathy, choroiditis
Toxoplasma gondii	Brain, eye, heart, adrenal, disseminated	Meningoencephalitis, chorioretinitis, myocarditis
Cryptosporidium	Intestine, gallbladder, bile ducts, respiratory epithelium	Diarrhea, cholecystitis, sclerosing cholangitis
Isospora belli	Intestine, lymph node	Diarrhea, lymphadenopathy
Entamoeba histolytica	Intestine	Diarrhea
Giardia lamblia	Intestine	Diarrhea
Acanthamoeba	Brain	Meningoencephalitis
Fungi		
Candida	Oropharynx, esophagus, trachea, bronchi, lung	Thrush, esophagitis, tracheobronchitis, pneumonia
Cryptococcus neoformans	Brain, lung, lymph node, bone marrow, skin, blood, urine, disseminated	Meningoencephalitis, pneumonia, lymphadenopathy, fungemia
Histoplasma capsulatum	Lung, liver, spleen, lymph node, adrenal, bone marrow, eye, skin, blood, urine, disseminated	Pneumonia, hepatosplenomegaly, lymphadenopathy, chorioretinitis, pancytopenia, fungemia
Coccidioides immitis	Lung, brain, lymph node, liver, spleen, skin, blood, urine, disseminated	Pneumonia, meningoencephalitis, hepatosplenomegaly, lymphadenopathy, fungemia
Sporothrix schenckii	Skin, joint, lung, liver, spleen, disseminated	Cutaneous lesions, tenosynovitis, arthritis, pneumonia
Bacteria		
Mycobacterium avium-intracellulare, tuberculosis, and kansasii	Lymph node, liver, spleen, bone marrow, intestine, lung, skin, adrenal, blood, urine, disseminated	Lymphadenopathy, hepatosplenomegaly, pancytopenia, pneumonia, diarrhea, mycobacteremia
Nocardia spp	Lung, pleura, pericardium, soft tissues, bone, brain, lymph node, spleen, kidney, disseminated	Pneumonia, empyema, pericarditis, retropharyngeal or subcutaneous abscess, draining sinus tract, encephalitis
Legionella spp	Lung	Pneumonia
Campylobacter spp	Intestine, blood	Diarrhea, bacteremia
Salmonella spp	Intestine, blood	Diarrhea, bacteremia
Shigella spp	Intestine, blood	Diarrhea, bacteremia
Listeria monocytogenes	Meninges, blood	Meningitis, bacteremia
Cat-scratch disease bacillus	Lymph node, skin	Lymphadenopathy, cutaneous lesions
Treponema pallidum	Lymph node, testis, brain	Lymphadenopathy, orchitis, neurosyphilis
Viruses		
Cytomegalovirus	Lung, adrenal, eye, brain, peripheral nerve, intestine, liver, seminal vesicle, blood, disseminated	Pneumonia, chorioretinitis, meningoencephalitis, radiculitis with polyneuropathy, diarrhea, viremia
Herpes simplex	Mucocutaneous, esophagus, bronchus, lung, disseminated	Ulcerative mucocutaneous lesions, esophagitis, bronchitis, pneumonia, encephalitis
Herpes zoster	Mucocutaneous, disseminated	Multiple dermatomal zoster, Herpes zoster ophthalmicus
Epstein–Barr	Lymph node, tongue, blood	EBV-positive non-Hodgkin's lymphomas, oral hairy leukoplakia
Hepatitis B	Liver	Antigenemia
Polyomavirus	Brain	Progressive multifocal leukoencephalopathy
Poxvirus	Mucocutaneous	Molluscum contagiosum
Papillomavirus	Mucocutaneous	Condyloma accuminatum, oral hairy leukoplakia
Helminths		
Strongyloides stercoralis	Intestine, lung, brain, disseminated	Diarrhea, pneumonia, meningoencephalitis, recurrent poly-microbial bacteremias
Arthropods		
Sarcoptes scabiei (burrowing mange mite)	Skin, disseminated	Norwegian scabies, secondary bacteremias

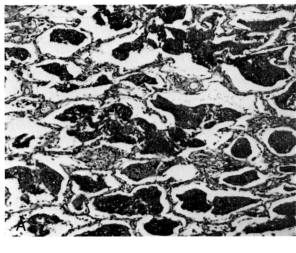

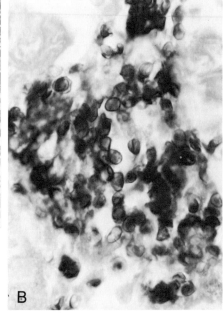

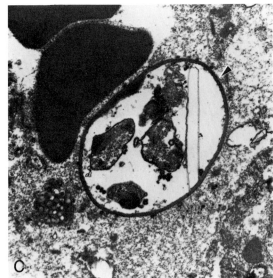

FIG. 10-8. (*A*) *Pneumocystis carinii* pneumonia with abundant intra-alveolar exudates (H&E stain; see Color Plate 10-3). (*B*) Oval, round, and cup-shaped cysts of *P. carinii* within intra-alveolar exudates are well demonstrated by silver stains (methenamine silver stain, ×1260). (Reichert CM, O'Leary TJ, Levens DL et al: Autopsy pathology in the acquired immune deficiency syndrome. Am J Pathol 112:357, 1983). (*C*) Cyst of *P. carinii* (*arrow*) with internal sporozoites. Compare size of the protozoan to the adjacent erythrocyte. (Electron micrograph courtesy of Dr. Timothy J. Triche)

spleen weighed 2000 g and contained grey-white nodules; microscopic examination revealed foci of eosinophilic foamy necrosis containing cysts of *P. carinii*. He died 1 month later and postmortem examination revealed similar necrotic foci containing *P. carinii* in lymph nodes, liver, kidneys, ureter, jejunum, omentum, mesentery, appendices epiploicae, pancreas, adrenals, heart, thyroid, bone marrow, choroid, and lung.[36] Two additional patients with AIDS had disseminated *P. carinii* infections involving spleen, lymph nodes, and lung. Therefore, although infection caused by *P. carinii* in the immunodeficient host is typically confined to alveoli of lung, it may disseminate. Splenomegaly and lymph-

adenopathy, not infrequent findings in patients with AIDS, may be caused by disseminated extrapulmonary *P. carinii* infections.

Toxoplasma gondii

In patients with AIDS, toxoplasmosis usually presents as an acute, subacute, or chronic encephalitis with fever and focal neurologic signs and/or chorioretinitis.[67,68] Patients with AIDS who develop neurologic deficits and single or multiple contrast-enhancing defects on computed tomographic (CT) scans frequently have toxoplasmal encephalitis,[69-71] although lesions caused by *Cryptococcus neoformans,* mycobacteria, *Nocardia* spp, cytomegalovirus, non-Hodgkin's lymphoma, and other processes must also be considered in the differential diagnosis.[72,73] Immunoglobulin G (IgG) toxoplasmal titers are frequently elevated in afflicted patients, reflecting past exposure; however, a low IgG titer does not rule out the diagnosis in immunosuppressed patients.[74] Furthermore, IgM titers may be negative despite active disease.[75-77] These serologic findings suggest that in patients with AIDS, central nervous system toxoplasmosis results from reactivation rather than from primary infection.

Definitive diagnosis requires visualization of the characteristic 2 × 6-μm tachyzoites or cysts on hematoxylin and eosin stained biopsy specimens or Wright-Giemsa stained smears.[77] Although tachyzoites are crescentic in fresh tissue (Greek *toxon* = arc) they appear rounded in fixed tissue sections. During acute infection the tachyzoites multiply asexually within engorged human host cells, which eventually rupture, releasing tachyzoites that infect additional cells. The destruction of parasitized cells results in foci of necrotic intracerebral lesions that may be detected grossly and microscopically. Histopathologically, large areas of vasculitis and necrotizing encephalitis may be present. There is a predilection for involvement of deep gray matter.[78] Encysted forms with their internal punctate bradyzoites are most often seen at the periphery of the necrotic foci. Free tachyzoites are most easily detected at the interface between viable and necrotic tissues (Fig. 10-9*A, B*). Central areas of necrosis contain few organisms (Fig. 10-9*C*). Histopathologic confirmation of intracerebral toxoplasmosis can at times be difficult, inasmuch as the organisms are small and can easily be confused with necrotic debris. When numbers of tachyzoites are too few for direct visualization, the organisms may be detected by the inoculation of suspected material into uninfected mice or through the use of specific immunoperoxidase stains.[79]

In our experience, many AIDS patients with toxoplasmal encephalitis also have disseminated toxoplasmosis. Histopathologically, one may find toxoplasmal

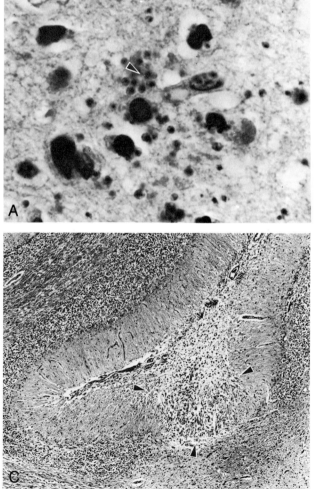

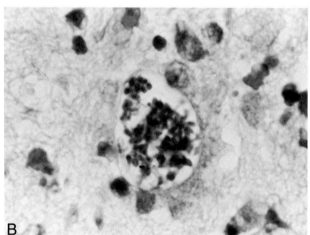

FIG. 10-9. (*A*) Extracellular toxoplasma tachyzoites (*arrow points to cluster of organisms*) in biopsied brain tissue of a patient with AIDS (H&E stain). (*B*) A group of spherical and arc-shaped tachyzoites in the biopsied brain of a patient with AIDS (H&E stain). (*C*) Necrotizing toxoplasma encephalitis (*arrows*) within the cerebellum of the same patient at autopsy. Following therapy, neither cyst forms nor tachyzoites could be detected histologically; however, small numbers of organisms were still present, inasmuch as toxoplasmosis was transmitted to mice through intraperitoneal injection of autopsy brain tissue (H&E stain). (*B* and *C* from Reichert CM, O'Leary TJ, Levens DL et al: Autopsy pathology in the acquired immune deficiency syndrome. Am J Pathol 112;357, 1983)

meningitis, chorioretinitis, myocarditis, pneumonitis, adrenalitis, pancreatitis, orchitis, and so forth. As in the brain, *Toxoplasma gondii* may cause extensive necrosis in these organs as well.

Cryptosporidium

Cryptosporidium is a protozoal coccidian first reported as a parasite of the intestinal tracts of many vertebrates, including reptiles, birds and mammals; these infected animals may be asymptomatic or may suffer from chronic enteritis, poor growth, and loss of vigor. As a zoonosis, cryptosporidium may pass to humans from calves and other animals. The first case of human infection with *Cryptosporidium* was reported in 1976 and occurred in an immunosuppressed patient.[80] We now know that *Cryptosporidium* may cause self-limited diarrhea (traveller's diarrhea) for 1 to 2 weeks even in those with intact immunity. In immunodeficient hosts, however, cryptosporidiosis may be fulminant and intractable.

Infection begins when *Cryptosporidium* attaches to the surface of the epithelial cells lining the small and large intestine. There is chronic, profuse, watery diarrhea in patients with AIDS.[81] Diagnosis is confirmed by identifying oocysts in stool. These are 2 to 6 μm across and are demonstrated in stool specimens using a modified Sheather's sucrose flotation technique.[82] In brief, after centrifugation of 0.5 g of stool specimen in a su-

crose solution, the oocysts accumulate on the surface; the oocysts are then transferred with a wire loop to a slide and examined by phase contrast microscopy. *Cryptosporidium* oocysts are distinguished from yeasts by their bright refractile quality. Because the oocysts are acid fast, the diagnosis may also be established by a modified Ziehl–Neelsen stain (Fig. 10-10*A*; Color Plate 10-4),[83,84] or by a fluorescent auramine stain of either fecal smear or formalin-ether and formalin concentrates of stool.[85]

Histopathologically, sections of small intestine stained by hematoxylin and eosin demonstrate rows of basophilic spherical cryptosporidia on the brush borders of intestinal villi. The villi may be blunted[86] or normal. Cryptosporidia may also lie free in the crypts. Cryptosporidia may also attach to the mucosal epithelium of the large intestine and appendix but do not invade the lamina propria. Cryptosporidiosis also occurs in the stomach and may lead to gastric outlet obstruction during the course of severe diarrheal disease. *Cryptosporidium* may also attach to respiratory epithelium.[87–89]

Transmission electron microscopy has demonstrated several different stages of the parasite, including trophozoite, schizont, oocyst, macrogametocyte, and merozoite.[90,91] The mechanism of cryptosporidial diarrhea is unknown. The typical absence of significant changes by light microscopy—inflammation and necrosis, for instance—suggests the elaboration of a toxin.

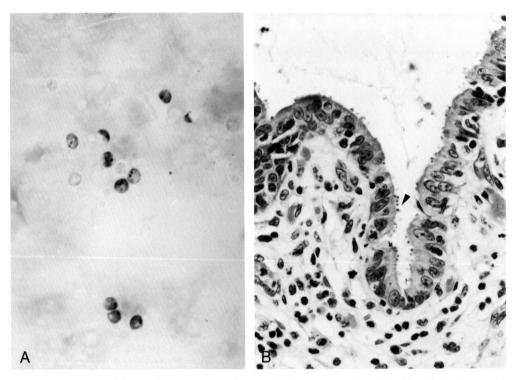

FIG. 10-10. (*A*) Acid-fast cryptosporidia in a fecal concentrate (modified Ziehl–Neelsen stain; sucrose flotation technique; see Color Plate 10-4). (*B*) Cryptosporidia aligned along the luminal border of the gallbladder mucosa (*arrow*) (H&E stain).

Cryptosporidium may also infect the gallbladder, as well as extrahepatic and intrahepatic bile ducts of patients with AIDS.[92-94] We studied two patients with AIDS who presented with right upper-quadrant abdominal pain caused by cryptosporidial cholecystitis and sclerosing cholangitis. Microscopic examination of the two gallbladder specimens revealed acute and chronic cholecystitis with numerous hematoxylinophilic spherical cryptosporidia attached in rows to the mucosal epithelium (Fig. 10-10*B*). Sections of liver revealed acute and chronic cholangitis as well as periductal lamellar fibrosis. Numerous cryptosporidia were attached to the epithelium of interlobular bile ducts. Cryptosporidial cholecystitis and cholangitis probably result from retrograde bile duct passage of organisms from the gastrointestinal tract.

Abdominal pain in the patient infected with HIV is a diagnostic problem that increasingly elicits surgical consultation. Surgical evaluation and intervention will be required more frequently as the number of HIV-infected cases continues to escalate. A thorough knowledge of the unusual infections and malignant processes that may be present in the patient with AIDS is mandatory for the physicians involved in the management of a patient with established or suspected AIDS.

Isospora belli

In addition to *Cryptosporidium,* another coccidial protozoan that causes chronic diarrhea in patients with AIDS is *Isospora belli.* In reported cases of human isosporiasis in non-AIDS patients, these protozoa have been demonstrated as intracellular parasites in the epithelium of the intestine. In patients with AIDS, however, enteric infections with *I. belli* may disseminate beyond the intestinal wall. In a case we studied,[35] intracellular and extracellular *I. belli* organisms were present in the mucosa and lamina propria of the small and large intestine, as well as in mesenteric and tracheobronchial lymph nodes. Lymphadenopathy, not an infrequent finding in patients with AIDS, may be caused by disseminated extraintestinal lymphadenopathic isosporiasis.

Other Enteric Pathogens

Chronic diarrhea in patients with AIDS may result from a variety of microorganisms, ranging from bacteria such as *Salmonella* spp, *Shigella* spp, and *Campylobacter* spp, to protozoans such as *Entamoeba histolytica* and *Giardia lamblia* (Fig. 10-11). Furthermore, patients with AIDS and chronic diarrhea may present with recurrent bacteremias caused by *Salmonella* spp, *Shigella* spp, and *Campylobacter* spp.[95]

Acanthamoeba

The free-living amoebas of the Hartmannella-Acanthamoeba group are known to infect immunosuppressed individuals and cause a meningoencephalitis.[96] We studied the case of a patient with AIDS who presented with numerous contrast-enhancing intracerebral lesions that were clinically thought to represent toxoplasmal encephalitis. Microscopic sections of brain stained by hematoxylin and eosin revealed multiple areas of vasculitis with acute and chronic inflammation and necrosis suggestive of toxoplasmosis. However, we did not see cysts or tachyzoites of *T. gondii.* Instead, there were numerous trophozoites, 10 to 25 μm across, each with a sharply outlined nucleus and a dense nucleolus. Sections stained by methenamine silver revealed cyst forms as well. These findings are characteristic of amebic meningoencephalitis caused by the Hartmannella-Acanthamoeba group.

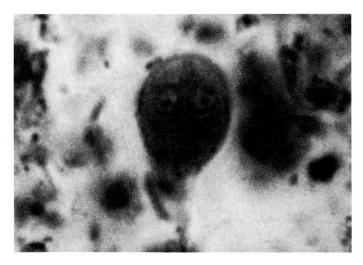

FIG. 10-11. *Giardia lamblia* in stool specimen (iron-hematoxylin stain).

Fungi

Candida *Species*

Oral candidiasis (thrush) frequently occurs in patients at risk for the development of AIDS. Otherwise, it is an uncommon infection in previously healthy persons who have not received prior antibiotic, hormonal, or immunosuppressive therapy. The presence of oral candidiasis in patients infected with HIV is highly predictive for the subsequent development of AIDS.[97] The diagnosis of thrush is established by the presence of characteristic intraoral white "cheesy" mucosal lesions; microscopic examination of unstained wet-mounted or Gram's-stained mucosal scrapings reveal budding yeasts and pseudohyphae characteristic of *Candida* spp (Fig. 10-12).

Patients with *Candida* esophagitis frequently complain of odynophagia, and mucosal ulcerations may be demonstrated by esophagoscopy or barium swallow esophagrams. Although the fungi can be microscopically detected in sections stained by hematoxylin and eosin, they can be easily overlooked. They are much more apparent in sections stained by periodic acid-Schiff or methenamine silver as 3- to 4-μm budding yeasts and pseudohyphae invading partially ulcerated epithelium. Candidiasis of the trachea, bronchi, and lungs also occur, particularly in pediatric patients with AIDS. Although candidiasis is often a life-threatening disseminated disease in immunosuppressed non-AIDS patients, in patients with AIDS, widespread visceral dissemination is infrequent.

Cryptococcus neoformans

Cryptococcus neoformans is a common cause of meningitis and disseminated disease in patients with AIDS.[98] Analysis of cerebrospinal fluid usually reveals a mild pleocytosis, hypoglycorrhachia, and elevated protein; however, any or all of these parameters may be normal. The India ink test, cryptococcal antigen, and fungal cultures are almost always positive. Patients with AIDS may also present with localized or disseminated extrameningeal disease, with or without an accompanying meningitis. Pneumonitis, lymphadenitis, peritonitis, thyroiditis, and retinitis caused by *C. neoformans* also occur. Blood cultures are often positive in these patients. In postmortem examinations we have demonstrated disseminated infections in the central nervous system (Fig. 10-13*A*), eye, lung, lymph node, bone marrow, liver, spleen, heart, adrenal gland, kidney, prostate, thyroid, intestine, pancreas, skin, and ovary.

Encapsulated narrow-pored budding yeasts within the cerebrospinal fluid may be detected by India ink wet-mount preparations. Microscopic examination of biopsied tissue sections stained by hematoxylin and eosin reveal the pale cell walls of encapsulated yeasts, 4 to 7 micrometers in diameter, amidst minimal to absent inflammation. Silver and periodic acid-Schiff stains are commonly used to demonstrate the yeasts (Fig. 10-13*B*). Positive capsular staining by mucicarmine distinguishes cryptococcal yeasts from those of *Blastomyces dermatitidis* and *Histoplasma capsulatum*.

Histoplasma capsulatum

Disseminated histoplasmosis occurs in patients with AIDS.[99,100] These patients may present with fever, pneumonia, hepatosplenomegaly, abnormal liver function tests, lymphadenopathy, pancytopenia, chorioretinitis, meningitis, and endocarditis. Most of these patients are fungemic, and both extracellular and intracellular narrow-pored budding yeasts may be seen on Wright–Giemsa stained smears of their peripheral blood. In postmortem examinations we have demonstrated disseminated infections in lung, central nervous system, eye, liver, spleen, lymph node, adrenal, kidney, heart, intestine, appendix, pancreas, testis, prostate, bone marrow, and thyroid.

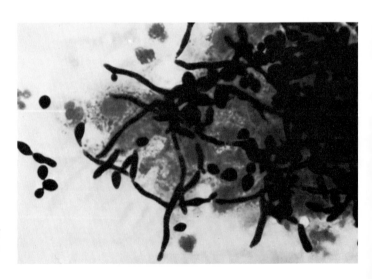

FIG. 10-12. Budding yeasts and pseudohyphae of *Candida albicans* scraped from the oropharynx of a patient with AIDS and oral thrush (Gram's stain).

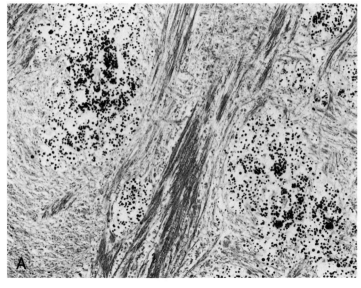

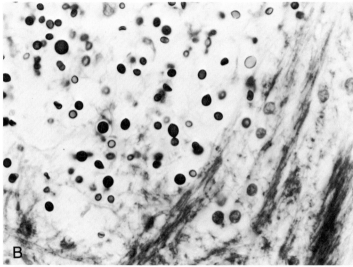

FIG. 10-13. (*A*) Microabscesses of *Cryptococcus neoformans* in the brain (methenamine silver stain, ×100). (*B*) Narrow-pore budding yeasts of *C. neoformans* in the brain (methenamine silver stain, ×860). (Reichert CM, O'Leary TJ, Levens DL et al: Autopsy pathology in the acquired immune deficiency syndrome. Am J Pathol 112:357, 1983)

In sections of biopsied tissue stained by hematoxylin and eosin, periodic acid-Schiff, and methenamine silver, characteristic oval 2- to 4-μm, narrow-pored budding yeasts of *Histoplasma capsulatum* are typically found within and expanding the cytoplasm of histiocytes. In some cases, there may be foci of caseation necrosis, and staining with periodic acid-Schiff and methenamine silver demonstrates the yeasts (Fig. 10-14). The areas of caseation necrosis are surrounded by minimal to absent granulomatous inflammation; multinucleated giant cells are infrequently seen. The histiocytic infiltrates, as well as the non-granulomatous areas of caseation necrosis, represent "anergic" host responses to their histoplasmal infections. Such anergic histopathologic reactions are also seen in the tissues of AIDS patients with disseminated infections caused by *Mycobacterium tuberculosis* (non-granulomatous caseation necrosis) and *M. avium-intracellulare* (histiocytic inflammation).

The numbers of AIDS patients with histoplasmosis will undoubtedly rise as cases of AIDS from areas where histoplasmosis is endemic continue to increase.

Coccidioides immitis

Coccidioides immitis is endemic in the soils of the southwestern United States and is frequently found as a disseminated opportunistic infection in patients with AIDS from this area.[101,102] Patients may present with pneumonia, meningoencephalitis, hepatosplenomegaly, lymphadenopathy, arthritis, osteomyelitis, and cutaneous lesions. In postmortem examinations we have seen disseminated infections in lung, brain, lymph node, liver, spleen, skin, bone, adrenal, kidney, prostate, and

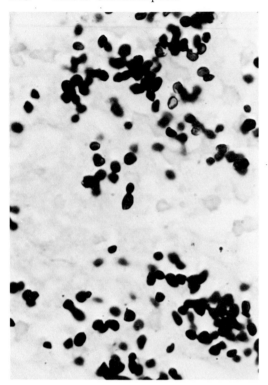

FIG. 10-14. *Histoplasma capsulatum* in the spleen of an AIDS patient with disseminated, clinically unsuspected histoplasmosis (methenamine silver stain, ×1260). Compare these oval budding yeasts with the non-budding cysts of *P. carinii,* with which they are frequently confused.

thyroid. Sections of tissue stained with hematoxylin and eosin reveal hematoxylinophilic, thick-walled, 30- to 60-μm spherules containing internal endospores; the spherules may be found within foci of caseation necrosis surrounded by minimal granulomatous inflammation.[103]

Sporothrix schenckii

Disseminated sporotrichosis also occurs as an opportunistic infection in patients with AIDS.[104] Patients may present with cutaneous lesions, tenosynovitis, arthritis, and pneumonia. Postmortem examinations have revealed disseminated infections in lung, liver, spleen, skin, and bone. Sections stained with periodic acid-Schiff and methenamine silver reveal elongated budding yeasts characteristic of *S. schenckii.*

Bacteria

Mycobacterium avium-intracellulare *(MAI),* M. tuberculosis, M. kansasii

Prior to the advent of AIDS, the ubiquitous, atypical, acid-fast bacillus of MAI was an infrequent cause of disseminated disease in immunosuppressed patients. Now patients with AIDS frequently develop disseminated MAI infections and present with lymphadenopathy, hepatosplenomegaly, pancytopenia, pneumonia, diarrhea, and mycobacteremia.[105–107] Postmortem examinations have revealed disseminated MAI infections in lymph node, liver, spleen, bone marrow, intestine, pancreas, lung, skin, adrenal, kidney, prostate, heart, brain, eye, and thyroid. In contrast to the caseating granulomas and giant-cell reactions that are classically observed in mycobacterial infections, histologic sections of MAI-infected tissues of patients with AIDS commonly reveal sheets of foamy histiocytes with otherwise minimal inflammation and poorly formed or absent granulomas. For this reason, overwhelming MAI infections may go undetected unless special stains are performed. Acid-fast stains (Ziehl–Neelsen, Fite) of affected tissues frequently reveal surprisingly large numbers of mycobacteria within the cytoplasm of histiocytes (Fig. 10-15; Color Plate 10-5), reminiscent of the "globi" seen in patients with lepromatous leprosy. Involvement of the small intestine may mimic Whipple's disease. In some cases it may be difficult to demonstrate the acid-fast organisms in histologic sections of culture-positive specimens. We suspect that the absence of demonstrable organisms at these sites may be more indicative of the patient's mycobacteremic state than of tissue-destructive infection by numbers of organisms too small to be reliably demonstrated histologically.

Disseminated infections by *M. tuberculosis* and *M. kansasii* also occur in patients with AIDS.[108,109] Histopathologically, one finds aggregates of histiocytes as well as areas of caseation necrosis surrounded by minimal to absent granulomatous inflammation, since multinucleated giant cells are not frequently seen.

Nocardia *species*

Patients with AIDS may develop disseminated nocardiosis.[110,111] *Nocardia* spp are aerobic actinomycetes, and as soil saprophytes, they are distributed throughout the world. Nocardiosis may present as an acute, subacute, or chronic infection, most often beginning in the lung. Clinical presentations in patients with AIDS have included pneumonitis, pleural effusion (empyema), purulent pericarditis, cervical osteomyelitis, retropharyngeal abscess, subcutaneous abscess, draining sinus tract, and brain abscess. Unlike pneumonia caused by *P. carinii,* pulmonary nocardiosis often presents with a productive cough. The initial illness may resemble a bacterial pneumonia, but slow radiologic progression continues despite antibiotic therapy, often with cavitation of radio-dense central areas. Contiguous spread causes pleural, pericardial, bone, and subcutaneous lesions. Lymphohematogenous dissemination to brain and subcutaneous tissue is frequent in nocardiosis.

Sputum, pus, or bronchial lavage/washing specimens should be examined by Gram's and modified acid-fast stains. The organisms appear as Gram-variable, weakly acid fast, filamentous, beaded, branching bacilli.

Conventional acid-fast staining procedures such as Ziehl–Neelsen or a fluorochrome do not stain *Nocardia* spp. In sections of tissue, *Nocardia* bacilli are found within foci of suppurative necrosis.

Other Bacteria

In patients with AIDS, *Listeria monocytogenes* may cause meningitis and bacteremia.[112] *Legionella* spp may cause pneumonia and disseminated infections.[113] *Treponema pallidum* may cause lymphadenitis, orchitis, and relapsing neurosyphilis; microscopic sections of lymph nodes and testes reveal unusually large numbers of spirochetes. Cat-scratch disease (CSD) is appearing as lymphadenitis and/or dermatitis with innumerable CSD bacilli found within blood vessels and areas of suppurative necrosis, without granulomatous inflammation. This anergic nongranulomatous form of CSD with prominent vascular proliferation may be misinterpreted as Kaposi's sarcoma. Other bacteria (e.g., *Streptococcus* spp., *Hemophilus influenzae,* etc.) may also cause serious infections (e.g., pneumonia, meningitis, bacteremia), particularly in children with AIDS.[114]

Viruses

Cytomegalovirus

Many patients with AIDS have persistent cytomegaloviremia, and cytomegalovirus (CMV) is a major cause of dysfunction in a variety of organs.[4] Patients may present with pneumonia, blinding chorioretinitis, esophagitis, colitis with extensive ulcerations and perforation, meningoencephalitis, radiculitis with polyneuropathies, and hepatitis. Diagnosis may be established by typical cytopathic changes observed in viral tissue cultures or by histologic detection of the characteristic viral inclusion cells in biopsy or necropsy specimens. The virus induces cellular gigantism (cytomegaly) with characteristic intranuclear and intracytoplasmic viral inclusions. In sections stained with hematoxylin and eosin, the enlarged nucleus of an infected cell possesses a large eosinophilic inclusion with a peripheral clear halo; within the cytoplasm of an infected cell are numerous puntate inclusions, which are also stained by periodic acid-Schiff and methenamine silver techniques.

Cytomegaloviral infection of lung results in focal and diffuse hemorrhagic interstitial pneumonitis (Fig. 10-16; Color Plate 10-6). Sections of adrenal gland infected by CMV may reveal massive bilateral hemorrhagic necrosis. Many male homosexuals shed CMV in their semen and urine, and it may be detected histologically within the male genitourinary system, especially in seminal vesicles and epididymis, where it may produce symptomatic epididymitis. Gastrointestinal involvement by CMV is characterized by ulceration in sites ranging from the esophagus to the rectum.[115] There is a reported predilection of CMV ulcers for involvement of the

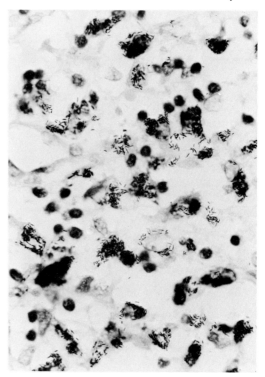

FIG. 10-15.   Lymph node with innumerable acid-fast bacilli, identified by culture as *Mycobacterium avium-intracellulare* (Fite stain, ×860; see Color Plate 10-5).

cecum, and these may provide a portal of entry into the bloodstream for a variety of enteric organisms. In CMV retinitis, affected retinas show varying degrees of perivascular exudative hemorrhagic lesions and histologic sections reveal foci of necrosis and characteristic viral inclusions within retinal, choroidal, and optic nerve tissues.[116] Within the central nervous system, CMV may produce a destructive meningoencephalitis[117] or a subacute encephalitis with microglial nodules; rarely, a CMV inclusion cell may be seen centrally within a microglial nodule (Fig. 10-17; Color Plate 10-7). In patients with polyneucropathies and abnormal cerebrospinal fluids, sections of spinal nerve roots may reveal multiple prominent foci of perivascular acute and chronic inflammation with necrosis and CMV inclusion cells.

Epstein–Barr Virus

A herpes group DNA virus, the Epstein–Barr virus (EBV) has been implicated in EBV-associated non-Hodgkin's lymphomas and oral hairy leukoplakia (see below).

Herpes Simplex and Zoster

Both herpes simplex and herpes zoster may cause severe infections in patients with AIDS.[118,119] Herpes simplex may produce ulcerative mucocutaneous lesions,

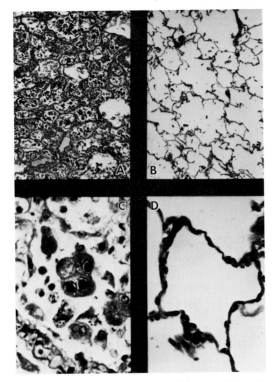

FIG. 10-16. (*A*) Massive consolidation of lung in an AIDS patient with terminal cytomegaloviral pneumonitis. (*B*) Normal lung control. (*C*) Cytomegaly of desquamated alveolar lining cells, containing large intranuclear viral inclusions with peripheral clear haloes. Intracytoplasmic inclusions are also apparent. (*D*) Normal pulmonary alveoli, provided for comparison (H&E stains; see also Color Plate 10-6).

esophagitis, bronchitis, pneumonitis, and/or encephalitis. Herpes zoster may present as multiple dermatomal lesions. Histopathologically, the characteristic mucocutaneous herpetic lesion consists of an intraepidermal vesicle produced by marked acantholysis and ballooning degeneration of epithelial cells. Eosinophilic viral inclusion bodies may be detected in the center of the enlarged nuclei of balloon cells. Infected cells may coalesce to form syncytial multinucleated inclusion cells.

Polyomavirus

Progressive multifocal leukoencephalopathy (PML) is a central nervous system demyelinating disorder caused by polyomaviruses of the papova family. Infections develop in adults who are immunologically suppressed, and PML occurs in patients with AIDS.[120,121] CT scans of the brain usually show focal hypodense white-matter lesions without contrast enhancement or mass effect.

Gross pathologic examination reveals a granular softening of white matter. Histopathologically, there are patchy areas of demyelination, necrosis, and gliosis. The plaques of demyelination are especially well seen by myelin stains. In sections stained with hematoxylin and eosin, within these areas are scattered oligodendroglia whose nuclei are filled with eosinophilic to amphophilic viral inclusions, gigantic bizarre astrocytes, and numerous foamy macrophages. Polyomavirus inclusions can be demonstrated by immunohistochemical staining, employing a polyclonal antibody with reactivity among JC, SV40, and BK types of polyomaviruses (Fig. 10-18; Color Plate 10-8).

An idiopathic demyelinating disorder that is not attributable to polyomavirus infection (either by immunocytochemistry or viral DNA extraction procedures) is also seen in patients with AIDS. Microglial nodules are also observed in these lesions (Fig. 10-19; Color Plate 10-9) (See Idiopathic Neurologic Lesions under Special Problems).

Hepatitis B

In addition to being at risk for the development of AIDS, male homosexuals and intravenous drug abusers are also at risk for developing hepatitis B infections. We have studied a number of hepatic tissue specimens from patients with AIDS who are antigenemic for hepatitis B. Although immunohistochemical staining for hepatitis B core antigen reveals numerous infected hepatocytes, there is usually minimal to absent associated inflammation. Perhaps patients with AIDS lack the effector cells

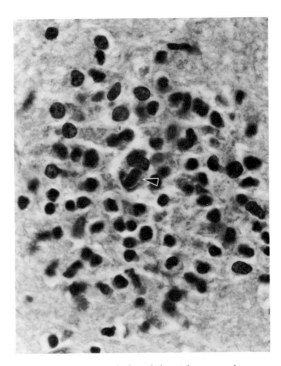

FIG. 10-17. Microglial nodule with a central cytomegaloviral inclusion cell (*arrow*) in the brain of a patient with AIDS (H&E stain; see also Color Plate 10-7).

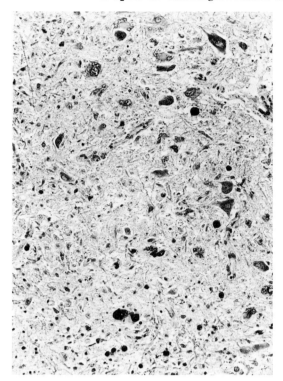

FIG. 10-18. Progressive multifocal leukoencephalopathy in a patient with AIDS. Plaque of demyelination demonstrating gliosis, bizarre giant astrocytes, and oligodendroglia that are positive for the antigens of polyoma virus. (Immunoperoxidase stain, courtesy of Drs. P. H. Howley and D. L. Levens; see Color Plate 10-8). (Reichert CM, O'Leary TJ, Levens DL et al: Autopsy pathology in the acquired immune deficiency syndrome. Am J Pathol 112:357, 1983)

responsible for the damaging sequelae of hepatitis B infection.[122]

Molluscum contagiosum

Molluscum contagiosum is a DNA virus of the poxvirus group. Infections in patients with AIDS typically appear as multiple 2- to 4-mm dome-shaped, umbilicated cutaneous papules distributed over the face and chest. The lesions possess central craters and discharge a curdlike material. Histopathologically, the lesions exhibit the following features:

1. Downward proliferation of the epidermis in a lobular configuration.
2. Numerous intracytoplasmic eosinophilic inclusions (molluscum bodies) within the epidermal cells of the stratum malpighii (excluding the basal layer).
3. Expansion of the epidermal cell with compression of the nucleus by proliferating viral particles.
4. Release of molluscum bodies into the central crater.

Condyloma Acuminatum

Condylomata acuminata are soft, verrucous mucocutaneous lesions caused by a DNA papillomavirus. In patients with AIDS, these lesions may occur in a perianal, genital, or perioral distribution. Histopathologically, the lesions exhibit papillomatosis and acanthosis. The diagnostic feature is the presence of vacuolated epithelial cells with hyperchromatic, basophilic intranuclear inclusions, which may be shown to contain the papillomavirus by immunohistochemical stains.

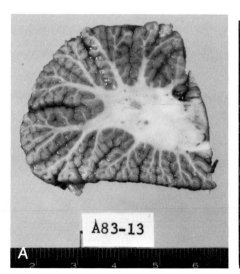

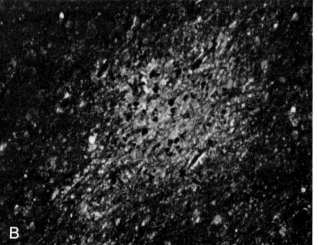

FIG. 10-19. (*A*) Multifocal demyelination of undetermined etiology, shown within the cerebellum of a patient with AIDS. (*B*) Plaques of demyelination, same case. (Luxol fast-blue-PAS myelin stain; see Color Plate 10-9). (Reichert CM, O'Leary TJ, Levens DL et al: Autopsy pathology in the acquired immune deficiency syndrome. Am J Pathol 112:357, 1983)

Helminths

Strongyloides stercoralis

The threadworm, *Strongyloides stercoralis,* may cause chronic diarrhea in patients with AIDS.[123] Although healthy individuals tolerate strongyloidiasis well, immunoincompetent patients may develop "hyperinfections." In patients with hyperinfection strongyloidiasis, a progressive internal recycling accumulates large numbers of adult worms and migratory larvae that mechanically damage the absorptive surface of the intestine, causing enteritis and malabsorption. Gastrointestinal symptoms are often severe and include nausea, vomiting, diarrhea, and fever. Overwhelming numbers of worms cause ulcerations of the small and large intestine, paralytic ileus, and even perforation. Migrating larvae introduce intestinal flora into the bloodstream and cause polymicrobial bacteremia. The migration of scores of larvae through the lungs causes pneumonitis with cough, hemoptysis, and dyspnea. Involvement of the central nervous system causes meningitis, brain abscess, and infarction. Septicemia, pneumonia, and meningitis are complications that tend to recur even after antibiotic treatment, unless the underlying strongyloidiasis is also cured. In cases of hyperinfection strongyloidiasis, death may be a consequence of respiratory failure, central nervous system damage, peritonitis caused by a perforated bowel, or persistent bacteremia.

Histopathologically, adult worms, embryonated eggs, and larvae are found burrowed within intestinal mucosal crypts. In severe infections the lamina propria is heavily infiltrated, mucosal villi are blunted, lacteals are dilated, and there is widespread mucosal edema. With hyperinfection, there is often mucosal ulceration of the small intestine; the invasive filariform larvae are found in submucosal lymphatics and blood vessels surrounded by inflammation. In the colon, filariform larvae are in the submucosa and muscularis, provoking focal accumulations of lymphoid cells and macrophages but rarely well-defined epithelioid cell granulomas. Penetration of the bowel by innumerable larvae promotes the secondary bacterial infections caused by intestinal "flora" (e.g., polymicrobial septicemia, meningitis, pneumonitis). Migrating filariform larvae may appear in any organ but are most frequently seen in the lung, liver, and brain. Larvae in tissues may cause no reaction or may provoke a mixed inflammatory cell infiltrate including eosinophils, neutrophils, lymphocytes, plasma cells, histiocytes, and giant cells.

Arthropods

Sarcoptes scabiei

Homosexual men are at increased risk of acquiring sexually transmitted diseases, including scabies. Furthermore, homosexual men with AIDS are susceptible to developing the more virulent "Norwegian" scabies.

Scabies is infection of man with *Sarcoptes scabiei,* the burrowing mange mite. The mites burrow tunnels in the epidermis, where they feed, defecate, and deposit eggs from which larvae hatch. Vesiculation and intense itching characterizes scabies. The mites prefer skin with few pilosebaceous follicles (e.g., interdigital folds, small of the back, nipples, penis, scrotum, and lower buttocks).

To diagnose scabies, skin scrapings are treated with 10% potassium hydroxide and examined microscopically to reveal characteristic mites and eggs. Histopathologic examination of a biopsy specimen reveals mites and eggs within tunnels in acanthotic epidermis. Underlying dermis may be heavily inflamed with eosinophils, lymphocytes, plasma cells, histiocytes, and, with secondary bacterial infection, neutrophils. Mites have a chitinous exoskeleton, striated muscle, characteristic spines on the dorsal surface of the cuticle, and a diameter less than 500 μm but usually more than 100 μm.

A more severe form of scabies, "Norwegian" scabies, is characterized by extraordinary numbers of *S. scabiei* without itching. It was first described in Norwegians with leprosy. Norwegian scabies is highly contagious because of the many mites present on the affected individual. A patient with ordinary scabies may have only a few dozen mites, but the patient with Norwegian scabies may have millions of mites. Failure to recognize Norwegian scabies in patients has caused several epidemics in hospitals.

Norwegian scabies afflicts debilitated and immunocompromised patients. In immunocompetent patients with ordinary scabies, cellular and humoral immune mechanisms are believed to control the number of mites and cause the intolerable itch. On the other hand, immunosuppressed patients with Norwegian scabies have enormous numbers of mites and minimal itching. Glover and others[124] reported the first case of Norwegian scabies in a male homosexual with AIDS. The patient's extensive cutaneous lesions became secondarily infected and caused a bacteremia from which he died.

NEOPLASMS

Kaposi's Sarcoma

In 1872, Dr. Moriz Kaposi described a condition, "sarcoma idiopathicum multiplex hemorrhagicum" (multiple idiopathic hemorrhagic sarcoma), that now bears his name.[125] Prior to the appearance of Kaposi's sarcoma (KS) in patients with AIDS, most cases of this relatively rare multifocal cutaneous vascular neoplasm were localized to the lower extremities of older men of Mediterranean descent.[126] Kaposi's sarcoma was also reported in iatrogenically immunosuppressed organ transplant recipients[127] and among young blacks in regions of equatorial Africa, where it is endemic.[128]

KS is considered an angioproliferative disorder and

differs from other neoplasms in that its pattern of dissemination suggests multicentric origin rather than hematogenous metastatic spread from a single primary site. It is not known whether under certain conditions HIV is capable of inducing KS, or if, as is thought more likely, KS has a different etiologic basis that is permitted expression in immunosuppressed patients.

In patients with AIDS, KS most frequently presents in one or more mucocutaneous sites. Within the oral cavity, lesions may appear on the lips, gingiva, buccal mucosa, palate, tonsils, tongue, oropharynx, and epiglottis.[129] Depending on the time course of the disease process, the erythematous to violaceous mucocutaneous lesions, which range from several millimeters to several centimeters in diameter, may appear as macules, infiltrative plaques or nodules. As first proposed by Kaposi, "the striking pigmentation is caused, perhaps entirely, but certainly preponderantly, by the large amount of blood and hemorrhage within the tumors." The hue of older Kaposi's sarcoma lesions may also be modified by hemosiderin deposition.

Lymph node involvement by KS is common. Although nodal disease usually accompanies mucocutaneous lesions, occasionally only lymph nodes are involved.[130] Grossly and microscopically, lymph nodes involved by Kaposi's sarcoma exhibit hemorrhagic lesions in capsular, subcapsular, sinusoidal, and hilar locations. Lesions may be subtle, and small foci may be missed unless serial sections are taken.[131]

Visceral lesions almost always appear in association with generalized mucocutaneous disease, although exceptions have been reported.[132] On gross examination of visceral lesions, the tumors appear as areas of petechiae or hemorrhage, usually first appearing in connective tissue surrounding blood vessels. This perivascular predilection is well demonstrated in the heart, where KS is often confined to the distribution of the epicardial coronary arteries (Fig. 10-20)[133] and in the liver, where tumor exhibits a striking predilection for portal tracts (Fig. 10-21). In the lungs KS grossly appears as erythematous plaques and nodules, localized to the pleura, to perivascular sites along bronchi and interlobular septae, and to the submucosa of the tracheobronchial tree. Serosanguinous pleural effusion may accompany pleural involvement by KS. At autopsy we have observed pulmonary nodules of KS as large as 3 cm in diameter. Diffuse pulmonary KS may result in massive intra-alveolar hemorrhage and death. Kaposi's sarcoma lesions within the gastrointestinal tract arise within the esophagus, stomach (Fig. 10-22), small and large intestine, appendix, and rectum and appear as flat to nodular vascular lesions, characteristically originating within the submucosa. Lesions frequently extend into the lamina propria and may produce mucosal ulcerations. Other sites of involvement by KS include spleen, gallbladder, pancreas, kidney, testis, epidydimis, palpebral conjunctivae,[134] adventitia of aorta and large vessels, and perineural connective tissue. The typical pattern of organ and tissue involvement by KS may reflect disparate abil-

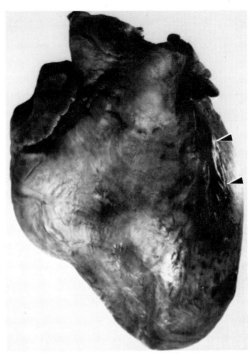

FIG. 10-20. Perivascular Kaposi's sarcoma following the distribution of the left anterior descending coronary artery (*arrows*) in a patient with AIDS.

ity of the etiologic agent of KS to permeate certain vascular barriers or to stimulate angiogenesis within selected tissue sites. Although we have not seen KS within the bone marrow or brain, involvement at these sites has been referred to in isolated case reports by others.[135–137]

Histopathologically, there is no difference between KS of AIDS patients and lesions from older, presumably heterosexual men and women with classic KS;[138] nor are there differences between the lesions of black Africans and caucasians.[139] The histologic spectrum of the lesions of KS may progress from angiomatous (early) to sarcomatous (late) forms. Histologic features of typical KS include (1) proliferation of bland-appearing spindle cells (Fig. 10-23; Color Plate 10-11); (2) arrangements of some of the neoplastic cells into small slit-like vascular spaces; (3) scattering of erythrocytes and variable hemosiderin deposition within and around the lesions; (4) identification of peculiar intracellular hyaline, periodic acid-Schiff positive, diastase-resistant globules in many of the specimens (Color Plate 10-12); and (5) a variable accompaniment of plasma cells and lymphocytes. Mitotic figures are few, and there is mild nuclear atypia. Early lesions are frequently angiomatous (telangiectatic), consisting of haphazardly arranged vascular channels with lumina that are either empty (with lymphatic channel-like appearance) or contain erythrocytes (Fig. 10-24; Color Plate 10-10). Lesions of KS are most likely to be confused with fibrous histio-

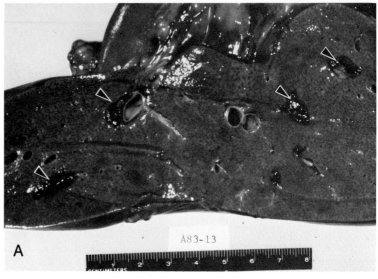

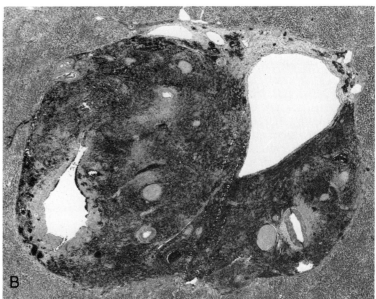

FIG. 10-21. (*A*) Hemorrhagic periportal Kaposi's sarcoma (*arrows*) of the liver in a patient with AIDS. (*B*) Microscopic detail showing expansion of a portal tract by Kaposi's sarcoma (H&E stain). (Reichert CM, O'Leary TJ, Levens DL et al: Autopsy pathology in the acquired immune deficiency syndrome. Am J Pathol 112:357, 1983)

cytomas, pyogenic granuloma, stasis dermatitis, telangiectasias, angiosarcoma, and florid granulation tissue (particularly in ulcerated mucosal and gastrointestinal lesions). In skin biopsies KS dissects through the collagen of the mid-dermis and exhibits a predilection for perivascular areas and the loose connective tissue surrounding adnexal structures. The overlying epidermis may become attenuated in nodular lesions. Nodular lesions are typically more cellular, with spindle cells arranged in interweaving fascicles (Fig. 10-26). As indicated previously, there is a histologic spectrum of KS lesions, and on occasion we and others[140] have seen lesions that are frankly sarcomatous, possessing a higher degree of cellularity, increased mitotic activity, and greater nuclear atypia than angiomatous forms. We have also studied specimens of skin that simultaneously showed angiomatous, intermediate, and sarcomatous stages of KS. After therapy, residual KS lesions may lose much of the spindle cell component, appearing as ectatic vascular channels with scattered hemosiderin deposits.

KS lesions most likely to come to the attention of a surgical pathologist include (1) skin biopsies, which are often obtained to establish the diagnosis of AIDS; (2) endoscopically obtained biopsies of the gastrointestinal tract (and oropharynx), which are usually biopsied to investigate complaints of anorexia, weight loss, nausea, pain, diarrhea, and bleeding; and (3) lung biop-

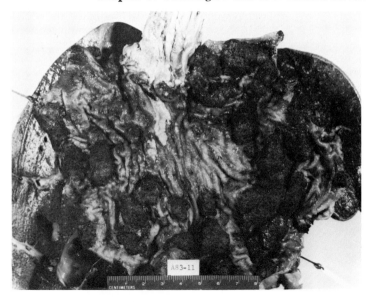

FIG. 10-22. Exophytic nodules of Kaposi's sarcoma in the stomach of a patient with AIDS. (Reichert CM, O'Leary TJ, Levens DL et al: Autopsy pathology in the acquired immune deficiency syndrome. Am J Pathol 112:357, 1983)

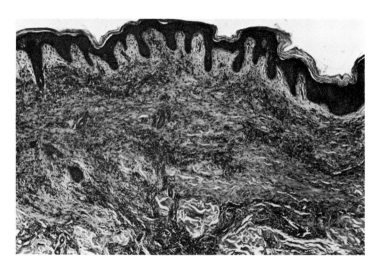

FIG. 10-23. Typical histologic appearance of cutaneous Kaposi's sarcoma in a patient with AIDS. Note dermal proliferation of spindle cells (H&E stain; see Color Plate 10-11).

sies, which generally have been performed to rule out opportunistic infections or to investigate hemoptysis.

Lymphomas

In addition to KS, patients with AIDS have an increased incidence of non-Hodgkin's lymphomas.[216,217] These frequently present in extranodal locations, a feature also seen in Burkitt's lymphomas and lymphomas in immunosuppressed (e.g., post-transplant) individuals. Notably, like Burkitt's lymphoma in Africa but unlike the nonendemic form, these neoplasms are frequently EBNA-positive. Cytogenetic analyses of several undifferentiated lymphomas in patients with AIDS have revealed chromosomal translocations typical of Burkitt's lymphoma involving the long arm of chromosome 8

and one of the chromosomes containing immunoglobulin genes, either 14 (heavy chains) or 22 (lambda light chains).[143-145]

These extranodal lymphomas may present within the central nervous system (Fig. 10-27),[146] orbit,[147] pharynx and jaw,[148] intestine,[142] liver (Fig. 10-28), kidney,[110] bone marrow, and muscle.[4] Tumors may remain localized or they may disseminate widely. Systemic sites of involvement include spleen, pleura, and peripheral blood. Architecturally these lymphomas are diffuse (as opposed to nodular) and histologically most often of the undifferentiated small non-cleaved (Burkitt's and non-Burkitt's) or of the large-cell (histiocytic) subtypes. The undifferentiated lymphocytes possess non-cleaved nuclei that approximate the nuclear size of macrophages, multiple small nucleoli, and scanty cytoplasm; a starry-sky architectural pattern (composed of tingible body macrophages) is often present, indicative of a high rate of cellular turnover. Large-cell lymphomas most commonly belong to the high-grade, immunoblastic or to the intermediate-grade, diffuse large-cell categories. Plasmacytomas have also been reported. When immunohistochemistry has been performed in cases of AIDS-related lymphomas, these tumors have been determined to be of B-cell lineage, with expression of either a kappa or lambda light chain and a heavy chain, most commonly IgM.

Although these lymphomas may be the initial manifestation of AIDS, they may also follow the diagnosis of KS or they may develop subsequent to the emergence of the unusual opportunistic infections that characterize AIDS. Occasionally, they are first discovered at autopsy.

Other Malignancies

The male homosexual population is at increased risk for the development of squamous-cell carcinoma of the oropharynx and cloacogenic or intraepithelial carcinoma of the anorectum.[149]

Several cases of small-cell undifferentiated (oat-cell) carcinoma have been reported in patients with AIDS.[150–152] Small-cell carcinomas are primitive neuroendocrine tumors that are most common in the lung, but can occur in many sites including the gastrointestinal tract and pancreas. Sites of origin in patients with AIDS have included the rectosigmoid, pancreas, and lung.

SPECIAL PROBLEMS

Pulmonary Lymphoid Hyperplasia/ Lymphoid Interstitial Pneumonitis

Patients with AIDS, particularly pediatric patients, may develop pulmonary infiltrates and pulmonary insufficiency caused by the complex of pulmonary lymphoid

hyperplasia/lymphoid interstitial pneumonitis (PLH/LIP).[153,154] In these cases, there are prominent nodular peribronchiolar and perivascular lymphoid aggregates with germinal centers, and mild to moderately severe lymphocytic infiltration of the surrounding alveolar septae. No viral inclusion cells are seen, and special

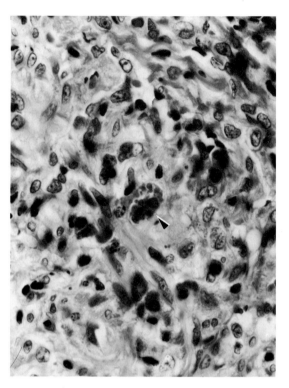

FIG. 10-24. Kaposi's sarcoma within the subcapsular sinus of a lymph node. Note spindle-shaped cells, intracytoplasmic hyaline globules (*arrow*), erythrocytes, and plasma cells. (PAS stain with diastase, ×860; see Color Plate 10-12). (Reichert CM, O'Leary TJ, Levens DL et al: Autopsy pathology in the acquired immune deficiency syndrome. Am J Pathol 112:357, 1983)

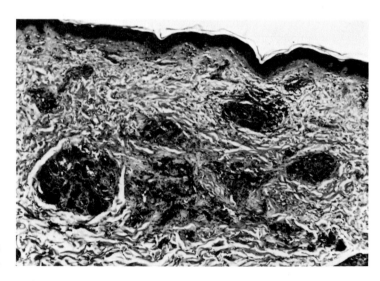

FIG. 10-25. Early angiomatous form of cutaneous Kaposi's sarcoma (H&E stain; see Color Plate 10-10).

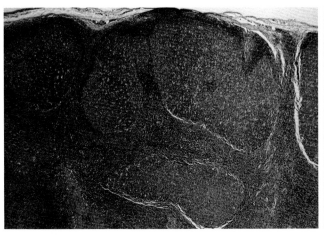

COLOR PLATE 10-1. Lymph node. Florid follicular hyperplasia with irregular prominent germinal centers in a patient with ARC (H&E stain).

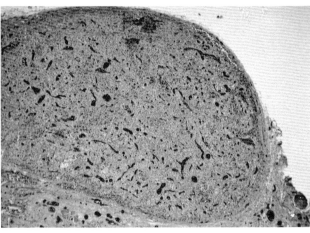

COLOR PLATE 10-2. Lymph node. Depletion (burn-out) of lymphocytes in a patient with AIDS (H&E stain).

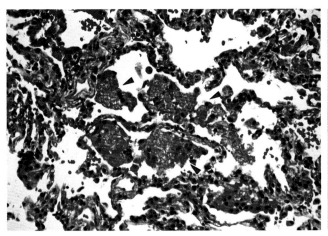

COLOR PLATE 10-3. Lung. Eosinophilic intra-alveolar exudates (*arrows*) of *Pneumocystis carinii* pneumonia in a patient with AIDS (H&E stain).

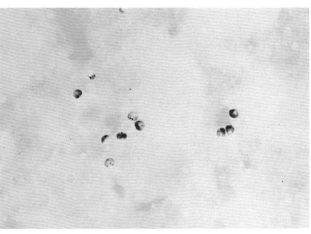

COLOR PLATE 10-4. Acid-fast cryptosporidia in a fecal concentrate (modified Ziehl–Neelsen stain, sucrose flotation technique).

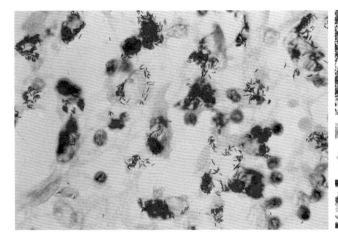

COLOR PLATE 10-5. Lymph node. Innumerable acid-fast bacilli of *Mycobacterium avium-intracellulare* (Fite stain, ×860).

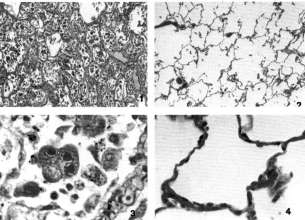

COLOR PLATE 10-6. Lung. (*1*) Cytomegaloviral pneumonitis with massive consolidation, resulting in the death of this patient with AIDS. (*2*) Normal lung control. (*3*) Cytomegaly of desquamated alveolar lining cells, containing intranuclear haloed as well as intracytoplasmic inclusions. (*4*) Normal pulmonary alveoli (H&E stain).

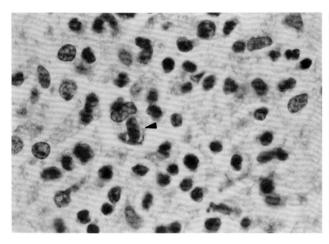

COLOR PLATE 10-7. Brain. Microglial nodule with a central cytomegaloviral inclusion cell (*arrow*) in a patient with AIDS (H&E stain).

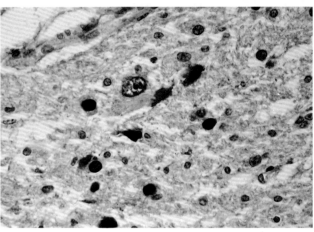

COLOR PLATE 10-8. Brain. Progressive multifocal leukoencephalopathy with plaque of demyelination showing gliosis, bizarre giant astrocytes, and oligodendroglia that are positive (*brown*) for the antigens of polyoma virus (Immunoperoxidase stain; courtesy of Drs. P. M. Howley and D. L. Levens).

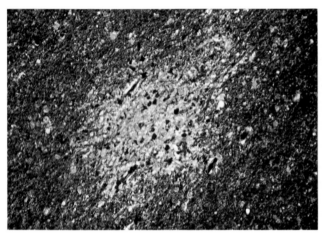

COLOR PLATE 10-9. Brain. Demyelination of unknown etiology in a patient with AIDS (Luxol fast-blue-PAS myelin stain).

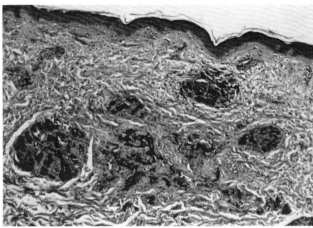

COLOR PLATE 10-10. Skin. Early angiomatous form of cutaneous Kaposi's sarcoma in a patient with AIDS (H&E stain).

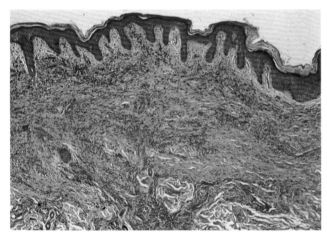

COLOR PLATE 10-11. Skin. Typical dermal proliferation of spindle cells in an AIDS patient with Kaposi's sarcoma (H&E stain).

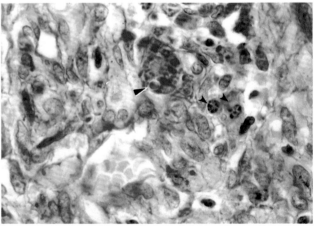

COLOR PLATE 10-12. Lymph node. Intracytoplasmic PAS-positive, diastase-resistant hyaline globules (*arrow*) and plasma cells (*smaller arrows*) within a lesion of Kaposi's sarcoma (PAS with diastase stain).

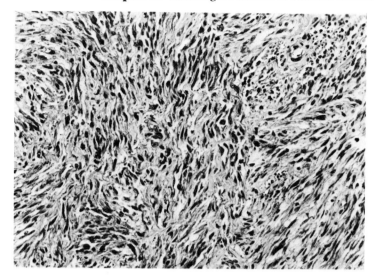

FIG. 10-26. Interlacing fascicles of spindle cells in the nodular phase of a Kaposi's sarcoma lesion (H&E stain).

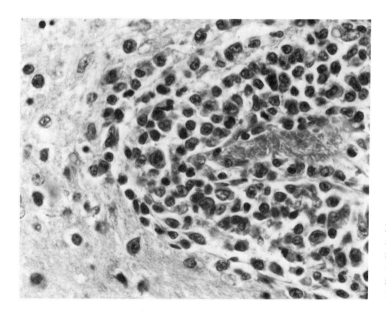

FIG. 10-27. Malignant lymphoma, undifferentiated small noncleaved (Burkitt's-like), within the brain of a patient with AIDS (H&E stain, ×520). (Reichert CM, O'Leary TJ, Levens DL et al: Autopsy pathology in the acquired immune deficiency syndrome. Am J Pathol 112:357, 1983)

stains including Grocott methenamine silver and acid-fast techniques reveal no microorganisms. Persistent generalized lymphadenopathy, PLH/LIP, and B-cell lymphomas may represent a continuum or spectrum of lymphoid lesions. Patients with AIDS are profoundly immunoincompetent, and the lymphoid lesions in PLH/LIP may represent a host response to yet another unrecognized opportunistic viral infection.

Oral Hairy Leukoplakia

Most cases of oral hairy leukoplakia (OHL) have been diagnosed in homosexual men who are seropositive for HIV. The lesion of OHL is a slightly raised, poorly demarcated, asymptomatic plaque measuring from a few millimeters to 2.0 × 3.5 cm. On gross inspection, the lesion has a corrugated or "hairy" surface. A review of 36 cases by Eversole and co-authors[155] found 86% of the lesions localized to the tongue with 72% involving the lateral border and 14% involving the ventral surface. Other sites of involvement include the buccal mucosa, floor of the mouth, palate, and dorsal tongue. Occasionally, the lesions are bilateral.

The diagnosis of OHL requires clinicopathologic correlation.[156] The histologic findings, while nonspecific, are nevertheless characteristic for OHL. There is acanthosis and marked hyperkeratosis with projections of keratin. In the prickle cell layer (stratum spinosum) there are koilocytotic changes with ballooned cells containing pyknotic nuclei and a perinuclear halo. These koilocytotic changes may involve only scattered cells or involve 3 to 5 layers of cells. In 88% of the biopsies of OHL in Eversole's series, there also were yeasts and pseudohyphae of *Candida* spp penetrating the parakeratin layer. Nevertheless, the plaques were firmly adherent to the mucosa, did not rub off, and did not resolve with antifungal therapy.

Using immunohistochemical techniques, Greenspan and others[157] reported that 73% of OHL-biopsied tissues showed evidence of papillomavirus within the nuclei of koilocytes and other prickle cells. Ultrastructurally, papilloma-like viral particles were seen in all 25 cases studied, and herpes-like virions were observed in 23 of the 25 cases. Using immunofluorescent antisera and DNA probes, the herpes-like virions were subsequently identified as EBV. In some specimens both papilloma-like and herpes-like particles were seen in the same cell. While both EBV and human papillomavirus

are found in OHL, the histologic features, specifically the koilocytes, are similar to those seen in condylomas involving other mucocutaneous sites caused by papillomavirus.

Testicular Atrophy

Postmortem examination of testis in patients with AIDS may reveal a moderate to striking degree of atrophy and spermatic maturation arrest (Fig. 10-29).[4] The basement membranes of the seminiferous tubules appear thickened, and fibrous scars may be present. The etiology of these histopathologic changes is unknown; these findings appear to be present independent of various known

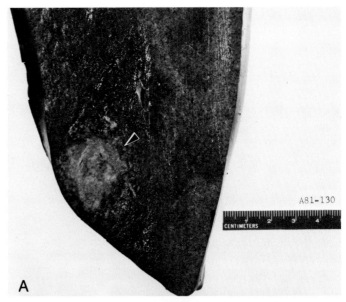

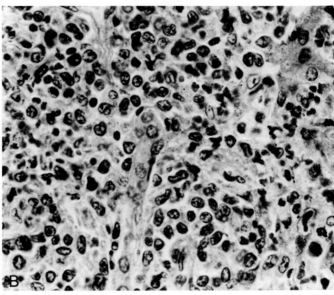

FIG. 10-28. (*A*) Primary lymphoma of the liver (*arrow*), first discovered at autopsy in a patient with AIDS. (*B*) Large-cell lymphomatous infiltrate in the liver (H&E stain). (Reichert CM, O'Leary TJ, Levens DL et al: Autopsy pathology in the acquired immune deficiency syndrome. Am J Pathol 112:357, 1983)

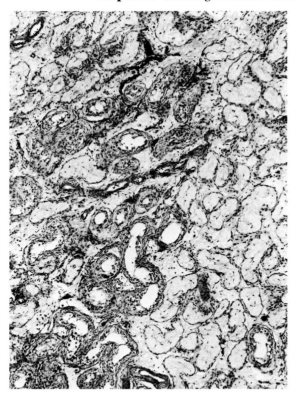

FIG. 10-29. Testis. Spermatic maturation arrest, atrophy, and focal fibrosis are seen to varying degrees in the autopsy testes of patients with AIDS (H&E stain). (Reichert CM, O'Leary TJ, Levens DL et al: Autopsy pathology in the acquired immune deficiency syndrome. Am J Pathol 112:357, 1983)

infectious and neoplastic manifestations of AIDS, and they occur in the absence of chemotherapy for KS or B-cell lymphomas.

Idiopathic Myocarditis

Cardiac complications in patients with AIDS include the aforementioned opportunistic infections and neoplasms. In addition, we have studied AIDS patients in whom clinical, echocardiographic, and morphologic findings of dilated cardiomyopathy were associated with cardiac insufficiency and death; postmortem examinations revealed focal myocarditis with diffuse myofibrillar loss and myocyte atrophy in the absence of identifiable microorganisms, viral inclusion cells, or tumors.[158]

Idiopathic Neurologic Lesions

Neurologic disease complicates the clinical course of over one-third of patients with AIDS. In addition to the aforementioned opportunistic infections and neoplasms involving the central nervous system, patients infected with HIV have a propensity for developing idiopathic subacute encephalitis,[159] aseptic meningitis,[160] vacuolar myelopathy,[161] and peripheral neuropathy.[162] Neuropathologic findings in cases of subacute encephalitis with dementia include microglial nodules predominantly in gray matter, with or without foci of demyelination in white matter; the microglial nodules may also contain multinucleated giant cells.

POSTSCRIPT

In the future, the pathology of AIDS will undoubtedly expand to include additional opportunistic infections, neoplasms, and unusual entities.

REFERENCES

Review Articles

1. Jaffe ES, Katz DA, Macher A et al: Pathology of AIDS. In AIDS: Modern Concepts and Therapeutic Challenges, p 143. Broder S (ed): New York, Marcel Dekker, 1987
2. Guarda LA, Luna MA, Smith JL et al: Acquired immune deficiency syndrome: Postmortem findings. Am J Clin Pathol 81:549, 1984
3. Hui AN, Koss MN, Meyer PR: Necropsy findings in acquired immunodeficiency syndrome. Hum Pathol 15:670, 1984
4. Reichert CM, O'Leary TJ, Levens DL et al: Autopsy pathology in the acquired immune deficiency syndrome. Am J Pathol 112:357, 1983

Handling of Tissues

5. Bauer S, Alpert LI, Carski TR et al: Guidelines for Protection of Laboratory Workers from Infectious Disease Transmitted by Blood and Tissue. National Committee for Clinical Laboratory Standards. NCCLS Document M29-P. Vol 7, No 9, 1987
6. Centers for Disease Control: Recommendations for prevention of HIV transmission in health care settings. Morbid Mortal Week Rep [Suppl] 2S:2S, 1987
7. Bradshaw A, Lines RW: The instability of sodium hypochlorite solutions. Lab Pract 36:4, 1987
8. Centers for Disease Control: Update: Human immunodeficiency virus infections in health care workers exposed to blood of infected patients. Morbid Mortal Week Rep 36:285, 1987
9. Gerberding JL (University of California—San Francisco Task Force on AIDS): Recommended infection-control policies for patients with human immunodeficiency virus infection. N Engl J Med 315:1562, 1986
10. Gerberding JL, Bryant LeBlanc CE, Nelson K et al: Risk of transmitting the human immunodeficiency virus, cytomegalovirus, and hepatitis B virus to health care workers exposed to patients with AIDS and AIDS-related conditions. J Infect Dis 156:1, 1987
11. Gerberding JL, Sande MA: Infection control policies and AIDS. N Engl J Med 316:1479, 1987

12. Henderson DK, Saah AJ, Zak BJ et al: Risk of nosocomial infection with human T-cell lymphotropic virus type III/lymphadenopathy-associated virus in a large cohort of intensively exposed health care workers. Ann Intern Med 104:644, 1986

13. MacArthur S, Schneiderman H: Infection control and the autopsy of persons with human immunodeficiency virus. Am J Infect Control 15:172, 1987

14. McCray E: Occupational risk of the acquired immunodeficiency syndrome among health care workers. N Engl J Med 314:1127, 1986

15. McEvoy M, Porter K, Mortimer P et al: Prospective study of clinical laboratory and ancillary staff with accidental exposures to blood or body fluids from patients infected with HIV. Br Med J 294:1595, 1987

16. Martin LS, McDougal JS, Loskoski SL: Disinfection and inactivation of the human T lymphotropic virus type III/lymphadenopathy-associated virus. J Infect Dis 152:400, 1985

17. Resnick L, Veren K, Salahuddin SZ et al: Stability and inactivation of HTLV-III/LAV under clinical and laboratory environments. JAMA 255:1887, 1986

18. Spire B, Barre–Sinoussi F, Montagnier L et al: Inactivation of a new retrovirus (lymphadenopathy-associated virus) by various agents (chemical disinfectants). Lancet 2:899, 1984

19. Spire B, Barre–Sinoussi F, Montagnier L et al: Inactivation of lymphadenopathy-associated virus by heat, gamma rays and ultraviolet light. Lancet 1:188, 1985

20. Tierno PM, Jr: Preventing acquisition of human immunodeficiency virus in the laboratory: Safe handling of AIDS specimens. Lab Med 17:696, 1986

21. Vlahov D, Polk BF: Transmission of human immunodeficiency virus within the health care setting. Occupat Med 2:429, 1987

22. Anonymous: Needlestick transmission of HTLV-III from a patient infected in Africa. Lancet 2:1376, 1984

23. Neisson–Verrant C, Mathez D, Leibowitch J et al: Needlestick HIV seroconversion in a nurse. Lancet 2:814, 1986

24. Oskenhendler E, Harzic M, Roux JM et al: HIV infection with seroconversion after a superficial needlestick injury to the finger. N Engl J Med 315:582, 1986

25. Stricof RL, Morse DL: HTLV-III/LAV seroconversion following deep intramuscular needlestick injury. N Engl J Med 314:1115, 1986

Morphologic Manifestations of Immunologic Impairment

26. Centers for Disease Control. Persistent generalized lymphadenopathy among homosexual males. Morbid Mortal Week Rep 31:249, 1982

27. Morris L, Distenfield A, Amorosi E et al: Autoimmune thrombocytopenic purpura in homosexual men. Ann Intern Med 96:714, 1982

28. McGinniss M, Macher A, Rook A et al: Red cell autoantibodies in patients with acquired immune deficiency syndrome. Transfusion 26:405, 1986

29. Ioachim HL, Lerner CW, Tapper ML: Lymphadenopathies in homosexual men. JAMA 250:1306, 1983

30. Ioachim HL, Lerner CW, Tapper ML: The lymphoid lesions associated with the acquired immunodeficiency syndrome. Am J Surg Pathol 7:543, 1983

31. Guarda LA, Butler JJ, Mansell P et al: Lymphadenopathy in homosexual men: Morbid anatomy with clinical and immunologic correlations. Am J Clin Pathol 79:559, 1983

32. Domingo J, Chin NW: Lymphadenopathy in a heterogeneous population at risk for the acquired immunodeficiency syndrome (AIDS): A morphologic study. Am J Clin Pathol 80:649, 1983

33. Macher A, De Vinatea M, Howell RS et al: AIDS case for diagnosis. Milit Med 151:M65, 1986

34. De Vinatea M, Macher A, Sbaschnig RJ et al: AIDS case for diagnosis. Milit Med 152:M57, 1987

35. Restrepo C, Macher A, Radany E: Disseminated extraintestinal isosporiasis in a patient with acquired immune deficiency syndrome. Am J Clin Pathol 87:536, 1987

36. Steigman CK, Pastore L, Park CH et al: AIDS case for diagnosis. Milit Med 152:M1, 1987

37. Modlin RL, Meyer PR, Hofman FM et al: T lymphocyte subsets in lymph nodes from homosexual men. JAMA 250:1302, 1983

38. Mangkornkanok–Mark M, Mark AS, Dong J: Immunoperoxidase evaluation of lymph nodes from acquired immune deficiency patients. Clin Exp Immunol 55:581, 1984

39. Said JW, Shintaku IP, Teitelbaum A et al: Distribution of T-cell phenotypic subsets and surface immunoglobulin-bearing lymphocytes in lymph nodes from male homosexuals with persistent generalized adenopathy. Hum Pathol 15:785, 1984

40. Elie R, Laroche CA, Arnoux E et al: Thymic dysplasia in acquired immunodeficiency syndrome. N Engl J Med 301:831, 1983

41. Spiers ASD, Robbins CL: Cytomegalovirus infection simulating lymphoma in a homosexual man. Lancet 1:1248, 1982

42. Abrams DI, Chinn EK, Lewis BJ et al: Hematologic manifestations in homosexual men with Kaposi's sarcoma. Am J Clin Pathol 81:13, 1984

43. Berner YN, Berrebi A, Green L et al: Erythroblastopenia in acquired immunodeficiency syndrome (AIDS). Acta Haematol 70:273, 1983

44. Pasternak J, Bolivar R: Bone marrow examination and culture in the diagnosis of acquired immunodeficiency syndrome (AIDS). Arch Intern Med 143:1495, 1983

45. Mead JH, Mason TE: Lymphoma versus AIDS. Am J Clin Pathol 80:546, 1983

Ultrastructural Studies

46. Sidhu GS, Stahl RE, El-Sadr W et al: Ultrastructural markers of AIDS. Lancet 1:990, 1983

47. Orenstein JM: Ultrastructural markers in AIDS. Lancet 2:284, 1983

48. Ewing EP, Spira TJ, Chandler FW et al: Ultrastructural markers in AIDS. Lancet 2:285, 1983

49. Shamoto M, Marakami S, Zenke T: Adult T-cell leukemia in Japan: An ultrastructural study. Cancer 47:1804, 1981

50. Jackson D, Tabor E, Gerety RJ: Acute non-A, non-B hepatitis: Specific ultrastructural alterations in endoplasmic reticulum of infected hepatocytes. Lancet 1:1249, 1979

51. Shimizu YK, Feinstone SM, Purcell RH et al: Non-A, non-B hepatitis: Ultrastructural evidence for two agents in experimentally infected chimpanzees. Science 205:197, 1979

52. Burrage TG, Andiman WA, Katz BZ et al: Virus-like rods

in a lymphoid line from an infant with AIDS. N Engl J Med 310:1460, 1984

53. Gyorkey F, Sinkovics JG, Gyorkey P: Tubuloreticular structures in Kaposi's sarcoma. Lancet 2:984, 1982

54. Kostianovsky M, Kang YH, Grimley PM: Disseminated tubuloreticular inclusions in acquired immunodeficiency syndrome (AIDS). Ultrastruct Pathol 4:331, 1983

55. Grimley PM, Kang Y, Frederick W et al: Interferon-related leukocyte inclusions in acquired immune deficiency syndrome: Localization in T cells. Am J Clin Pathol 81:147, 1984

56. Rutsaert J, Melot C, Ectors M et al: Infectious pulmonary and neurologic complications of Kaposi's syndrome: Anatomoclinical correlations with ultrastructural study. Ann Anat Pathol (Paris) 25:125, 1980

57. Grimley PM, Kang YH, Masur H et al: Tubuloreticular inclusions in patients with AIDS: Interferon related effect in circulating T cells and monocytes. In Friedman–Kien AE, Laubenstein LJ (eds): AIDS: The Epidemic of Kaposi's Sarcoma and Opportunistic Infections, p 181. New York, Masson Publishing, 1984

58. Schaff Z, Barry DW, Grimley PM: Cytochemistry of tubuloreticular structures in lymphocytes from patients with systemic lupus erythematosus and in cultured human lymphoid cells. Lab Invest 29:577, 1987

59. Grimley PM, Schaff Z: Significance of tubuloreticular inclusions in the pathobiology of human disease. In Ioachim HL (ed): Pathobiology Annual, p 221. New York, Appleton-Century-Crofts, 1976

60. Ewing EP, Spira TJ, Chandler FW et al: Unusual cytoplasmic body in lymphoid cells of homosexual men with unexplained lymphadenopathy. N Engl J Med 308:819, 1983

Infections

61. Fauci AS, Macher AM, Longo DL et al: Acquired immune deficiency syndrome. Ann Intern Med 100:92, 1984

62. Lobenthal SW, Hajdu SI, Urmacher C: Cytologic findings in homosexual males with acquired immunodeficiency syndrome. Acta Cytol 27:597, 1983

63. Masur H, Michelis MA, Greene JB et al: An outbreak of community-acquired Pneumocystis carinii pneumonia: Initial manifestation of cellular immune dysfunction. N Engl J Med 305:1431, 1981

64. Murray JF, Felton CP, Garay SM et al: Pulmonary complications of the acquired immunodeficiency syndrome. N Engl J Med 310:1682, 1984

65. Macher A, Shelhamer J, MacLowry J et al: *Pneumocystis carinii* identified by Gram stain of lung imprints. Ann Intern Med 99:484, 1983

66. Domingo J, Waksal HW: Wright's stain in rapid diagnosis of *Pneumocystis carinii.* Am J Clin Pathol 81:511, 1984

67. Wong B, Gold JW, Brown AE et al: Central nervous system toxoplasmosis in homosexual men and parenteral drug abusers. Ann Intern Med 100:36, 1984

68. Handler M, Ho V, Whelan M et al: Intracerebral toxoplasmosis in patients with acquired immune deficiency syndrome. J Neurosurg 59:994, 1983

69. Pitchenik AE, Finch MA, Walls KW: Evaluation of cerebral mass lesions in acquired immune deficiency syndrome. N Engl J Med 308:1099, 1983

70. Chan JC, Moskowitz LB, Olivella J et al: Toxoplasma encephalitis in recent Haitian entrants. South Med J 76:1211, 1983

71. Post JD, Chan JC, Hensley GT et al: Toxoplasma encephalitis in Haitian adults with acquired immunodeficiency syndrome: A clinical-pathologic CT correlation. Am J Roentgenol 140:861, 1983

72. Levy RM, Pons VG, Rosenblum ML: Intracerebral mass lesions in the acquired immunodeficiency syndrome. N Engl J Med 309:1454, 1983

73. Snider WD, Simpson DM, Nielson S et al: Neurologic complications of acquired immune deficiency syndrome: Analysis of 50 patients. Ann Neurol 14:403, 1983

74. Anderson SE, Remington JS: The diagnosis of toxoplasmosis. South Med J 68:1433, 1975

75. Pitchenik AE, Fischl MA, Dickinson GM et al: Opportunistic infections and Kaposi's sarcoma among Haitians: Evidence of a new acquired immunodeficiency state. Ann Intern Med 98:277, 1983

76. Hauser WE, Luft BJ, Conley FK et al: Central nervous system toxoplasmosis in homosexual and heterosexual adults. N Engl J Med 307:498, 1982

77. Horowitz SL, Bentson JR, Benson DF et al: CNS toxoplasmosis in acquired immune deficiency syndrome. Arch Neurol 40:649, 1983

78. Alonzo R, Heiman–Patterson T, Mancall EL: Cerebral toxoplasmosis in acquired immune deficiency syndrome. Arch Neurol 41:321, 1984

79. Moskowitz LB, Hensley GT, Chan JC et al: The neuropathology of acquired immune deficiency syndrome. Arch Pathol Lab Med 108:867, 1984

80. Meisel JL, Perera DR, Meligro C et al: Overwhelming watery diarrhea, associated with a cryptosporidium in an immunosuppressed patient. Gastroenterology 70:1156, 1976

81. Centers for Disease Control: Cryptosporidiosis: Assessment of chemotherapy of males with acquired immunodeficiency syndrome (AIDS). Morbid Mortal Week Rep 31:589, 1982

82. Current WL, Reese NC, Erust JV et al: Human cryptosporidiosis in immunocompetent and immunodeficient persons. N Engl J Med 308:1252, 1983

83. Henriksen SA, Pohlenz JFL: Staining of cryptosporidia by a modified Ziehl–Neelsen technique. Acta Vet Scand 22:594, 1981

84. Current WL: Human cryptosporidiosis. N Engl J Med 309:1326, 1983

85. Payne P, Lancaster LA, Heinzman M et al: Identification of *Cryptosporidium* in patients with the acquired immune deficiency syndrome. N Engl J Med 309:613, 1983

86. Vetterling JM, Jervis HR, Merrill TG et al: *Cryptosporidium wrairi* sp. from the guinea pig *Cavia porcellus,* with an emendation of the genus. J Protozool 18:243, 1971

87. Forgacs P, Tarshis A, Ma P et al: Intestinal and bronchial cryptosporidiosis in an immunodeficient homosexual man. Ann Intern Med 99:793, 1984

88. Brady EM, Margolis ML, Korzeniowski OM: Pulmonary cryptosporidiosis in acquired immune deficiency syndrome. JAMA 252:89, 1984

89. Ma P, Villanueva TG, Kaufman D et al: Respiratory cryptosporidiosis in the acquired immune deficiency syndrome. JAMA 252:1298, 1984

90. Lefkowitch JH, Krumholz S, Feng–Chen K et al: Cryptosporidiosis of the human small intestine: A light and electron microscopic study. Hum Pathol 15:746, 1984

91. Chiampi NP, Sandberg RD, Klompus JP et al: Cryptosporidial enteritis and pneumocystic pneumonia in a homosexual man. Hum Pathol 14:734, 1983

92. Kahn D, Garfinkle J, Rabin L et al: AIDS case for diagnosis. Milit Med 152:M81, 1987

93. Pitlick SD, Fainstein V, Rios A et al: Cryptosporidial cholecystitis. N Engl J Med 308:967, 1983

94. Blumbert RS, Kelsey P, Perrone T et al: Cytomegalovirus and *Cryptosporidium* associated acalculous gangrenous cholecystitis. Am J Med 76:1118, 1984

95. Smith P, Macher A, Bookman M et al: *Salmonella typhimurium* enteritis and bacteremia in the acquired immune deficiency syndrome. An Intern Med 102:207, 1985

96. Culbertson CG: Amebic meningoencephalitides. In Binford CH, Connor DH (eds): Pathology of Tropical and Extraordinary Diseases, p 317. Washington, DC, Armed Forces Institute of Pathology, 1976

97. Klein RS, Harris CA, Small CB et al: Oral candidiasis in high-risk patients as the initial manifestation of the acquired immune deficiency syndrome. N Engl J Med 311:354, 1984

98. Kovacs J, Kovacs A, Polis M et al: Cryptococcosis in patients with the acquired immune deficiency syndrome. Ann Intern Med 103:533, 1985

99. Macher A, Rodrigues M, Kaplan W et al: Disseminated bilateral chorioretinitis due to *Histoplasma capsulatum* in a patient with the acquired immunodeficiency syndrome. Ophthalmology 92:1159, 1985

100. Pasternak J, Bolivar R: Histoplasmosis in acquired immunodeficiency syndrome (AIDS): Diagnosis by bone marrow examination. Arch Intern Med 143:2024, 1983

101. Kovacs A, Kovacs JA, Overturf GD: Disseminated coccidioidomycosis in a patient with acquired immune deficiency syndrome. West J Med 140:447, 1984

102. Abrams DI: Disseminated coccidioidomycosis in AIDS. N Engl J Med 310:986, 1984

103. Macher A, De Vinatea M, Koch Y et al: AIDS case for diagnosis. Milit Med 151:M57, 1986

104. Lipstein–Kresch E, Isenberg H, Singer C et al: Disseminated *Sporothrix schenckii* infection with arthritis in a patient with acquired immunodeficiency syndrome. J Rheumatol 12:805, 1985

105. Zalowski P, Fligiel S, Berlin GW et al: Disseminated *Mycobacterium avium-intracellulare* infection in homosexual men dying of acquired immunodeficiency syndrome. JAMA 248:2980, 1982

106. Sohn CC, Schroff RW, Kliewer KE et al: Disseminated *Mycobacterium avium-intracellulare* infection in homosexual men with acquired cell-mediated immunodeficiency: a histologic and immunologic study of two cases. Am J Clin Pathol 79:247, 1983

107. Green JB, Sidhu GS, Lewin S et al: *Mycobacterium avium-intracellulare:* A cause of disseminated life-threatening infection in homosexuals and drug abusers. Ann Intern Med 97:539, 1982

108. Pitchenik A, Cole C, Russell B et al: Tuberculosis, atypical mycobacteriosis, and the acquired immunodeficiency syndrome among Haitian and non-Haitian patients in south Florida. Ann Intern Med 101:641, 1984

109. Lasala G, Rivera I, Climent C et al: AIDS case for diagnosis. Milit Med 151:M65, 1987

110. Macher A, De Vinatea M, Daly M et al: AIDS case for diagnosis. Milit Med 151:M73, 1986

111. Nelson A, Macher A, Neafie R et al: AIDS case for diagnosis. Milit Med 151:M81, 1986

112. Koziol K: *Listeria monocytogenes* meningitis in AIDS. Can Med Assoc J 135:43, 1986

113. Murray JF, Felton CP, Garay SM et al: Pulmonary complications of the acquired immunodeficiency syndrome. N Engl J Med 310:1682, 1984

114. Garbowit DL: Letter: *Hemophilus influenzae* bacteremia in a patient with immunodeficiency caused by HTLV-III. N Engl J Med 314:56, 1986

115. Knapp AB, Horst DA, Eliopoulos G et al: Widespread cytomegalovirus gastroenterocolitis in a patient with acquired immunodeficiency syndrome. Gastroenterology 85:1399, 1983

116. Palestine AG, Rodrigues MM, Macher AM et al: Ophthalmic considerations in acquired immune deficiency syndrome. Ophthalmology 91:1092, 1984

117. Hawley DA, Schaefer JF, Schulz DM et al: Cytomegalovirus encephalitis in acquired immunodeficiency syndrome. Am J Clin Pathol 80:874, 1983

118. Quinnan GV, Masur H, Rook AH et al: Herpes virus infections in the acquired immunodeficiency syndrome. JAMA 252:72, 1984

119. Siegal FP, Lopez C, Hammer GS et al: Severe acquired immunodeficiency in male homosexuals, manifested by chronic perianal ulcerative herpes simplex lesions. N Engl J Med 305:1439, 1981

120. Bedri J, Weinstein W, De Gregorio P et al: Progressive multifocal leukoencephalopathy in acquired immunodeficiency syndrome. N Engl J Med 309:492, 1983

121. Macher A, Parisi J, Aksamit A et al: AIDS case for diagnosis. Milit Med 151:M25, 1986

122. Rustgi V, Hoofnagle J, Masur H et al: Serological markers and clinical evidence of chronic hepatitis B virus infection in patients with AIDS. Gastroenterology 86:1226, 1984

123. Baird J, De Vinatea M, Macher A et al: AIDS case for diagnosis. Milit Med 152:M17, 1987

124. Glover R, Young L, Goltz R: Norwegian scabies in acquired immunodeficiency syndrome: Report of a case resulting in death from associated sepsis. J Am Acad Dermatol 16:396, 1987

Kaposi's Sarcoma

125. Braun M: Classics in Oncology: Moriz Kaposi, M.D.; Idiopathic multiple pigmented sarcoma of the skin. Cancer 32:340, 1982

126. Cox FH, Helwig EB: Kaposi's sarcoma. Cancer 12:289, 1959

127. Penn I: Kaposi's sarcoma in organ transplant recipients: Report of 20 cases. Transplant 27:8, 1979

128. Taylor JF, Templeton AC, Vogel CL et al: Kaposi's sarcoma in Uganda: A clinicopathological study. Int J Cancer 8:122, 1971

129. Patow C, Steis R, Longo D et al: Kaposi's sarcoma of the head and neck in the acquired immune deficiency syndrome. Otolaryngol Head Neck Surg 92:255, 1984

130. Friedman–Kien AE, Laubenstein LJ, Rubenstein P et al: Disseminated Kaposi's sarcoma in homosexual men. Ann Intern Med 96:693, 1982

131. Boyko WJ, Sharp F, Jeffries E et al: Small foci of Kaposi's sarcoma in lymph nodes may be missed without serial sections. Lancet 1:158, 1984

132. Kornfeld HJ, Axelrod JL: Pulmonary presentations of Ka-

posi's sarcoma in a homosexual patient. Am Rev Resp Dis 127:248, 1983

133. Silver MA, Macher AM, Reichert CM et al: Cardiac involvement by Kaposi's sarcoma in acquired immunodeficiency syndrome (AIDS). Am J Cardiol 53:983, 1984

134. Macher AM, Palestine A, Masur H et al: Multicentric Kaposi's sarcoma of the conjunctiva in a male homosexual with the acquired immunodeficiency syndrome. Ophthalmology 90:879, 1983

135. Krigel RL, Laubenstein LJ, Muggia FM: Kaposi's sarcoma: A new staging classification. Cancer Treat Rep 67:531, 1983

136. Gottlieb MS, Groopman JE, Weinstein WM et al: The acquired immunodeficiency syndrome. An Intern Med 99:208, 1983

137. Kelly WM, Brant-Zawadzki M: Acquired immunodeficiency syndrome: Neuroradiologic findings. Radiology 149:485, 1983

138. Gottlieb GJ, Ackerman AB: Kaposi's sarcoma: An extensively disseminated form in young homosexual men. Human Pathol 13:882, 1982

139. Murray JF, Lothe F: The histopathology of Kaposi's sarcoma. Acta Un Int Cancer 18:413, 1962

140. Safai B, Parris A, Urmacher C: Histopathology of Kaposi's sarcoma and other neoplasms. In Ebbesen P, Biggar RJ, Melbye M (eds): AIDS: A Basic Guide for Clinicians, p 113. Copenhagen, Munksgaard, 1984

Lymphomas and Other Malignancies

141. Centers for Disease Control: Diffuse, undifferentiated non-Hodgkin's lymphoma among homosexual males: United States. Morbid Mortal Week Rep 31:277, 1982

142. Ziegler JL, Beckstead JA, Volberding PA et al: Non-Hodgkin's lymphoma in 90 homosexual men. N Engl J Med 311:565, 1984

143. Andiman W, Gradoville L, Heston L et al: Use of cloned probes to detect Epstein–Barr viral DNA in tissues of patients with neoplastic and lymphoproliferative disease. J Infect Dis 148:967, 1983

144. Chaganti RS, Jhanovau SC, Koziner B et al: Specific translocations characterize Burkitt's-like lymphoma of homosexual men with the acquired immune deficiency syndrome. Blood 61:1265, 1983

145. Whang–Peng J, Lec EC, Sieverts H et al: Burkitt's lymphoma in AIDS: Cytogenetic study. Blood 63:818, 1984

146. Snider WD, Simpson DM, Aroynk KE et al: Primary lymphoma of the central nervous system associated with acquired immune deficiency syndrome. N Engl J Med 308:45, 1983

147. Doll DC, List AF: Burkitt's lymphoma in a homosexual. Lancet 1:1026, 1982

148. Figlin RA, Morisuchi JD, Coffey RA et al: Kaposi's sarcoma and immunoblastic sarcoma in the acquired immune deficiency syndrome. JAMA 251:342, 1984

149. Cooper HS, Patchefsy AJ, Marks G: Cloacogenic carcinoma of the anorectum in homosexual men: An observation of four cases. Dis Colon Rectum 22:557, 1979

150. Read EJ, Orenstein JM, Chorba TL et al: *Listeria monocytogenes* sepsis and small cell carcinoma of the rectum: An unusual presentation of the acquired immunodeficiency syndrome. Am J Clin Pathol 83:385, 1985

151. Nusbaum NJ: Letter: Metastatic small cell carcinoma of the lung in a patient with AIDS. N Engl J Med 312:1706, 1985

152. Moser RJ, Tenholder MF, Ridenour R: Letter: Oat cell carcinoma in transfusion-associated acquired immunodeficiency syndrome. Ann Intern Med 103:478, 1985

Special Problems

153. Joshi V, Oleske J: Pulmonary lesions in children with the acquired immunodeficiency syndrome: A reappraisal based on data in additional cases and follow-up study of previously reported cases. Human Pathol 17:641, 1986

154. Anderson DW, De Vinatea M, Macher A et al: AIDS case for diagnosis. Milit Med 152:M25, 1987

155. Eversole L, Jacobsen P, Stone C et al: Oral condyloma planus (hairy leukoplakia) among homosexual men: A clinicopathologic study of thirty-six cases. Oral Surg 61:249, 1986

156. Lewis D, Petersen–Carter W, Anderson DW et al: AIDS case for diagnosis. Milit Med 152:M49, 1987

157. Greenspan D, Greenspan J, Conant M et al: Oral hairy leukoplakia in male homosexuals: Evidence of association with both papillomavirus and a herpes group virus. Lancet 2:831, 1984

158. Cohen I, Anderson D, Virmani R, et al: Congestive cardiomyopathy in association with the acquired immunodeficiency syndrome. N Engl J Med 315:628, 1986

159. Nielsen SL, Petito CK, Urmacher CD et al: Subacute encephalitis in acquired immune deficiency syndrome: A postmortem study. Am J Clin Pathol 82:678, 1984

160. Ho DD, Rota TR, Schooley RT et al: Isolation of HTLV-III from cerebrospinal fluid and neural tissues of patients with neurologic syndromes related to the acquired immunodeficiency syndrome. N Engl J Med 313:1493, 1985

161. Petito CK, Navia BA, Cho E–S, et al: Vacuolar myelopathy resembling subacute combined degeneration in patients with the acquired immunodeficiency syndrome. N Engl J Med 312:874, 1985

162. Lipkin I, Parry G, Kiprov D et al: Inflammatory neuropathy in homosexual men with lymphadenopathy. Neurology 35:1479, 1985

Central and Peripheral Nervous System Complications of HIV Infection and AIDS

Bruce Brew
Marc Rosenblum
Richard W. Price

11

The neurologic complications of HIV infection, and particularly its late phase, AIDS, are both common and varied, and contribute importantly to patient morbidity and mortality. Both the central nervous system (CNS) and peripheral nervous system (PNS) are affected by a spectrum of disorders, some of which can occur as early as the period of acute HIV infection, although most occur as infection progresses to its terminal stages (Table 11-1). The etiologies and pathogenetic processes underlying these neurologic disorders are diverse and, as with systemic AIDS, include both opportunistic infections and neoplasms. Additionally, they include the consequences of direct nervous system infection by HIV, and, at least in the case of the PNS, likely autoimmune disorders as well. Because specific therapies are effective in reversing many of these conditions, vigorous workup and precise neurologic diagnosis are critical to patient management.

This chapter provides an overview of the neurologic complications of HIV infection and AIDS. It is subdivided into sections dealing in turn with

Disorders known or suspected to be due to direct infection of the CNS by HIV, emphasizing the AIDS dementia complex
CNS opportunistic infections
CNS opportunistic neoplasms
Other CNS disorders
PNS and skeletal muscle disorders

DIRECT HIV INFECTION OF THE CNS: KNOWN AND PRESUMED CLINICAL MANIFESTATIONS

Although it is now clear that HIV can directly infect the CNS, understanding is still limited regarding the nature of this infection, including its frequency, timing, patho-biology, and clinical manifestations. Accumulating clinical and laboratory observations are beginning to clarify these issues and have allowed at least a partial definition of what may be considered overlapping phases or clinical sequelae, which include (1) asymptomatic infection, (2) CNS disorders occurring in the context of acute HIV infection, (3) aseptic meningitis, and (4) the AIDS dementia complex.

Asymptomatic HIV Infection of the CNS

Evidence is now accumulating that early asymptomatic HIV infection of the CNS, or at least of the leptomeninges, is common and may, in fact, be the rule. This early infection has been demonstrated in asymptomatic seropositive patients by cerebrospinal fluid (CSF) evaluations showing abnormalities of "routine" studies including cell count, protein, and immunoglobulin; local, "intra–blood-brain barrier" synthesis of anti-HIV antibody; and isolation of virus.[1-11] Although data are limited, it may be that even asymptomatic patients experience an acute phase of CNS HIV infection with detectable virus and CSF pleocytosis, followed by reduced or absent detectable virus, return to minimal or no cells, and the residual presence of locally produced antiviral antibodies in the CSF. These observations not only have biologic implications vis-à-vis the extent of dissemination of HIV in the host, but also have practical application with respect to the use of the CSF in neurologic diagnosis. Early or persistent asymptomatic HIV infection may result in later "incidental" abnormalities in protein, immunoglobulin, oligoclonal bands, or even HIV recovery. Such abnormalities must be taken into account when interpreting CSF results obtained for other diagnostic purposes.

Table 11-1
Neurological Complications in HIV-Infected Patients

Brain
Predominantly Nonfocal
  AIDS dementia complex
  Metabolic encephalopathies
  CMV encephalitis
  Herpes encephalitis
  Acute HIV-related encephalitis
Predominantly Focal
  Cerebral toxoplasmosis
  Primary CNS lymphoma
  Progressive multifocal leukoencephalopathy (PML)
  Tuberculous brain abscess/tuberculoma cryptococoma
  VZV encephalitis
  Vascular disorders
Spinal Cord
  Vacuolar myelopathy
  VZV myelitis (herpes zoster)
  Spinal epidural or intradural lymphoma
Meninges
  Aseptic meningitis (HIV)
  Cryptococcal meningitis
  Lymphomatous meningitis (metastatic)
  Tuberculous meningitis (*M. Tuberculosis*)
Peripheral Nerve and Root
  Chronic sensory-motor polyneuropathy
  Acute and chronic demyelinating neuropathies
  Mononeuropathy associated with aseptic meningitis
  Mononeuropathy secondary to lymphomatous meningitis
  Mononeuritis multiplex
  Autonomic neuropathy
  Herpes zoster
  CMV polyradiculopathy
Muscle
  Polymyositis and other myopathies

"Early" CNS Manifestations: Acute and Subacute Syndromes

A variety of CNS disorders have now been described early in the course of HIV infection, although these are not yet well characterized, having been described only as individual case reports.[12-16] These have occurred in association with seroconversion, or, less commonly, somewhat later during the asymptomatic or latent phase of systemic disease. Neurologic involvement has occurred within days to several weeks of the seroconversion-related illness that resembles mononucleosis, and may take the form of an encephalitis, meningitis, ataxia, or myelopathy, either alone or together with PNS abnormalities including brachial plexopathy or neuropathy. The course of these disorders is monophasic and most patients have recovered within a number of weeks. The CSF usually shows a minor lymphocyte-predominant pleocytosis with a modest rise in protein. Computed tomographic (CT) brain scan has been normal, but the electroencephalogram may be focally or diffusely slow.

Although these early syndromes are apparently uncommon, it is possible that their incidence is underappreciated. Clinically, they are indistinguishable from other acute viral or postinfectious encephalitides, most of which never achieve specific diagnosis. There may be no background systemic illness to engender suspicion of HIV infection, and even when present the acute systemic manifestations of HIV may be disregarded when neurologic disease is prominent. If the patient is not a high risk-group member or if serologic testing is not done, there may be no clue as to the etiologic diagnosis. Moreover, in those serotested in the acute phase, HIV antibodies may not be detected. Immunologic assessment will likewise also usually be unrewarding since T-lymphocyte subsets are often normal or include only transient elevation of the CD8$^+$ subset, but usually without depression of the CD4$^+$ subset. Consequently, acute and convalescent (extended to 6–12 weeks or longer) serologic data in these encephalitides are needed, and in some patients virus isolation or antigen detection may be required for diagnosis.

Aseptic Meningitis

Aseptic meningitis may occur acutely, accompanying the seroconversion-related illness described above, but is more common later in the course of HIV infection either in otherwise asymptomatic seropositives or in those with pre-AIDS symptomatology.[17-19] Hollander has segregated aseptic meningitis into two clinical types, an acute and a chronic form.[19] Both are accompanied by meningeal symptoms including headache, but meningeal signs are confined to the acute group. Cranial nerve palsies may also complicate the course, most often affecting cranial nerves V, VII, or VIII with Bell's palsy sometimes recurring. The CSF shows a mononuclear pleocytosis usually with normal glucose and slightly elevated protein. The syndrome itself is benign, although affected patients may have an overall poor prognosis because of other HIV complications. Present data suggest that these patients are neither more nor less likely to develop the AIDS dementia complex. The meningitis is presumed to relate to direct HIV infection as the virus can be readily isolated from the CSF.

AIDS Dementia Complex

In the later stages of HIV infection patients may develop a particular neurologic disorder, the AIDS dementia complex (ADC), characterized by cognitive, motor, and behavioral dysfunction.[20] This is, in fact, the most common CNS complication of HIV infection, and likely eventually afflicts the majority of AIDS patients.[20,21] Characteristically this disorder manifests after patients develop major opportunistic infections or neoplasms that define systemic AIDS. However, clearly patients can present with this syndrome prior to these major systemic complications, when they do not yet fulfill previous formal criteria for the diagnosis of AIDS on the basis of their systemic disease.[22] Recognition of this early presentation has resulted in the addition of ADC to the diagnostic criteria for AIDS.[23] It should be emphasized that although a substantial number of patients exhibit ADC before systemic AIDS, almost always these patients have already evidenced minor complications of HIV infection such as lymphadenopathy, malaise, weight loss, or oral candidiasis. It is only a very small number of patients who develop dementia when they are otherwise medically well and systemically asymptomatic, and even these patients are characteristically immunosuppressed by laboratory criteria.

Clinical Features

ADC has been recognized almost since the very beginning of the AIDS epidemic, and a variety of terms have been used to describe it including *subacute encephalitis, subacute encephalopathy,* and *AIDS encephalopathy.*[24-26] Because of the prominence of cognitive dysfunction in the disorder and the frequency of motor and behavioral signs that in some cases predominate, we now prefer the term *AIDS dementia complex.*[20,27,28] Patients with this disorder present with a variable, yet characteristic, constellation of clinical abnormalities. Perhaps the salient aspect of the disorder is slowing and loss of precision in both mentation and motor control.

The clinical features of ADC are briefly summarized in Table 11-2 and have been described in more detail elsewhere.[20,28] Patients' earliest symptoms usually consist of difficulties with concentration and memory. They begin to lose track of their train of thought or conversations, and many complain of "slowness" in thinking. Complex tasks become more difficult and take longer to complete, while memory impairment or difficulty in concentration lead to missed appointments and the need to keep lists. If patients require a high level of concentration or organization for their occupation or activities at home, ADC may make its effects known quite early. In other instances, a friend or family member may be the first to notice subtle cognitive and personality changes as the patient begins to withdraw socially and appears apathetic and unusually quiet.

Those with motor dysfunction early in the course of the disease most often complain of poor balance or incoordination. They may drop things more frequently, or become slower and less precise with hand activities, such as eating or writing. Similarly, gait incoordination may result in more frequent tripping or falling, or a perceived need to exercise new care in walking. Psychological depression is surprisingly infrequent in these patients, but may be difficult to differentiate clinically. In a minority a more agitated organic psychosis may be the presenting or predominant aspect of the illness. Such

Table 11-2
Clinical Manifestations of ADC

Early Manifestations
Symptoms
  Cognition
    Impaired concentration
    Memory loss
    Mental slowing
  Motor
    Unsteady gait
    Leg weakness
    Loss of coordination, impaired handwriting
    Tremor
  Behavior
    Apathy, withdrawal, "depression"
    Agitation, confusion, hallucinations
Signs
  Mental Status
    Psychomotor slowing
    Impaired serial 7s or reversals
    Organic psychosis
  Neurologic Examination
    Release reflexes (snout, glabellar, grasp)
    Impaired rapid movements (limbs, eyes)
    Gait ataxia (impaired tandem gait, rapid turns)
    Hyperreflexia
    Tremor (postural)
    Leg weakness
Late Manifestations
  Mental Status
    Global dementia
    Psychomotor slowing: verbal responses delayed, near or absolute mutism, vacant stare
    Unawareness of illness, disinhibition
    Confusion, disorientation
    Organic psychosis
  Neurologic Signs
    Weakness (legs ⩾ arms)
    Ataxia
    Pyramidal tract signs: spasticity, hyperreflexia, extensor plantar responses
    Urinary and fecal incontinence
    Myoclonus

patients are irritable and hyperactive and may become overtly manic.

Early in the evolution of the illness, formal bedside mental status testing may be remarkably normal, although responses are characteristically slow even when their content is accurate. As the disease progresses, patients perform poorly on tasks requiring concentration and attention such as word and digit reversals and serial 7s. With increasing severity, a larger array of mental status tests becomes abnormal. Slowing remains prominent, and afflicted individuals often appear apathetic, have poor insight, and are indifferent to their illness.

Motor abnormalities can usually be detected early in the course of the disease. These include pathologic reflexes with development of snout, glabellar and, less commonly, grasp responses, along with generalized hyperreflexia, including the jaw jerk. Slowing of rapid successive and alternating movements of the fingers, wrists, or feet, as well as impaired ocular motility with interruption of smooth pursuits and slowing or inaccuracy of saccades are common early findings. As the disease evolves, ataxia, which at first affects only rapid turns or tandem gait, may become disabling, although usually as patients worsen their leg weakness increases and paraparesis limits walking. A few patients will exhibit myoclonus as well. Bladder and bowel incontinence are common in the late stages of the disease. In the end stage affected patients become nearly vegetative, lying in bed with a vacant stare, incontinent and unable to ambulate. However, with the exception of occasional hypersomnolence, the level of arousal is usually preserved, unless intercurrent illness develops.

In children, the disorder has the same general features, although the course may vary somewhat and present in either a progressive or static form.[29,30] The progressive form is characterized by the gradual loss of previously acquired motor skills in conjunction with the evolution of motor abnormalities ranging from spastic paraparesis to quadriplegia with pseudobulbar palsy and rigidity. Acquired microcephaly is almost universal. The CDC surveillance criteria and classification for childhood AIDS now includes neurologic disease with one or more of the following progressive findings: (1) loss of developmental milestones or intellectual ability, (2) impaired brain growth (acquired microcephaly and/or brain atrophy) demonstrated on computed tomographic (CT) scan or magnetic resonance imaging (MRI), or (3) symmetrical motor deficits manifested by two or more of the following: paresis, abnormal tone, pathologic reflexes, ataxia, or gait disturbance.[31]

Neuropsychological Test Profile

Neuropsychological studies quantitatively support these clinical findings and are useful in establishing the degree of impairment and in serially following the course of disease or response to therapy. The characteristic abnormalities include difficulty with complex sequencing, impairment of fine and rapid motor movement, and slowed verbal fluency.[32,33] In general, the neuropsychological tests most sensitive to ADC require some or all of the following: performance under time pressure, problem solving, visual scanning, visual-motor integration and alternation between two performance rules or stimulus sets.

Neurodiagnostic Studies

Two types of neurodiagnostic study, neuroimaging procedures and CSF examination, are essential to the evaluation of AIDS patients with CNS dysfunction and are useful both in establishing the diagnosis of ADC and, perhaps even more importantly, in excluding other neurologic conditions complicating AIDS. Such studies also provide a view into certain aspects of the disease pathobiology.

Neuroradiologic abnormalities in ADC include the nearly universal finding of cerebral atrophy.[20] Additionally, in some patients abnormalities in the hemispheric white matter and, less commonly, in the basal ganglia or thalamus are noted on MRI, with either patchy or diffusely increased signal in T2-weighted images, consistent with increased water content.[20,34,35] Children with AIDS-related dementia often have basal ganglia calcification in addition to atrophy.[36]

Routine examination of the CSF reveals a mildly elevated protein in approximately two-thirds of demented patients and a mild mononuclear pleocytosis in nearly one-quarter.[20] Additionally, HIV can be directly isolated from the CSF of many.[18,37] However, as noted above, it should be recognized that HIV can also be isolated from CSF in a variety of infected patients, including those who are asymptomatic or suffering aseptic meningitis, as well as those with overt dementia. Thus, at present the diagnostic and prognostic significance of various chemical abnormalities or viral detection have yet to be defined. More recently, HIV antigens, principally p24, have been directly assessed in CSF and may offer an accurate and convenient method of quantitating infection for future therapeutic trials.[38]

Epidemiology and Natural History

The epidemiology and natural history of ADC are currently imprecisely defined. Clinically based series such as our own[20] cannot accurately represent the broader population at risk for this complication, and a more accurate picture awaits the findings of prospective longitudinal studies. We have attempted to derive crude estimates of the prevalence of the ADC at different points in the course of HIV infection and AIDS based on our autopsy study, preliminary prospective clinical and neuropsychological studies of newly diagnosed AIDS patients, and an inpatient survey of patients with AIDS.[20,28] Our experience suggests that early in the course of systemic AIDS perhaps one-third of patients exhibit moderate-to-severe dementia and another quarter may suffer subclinical or mild cognitive loss that can be documented by careful examination. Late in the course of the disease, as many as two-thirds of all AIDS patients may exhibit moderate-to-severe dementia, and an additional one-quarter of patients may suffer subclinical impairment. One of the fundamental questions yet to be clearly answered relates to the prevalence of ADC in otherwise asymptomatic seropositives or in those with early or mild systemic symptomatology. We and others are currently attempting to define these figures more precisely, both in the clinical setting and in larger populations at risk.

Neuropathology

Histologic abnormalities in demented AIDS patients are most prominent in the subcortical structures: the central white matter, deep gray structures including the basal ganglia and thalamus, the brain stem and the spinal cord, with relative sparing of the cortex.[21,39,40] These abnormalities can be segregated into three seemingly discontinuous, but overlapping, sets: diffuse white-matter pallor, multinucleated cell encephalitis, and vacuolar myelopathy;[21] a less common additional finding is diffuse or focal spongiform change of the cerebral white matter. The most common of these is diffuse white-matter pallor accompanied by astrocytic reaction and involves particularly the central and periventricular white matter. The prominence of this diffuse pallor generally parallels the severity of neurologic symptomatology, but can also be identified to a mild extent in an appreciable number of patients without overt neurologic dysfunction. When simple pallor is present without multinucleated cells, inflammation is characteristically scant, consisting of a few perivascular lymphocytes and brown-pigmented macrophages accompanying the astrocytosis.

Multinucleated cells are found in a subgroup of patients with more severe clinical disease. In these brains reactive infiltrates are more prominent and consist of perivascular and parenchymal foamy macrophages, microglia, and lymphocytes, along with the multinucleated cells. Because of the association of these findings with direct HIV brain infection as described below, this pathologic subset has been termed *HIV encephalitis* by some.[39] The characteristic multinucleated cell and macrophage infiltrates are most often concentrated in the white matter and deep gray structures. In the white matter, they are frequently surrounded by focal rarefaction, and less commonly by frank demyelination.

Although inflammation with multinucleated cells may also affect the spinal cord, in our own experience a vacuolar myelopathy is more common.[20,39,41] The latter pathologically resembles subacute combined degeneration resulting from vitamin B_{12} deficiency, but levels of this vitamin are normal in serum. Although there is a general correlation between the incidence of vacuolar myelopathy and the other pathologic abnormalities found in the brain, the myelopathy can occur in the absence of the multinucleated cell-associated changes, and vice versa. These discrepancies leave open the question of whether vacuolar myelopathy is a variant of the process causing the multinucleated cell formation and other brain changes or whether it is etiopathogenetically independent.

Etiology and Pathogenesis

Accumulating evidence from clinical observations, animal precedent and direct demonstration of the virus supports the hypothesis that ADC is due to direct brain infection by HIV, at least in a subset of patients. This has now been shown by a variety of techniques, beginning with studies using Southern blot analysis which showed a high frequency of proviral DNA (comparable to that of lymphatic tissue) and high copy number in the brains of some patients with ADC.[42] Both integrated and nonintegrated forms of the genome have been found. *In situ* studies have also detected the presence of viral DNA and RNA within these brains,[42–45] and HIV has been cultured directly from both the brain and CSF of demented patients.[18,37] In addition, HIV antigens have been observed in brain using immunohistochemical techniques,[43,45–48] and HIV virions have been identified by electron microscopy.[49,50]

Although there remains some controversy concerning the cell types involved in productive brain infection, a consensus is emerging that macrophages and multinucleated cells derived from macrophages are principal participants.[43,47,48,51] Although not an invariant finding in HIV-infected brains, the multinucleated cells are histologic markers of productive HIV brain infection, and indeed the multinucleation almost certainly results from direct virus-induced cell fusion occurring *in vivo*. Viral antigens have also been detected in other cells that exhibit cellular processes, and recent studies have identified many of these morphologically and histochemically as microglia.[47,52] Microglia likely also participate in the formation of multinucleated forms. Whether other cell types in the brain, including the native astrocytes, oligodentrocytes, and neurons, are also infected is less clear and requires further investigation. Cell culture studies have demonstrated low-level infection of astrocytic tumor cell lines.[53–55]

Management and Therapy of CNS HIV Infection and ADC

The evidence that direct HIV brain infection likely causes ADC, combined with the knowledge that the brain becomes infected early in the course of systemic HIV disease and therefore might serve as a "sanctuary" for the virus, has stimulated efforts to find antiviral drugs that can penetrate the blood–brain and blood–CSF barriers.[56] The observation that productive brain infection is confined principally to macrophages and microglia rather than to other glial elements or neurons, and the speculation that toxic products of infected or noninfected cells might interfere with normal cell function,[57–59] provide hope that effective antiviral therapy might not only halt progression of disease, but also restore brain function. The rapid response to zidovudine therapy of neurologic impairment noted in the initial study reported by Yarchoan and colleagues[56] provides further foundation for such a hope, and, of course, anecdotal evidence that ADC is amenable to antiviral treatment. Further studies are now needed to confirm these findings and to establish the overall impact of such therapy on the disease.

OPPORTUNISTIC CNS INFECTIONS

A variety of infections of the CNS complicate AIDS and may be the initial AIDS-defining disorder. Specific diagnosis of these infections is important since several can be effectively treated. We consider here the more common and clinically most important of these.

Cerebral Toxoplasmosis

Cerebral toxoplasmosis is the most frequent of the CNS opportunistic infections occurring in AIDS, complicating the course in 5% to 15% of patients, depending somewhat on geographic origin.[60,61] It characteristically presents as a subacute illness in which focal cerebral dysfunction predominates but is often combined with nonfocal, "encephalitic" symptoms. Focal manifestations usually relate to hemispheric lesions, but less commonly, cerebellar or even brain stem abnormalities may be prominent. The nonfocal aspects include general confusion and altered consciousness with lethargy or, at times, coma. Headache and fever are relatively common.

Pathologically, the disease is characterized by a variable number of *toxoplasma gondii* cerebral abscesses.[60] In the acute encephalitic form of the disease the brain may exhibit numerous small lesions with little in the way of cellular reaction. More slowly developing lesions are often larger with mononuclear cell reaction, surrounding edema, and at times vascular occlusion or an element of microscopic hemorrhage. Chronic healed lesions exhibit minor fibrotic changes. Untreated disease is characterized by the presence of free forms of *t. gondii,* whereas after treatment these are no longer seen, although encysted forms may persist.

In evaluating AIDS patients with suspected toxoplasmosis or other focal disorders, neuroimaging techniques, particularly CT and more recently MRI, are critical both to confirm the presence of macroscopic focal disease and to determine the nature of the abnormalities. Multiple lesions involving the cortex or deep brain nuclei (thalamus, basal ganglia) surrounded by edema strongly favor cerebral toxoplasmosis. In most cases toxoplasma abscesses exhibit ring-like contrast enhancement on CT scan, but either homogeneous contrast enhancement or nonenhancing hypodense lesions may be noted. Double-dose contrast CT studies, or preferably MRI, may more clearly define these lesions or show additional spherical lesions characteristic of the disease. Only rarely will the CT scan be normal.

The major differential diagnosis to be considered in AIDS patients suspected to suffer toxoplasmosis is cerebral lymphoma, which may produce a similar CT appearance, although the lesions of lymphoma commonly exhibit more diffuse or less clear-cut contrast enhancement, tend to be radiologically less numerous, and are more often located in the white matter adjacent to the lateral ventricles. Toxoplasma serology is of ad-

ditional help if appropriately interpreted. Since the disease is due to reactivation of the organism, patients with cerebral toxoplasmosis rarely have negative serum IgG antibody titers.[60] However, these titers may be low (occasionally an apparently negative titer will be positive when a more concentrated specimen, such as a 1:4 dilution, is tested) and frequently do not rise during the course of the disease.

To establish the diagnosis of cerebral toxoplasmosis, we rely principally on a *therapeutic trial* and reserve brain biopsy for treatment failures or clinically atypical patients, such as those who are seronegative or have an uncharacteristic CT or MRI study. When treated promptly, toxoplasmosis responds with clear clinical and CT improvement within 1 to 2 weeks. In fact, many patients are clinically better within 24 to 48 hours.

Treatment of toxoplasmosis is initiated with a loading dose of 50 mg of pyrimethamine followed by a single oral daily dose of 25 mg thereafter, together with a sulfa drug, usually sulfadiazine (2–6 g daily in four divided doses). Patients also receive folinic acid, 10 mg daily, as a single oral dose. Adverse reactions to sulfa, including allergy and bone marrow depression, may necessitate substitution with clindamycin at an oral dose of 600 mg qid. In our experience this has not resulted in adverse consequences, but the efficacy of clindamycin has not been established by controlled study.[60,62] If possible, treatment should be continued *indefinitely,* since stopping combined therapy or lowering the dose often leads to relapse.

In treating cerebral toxoplasmosis, and indeed in treating any AIDS patient, corticosteroids should be avoided when possible. This is particularly important when considering a therapeutic trial to differentiate between toxoplasmosis and CNS lymphoma. Since the latter may respond symptomatically to corticosteroids alone, clinical or CT improvement on combination antibiotic and steroid treatment is difficult to interpret. More generally, corticosteroids intensify the impairment of immune defenses in AIDS patients, potentially worsening not only toxoplasmosis but also other systemic opportunistic infections. However, if cerebral edema threatens brain herniation, then judicious short-term use of corticosteroids may be instituted along with appropriate specific therapy, and subsequently must be tapered rapidly once the patient improves.

Cryptococcal Meningitis

Cryptococcal meningitis is the most common CNS fungal infection in AIDS patients,[63,64] and most frequently presents as a subacute meningitis or meningoencephalitis with headache, nausea, vomiting, confusion, and lethargy, just as in non-AIDS patients. However, in some patients symptoms are remarkably mild or even absent. Likewise, the CSF formula may be bland, with few or no cells and little or no perturbation in glucose or protein levels. Accordingly, one should routinely obtain

India ink preparations, CSF cryptococcal antigen titers, and fungal cultures on all AIDS patients at lumbar puncture. Treatment of cryptococcal meningitis follows the guidelines used in other patients and relies on intravenous amphotericin B with or without 5-flucytosine; AIDS patients may be particularly vulnerable to the bone marrow suppression associated with the latter. In patients who fail systemic therapy, intrathecal amphotericin B can be added. Although therapy may relieve symptoms and induce an initial laboratory improvement, patients may relapse, and it may be difficult to sterilize the CSF. Weekly maintenance therapy with amphotericin sometimes proves effective in such instances.[64] High-dose oral ketoconazole has also been reported to provide effective maintenance therapy.[65]

Cytomegalovirus Infection

Systemic cytomegalovirus CMV infection is common in AIDS patients, and evidence of minor brain CMV infection in the form of isolated inclusion-bearing cells within an occasional microglial nodule can be found at autopsy in as many as one-third of patients.[21,39,66] Although some uncertainty remains regarding the contribution of this type of CMV infection to neurologic symptoms and signs in AIDS patients, the clinical effect is likely minor and in most patients is overshadowed by ADC. Only in an occasional patient does severe CMV infection result in symptomatic subacute brain dysfunction, clouded consciousness, seizures, or radiculomyelitis. Ventricular ependymitis with local contrast enhancement may be detected on CT scan or MRI. The clinical diagnosis of brain CMV infection, however, is difficult. Anti-CMV antibody titers in blood are commonly chronically elevated in AIDS and therefore are not useful in neurologic diagnosis, and CSF cultures are usually negative except in patients with radiculomyelitis.[66]

In cases where CMV infection of the brain is strongly suspected, specific antiviral therapy using gancyclovir can be considered, although the efficacy of this drug in CNS CMV infection, other than retinopathy, has not yet been adequately tested.

Progressive Multifocal Leukoencephalitis

Progressive multifocal leukoencephalitis (PML) is an opportunistic infection caused by a human papovavirus, JC.[67] The disease is characterized by selective demyelination.[63,68] The pathologic lesions begin as small foci in the subcortical white matter, which then coalesce to form larger lesions. The microscopic appearance includes inclusion-bearing swollen oligodendrocyte nuclei and pleomorphic, hyperchromatic astrocytes. The oligodendrocyte inclusions relate to the presence of JC virus nucleocapsids, which can be identified by electron microscopy, and the demyelinating lesions are caused by the death of these cells with secondary degeneration of their myelin-forming processes. Inflammation is inconspicuous in the majority of cases.

Clinical evolution of PML is usually more protracted than that of either toxoplasmosis or CNS lymphoma, and altered consciousness related to brain swelling is not a feature of the disease. Neither serum nor CSF serology is useful, and definitive diagnosis is made only by brain biopsy or autopsy, although suspicion is aroused by the clinical history and an examination suggesting more than one cerebral focus, along with a CT scan or MRI demonstrating white-matter lesions, without mass effect or contrast enhancement.[69,70] There is no proven effective therapy for the disease. Individual reports of non-AIDS patients suggest that cytosine arabinoside may be helpful in some cases,[71] although there has been no controlled trial, and favorable experience has not yet accumulated with AIDS patients. Spontaneous sustained remission of PML in two AIDS patients has recently been reported.[72]

Cerebral Tuberculosis

Although not strictly an opportunistic pathogen, *Mycobacterium tuberculosis* infections appear to be more common and perhaps more severe in HIV-infected individuals. The development of *M. tuberculosis* is additionally influenced by socioeconomic factors, and currently predominantly affects intravenous drug abusers rather than patients with homosexuality or transfusion as AIDS risk factors.[73,74] Even in AIDS patients with systemic tuberculosis, CNS involvement is uncommon, but can occur in the context of seemingly more aggressive infection. Anergy may make diagnosis difficult, and CSF smear and culture are still the best methods of diagnosis. Brain biopsy may be necessary to diagnose tuberculous abscesses. Treatment should include three drugs, at least initially. A recommended regimen includes isoniazid, rifampin and either ethambutol or pyrazinamide. A fourth drug may be needed. Treatment should continue for at least 6 months after culture conversion and may need to exceed nine months.[75,76] Although systemic atypical mycobacteria, especially *Mycobacterium avium-intracellulare,* commonly infect AIDS patients, they do not appear to constitute important CNS pathogens. While these organisms have been isolated from CSF and even from brain, they have not been shown to infiltrate the brain parenchyma or cause clinical dysfunction.[24]

Varicella Zoster Virus and Herpes Simplex Virus Infections

Although unusual, varicella zoster virus (VZV) and, to a lesser extent, the herpes simplex viruses HSV-1 and HSV-2 have been reported to cause CNS disease in AIDS patients. VZV infections are of three types: (1) multifocal direct brain infection affecting principally the white matter and partially mimicking PML,[77-79] (2) cerebral vasculitis that characteristically occurs in the setting of ophthalmic herpes zoster and causes contralateral hemiplegia,[80,81] and (3) myelopathy complicating herpes zoster.[82] Both HSV-1 and HSV-2 have been identified in the brains of some AIDS patients, but the clinical correlates of these infections have not yet been wholly delineated.[83,84]

Because of the relative rarity of these herpesvirus infections of the CNS and difficulty in their diagnosis, the effects of therapy generally have not been defined. Nonetheless, when clinically recognized and documented by biopsy or viral culture, they should be treated with acyclovir, probably at a dose of approximately 10 mg/kg IV q8h, as recommended in herpes encephalitis in the nonimmunosuppressed. However, therapy may need to be continued beyond the usual 10 days recommended for the latter, and higher doses may be needed for VZV treatment.

OPPORTUNISTIC CNS NEOPLASMS

The CNS is also subject to the development of opportunistic neoplasms, and in particular to lymphomas that either arise in the brain itself or metastasize from extraneural sites. Although Kaposi's sarcoma involving the brain has been reported,[83] it is so exceedingly rare that it does not warrant general consideration in differential diagnosis of brain disease.

Primary CNS Lymphoma

Primary CNS lymphomas of B-cell origin are opportunistic neoplasms that complicate the course of AIDS in approximately 5% of patients, although this estimate includes lymphomas noted incidentally at autopsy.[39,85] The incidence of primary CNS lymphoma in non-AIDS patients is increasing,[86] and our own recent experience suggests that this trend may now be reflected in AIDS patients as well. When symptomatic, primary brain lymphomas present with progressive focal or multifocal neurologic deficits similar to toxoplasmosis, although the tempo of disease evolution is usually slower. Neuroradiologic studies are usually sensitive in detecting primary brain lymphomas but do not establish definitive diagnosis. Characteristically these tumors are multicentric but most often show only one or two lesions on CT scan or MRI. Their location is characteristically deep in the brain, surrounding the ventricles, and most often in the white rather than gray matter. On CT scan they may enhance after contrast administration, but very often such enhancement is either weak or absent. Indeed, delineation of lymphomas by CT may be vague, and MRI scanning is more sensitive. Unfortunately, CSF cytology is frequently negative, and final diagnosis relies on brain biopsy. As discussed earlier, we usually un-

dertake brain biopsy when antitoxoplasmosa therapy fails to relieve a focal CNS lesion.

Current standard therapy for lymphoma in AIDS patients includes whole-brain radiation. The role of systemic chemotherapy is uncertain. Because some AIDS patients with systemic lymphoma have been successfully treated with chemotherapy, it may be that the same will prove true for primary brain lymphoma. However, primary lymphomas usually occur later in the course of HIV infection when systemic disease is more advanced and patients are more vulnerable to the toxic effects of corticosteroids and cytoreductive drugs.

Metastatic Lymphoma

Systemic lymphoma complicating HIV infection secondarily involves the CNS with some regularity. Unlike primary brain lymphomas, metastatic lymphomas most frequently involve the meninges rather than the brain parenchyma and may present with cranial nerve palsies, headaches, or increased intracranial pressure.[24] However, metastatic parenchymal brain disease may also occur, and in some cases the course may be fulminant. Otherwise the clinical and diagnostic features resemble non-AIDS lymphomas. Therapeutic regimens have not been clearly defined, but include whole-brain irradiation and intrathecal chemotherapy as adjuncts to systemic chemotherapy.[86]

OTHER CNS DISORDERS

Cerebrovascular Complications

Some AIDS patients suffer transient ischemic attacks or even strokes leaving residual brain injury. The incidence of such vascular episodes is not yet clearly defined, but our experience suggests that they are not rare. In most cases the pathogenesis of these events is unclear, but fortunately, most have a benign outcome. Less common are more severe, usually agonal, vascular episodes, including cerebral hemorrhage related to thrombocytopenia, cerebral infarction from nonbacterial thrombotic endocarditis, and dural sinus or cerebral venous occlusion.[24,83] Of interest also are reports of blood vessel changes, possibly directly related to HIV infection.[87,88]

Metabolic Diseases

It is important to be aware that patients with AIDS are subject to a constellation of metabolic brain disorders as a result of their complex systemic illnesses. These include encephalopathies related to hypoxia and pulmonary disease, to sepsis and, less commonly, to renal failure. Likewise, toxic encephalopathies may relate to various therapies with CNS side effects. Such metabolic and toxic influences will frequently exacerbate or unmask ADC, leading to abrupt functional deterioration. The diagnostic approach and treatment of these disorders parallels that in patients without AIDS.

PERIPHERAL NERVOUS SYSTEM AND MUSCLE

Peripheral Neuropathies

Peripheral neuropathies may complicate HIV infection at virtually each of its stages. During the earliest stage, at or near the time of seroconversion, a variety of neuropathies have been described, although their incidence appears to be very low. These have included brachial plexopathy, mononeuritides involving either peripheral or cranial nerves, and polyneuropathy.[16,89] Each appears to be self-limiting with good general recovery.

Apparently much more common is the development of demyelinating neuropathies during the asymptomatic or latent phase of HIV infection.[90] These resemble Guillain-Barré syndrome or chronic inflammatory demyelinating polyneuropathy (IDPN) seen in other contexts with the exception that the CSF often exhibits an uncharacteristic yet mild pleocytosis. These patients are usually otherwise well. Likely the pathophysiology of their neuropathy parallels that of the disorder in other settings and has an autoimmune basis. They respond favorably to plasmapheresis or corticosteroids, and plasmapheresis is now tentatively recommended as the treatment of choice.

In the setting of ARC, and more commonly AIDS, several other neuropathies have been described. These include the infectious neuropathies caused by a varicella-zoster virus (i.e., herpes zoster), and an ascending polyradiculopathy caused by CMV.[91] Cranial mononeuritides may also complicate both the aseptic meningitis presumably related to HIV infection and metastatic lymphomatous meningitis as described above. Mononeuritis multiplex has also been described in patients at this stage of systemic disease. Biopsy has shown an axonal degeneration, sometimes with an accompanying segmental demyelination.[92] Inflammatory cells are present, but evidence of a vasculitis in the form of vasonecrosis with or without fibrosis has thus far been lacking in the documentation. Treatment with steroids has been disappointing, although a favorable response to plasmapheresis has been reported.

However, the most common neuropathy is a distal, predominantly sensory and axonal neuropathy most often encountered in patients with AIDS.[24,92–94] Characteristically, the sensory symptoms far exceed either sensory or motor dysfunction. The incidence of this disorder is uncertain but likely in mild form it is probably quite common. A variant of this is a less common but clinically very important sensory polyneuropathy with severe "burning feet" clinically reminiscent of severe alcoholic or diabetic neuropathy. Even in these patients sensory loss and motor weakness are usually mild, but the painful parasthesias and burning may cause sufficient dis-

ability to prevent walking. The pathogenesis of this disorder is uncertain, but it has been suggested that it may be related to direct HIV infection of nerve or dorsal root ganglion, although this has not yet been clearly documented.[37,95] Treatment is symptomatic using tricyclic antidepressants or, if there is a tic-like component to the pain, carbamazapain or phenytoin.

Autonomic neuropathy has also been reported in AIDS patients, occasionally in conjunction with a more general peripheral neuropathy.[96,97] The clinical features have ranged from positional hypotension to cardiovascular collapse in the setting of invasive procedures such as lung biopsy.

Myopathies

As with the neuropathies, myopathies may also occur at several stages of HIV infection, although they are less common and less well characterized. Accumulating data suggest that there may be a wide range of presentations, extending from asymptomatic creatine kinase elevation to progressive proximal weakness.[24,98–101] A polymyositis or dermatomyositis-like illness has been described in AIDS and pre-AIDS patients, but as with the other myopathies the pathogenesis is not clear. Viral antigens have been found in the inflammatory lymphoid cells but not in myocytes, and one recent report has identified multinucleated giant cells in the inflammatory muscle infiltrate.[98]

GENERAL APPROACH TO DIAGNOSIS AND MANAGEMENT OF NERVOUS SYSTEM COMPLICATIONS

The approach to the diagnosis of CNS disease in patients with HIV infection or AIDS follows that of neurologic diagnosis in general but takes into account the particular vulnerabilities of these patients enumerated above (Table 11-3). It is, of course, important to establish a diagnosis of systemic HIV infection in order to confirm the arena of diagnosis. This becomes paramount in patients who first present with neurologic disease. In addition to serologic or virologic confirmation of HIV infection, it also is important to establish the "stage" of HIV infection in each patient since the spectrum of neurologic disease varies with the changing immunologic and virologic status as tentatively outlined in Table 11-4. An additional consideration in the late phase of HIV infection is that patients may develop more than one neurologic disease, and thus evaluation of concomitant or serially occurring diseases may be needed.

As in the non-AIDS patient, approach to specific neurologic diagnosis begins with the *neurologic history,* which establishes the background setting of the illness and its temporal profile, and usually provides an initial impression of its anatomic localization. The tempo of neurologic disease is a critical factor in differential diagnosis, allowing separation of acute events (vascular episodes or seizures) from those with slower evolution over days (toxoplasmosis) or weeks (ADC). The *neurologic examination* serves to refine this localization and uncover additional asymptomatic abnormalities. Anatomic-physiological diagnosis segregates diffuse brain disease with concomitant depressed alertness (e.g., metabolic encephalopathies), diffuse brain disease with preserved alertness (ADC), focal brain diseases (e.g., toxoplasmosis, primary CNS lymphoma, PML), meningitidites (e.g., aseptic or cryptococcal meningitis), myelopathies, peripheral neuropathies, and myopathies (see Table 11-1). *Neuroimaging studies* using CT or MRI, and less commonly myelography or angiography, add further precision to anatomic localization and also narrow the range of possible underlying pathologic processes. Thus, ADC is typically marked by cerebral atrophy, at times accompanied by white-matter abnormalities by MRI, while the predominantly focal brain diseases show mass lesions (e.g., toxoplasmosis or primary lymphoma) or demyelination (PML). *Electrodiagnosis* using electroencephalography (EEG) or evoked potentials may also be helpful in delineating and localizing physiologic dysfunction (e.g., metabolic encephalopathies or myelopathies), and nerve conduction studies and electromyography can similarly refine diagnosis of neuromuscular disorders. Examination of the CSF provides a direct view of inflammatory reactions in the meninges and can precisely diagnose invading or-

Table 11-3

Diagnosis of Neurologic Disease in HIV-Infected and AIDS Patients: Approach and Methods

Diagnosis and staging of HIV infection
  Serostatus
  Systemic disease record, immune status, virus load
Neurological history
  Temporal profile of evolution
  Provisional anatomic localization
  Functional severity
Neurological examination
  Refined anatomic localization
Neuroimaging (CT, MRI, less commonly myelography, angiography)
  Refined anatomic localization
  Preliminary etiologic diagnosis
CSF analysis
  Etiologic diagnosis (culture, cytology)
Neuropsychological testing
  Staging ADC
Electrodiagnosis (EEG, evoked potentials, EMG, nerve conduction)
  Physiological diagnosis and localization
Therapeutic trial
  Targeted to toxoplasmosis
Brain biopsy
  Diagnosis of focal brain lesions

Table 11-4

Timing Estimates of the CNS and PNS Complications of HIV Infection in Relation to Stage of Systemic Disease

Complication	Systemic Disease Stage*			
	Early	*Latent*	*Early–Late*	*Late*
Central Nervous System				
Asymptomatic infection	←———————————————————→			
Acute encephalitis	←————————→			
Aseptic meningitis	←————————→		←———————————→	
ADC			←——————————→	
Opportunistic CNS infections				←→
Primary CNS lymphoma			←——————————→	
Metastatic systemic lymphoma			←——————————→	
Peripheral nervous system				
Acute demyelinating polyneuropathy	←———————————————→			
Chronic demyelinating polyneuropathy		←———————————→		
Mononeuropathies	←———————————————→			
Mononeuropathy			←——————————→	
Sensorimotor polyneuropathy		←———————————————————→		

* Definitions
  Early: Time of acute HIV infection with early viremia, primary immune response, and seroconversion
  Latent: Period of asymptomatic infection or chronic persistent lymphadenopathy without constitutional symptoms
  Early–late: Beginning of constitutional symptoms, Kaposi's sarcoma, or "minor" opportunistic infections (late ARC)
  Late: Time of marked immunosuppression and development of AIDS-defining opportunistic infections

ganisms (HIV, cryptococcus) or neoplasms (lymphoma). *Therapeutic trial* (toxoplasmosis) and *brain biopsy* (brain lymphoma, PML) are coordinated for exact diagnosis of focal brain disease.

These evaluations, when pursued with a background understanding of the spectrum of neurologic disorders affecting these patients, allows exact neurologic diagnosis in the majority of HIV-infected and AIDS patients. As with other aspects of AIDS, this is an important and often fruitful exercise, since a number of these disorders can be treated with gratifying relief of morbidity and prevention of death.

REFERENCES

1. Resnick L, DiMarzo-Veronese F, Schupbach J et al: Intra-blood brain-barrier synthesis of HTLV-III specific IgG in patients with neurologic symptoms associated with AIDS or AIDS-related complex. N Engl J Med 313:1498, 1985
2. Goudsmit J, Wolters EC, Bakker M et al: Intrathecal synthesis of antibodies to HTLVIII in patients without AIDS or AIDS related complex. Brit Med J 292:1231, 1986
3. Resnick L, Berger JR, Shapshak P et al: Early penetration of the blood-brain-barrier by HTLV-III/LAV. Neurology (in preparation)
4. Appelman ME, Brey RL, Marshall DW et al: Cerebrospinal fluid (CSF) findings in HIV positive patients (pts) without AIDS. [abstr] III International Conference on AIDS, Washington DC, June 1–5, 1987
5. Clotet B, Barrera JM, Ercilla G et al: Asymptomatic neurologic infection in persistent generalized lymphadenopathy syndrome associated to HIV infection. [abstr] III International Conference on AIDS, Washington DC, June 1–5, 1987
6. Collier AC, Coombs RW, Nikora B et al: Cerebrospinal fluid findings in HIV infected persons without clinically evident neurologic disease. [abstr] III International Conference on AIDS, Washington DC, June 1–5, 1987
7. Hutto C, Scott GB, Parks ES et al: Cerebrospinal fluid (CSF) studies in adult and pediatric HIV infections. [abstr] III International Conference on AIDS, Washington DC, June 1–5, 1987
8. Katalama C, Rey MA, Salmon RD et al: Cerebrospinal fluid study in forty four HIV infected patients: Clinical correlation with virus isolation and intrathecal specific antibody synthesis. [abstr] III International Conference on AIDS, Washington DC, June 1–5, 1987
9. Elovaara I, Iivanainen M, Sirkka–Liisa V et al: CSF protein and cellular profiles in various stages of HIV infection related to neurological manifestations. J Neurol Sci 78:331, 1987
10. McArthur JC, Cohen BA, Farzadegan H, et al: Cerebrospinal fluid abnormalities in homosexual/ men with and without neuropsychiatric symptoms. Ann Neurol 23 (Suppl):534, 1988
11. Vittecco D, Harzick M, Ferchal F et al: Isolation of HIV from cerebrospinal fluid of patients with AIDS related disorders. [abstr] III International Conference on AIDS, Washington DC, June 1–5, 1987
12. Carne CA, Smith A, Elkington SG et al: Acute encepha-lopathy coincident with seroconversion for anti HTLVIII. Lancet 2:1206, 1985
13. Ho DD, Sarngadharan MG, Resnick L et al: Primary human T lymphotropic virus type III infection. Ann Intern Med 103:880, 1985
14. Piette AM, Tusseau F, Vignon D et al: Letter: Lancet 1: 852, 1986
15. Denning DA, Anderson J, Rudge P et al: Acute myelopathy associated with primary infection with human immunodeficiency virus. Brit Med J 294:143, 1987
16. Brew BJ, Cooper DA, Perdices MJ et al: The neurological complications of HIV infection in the absence of significant immunodeficiency. [abstr] III International Conference on AIDS, Washington DC, June 1–5, 1987
17. Bredesen DE, Lipkin WI, Messing R: Prolonged, recurrent aseptic meningitis with prominent cranial nerve abnormalities: A new epidemic in gay men? [abstr] Neurology 33:85, 1983
18. Levy JA, Shimabukuro J, Hollander H et al: Isolation of AIDS associated retroviruses from cerebrospinal fluid and brain of patients with neurological symptoms. Lancet 2: 586, 1985
19. Hollander H, Stringari S: Human immunodeficiency virus-associated meningitis: Clinical course and correlations. Am J Med 83:813, 1987
20. Navia BA, Jordan BD, Price RW: The AIDS dementia complex: I. clinical features. Ann Neurol 19:517, 1986
21. Navia BA, Cho ES, Petito CK et al: The AIDS dementia complex: II. neuropathology. Ann Neurol 19:525, 1986
22. Navia BA, Price RW: The acquired immunodeficiency syndrome dementia complex as the presenting or sole manifestation of human immunodeficiency virus infection. Arch Neurol 44:65, 1987
23. Centers for Disease Control: Revision of the CDC surveillance case definition for acquired immunodeficiency syndrome. Morbid Mortal Week Rept 36:1S, 1987
24. Snider WD, Simpson DM, Nielsen S et al: Neurological complications of acquired immune deficiency syndrome: Analysis of 50 patients. Ann Neurol 14:403, 1983
25. Britton CB, Miller JR: Neurologic complications in acquired immunodeficiency syndrome (AIDS). Neurol Clin 2:315, 1984
26. Price RW, Navia BA, Cho ES: AIDS encephalopathy. Neurol Clin 4:285, 1986
27. Price RW, Sidtis JJ, Rosenblum M: The AIDS dementia complex: Some current questions. Ann Neurol 23 (Suppl):527, 1988
28. Price RW, Sidtis JJ, Navia BA et al: AIDS Dementia Complex. In Rosenblum ML, Levy RM, Bredesen DE (eds): AIDS and the Nervous System, New York, Raven Press 1988
29. Epstein LG, Sharer LR, Joshi V et al: Progressive encephalopathy in children with acquired immune deficiency syndrome. Ann Neurol 17:488, 1985
30. Belman AL, Ultmann MH, Horoupian D et al: Neurological complications in infants and children with acquired immune deficiency syndrome. Ann Neurol 18:560, 1985
31. Centers for Disease Control: Classification system for human immunodeficiency virus (HIV) infection in children under 13 years of age. Morbid Mortal Week Rept 36:225, 1987
32. Sidtis JJ, Amitai H, Ornitz D et al: The brief neuropsychological examination for AIDS dementia complex: Correlations with functional status scales and other neu-

ropsychological tests. [abstr] III International Conference on AIDS, Washington DC, June 1–5, 1987

33. Tross S, Price RW, Navia BA et al: Neuropsychological characterization of the AIDS dementia complex: A preliminary report. AIDS (in press)

34. Shabas D, Gerard G, Cunha B et al: MRI appearance of AIDS subacute encephalopathy. Comput Radiol 11:69, 1987

35. Jarvik J, Hesselink J, Kennedy C et al: Patterns of magnetic resonance brain scanning of lesions in AIDS and ARC patients. [abstr] III International Conference on AIDS, Washington DC, June 1–5, 1987

36. Belman AL, Lantos G, Horoupian D et al: Calcification of the basal ganglia in infants and children. Neurology 36:1192, 1986

37. Ho DD, Rota TR, Schooley RT et al: Isolation of HTLV-III from cerebrospinal fluid and neural tissues of patients with neurologic syndromes related to the acquired immunodeficiency syndrome. N Engl J Med 313:1493, 1985

38. Goudsmit J, deWolf F, Paul DA et al: Expression of human immunodeficiency virus antigen (HIV-Ag) in serum and cerebrospinal fluid during acute and chronic infection. Lancet 2:177, 1986

39. Petito CK, Cho ES, Lemann W et al: Neuropathology of acquired immunodeficiency syndrome (AIDS): An autopsy review. J Neuropathol Exp Neurol 45:635, 1986

40. Kato T, Hirano A, Llena JF et al: Neuropathology of acquired immune deficiency syndrome (AIDS) in 53 autopsy cases with particular emphasis on microglial nodules and multinucleated giant cells. Acta Neuropathol 73:287, 1987

41. Petito CK, Navia BA, Cho ES et al: Vacuolar myelopathy pathologically resembling subacute combined degeneration in patients with acquired immunodeficiency syndrome (AIDS). N Engl J Med 312:874, 1985

42. Shaw GM, Harper ME, Hahn BH et al: HTLV-III infection in brains of children and adults with AIDS encephalopathy. Science 227:177, 1985

43. Koenig S, Gendelman HE, Orenstein JM et al: Detection of AIDS virus in macrophages in brain tissue from AIDS patients with encephalopathy. Science 233:1089, 1986

44. Stoler MH, Eskin TA, Benn S et al: Human T cell lymphotropic virus type III infection of the central nervous system: A preliminary in situ analysis. JAMA 256:2360, 1986

45. Wiley CA, Schrier RD, Nelson JA et al: Cellular localization of human immunodeficiency virus infection within the brains of acquired immune deficiency syndrome patients. Proc Natl Acad Sci 83:7089, 1986

46. Gabuzda DH, Ho DD, De La Monte SM et al: Immunohistochemical identification of HTLVIII antigen in brains of patients with AIDS. Ann Neurol 20:289, 1986

47. Vazeux R, Brousse N, Jarry A et al: AIDS subacute encephalitis: Identification of HIV-infected cells. Am J Pathol 126:403, 1987

48. Pumarola–Sune T, Navia BA, Cordon–Cardo C et al: HIV antigen in the brains of patients with the AIDS dementia complex. Ann Neurol 21:490, 1987

49. Epstein LG, Sharer LR, Cho ES et al: HTLVIII/LAV like retrovirus particles in the brains of patients with AIDS encephalopathy. AIDS Res 1:447, 1985

50. Gyorkey F, Melnick JL, Gyorkey P: Human immunodeficiency virus in brain biopsies of patients with AIDS and progressive encephalopathy. J Infect Dis 155:870, 1987

51. Gartner S, Markovits P, Markovits DM et al: Virus isolation from an identification of HTLVIII/LAV producing cells in brain tissue from a patient with AIDS. JAMA 256:2365, 1986

52. Michaels J, Price RW, Rosenblum MK: Microglia in the human immunodeficiency virus encephalitis of acquired immune deficiency syndrome: Proliferation, infection and fusion. Acta Neuropathol (in press)

53. Cheng–Mayer C, Rutka JT, Rosenblum ML et al: Human immunodeficiency virus can productively infect cultured human glial cells. Proc Natl Acad Sci 84:3526, 1987

54. Dewhurst S, Bresser J, Stevenson M et al: Susceptibility of human glial cells to infection with human immunodeficiency virus (HIV). Ann Neurol 213:138, 1987

55. Weber J, Robey E, Axel R et al: In vitro infection of glial cells with diverse HIV isolates. [abstr] III International Conference on AIDS, Washington DC, June 1–5, 1987

56. Yarchoan R, Berg G, Brouwers P et al: Response of human immunodeficiency virus associated neurological disease to 3'-azido-3'-deoxythymidine. Lancet 1:132, 1987

57. Price RW, Brew B: Infection of the central nervous system by human immunodeficiency virus: Role of the immune system in pathogenesis. Ann NY Acad Sci (in preparation).

58. Price RW, Brew B, Sidtis J et al: The brain in AIDS: Central nervous system HIV-1 infection and the AIDS dementia complex. Science 239:586, 1988

59. Lee MR, Ho DD, Gurney ME: Functional interaction and partial homology between human immunodeficiency virus and neuroleukin. Science 237:1047, 1987

60. Navia BA, Petito CK, Gold JWM et al: Cerebral toxoplasmosis complicating the acquired immune deficiency syndrome: Clinical and neuropathological findings in 27 patients. Ann Neurol 19:224, 1986

61. Haverkos H: Assessment of therapy for toxoplasma encephalitis. Am J Med 82:907, 1987

62. Rolston KVI, Hoy J: Role of clindamycin in the treatment of central nervous system toxoplasmosis. Am J Med 83:551, 1987

63. Kovacs JA, Kovacs AA, Polis M et al: Cryptococcosis in the acquired immunodeficiency syndrome. Ann Intern Med 103:533, 1985

64. Zuger A, Louie E, Holzman RS et al: Cryptococcal disease in patients with the acquired immunodeficiency syndrome. Ann Intern Med 104:234, 1986

65. Mess TP, Hadley WK, Wofsky CB: Use of high dose oral ketoconazole in AIDS patients for prevention of relapse in cryptococcal meningitis. [abstr] III International Conference on AIDS, Washington DC, June 1–5, 1987

66. Morgello S, Cho ES, Nielsen S et al: Cytomegalovirus encephalitis in patients with acquired immunodeficiency syndrome. Hum Pathol 18:289, 1987

67. Padgett BL, Walker DL, Zu Rhein GM et al: JC papovavirus in progressive multifocal leukoencephalopathy. J Infect Dis 133:686, 1976

68. Richardson EP: Progressive Multifocal Leukoencephalopathy. In Vinken PJ, Bruyn GW (eds): Handbook of Clinical Neurology, vol 34, p 307. Amsterdam, Elsevier, 1978

69. Krupp LB, Lipton RB, Swerdlow ML et al: Progressive multifocal leukoencephalopathy: Clinical and radiographic features. Ann Neurol 17:344, 1985

70. Berger JR, Kaszovitz B, Post JD et al: Progressive multifocal leukoencephalopathy associated with human immunodeficiency virus infection. Ann Intern Med 107:78, 1987

71. Marriott PJ, O'Brien MD, MacKenzie ICK et al: Progressive

multifocal leukoencephalopathy remission with cytarabine. J Neurol Neurosurg Psychiatry 38:205, 1975

72. Berger JR, Mucke L: Neurological recovery and prolonged survival in progressive multifocal leukoencephalopathy with HIV infection. [abstr] III International Conference on AIDS, Washington DC, June 1–5, 1987

73. Sunderam G, McDonald RJ, Maniatis T et al: Tuberculosis as a manifestation of the acquired immunodeficiency syndrome (AIDS). JAMA 256:362, 1986

74. Guarner J, Del Rio C, Slade B: Tuberculosis as a manifestation of the acquired immunodeficiency syndrome. JAMA 256:3092, 1986

75. Centers for the Disease Control: Diagnosis and management of mycobacterial infection and disease in persons with human T-lymphotropic virus type III/lymphadenopathy-associated virus infection. Morbid Mortal Week Rept 35:448, 1986

76. Centers for Disease Control: Tuberculosis and acquired immunodeficiency syndrome—Florida. Morbid Mortal Week Rept 35:587, 1986

77. Horten B, Price RW, Jimenez D: Multifocal varicella-zoster virus leukoencephalitis temporally remote from herpes zoster. Ann Neurol 9:251, 1981

78. Ryder JW, Croen K, Kleinschmidt–De-Masters BK et al: Progressive encephalitis three months after resolution of cutaneous zoster in a patient with AIDS. Ann Neurol 19:182, 1986

79. Morgello S, Block GA, Price RW et al: Varicella-zoster virus leukoencephalitis and cerebral vasculopathy. Arch Pathol Lab Med 112:173, 1988

80. Hilt DC, Bucholz D, Krumholz A et al: Herpes zoster ophthalmicus and delayed contralateral hemiparesis caused by cerebral angiitis: diagnosis and management approaches. Ann Neurol 14:543, 1983

81. Eidelberg D, Sotrel A, Horoupian DS et al: Thrombotic cerebral vasculopathy associated with herpes zoster. Ann Neurol 19:7, 1986

82. Devinsky O, Cho ES, Petito CK et al: Herpes zoster myelitis. [abstr] Neurology 37(Suppl 1):319, 1987

83. Levy RL, Bredesen DE, Rosenblum ML: Neurological manifestations of the acquired immunodeficiency syndrome (AIDS): Experience at UCSF and review of the literature. J Neurosurg 62:475, 1985

84. Rhodes RH: Histopathology of the central nervous system in the acquired immunodeficiency syndrome. Hum Pathol 18:636, 1987

85. So YT, Beckstead JH, Davis RL: Primary central nervous system lymphoma in acquired immune deficiency syndrome: A clinical and pathological study. Ann Neurol 20:566, 1986

86. Levine AM: Non-hodgkin's lymphomas and other malignancies in the acquired immune deficiency syndrome. Semin Oncol 14(Suppl):34, 1987

87. Yankner BA, Skolnik PR, Shoukimas GM et al: Cerebral granulomatous angiitis associated with isolation of human T lymphotropic virus type III from the central nervous system. Ann Neurol 20:362, 1986

88. Cho ES, Sharer LR, Peress NS et al: Intimal proliferation of leptomeningeal arteries and brain infarcts in subjects with AIDS. J Neuropathol Exp Neurol 46:385, 1987

89. Elder G, Dalakas M, Pezeshkpour G et al: Letter. Lancet 2:1275, 1986

90. Cornblath DR, McArthur JC, Kennedy PGE et al: Inflammatory demyelinating peripheral neuropathies associated with human T-cell lymphotropic virus type III infection. Ann Neurol 21:32, 1986

91. Eidelberg D, Sotrel A, Vogel H et al: Progressive polyradiculopathy in acquired immune deficiency syndrome. Neurology 36:912, 1986

92. Lipkin WI, Parry G, Kiprov D et al: Inflammatory neuropathy in homosexual men with lymphadenopathy. Neurology 35:1479, 1985

93. Cornblath DR, McArthur J, Rance NE et al: Painful sensory neuropathy (psn) in patients with AIDS. [abstr] III International Conference on AIDS, Washington DC, June 1–5, 1987

94. Gastaut JA, Gastaut JL, Pelissier JF et al: Polyneuropathies in subjects infected with HIV. [abstr] III International Conference on AIDS, Washington DC, June 1–5, 1987

95. Rance NE, McArthur JC, Cornblath DC: Gracile tract degeneration in patients with sensory neuropathy and AIDS. Neurology 38:265, 1988

96. Craddock C, Pasvol G, Bull R et al: Cardiorespiratory arrest and autonomic neuropathy in AIDS. Lancet 2:16, 1987

97. Lin–Greenberg A, Taneja–Uppal N: Dysautonomia and infection with the human immunodeficiency virus. Ann Intern Med 106:167, 1987

98. Dalakas MC, Pezeshkpour GH, Gravell M et al: Polymyositis associated with AIDS retrovirus. JAMA 256:2381, 1986

99. Simpson DM, Bender AN: HTLV-III-associated myopathy. [abstr] Neurology 37(Suppl):319, 1987

100. Harrison WO, Berg SW, Counihan CM: Asymptomatic myositis in HIV antibody positive men. [abstr] III International Conference on AIDS, Washington DC, June 1–5, 1987

101. Bailey RO, Turok DI, Jaufmann BP et al: Myositis and acquired immunodeficiency syndrome. Hum Pathol 18:749, 1987

Opportunistic Infections

Joseph A. Kovacs
Henry Masur

12

Opportunistic infections are the major identifiable cause of morbidity and mortality of HIV-infected patients. When the primary cause of death is assessed at autopsy, most series report that 90% of fatalities are caused by infection, whereas the remaining 10% are caused by lymphoma, Kaposi's sarcoma, gastrointestinal bleeding, suicide, or other noninfectious processes.[1-5] Thus, until the underlying immunologic defect caused by HIV can be reversed, the most direct method for improving the quality and duration of patient survival is to emphasize the prevention and the expeditious therapy of opportunistic infections. Many patients and health-care providers are fatalistic about the outcome of HIV infection and cease to be prompt or diligent about evaluating new clinical problems. Once a patient has AIDS, death currently appears to be inevitable, but this inevitability should not discourage efforts to prolong the duration of reasonable-quality existence, however the patient wishes to define this term. Many of the diseases that health-care providers currently manage are incurable, including atherosclerotic heart disease, rheumatologic disorders, many cancers, and chronic lung diseases. Clinicians and patients invest considerable energy and resources into palliating these disorders and attempting to prolong survival. Advances in diagnosis and therapy of opportunistic infection can improve the quality and duration of survival for HIV-infected patients. These advances need to be brought to bear so that quality and duration of survival can be improved for HIV-infected patients as with these other currently incurable diseases, even if the maximum expected benefit will be measured in months or a few years.

HIV-infected patients are susceptible to community- and hospital-acquired infections prevalent among HIV-seronegative individuals as well as to opportunistic infections that take advantage of HIV-induced immunodepression. Thus, when an HIV-seropositive individual becomes infected with these pathogens, the health-care provider must consider common infectious agents as well as less ordinary opportunistic pathogens. Special consideration must focus on those nonopportunistic infections unique to relevant aspects of the patient's lifestyle such as homosexuality, drug abuse, or hemophilia. The relative susceptibility of HIV-infected individuals to opportunistic pathogens depends on the degree of HIV-induced immunosuppression. During the initial months after HIV infection, patients are probably at no enhanced risk of infection. Until their T4 lymphocyte count falls below 250/mm^3, patients do not appear to be susceptible to *Pneumocystis,* cytomegalovirus (CMV), or disseminated *Mycobacterium avium-intracellulare.* During this intermediate interval, however, it appears that tuberculosis, and probably fungal diseases such as histoplasmosis and coccidiomycosis, can occur.

The opportunistic infections that are common among HIV-infected patients are a unique constellation of pathogens that, as a group, are quite different from those seen with any other immunosuppressive disorder (Tables 12-1, 12-2). The specific infectious processes that occur are presumably a reflection of the unique qualitative and quantitative immunosuppression induced by HIV. The specific infections that occur are also a reflection of environmental exposure, which differs according to geographic location and life-style. Perirectal Herpes simplex is seen almost exclusively in homosexual AIDS patients in contrast to patients with other risk factors. Haitian AIDS patients are much more likely to have isosporiasis or tuberculosis than most life-long residents of the United States. Coccidioidomycosis and histoplasmosis are more common in areas endemic for these fungi. The opportunistic processes that occur in adults are primarily those that would be anticipated in patients with deficient T-cell number or function, although why certain infections such as *Listeria monocytogenes* do not occur is a mystery. In pediatric patients, pathogens such as *Pneumococcus* and *Hemophilus* occur that reflect B-cell dysfunction early in life before humoral defenses can be synthesized.

The uniqueness of the opportunistic infections in HIV-infected patients is also made apparent by the impressive frequency of certain pathogens and their clinical presentation. *Pneumocystis* has an attack rate in AIDS patients of 35% to 70% per year, whereas in most other immunodeficient adult populations attack rates are 1% or less.[6] Similarly, *M. avium-intracellulare* and *Cryptosporidia* rarely caused systemic infection or enteritis, respectively, in any immunologically normal or abnormal population before the advent of AIDS.[7,8] Fewer than 20 adult cases of disseminated *M. avium-intracellulare* were reported in the world's literature before 1979, yet since then probably 40% of the 50,000 AIDS cases in the United States have been recognized to be infected. Similarly, *Toxoplasma* encephalitis and mucocutaneous candidiasis are much more common among HIV-infected patients than among other groups of immunodeficient patients.[9]

Qualitatively, opportunistic infections often manifest clinically in a different form in AIDS patients compared to other immunodeficient populations. Pneumocystis pneumonia is a much more indolent and subtle disease in AIDS than in patients with lymphoma or those receiving corticosteroids.[6] Herpes simplex often manifests as perirectal ulceration in AIDS patients, but rarely is this lesion seen in homosexual men with other immunodeficiencies.[10] Thus, the immunologic lesion in AIDS patients influences clinical manifestations, as well as frequency, of infection.

The techniques for diagnosis of opportunistic infections in HIV-infected patients do not differ substantially from those used with other immunosuppressed patients. The large population of HIV-infected patients has provided an opportunity to develop new diagnostic techniques that are directed at the pathogens that are particularly common in AIDS and to take advantage of the large quantities of organisms that are characteristically present. Diagnostic techniques such as sputum induction for *Pneumocystis,* Giemsa's or monoclonal antibody staining for *Pneumocystis,* lysis-centrifugation ·blood cultures for mycobacteria, and modified acid-fast staining for *Cryptosporidia* are examples of new developments that are facilitating the speed, accuracy, and economy of diagnoses, and should continue to evolve rapidly.

Effective therapy is available for many of the opportunistic pathogens that occur commonly in HIV-infected patients. Therapy is not uniformly successful for any of the pathogens listed in Table 12-3, but in most cases a high percentage of cases will respond if therapy is instituted relatively early in the course of the infection. An important characteristic of each of the treatable opportunistic infections in HIV-infected patients, however, is that each has a high likelihood of recurring if specific therapy is discontinued (Table 12-4). Thus, after each infection is successfully treated, consideration needs to be given to a suppressive or prophylactic regimen that

Table 12-1
Opportunistic Infection in HIV-Infected Patients

Common
  Pneumocystis
  Cryptosporidia
  Toxoplasma
  Isospora
  Mycobacterium tuberculosis
  Mycobacterium avium-intracellulare
  Pneumococcus (children)
  Hemophilus (children)
  Salmonella
  Cryptococcus
  Histoplasma
  Coccidioides
  Candida
  CMV
  Herpes simplex
  Herpes zoster
  J–C virus
Uncommon
  Listeria
  Nocardia
  Aspergillus
  Systemic *Candida*
  Mucor

would be continued for life unless the underlying immunosuppression was cured. Whether the regimens used would have to be as intensive as the initial therapeutic regimen remains to be determined. The current practice, for instance, is to switch trimethoprim-sulfamethoxazole therapy for pneumocystis infection from 960 mg trimethoprim/4800 mg sulfamethoxazole daily to 320 mg trimethoprim/1600 mg sulfamethoxazole daily (or 2 or 3 consecutive days per week) in contrast to therapy for toxoplasmosis, which is maintained at full therapeutic daily doses.[11] Finding suppressive regimens that are effective, well tolerated, and economical is a major priority for this patient population.

Before HIV-infected patients develop opportunistic infection, it would be desirable to prevent infections by either reconstituting their immune systems or developing specific anti-infective prophylaxis. Since immune reconstitution of HIV-induced immunodepression is not currently possible, the latter strategy needs to be pursued, especially for those pathogens that produce life-threatening complications. Limiting exposure of patients to specific pathogens may be helpful in a few situations such as avoiding CMV-positive blood products or CMV-positive sexual contacts for a CMV-negative AIDS patient; avoiding exposure to Varicella for VZV-seronegative AIDS patients; and avoiding cat feces or rare lamb for *Toxoplasma*-seronegative AIDS patients. Avoiding respiratory contact with Pneumocystis pneumonia patients might conceivably be useful. Most of the opportunistic infections that develop in HIV-infected patients

Table 12-2
Characteristic Opportunistic Infections in HIV-Infected Patients in the United States

| Organism | Clinical Manifestations | |
	Common	Infrequent
Protozoa		
Pneumocystis carinii	Pneumonia	Otitis
		Dissemination
Toxoplasma	Encephalitis	Pneumonia
	Retino-choroiditis	Dissemination
Cryptosporidium	Enteritis	Cholangitis
		Bronchopleural
Isospora belli	Enteritis	
Fungi		
Candida sp.	Stomatitis	Proctitis
	Esophagitis	Vaginitis
		Dissemination
Cryptococcus neoformans	Meningitis	Pneumonitis
	Dissemination	
Histoplasma capsulatum	Dissemination	
Coccidioides immitis	Dissemination	
Bacteria		
Mycobacterium tuberculosis	Pneumonia	Meningitis
	Dissemination	
Mycobacterium avium-intracellulare	Dissemination	Pneumonia
		Diarrhea
Mycobacterium kansasii	Dissemination	Pneumonia
Streptococcus pneumoniae (esp. pediatric)	Upper respiratory	
	Pneumonia	
	Sepsis	
Hemophilus influenza (esp. pediatric)	Upper respiratory	
	Pneumonia	
	Sepsis	
Salmonella sp.	Diarrhea	
	Sepsis	
Treponema pallidum		Neurosyphilis
Viruses		
Cytomegalovirus	Retino-choroiditis	Adrenal necrosis
	Pneumonia	Encephalitis
	Colitis	Myelitis
Herpes simplex	Mucocutaneous (mouth, digit, rectum)	Pneumonia
		Encephalitis
Herpes zoster	Dermatomal skin	Encephalitis
		Disseminated skin
Epstein-Barr	Hairy leukoplakia	
	Neoplasia (?)	
J–C	Progressive multifocal leuko-encephalopathy	

appear to represent reactivation of latent infections that were acquired prior to the onset of HIV-induced immunosuppression, however. Thus, for most patients chemoprophylaxis against specific pathogens is a more logical strategy. No prophylactic regimen has been proved effective against any pathogen in HIV-infected patients. There is suggestive data, however, that tri-methoprim-sulfamethoxazole 2, 3, or 7 consecutive days per week is effective against *Pneumocystis* although the regimen is poorly tolerated. Pyrimethamine-sulfadoxine and aerosolized pentamidine are also promising. Prophylaxis against mycobacteria, *Toxoplasma,* CMV, and some fungi deserve high priority in certain geographic locations or among certain subpopulations as well, al-

Table 12-3
Therapeutic Options for Common Opportunistic Infections in HIV-Infected Patients

Clinical Manifestation and Etiologic Agent	Standard Therapy	Usual Adult Daily Dose (route, interval)	Investigational Alternatives (route)	Minimal Duration of Therapy
Protozoa				
Pneumocystis pneumonia	Pentamidine isethionate	4 mg/kg (IV, IM, qd)	Pentamidine isethionate (aerosol)	21 days
	Trimethoprim-sulfamethoxazole	15–20 mg/kg 75–100 mg/kg (IV, po, q6–8h)	Trimetrexate (IV) Difluoromethyl ornithine (IV)	
Toxoplasma encephalitis	Pyrimethamine plus	75 mg once, then 25 mg (po, qd)	Pyrimethamine (PO)	Indefinite
	Sulfadiazine	4–8 g (po, q6h)	Clindamycin (IV)	
Cryptosporidia colitis	None	—	Spiramycin (po)	Unknown
Isospora enteritis	Trimethoprim-sulfamethoxazole	640 mg 3.2 g (po, qid)	None	10 days, $\frac{1}{2}$ dose for 3 weeks (bid)
Fungi				
Candida stomatitis	Nystatin	3×10^6 units (po, qd)	Fluconazole	Indefinite
	Clotrimazole	50 mg (po, q4h)		
	Ketoconazole	400 mg (po, q12h)		
	Amphotericin B	0.6 mg/kg (IV, qd)		
Candida esophagitis	Ketoconazole	400 mg (po, q12h)	Fluconazole	14 days
	Amphotericin B	0.6 mg/kg (IV, qd)		
Cryptococcosis	Amphotericin B	0.6 mg/kg (IV, qd)	Fluconazole	Indefinite
	with or without flucytosine	150 mg/kg (po, q4h)		
Histoplasmosis	Amphotericin B	0.6 mg/kg (IV, qd)	Fluconazole	Indefinite
Coccidioidomycosis	Amphotericin B	0.6 mg/kg (IV, qd)	Fluconazole	Indefinite
Bacteria				
Mycobacterium tuberculosis	Isoniazid	300 mg (po, IM, qd)		Indefinite
	plus rifampin	600 mg (po, qd)		
	plus ethambutol	15 mg/kg (po, qd)		
Mycobacterium avium-intracellulare	None	—	Clofazimine and ansamycin plus conventional agents	Unknown
Salmonellosis	Ampicillin	2–12 g (po, IV, q6h)		14–21 days
	Trimethoprim-sulfamethoxazole	20 mg/kg 100 mg/kg (po, IV, q6–8h)		14–21 days
	Chloramphenicol	2–8 g (po, IV, q6h)		

Table 12-3
(*Continued*)

Clinical Manifestation and Etiologic Agent	Standard Therapy	Usual Adult Daily Dose (route, interval)	Investigational Alternatives (route)	Minimal Duration of Therapy
Bacteria (*continued*)				
	Cefotaxime	4–8 g (IV, q6h)		
Viruses				
Cytomegalovirus	Ganciclovir (DHPG)	10 mg/kg (IV, q12h)		Indeterminate
Herpes simplex	Acyclovir	15 mg/kg (po, q4h) (IV, q8h)		Indeterminate
Herpes zoster	Acyclovir	30 mg/kg (IV, q8h)		Indeterminate
Epstein–Barr	None	—	—	—
J–C	None	—	—	—

Table 12-4
Availability of Therapeutic Agents for Opportunistic Infections in HIV-Infected Patients

Pathogens for Which Effective Therapy is Available

Pneumocystis ⎫
Toxoplasma
Isospora
Herpes simplex
Herpes zoster   Recur with
CMV   high frequency
mycobacterium tuberculosis   when therapy
Salmonella   is discontinued
Cryptococcus
Candida
Histoplasma
Coccidioides ⎭

Pathogens for Which no Effective Therapy is Available

Cryptosporidia
Mycobacterium avium-intracellulare
J–C virus

though strategies for such efforts are not currently well formulated.

COMMON PATHOGENS

PNEUMOCYSTIS CARINII. Pneumocystis pneumonia is the most commonly recognized life-threatening opportunistic infection in HIV-infected patients. Pneumocystis pneumonia is the initial AIDS-defining process (infection or tumor) in 65% of HIV-infected patients and ultimately occurs in at least 80% of patients. Because of the frequency and lethality of this opportunistic infection, its diagnosis, therapy, and prevention are major issues in the management of an HIV-infected patient.

Pneumocystis carinii is a ubiquitous protozoan of mammals that appears to be transmitted by a respiratory route.[12] It is presumed (with very little evidence) that human infection occurs early in life, that humans acquire the infection from other humans, and that the infection remains latent until the host becomes significantly deficient in cell-mediated or humoral immunity. *Pneumocystis* has an unusual affinity for the lungs: organisms are rarely found elsewhere. Occasional reports have noted the presence of *Pneumocystis* in liver, spleen, lymph nodes, external auditory canals, skin, and less convincingly, in other organs.[13–15] It is extraordinarily unusual for *Pneumocystis* to cause clinical manifestations outside the lung.

In HIV-infected patients *Pneumocystis* ordinarily presents with some combination of fever, chest tightness, exercise intolerance, shortness of breath, cough, and chest radiographic abnormality. It is now well recognized that in HIV-infected patients, pneumocystis pneumonia can be impressively subtle in presentation and especially indolent in its progression.[6] Well-educated patients and health-care providers can facilitate prompt recognition and evaluation of symptoms. Such early diagnosis appears to improve the prognosis for each episode. Unfortunately the early clinical symptoms, signs, and radiographic abnormalities of pneumocystis pneumonia are indistinguishable from a wide array of trivial or serious upper respiratory and lower respiratory processes including common viral or Mycoplasma upper respiratory infections, influenza, nonspecific pneumonitis, CMV pneumonia, or pulmonary Kaposi's sarcoma. It is important for clinicians to recognize that the chest radiograph in particular may be normal, or may show any pattern of abnormalities including bilateral interstitial or alveolar infiltrates, upper lobe infiltrates, nodules, cavities, or asymmetry.

To establish the presence or absence of pneumocystis pneumonia, there is no cheap, noninvasive screening method. Human *Pneumocystis* cannot be cultivated from pulmonary material, and serologies are nonspecific. Chest radiographs, Gallium scans, pulmonary function tests, computed tomography (CT), and DTPA scanning can each demonstrate abnormalities of pulmonary structure or function.[16-18] None of these techniques is completely sensitive for the presence of histologically documentable pneumonia, however, and all are quite nonspecific, and each requires time and expense that could probably be more profitably directed elsewhere. The diagnosis of pneumocystis pneumonia depends on demonstrating the organism in pulmonary secretions or tissue.

Although bronchoscopy with bronchoalveolar lavage (sometimes with transbronchial biopsy) has become the standard method for obtaining samples for special stains, less invasive techniques are being developed that appear to be faster, safer, better tolerated, and less expensive.[19-21] Early clinical literature prior to the era of HIV infection indicated that patients with pneumocystis pneumonia rarely produced sputum and that analysis of available sputum samples was rarely productive.[23] Investigators from the University of Miami and San Francisco General Hospital have recently demonstrated that sputum can be induced from AIDS patients with pneumocystis pneumonia in most cases.[20,21] Careful evaluation of sputum using Giemsa's or methenamine silver staining techniques can demonstrate organisms in 50% to 60% of those patients ultimately shown to have pneumocystis pneumonia. The efficiency of sputum evaluation can be as high as 90% if sputum smears are processed uniformly and sensitive stains, especially immunofluorescent techniques using monoclonal antibodies against human organisms, are used. The most important variables determining the yield are the skill used to obtain an adequate sample and the expertise available to stain and to methodically survey the smear. Sputum evaluation appears to be useful for patients with subtle or severe clinical manifestations, although more detailed evaluation of these populations is needed. A variety of non-bronchoscopic lavage procedures have been described for obtaining samples.[24] Whether these techniques offer substantial improvements in sensitivity over sputum remains to be determined.

Bronchoalveolar lavage or transbronchial biopsy should demonstrate organisms in over 95% of cases if adequate material is obtained.[19,25] Unpublished studies on asymptomatic HIV-infected patients suggest that *Pneumocystis* is not ordinarily present in the absence of clinical manifestations. Thus demonstration of organisms should be presumptive evidence that *Pneumocystis* is causing pulmonary disease. Histology almost always shows intra-alveolar exudate and cellular infiltrate when *Pneumocystis* is present. The inflammatory response and the number of *Pneumocystis* are often quite impressive despite minimal symptoms and normal or only minimally abnormal chest radiographs.[6] Because Pneumocystis pneumonia is so readily diagnosed by sputum, bronchoalveolar lavage, or transbronchial biopsy, there is little role for open lung biopsy to establish this diagnosis in AIDS patients.

Trimethoprim-sulfamethoxazole (intravenous or oral) and pentamidine isethionate (intravenous) are equally effective therapeutic agents for pneumocystis pneumonia.[6,26,27] Patients may become clinically and radiographically worse during the first 3 or 4 days of therapy. Patients who ultimately survive often do not show convincing signs of improvement for 7 or even 10 days. A very few patients may begin to improve even later. The likelihood of survival depends on the immunologic status of the patient, the presence of concurrent medical problems, the patient's ability to tolerate therapy, and the severity of pulmonary dysfunction at the time therapy is initiated.[28] Severe chest radiographic abnormalities and alveolar–arterial oxygen gradients greater than 30 torr correlate most clearly with a poor prognosis.[28] In general, however, about 80% to 90% of patients with first episodes of pneumocystis pneumonia will survive with standard therapy, and about 60% to 70% of patients with all episodes will survive.[29-31] Patients who have been receiving azidothymide (also known as AZT or zidovudine) at the time pneumocystis pneumonia is documented probably have milder disease and a better prognosis.

The major difficulty associated with trimethoprim-sulfamethoxazole and pentamidine isethionate are the high frequencies of serious adverse effects.[6,26,27,29,32] As many as 70% to 100% of patients on either therapeutic regimen will have an adverse reaction.[26,30,32] Intravenous pentamidine in any patient population is associated with neutropenia, azotemia, hyperglycemia, hypoglycemia, and pancreatitis.[33] (Pentamidine should not ordinarily be given intramuscularly since intramuscular injections can be associated with substantial pain and sterile abscesses; despite previous reports to the contrary, slow intravenous infusion is quite safe and well tolerated.[34] Trimethoprim-sulfamethoxazole is associated with adverse effects that occur with unique and unexplained frequency in HIV-infected patients.[6,32] These include rash, fever, leukopenia, hepatitis, nausea, and nephritis. The leukopenia may correlate with higher trimethoprim levels and may respond to reductions in the dose of trimethoprim from 20 mg/kg/day to 15 mg/kg/day (with parallel reduction in sulfamethoxazole dose). Trimethoprim-sulfamethoxazole therapy can often be continued for the full 21-day course despite adverse effects since these can often be tolerated. As an indication of the frequency of serious adverse effects of standard therapy, however, in one small prospective study only 6 of 20 AIDS patients (30%) started on trimethoprim-sulfamethoxazole and 8 of 20 started on pentamidine were still alive and receiving their original drug 21 days after therapy was initiated.[26]

Because anti-pneumocystis therapy is often unsuccessful or poorly tolerated, several new therapeutic approaches have been developed. Dapsone-trimethoprim has been shown to be an effective oral regimen for patients with mild pulmonary disease.[35-37] Its efficacy relative to standard therapy has not been methodically tested. Adverse reactions to dapsone are very common, but they may not be as severe as those to sulfamethoxazole. Thus, the role for dapsone in the armamentarium of anti-*Pneumocystis* drugs has not been delineated.

To circumvent the systemic toxicity of pentamidine, this drug has been administered to AIDS patients with mild disease as an aerosol.[38-39] Preliminary trials have demonstrated that aerosolized pentamidine can be effective and well tolerated when delivered by this method. Little pentamidine was detected in the serum, and the only adverse reactions was cough. Whether aerosolized pentamidine is as effective as standard therapy for patients with mild disease or severe disease remains to be demonstrated. The ease of administration, low apparent toxicity, and preliminary efficacy results suggest that aerosolized pentamidine may become an important therapy for pneumocystis pneumonia if further trials confirm these early results.

Trimetrexate is a lipid-soluble analog of methotrexate that has much more potent activity against dihydrofolate reductase in *Pneumocystis* organisms than do trimethoprim or pyrimethamine.[40] Trimetrexate has potential antifol activity against both mammalian and protozoan dihydrofolate reductase, but leucovorin can bypass the enzymatic block, and only mammalian cells can transport leucovorin. Thus, leucovorin administered with trimetrexate can prevent mammalian toxicity without diminishing the antiprotozoan effect. Preliminary trials have demonstrated that intravenous trimetrexate with leucovorin is effective and well tolerated therapy.[30] Its major toxicity is granulocytopenia, which can be effectively managed in most cases by increasing the dose of leucovorin. Trimetrexate is clearly an alternative therapy for patients who cannot tolerate either standard therapy or who have failed both standard regimens. Whether trimetrexate is as effective as standard therapy and whether relapses will be more frequent awaits a rigorous comparative trial.

Difluoromethylornithine (DFMO) is an inhibitor of ornithine metabolism that is an effective agent against trypanosomes.[41-43] DFMO has been used successfully in patients who have failed conventional therapy. It has been used as the only therapy with success in a few AIDS patients as well. DFMO causes significant thrombocytopenia. Its role as an anti-*Pneumocystis* agent also remains to be determined.

Because *Pneumocystis* rarely involves organs other than the lung and because physiologic derangement in the lung is caused to a considerable extent by the inflammatory response *Pneumocystis* evokes, attempts to treat pneumocystis pneumonia with corticosteroids have recently been attempted for patients with severe disease.[44] In theory, the anti-inflammatory effects could permit improvement in gas exchange while concurrent administration of anti-*Pneumocystis* agents eradicated the protozoa. Small series have employed corticosteroids in patients with severe hypoxemia either at the time therapy was initiated or when it was clear that standard therapy was failing. Temporary improvement in symptoms, gas exchange, and chest radiograph can be shown, and there have been suggestions of improved survival. Rigorous studies need to define the optimal dose, duration, and timing of corticosteroids in studies designed to assess whether long-term survival is in fact improved.

Trimethoprim-sulfamethoxazole (intravenous or oral) or pentamidine isethionate (intravenous) remains the treatment of choice for pneumocystis pneumonia pending further studies. For patients who are deteriorating after 7 to 10 days of therapy, or for patients who are failing to improve, there are several options: (1) continue current therapy; (2) switch to the alternate standard therapy (trimethoprim-sulfamethoxazole to pentamidine or vice versa); (3) use both standard therapies simultaneously; (4) add corticosteroids; (5) switch to DFMO; or (6) switch to trimetrexate-leucovorin. Which of these options is most likely to be successful remains to be determined. For patients who cannot tolerate either standard therapy due to toxicity, switching to trimetrexate, DFMO, or aerosolized pentamidine can be successful.

A subsequent episode of symptomatic pneumocystis pneumonia will occur within 3 months of terminating therapy in 10% to 40% of patients. Whether these subsequent episodes represent relapse or reinfection is not clear.

Since pneumocystis pneumonia is such a common and potentially life-threatening complication of HIV infection, prevention is an important strategy for the optimal long-term management of patients. AZT can reduce the frequency and severity of pneumocystis pneumonia, but AZT does not eliminate morbidity or death due to this process. How well tolerated prophylactic regimens are when given with AZT remains to be determined. Trimethoprim-sulfamethoxazole (2.5 mg/kg trimethoprim 12.5 mg/kg sulfamethoxazole q12h) is effective prophylaxis in non-AIDS patients when given 7 days per week, or when given 2 or 3 consecutive days per week.[11,45] Anecdotally these regimens are effective in AIDS patients, as is sulfadoxine-pyrimethamine (500 mg and 25 mg respectively) once weekly.[46] These regimens are not tolerated by a substantial portion of HIV-infected patients, especially the former regimen. Aerosolized pentamidine shows promise as a well-tolerated and effective prophylactic agent. There may also be a role for chronic oral trimetrexate-leucovorin.

TOXOPLASMA GONDII. *T. gondii* is a primary cause of focal encephalitis in patients with AIDS, although occasionally it can cause retinochoroiditis and pneumonia.[47-49] The organism is a protozoon whose definitive host is the cat.[50] Man can acquire infection by ingesting infectious oocysts excreted in cat feces or by ingesting meat containing tissue cysts. In non-immunosuppressed patients, *T. gondii* usually causes asymptomatic infection, although it can cause a mononucleosis-like syndrome, characterized by lymphadenopathy, hepatosplenomegaly, and fever, which resolves spontaneously over a few weeks. Based on serologic studies, 20% to 90% of healthy adults have been infected with *T. gondii.*[51]

Although the specific incidence of toxoplasmosis in patients with HIV infection is unknown, at least 3% of patients with CDC-defined AIDS have had toxoplasmosis.[52] Based on serologic studies, in which the presence of anti-*Toxoplasma* antibodies has been demonstrated months prior to the development of toxoplasmosis, disease in most patients appears to represent reactivation rather than primary infection.[47] A much larger proportion of patients with AIDS have been previously infected with *T. gondii,* based on serologic studies, than develop disease. Of patients with AIDS or lymphadenopathy, 31% to 69% have been found to have anti-*Toxoplasma* antibodies, yet only a small proportion of these patients go on to develop reactivation.[49,53] The specific determinants of reactivation are currently unknown.

The primary clinical manifestations of toxoplasmosis in AIDS patients are usually symptoms attributable to focal encephalitis.[47–49] Symptoms often develop subacutely, over the course of a few weeks, and usually include focal neurologic abnormalities such as hemiparesis and seizures, which can be seen in 29% to 89% of patients.[47–49] Symptoms suggesting a diffuse encephalopathy can be seen in 14% to 63% of patients and frequently occur together with focal abnormalities. Headaches, which may be severe and unremitting, occur in about 50% of patients, and fevers are seen in only 60%. Meningismus is seen in less than 10% of cases.

Histopathologically the primary process in the brain is a focal necrotizing encephalitis characterized by a central area of necrosis surrounded by inflammatory cells, which may be associated with arteritis and thrombosis.[47–49] Multiple lesions, usually in the cerebral and cerebellar cortex, are seen at autopsy. To confirm that a necrotic process is indeed due to *T. gondii,* organisms must be identified in the involved area and are usually seen in the periphery, not the central necrotic area.

Occasionally disease manifestations of toxoplasmosis will be seen at other sites. Retinochoroiditis, pneumonitis, and orchitis due to *T. gondii* have all been reported in rare patients.[55–58] *T. gondii* have also been detected in heart, stomach, adrenals, pancreas, and muscle in addition to brain, eyes, and lung at autopsy, although specific symptoms are not always attributable to infections at the former sites.[59]

Routine laboratory evaluation in AIDS patients suspected of having toxoplasmosis is not usually helpful in making the diagnosis. Lumbar puncture yields an abnormal but nondiagnostic spinal fluid, characterized by an elevated protein, mild mononuclear pleocytosis, and normal or minimally depressed glucose levels.[47,48] CT scans are usually abnormal in patients with toxoplas-

mosis, but are nonspecific. Scans will often demonstrate one or more focal abnormalities that will usually enhance following contrast administration.[47,48] Ring enhancement is seen most often, but occasional enhancement in a homogenous pattern is seen. Rarely, a normal CT or absence of contrast enhancement of a hypodense lesion will be seen.[47,48] The sensitivity of CT scanning can be improved by using a double dose of contrast and delaying the scan for 1 hour. Although the role of magnetic resonance imaging (MRI) in toxoplasmosis has not been defined, anecdotal reports have suggested that it may be more sensitive than CT scanning.[47]

Definitive diagnosis of toxoplasmosis requires demonstration of the organisms histopathologically in an involved area or culturing the organism from a body fluid or involved tissue. Since this usually requires an invasive procedure, the diagnosis in immunocompetent hosts has usually been based on serologic studies, such as the Sabin–Feldman dye test or IgG ELISA, that demonstrate high titers of antibody or four-fold changes in titer.[60] More recently, assays to measure IgM, such as a double-sandwich ELISA technique, have been used with greater reliability.[61] Unfortunately, in AIDS patients serologic assays are of limited use in diagnosing toxoplasmosis. IgG assays are positive in virtually 100% of AIDS patients with toxoplasmosis, but, as noted previously, may be positive in up to 70% of patients without clinical evidence of toxoplasmosis.[53,54,59] Titers are elevated (greater than 1:1024) in only 20% of patients with active disease.[54] Moreover, specific anti-*Toxoplasma* IgM is found in less than 5% of patients with toxoplasmosis. In one study, only 1 of 37 AIDS patients with toxoplasmosis had detectable IgM antibodies.[54]

Given the lack of reliability of serologic studies, diagnosis must be based on detection of the organism. This is most commonly done by histopathologic detection of *T. gondii* in brain biopsy specimens. Although there is some risk associated with this procedure, recent innovations such as CT-scan–directed stereotactic needle biopsy have improved the safety of obtaining tissue.[48] *T. gondii* can be detected on hematoxylin and eosin stained specimens, although in one study the organism was not seen in over 50% of positive cases.[54] Immunoperoxidase staining techniques have been found to improve the sensitivity, and were positive in all specimens in one study, but in only 50% in another study.[48,54] Immunofluorescence using monoclonal antibodies or polyclonal serum has also been useful in detecting the organism in impression smears made from biopsy tissue.[62]

Culture of biopsy specimens in tissue culture or mice can also establish the diagnosis, although there may be a delay of a few weeks. *T. gondii* can also be cultured from other clinical specimens, such as blood and bronchoalveolar lavage fluid, although this has only rarely been reported.[63,64]

Therapy should be initiated following a specific diagnosis. In AIDS patients, if a biopsy is not feasible because of the underlying condition of the patient or the location of a lesion, empiric therapy is warranted, especially in a patient with an appropriate CT scan and positive IgG serology. *T. gondii* is the causative agent in a high percentage of contrast-enhancing mass lesions in this patient population. Other processes, however, such as lymphoma, Kaposi's sarcoma, and progressive multifocal leukoencephalopathy, may present with a similar clinical and radiographic picture, and thus a histopathologic diagnosis should be established if possible, especially if response to empiric antitoxoplasma therapy is not prompt. Delay in establishing the diagnosis may result in delay of therapy for other treatable processes.

Therapy of toxoplasmosis has traditionally utilized the toxoplasmastatic combination of pyrimethamine (75 mg for 1 dose, then 25 mg/day orally) plus sulfadiazine (1 g orally 4 times daily) for 4 to 6 weeks.[65] Although *in vitro* and animal data as well as anecdotal human data support the use of this combination, no controlled human studies have been performed in any patient population. This combination has been utilized successfully in a number of AIDS patients, as judged by improvement in clinical symptoms and disappearance of CT-scan-documented lesions.[47–49,66]

Over 80% of patients in two reports responded to this combination, usually within a few weeks.[48,66] However, as with many other infections in AIDS patients, recurrence is common following traditional courses of therapy. Relapses have been reported to occur in 50% to 100% of patients, usually within 2 to 12 weeks of stopping therapy.[47,48,66] Given the high incidence of relapse, therapy should be continued for prolonged periods, probably for life.

There is a high incidence of adverse reactions—approaching 60%—in AIDS patients treated with pyrimethamine plus sulfa drugs.[66] In half of these patients, therapy with these drugs must be discontinued. The most common reactions include neutropenia, fever, and rash, which are also seen in patients with AIDS and *P. carinii* pneumonia who are treated with trimethoprim-sulfamethoxazole. These reactions are probably caused by the sulfa component. Additionally, pyrimethamine, which interferes with folate metabolism, can be associated with leukopenia and thrombocytopenia due directly to bone marrow suppression. Concomitant administration of folinic acid (calcium leucovorin) can bypass the blockade of folate metabolism in mammalian cells without affecting anti-protozoan activity.[65,67] Folinic acid is usually given at a dose of 10 mg intravenously or orally 2 to 3 times a week, although higher doses can be given without complications.

If pyrimethamine plus sulfadiazine cannot be administered, no alternative regimens with well documented efficacy are available. Pyrimethamine alone was effective in only three of seven patients in one report although high doses with concurrent leucovorin rescue was not tried.[47] Clindamycin and spiramycin, two macrolide antibiotics, have been shown to be effective in animals.[68,69] Case reports suggest their efficacy in humans. Clindamycin can be given in doses of 300 mg to 450 mg orally four times daily (although high-dose intravenous therapy is more likely to be effective), and spiramycin 50 mg/kg/day in 2 to 4 divided doses.

Spiramycin has been reported to be ineffective in treating or preventing relapse in four AIDS patients with toxoplasmosis.[70] Trimethoprim-sulfamethoxazole has also been reported to be of use in treating toxoplasmosis, but offers no advantage over pyrimethamine plus sulfadiazine.[71] At least three patients have developed toxoplasmosis while receiving trimethoprim-sulfamethoxazole.[60]

Trimetrexate is an inhibitor of folate metabolism that is about 500 times more potent than pyrimethamine in inhibiting the dihydrofolate reductase (DHFR) of *T. gondii*.[67] Inhibition of mammalian DHFR can be bypassed by the concurrent administration of folinic acid. Tissue culture and animal studies have confirmed that trimetrexate is very active against *T. gondii*.[72] However, preliminary studies in humans with toxoplasmosis have shown that while trimetrexate does have anti-*Toxoplasma* activity, clinical deterioration is eventually seen following prolonged administration of one dosing regimen.[73]

Corticosteroids are frequently used in conjunction with antibiotics in treating patients with toxoplasmosis, primarily in patients with cerebral edema. Because of the concern of exacerbating immunosuppression in an already immunosuppressed patient, steroid use should be limited as much as possible. No significant beneficial or harmful effect has been clearly associated with the use of corticosteroids in patients with toxoplasmosis.

CRYPTOSPORIDIUM. Cryptosporidia have only recently been recognized to be human pathogens.[8] The first case of human disease caused by this veterinary pathogen was reported in 1976, and by 1982, only seven human infections were reported. As more laboratories have learned how to recognize this protozoan in stool specimens, cryptosporidiosis has been shown to be prevalent in heterosexual immunocompetent individuals, in immunocompetent homosexuals, and in AIDS patients. Cryptosporidiosis has particular importance in AIDS because it is in this disease more than any other immunodeficiency that cryptosporidiosis is likely to cause a persistent debilitating diarrhea.[74–76] In immunocompetent individuals who are exposed to this protozoan (i.e., veterinarians and slaughterhouse workers), which is spread by a fecal–oral route, the diarrhea is a mild, self-limiting process.

Cryptosporidiosis has been reported in nearly 4% of AIDS patients in the United States.[76] It occurs more frequently in homosexual or bisexual men than in other North American patients with AIDS. However, in Haiti, 50% of 131 AIDS patients with opportunistic infections were found to have cryptosporidiosis.[75] This difference is probably accounted for by environmental and sanitary conditions related to stool exposure.

The most common clinical presentation of *Cryp-*

tosporidium infection in AIDS patients is severe, watery diarrhea, ranging from a few soft stools daily to 10 to 20 stools per day, that may persist for many months.[76,77] Blood and mucus are usually not present. Crampy abdominal pain, nausea, and occasionally vomiting can also be seen. A profound weight loss ranging from 9 to 18 kg is common, being seen in all 13 patients in two reports.[76,77] Fever can be seen but is not a prominent finding; if present, it is usually under 39°C. Although the organism is primarily a small bowel pathogen, it has been seen in other parts of the gastrointestinal tract. One child with AIDS has been reported to have developed symptomatic *Cryptosporidium* esophagitis.[78]

Cryptosporidium has also been occasionally detected in other sites. Involvement of the gall-bladder and biliary tree has been seen, and has been associated with acalculous cholecystitis as well as biliary stenosis with biliary obstruction.[79,80] Pulmonary cryptosporidiosis has been reported in at least five patients.[81,82]

Cryptosporidia cannot usually be identified in stool by conventional techniques. They can be recognized in iodine-stained wet mounts or in acid-fast stains of stool smears.[83] They are concentrated by sucrose flotation, but not reliably by zinc. In biopsy specimens of gastrointestinal mucosa, they can be recognized by light microscopy or electron microscopy. They are easy to miss on autopsy specimens, since autolysis causes the organisms to separate from mucosal surfaces.

Therapy of cryptosporidiosis has been remarkably unsuccessful. In non-AIDS patients in whom immunosuppression was induced by drugs, clearing of the infection has been temporally associated with decreasing the immunosuppressive regimens. Unfortunately, attempts at immunomodulation in AIDS patients have been unsuccessful to date. Specific chemotherapy directed against cryptosporidia has also been disappointing, despite trials with most antiprotozoan agents.[84]

Spiramycin, a macrolide antibiotic with antitoxoplasma activity, has been reported to be effective in AIDS patients with chronic cryptosporidiosis. Of ten patients (9 with AIDS) treated with 1 g spriamycin three times daily for 1 to 16 weeks, six had complete resolution of diarrhea, and four had symptomatic improvement.[85] In five patients therapy resulted in eradication of the organism from stool specimens. Adverse effects of the spiramycin in this study were minimal, although nausea, vomiting, diarrhea, epigastric pain, and acute colitis have been reported previously. Although anecdotal experiences have not confirmed the efficacy of spiramycin, patients with chronic cryptosporidiosis and symptoms severe enough to require therapy should be considered for a trial of spiramycin (1 g 3 times daily); if the patient has a clinical response, the drug should be continued until there is clearing of the organism from the stool (up to 16 weeks). Supportive measures, including antidiarrheal agents and nutritional supplementation, are important adjuvants to therapy. Appropriate precautions should be observed to prevent transmission of the organism to other immunosuppressed patients.

ISOSPORA BELLI. *I. belli* is a coccidian that has occasionally been reported to cause chronic diarrhea in North American patients with AIDS. Although this organism has been seen in less than 0.2% of AIDS patients reported to the CDC, in Haiti it was seen in 15% (20/131) of patients in one study.[75] The reason for this difference is unknown, but is probably related to environmental factors. The organism is probably transmitted through the fecal-oral route. *I. belli* infection is frequently the initial opportunistic infection seen in HIV-infected patients in Haiti.[75] Clinical manifestations include chronic diarrhea, persisting for a mean of nearly 6 months in 1 study, weight loss, nausea, and crampy abdominal pain.[75] Fever and vomiting are uncommon, occurring in 5/15 and 3/15 patients, respectively, in one report.[75] Fecal leukocytes are rarely seen. Extraintestinal isosporiasis has rarely been seen, having been documented at autopsy to involve lymph nodes in one patient.[86]

Diagnosis of *I. belli* infection depends on demonstration of the organism in stools. *I. belli* can be detected by examining wet mounts of stool or by staining with a modified acid-fast method, techniques identical to those used to identify *Cryptosporidium*.[75] The oocysts of *I. belli* are readily distinguished from *Cryptosporidium* by their size, shape, and number of sporocysts.

Unlike *Cryptosporidium, I. belli* infection can be treated very effectively with trimethoprim-sulfamethoxazole. One regimen reported to be effective is 160 mg of trimethoprim plus 800 mg of sulfamethoxazole 4 times a day orally for 10 days, followed by twice daily therapy for 3 weeks.[75] Whether such a prolonged regimen is necessary is uncertain, since all 15 patients treated with this regimen responded with cessation of diarrhea and abdominal pain within 2 days of beginning therapy. All stool specimens examined while on therapy were negative for *I. belli* organisms after the second day of therapy. Although no evidence of recurrent infection was seen in half the patients during a mean of 5 months of follow-up, in half the patients recurrent symptomatic disease developed within a mean of 8 weeks of cessation of therapy.[75] Whether this recurrence represented relapse or reinfection could not be determined. It is possible that a prophylactic or suppressive regimen, such as lower doses of trimethoprim-sulfamethoxazole given chronically, may be effective in preventing recurrence. Occasional patients with isosporiasis have failed prolonged therapy with trimethoprim-sulfamethoxazole.[87]

Other protozoa rarely cause significant disease in patients with HIV infection. Both amebiasis and giardiasis are common pathogens in homosexual men, but do not appear to occur more frequently or to cause more severe disease in HIV-infected individuals. Rare cases of acanthamoeba meningoenchephalitis have been seen in AIDS patients.[88]

CRYPTOCOCCUS NEOFORMANS. *C. neoformans* is a fungus that is a common cause of meningitis and disseminated disease in patients with AIDS. Although cryptococcosis can occur in normal hosts, immunosuppressed patients, especially patients with defects in cell-mediated immunity, are at risk for developing this infection. In AIDS patients, cryptococcosis occurs in 7% of patients, based on data from the CDC.[52] It may be the presenting manifestation of AIDS (7/27 patients in one series), or may occur simultaneously with (4/27) or subsequent to (16/27) other opportunistic infections or tumors.[89]

The most common clinical presentation of cryptococcosis in AIDS patients, as in other immunosuppressed patients, is meningitis: 72% of 53 patients presented this way in two recent reports.[89,90] Meningitis in this population often presents in a subtle manner. Fever and headache are common, occurring in over 80% of patients. Nausea and vomiting may be seen in half the patients. However, stiff neck, photophobia, focal neurologic abnormalities, papilledema, and seizures are seen in less than 30% of patients. Occasional patients with meningitis will have no signs or symptoms directly referable to the central nervous system. Focal encephalitis due to *C. neoformans* can also be seen in the absence of meningeal involvement.[90]

Extraneural disease due to *C. neoformans* is common in patients with AIDS: 57% of patients (30/53) have been reported to have positive cultures from extraneural sites, and in 25% (13/53) no central nervous system infection could be documented.[89,90] Clinical manifestations of extraneural disease have included skin lesions, pneumonitis, pericarditis with cardiac tamponade, arthritis, retinitis, pleural effusion, and abdominal pain due to cryptococcal peritonitis.[89-94] Skin lesions have been common and include herpetiform lesions as well as lesions that have resembled *Molluscum contagiosum*.[91,92] Pneumonitis is characterized by cough, sputum production, and interstitial infiltrates on chest radiograph.[93] Occasionally patients are entirely asymptomatic but have cryptococcosis documented by positive cultures or serum cryptococcal antigen.[89] At autopsy, *Cryptococcus* has been identified in brain, lung, lymph nodes, adrenal gland, kidney, spleen, liver, bone marrow, and thyroid.[89]

Diagnosis of cryptococcosis requires documentation of the organism by culture or histopathology, or demonstration of cryptococcal antigen in body fluids. In patients with meningitis, lumbar puncture will yield CSF that has only minimal abnormalities: glucose and leukocyte count are normal in two-thirds of patients, and protein is normal in one-third.[89] In 16% of patients in one series, all three parameters were normal.[89] However, CSF India ink is positive in most, and CSF cryptococcal antigen as well as CSF culture are positive in virtually all patients with meningitis.[89,90]

In patients with extraneural disease, diagnosis is usually made by biopsy and culture of affected tissue. For patients with pneumonitis, bronchoscopy appears to be very useful in making the diagnosis. Transbronchial biopsy was positive in 6/8 patients (75%) in one series.[93] An interstitial pattern of dissemination of the organism is usually seen histopathologically. *Cryptococcus* was also identified in 5/8 (63%) bronchial brush specimens, 5/6 (83%) bronchoalveolar lavage specimens, and 7/7 (100%) cell blocks prepared from bronchoalveolar lavage fluid.[93]

Blood, bone marrow, and urine cultures are occasionally positive in the absence of symptoms or when fever alone has been noted.[89] Newer blood culture techniques have probably increased the ability of microbiology laboratories to detect the organism at an earlier point in the disease process. The lysis-centrifugation technique appears to be more sensitive than the radiometric technique. The latter technique has been reported to have failed in detecting *C. neoformans* fungemia in an AIDS patient.[95]

C. neoformans isolated from some patients with AIDS has been reported to differ morphologically from isolates obtained from non-AIDS patients.[96] Colonies may be nonmucoid and dry on primary isolation, and may be poorly encapsulated. Poor encapsulation may lead to confusion histopathologically with other yeast.[93]

Serum cryptococcal antigen is usually positive in patients with disseminated disease, and occasionally has established the diagnosis in the absence of positive cultures.[89,90] Serum cryptococcal antigen is positive in nearly all patients with cryptococcal meningitis.[89] Extraordinarily high titers of cryptococcal antigen have been reported in AIDS patients, from both serum and CSF. These titers have ranged up to 1:2,000,000 in serum, and 1:20,000 in CSF.[97]

Patients with an established diagnosis of cryptococcosis should receive therapy; this should include patients who may be asymptomatic but have positive cultures or cryptococcal antigen, because of the high risk for developing meningitis and disseminated disease.

Two regimens have been found to be effective in treating cryptococcal infection in non-AIDS patients: (1) amphotericin B (0.3–0.6 mg/kg/day) combined with flucytosine (150 mg/kg/day) for 6 weeks, and (2) high-dose amphotericin B (0.6 mg/kg/day) given for 10 weeks as a single agent. Both regimens have been utilized in AIDS patients. Neither regimen has clearly been more efficacious, though controlled studies are lacking.

As reported in two recent studies, only 54% of patients (28/52) who received therapy with amphotericin B alone or combined with flucytosine successfully completed a course of therapy.[89,90] Patients usually received 1 to 2 g of amphotericin B, although over 3 g was occasionally given. Adverse reactions to amphotericin B were common, and included fever, chills, and renal dysfunction, but did not require discontinuation of drug. Adverse reactions to flucytosine were common, and necessitated discontinuation of drug in 30% to 40% of patients. These reactions included bone marrow suppression and liver dysfunction. Recently recommendations for dosing and monitoring non-AIDS patients treated with flucytosine, based on experience obtained during a prospective study, have been published.[98]

Six of 53 patients in two studies received intrathecal amphotericin B in addition to intravenous therapy; only one patient survived.[89,90] At least three patients developed complications secondary to intrathecal therapy, including shunt infection and arachnoiditis. Although intrathecal amphotericin B appeared to be beneficial in a retrospective study of non-AIDS immunocompromised patients with cryptococcal meningitis, this experience cannot be extrapolated to patients with AIDS.[99]

Very few characteristics have been found to be predictive of response to therapy in AIDS patients. In one small study, a CSF cryptococcal antigen titer of at least 1:10,000 was found to be associated with 100% mortality (3/3 patients), compared to 22% (4/18) in patients with titers less than 1:10,000.[90] A positive CSF India ink test also appears to be associated with a poorer prognosis.[89,90] Other factors that have been associated with a poor prognosis in non-AIDS patients, such as low CSF leukocyte count, positive blood cultures, and the presence of *C. neoformans* at extraneural sites, are frequently seen in AIDS patients, but have not been useful in predicting outcome.[100] Relapse rates following cessation of therapy in AIDS patients with cryptococcosis are very high: in two recent studies, 56% (10/18) relapsed,[89,90] usually within a few months of discontinuing therapy. Relapse is associated with a poor prognosis: only 1 of 10 patients (10%) who relapsed responded to a second course of therapy. Because of the high relapse rate, patients who respond to treatment with 2 g of amphotericin B should be continued on suppressive antifungal therapy for prolonged periods, probably for life. The optimal suppressive regimen has not been determined. Amphotericin B given on an outpatient basis is currently most commonly used. Regimens of amphotericin B being evaluated include 100 mg once a week, and 25 mg three times a week.[90] Ketoconazole anecdotally does not appear to be an effective suppressive regimen. Fluconazole, a new imidazole that has efficacy against *C. neoformans* in animal models, is currently being evaluated as a suppressive agent in controlled studies.[101]

HISTOPLASMA CAPSULATUM. *Histoplasma capsulatum* is a fungus that has been recognized with increasing frequency in patients with HIV infection. The organism is a dimorphic fungus that can cause disease in immunocompetent as well as immunosuppressed patients. *H. capsulatum* is endemic to central and southern United States. Initially only rare cases of histoplasmosis were reported in patients with AIDS. This may have been due to the low number of HIV-infected individuals in endemic areas. As HIV infection has become more widespread, it has become clear that these patients are at great risk for developing disseminated histoplasmosis. Among the first 15 Indiana residents diagnosed with AIDS, 7 developed disseminated histoplasmosis.[102,103] Histoplasmosis has also been recognized in nonendemic areas such as New York City,

especially in patients from Puerto Rico as well as Central and South America.[104,105]

In immunocompetent patients, *H. capsulatum* usually causes asymptomatic infection, but may cause pulmonary infection that is usually self-limited. Disseminated disease in immunocompetent patients is distinctly unusual, occurring in less than 1% of infected patients and less than 5% of patients with clinical disease.[106] In AIDS patients, disseminated disease is the primary clinical presentation.[102–105] It may be the initial manifestation of AIDS, or may occur simultaneous with or subsequent to other opportunistic infections. Reactivation of latent disease rather than de novo infection with the organism appears to occur in at least some patients with AIDS.[105]

Presenting symptoms are non-specific and include fever, chills, sweats, weight loss, nausea, vomiting, and diarrhea.[102–105] Pneumonitis with diffuse or patchy reticulonodular infiltrates are also common. Skin lesions and lymphadenopathy have occasionally been the most prominent manifestation at presentation. Symptoms may be present for weeks to months before the correct diagnosis is made. Physical exam may show lymphadenopathy and hepatosplenomegaly. Laboratory evaluation will frequently show leukopenia and thrombocytopenia. Liver dysfunction, characterized by elevation of both alkaline phosphatase and transaminases, may be prominent. In a large number of patients, the chronic wasting syndrome may progress to a picture of septic shock, characterized by fungemia, refractory hypotension, renal, hepatic, and pulmonary failure, disseminated intravascular coagulation, and death.[102–105]

Diagnosis of histoplasmosis depends on documenting the organisms in clinical specimens by culture or histopathology. Serology may be positive and may provide early evidence of infection. In one report, all seven patients had positive serology, and in one patient therapy was instituted presumptively while cultures were pending.[102] In another report, however, serology was negative in all three patients tested.[105] The most rapid method of making the diagnosis is by detecting the organism on clinical specimens that are stained with hematoxylin and eosin, Giemsa's, or methenamine silver.[106] *H. capsulatum* has been seen in bone marrow, liver, lymph node, skin, and bronchoscopic lung biopsy specimens.[102–105] The organisms are usually seen inside macrophages; granuloma are occasionally but not always seen. In rare patients with AIDS, histoplasmosis has been diagnosed from peripheral blood smears, which can demonstrate both intracellular and extracellular organisms.[107]

Cultures of specimens in which the organism is detected by histopathology will almost invariably be positive. However, cultures will frequently be positive when the organism cannot be seen. Unfortunately, this may delay the diagnosis for a few weeks. Cultures of blood and bone marrow are most frequently positive. In one study 5/5 patients with histoplasmosis had positive blood cultures.[104] Although blood cultures obtained by standard techniques can be positive, recent studies suggest that the lysis-centrifugation technique may be positive more frequently and at an earlier time than standard techniques.[108] In one study of non-AIDS patients, blood cultures were positive in a mean of 8 days by the former technique, compared to 24 days by standard techniques.[109] The organism has also been found in lymph nodes, urine, bronchoscopy specimens, liver, skin, and CSF.

Therapy should be instituted based on histopathologic or culture documentation of histoplasmosis. Occasionally empiric therapy in an acutely ill patient who has been to an endemic area, and who has positive serology, may be warranted, as noted above.[102] Amphotericin B is the drug of choice in immunosuppressed patients with histoplasmosis. Although ketoconazole is effective in nonimmunosuppressed patients, in immunosuppressed patients it does not appear to be as effective as amphotericin B. Patients will often respond rapidly to institution of amphotericin B, with improvement in symptoms occurring in a few days.[102-105] Ten of 14 patients treated with amphotericin B responded clinically to therapy. Therapy should be continued until a total dose of 2 to 3 g has been given.

The relapse rate following cessation of therapy in AIDS patients with histoplasmosis is high: of 10 patients who responded to amphotericin B, 5 did not receive a suppressive drug regimen. All 5 relapsed, usually within a few months.[102-105] The remaining 5 patients received ketoconazole, usually 400 mg/day, as a suppressive regimen following discontinuation of amphotericin B. None of these five patients relapsed, with a follow-up period of up to 6 months. However, at least three patients have been reported to have failed chronic ketoconazole therapy.[110-111] Thus, while it is clear that a suppressive regimen is needed following successful treatment of histoplasmosis in AIDS patients, it is uncertain what regimen is best. An alternative to ketoconazole would be low dose amphotericin B, given intermittently in an outpatient setting.

COCCIDIOIDES IMMITIS. *C. immitis* is a fungus-like *H. capsulatum* that can cause disease in both non-immunosuppressed and immunosuppressed patients. Disease is seen primarily in endemic areas such as the southwestern United States, especially southern California and Arizona. Although this includes areas where HIV infection is common, coccidioidomycosis has rarely been reported in AIDS patients. However, recent reports suggest that patients with HIV infection are in fact at increased risk for disseminated coccidioidomycosis. In a retrospective study, of 27 patients with AIDS in Tucson, 7 (26%) developed coccidioidomycosis.[112] It was estimated in this study that coccidioidomycosis occurred at an annual rate of 27% in this population, or at a rate of 2.7% per year of lifetime exposure to the organism. Coccidioidomycosis can occur prior to or concurrent with other opportunistic infections.

In non-immunocompromised patients, infection with *C. immitis* is usually inapparent or self-limited.

Disseminated disease may develop, but it has been estimated to occur only in 1.2% of nonimmunocompromised patients who develop infection severe enough to require hospitalization.[112] In immunocompromised patients, however, especially in patients with AIDS, dissemination occurs much more frequently: all seven patients in one report presented with disseminated disease.[112] Although it is not clear in all cases whether disseminated disease represents reactivation of latent infection, or newly acquired infection, at least one case of reactivated disease has been documented in the literature.[113]

Clinical manifestations of coccidioidomycosis in AIDS patients may include a prodrome of fever, malaise, and weight loss, that may be present for up to 12 weeks.[112] Cough may be very prominent, and may be associated with bilateral reticulonodular or nodular infiltrates: five of seven patients in one series presented in such a manner.[112] Diagnosis is based on detection of the organism by culture or histopathology in clinical specimens. For patients with pulmonary infiltrates, sputum specimens are occasionally positive, but bronchoscopy with bronchoalveolar lavage, washings, and biopsy will frequently demonstrate the organism, being positive in 1/1, 3/5, and 3/4 specimens, respectively, in one series.[112] Other sites may also be positive: the organism has been isolated from blood, bone marrow, urine, liver, and lymph node biopsies.[112-114] Blood cultures may be positive using standard media, but the lysis-centrifugation technique appears to improve the yield.[115] At autopsy, the organism has also been found in the kidneys, spleen, brain, and thyroid.[112] Bone, joint, and skin infection, commonly seen in chronic dissemination, have not been reported in this population. Serology may play a role in diagnosis: in 5/7 patients in one study, serological tests were reactive at the time of diagnosis.[112]

Optimal therapy in AIDS patients with coccidioidomycosis has not been determined. Ketoconazole as initial therapy appears to be inadequate. Amphotericin B, in doses ranging up to 2500 mg, has been associated with gradual clinical improvement.[112] Ketoconazole following amphotericin B has been reported to control symptoms, although relapse can occur within three weeks of discontinuing ketoconazole therapy.[112] Based on limited published data and on the experience in other fungal infections in patients with AIDS, suppressive regimens should be continued following control of symptoms in AIDS patients with coccidioidomycosis. Whether ketoconazole is a more effective regimen than low dose amphotericin B has not been sufficiently evaluated to date.

***CANDIDA* SPECIES.** *Candida* species frequently cause annoying symptomatic mucosal disease in AIDS patients, but rarely do these yeasts cause life threatening processes. *Candida* infections ultimately occur in almost all patients with AIDS.

Candida infections of the oropharynx are very commonly the initial clinical manifestation of HIV infection.[116,117] Characteristic white plaques develop on the buccal mucosa, tongue, or palate and can be diagnosed either by their typical appearance or by a smear of the lesion. Oral candidiasis must be distinguished from the white mucosal lesions of hairy leukoplakia which may have some resemblance to candidiasis but will not show sheets of yeast on smear. Oral candidiasis so rarely occurs in an individual who is not diabetic, not receiving antibiotics, not receiving corticosteroids, and not known to be immunosuppressed that its occurrence in an apparently healthy individual without these risk factors should raise a high suspicion of HIV infection. If an HIV-infected individual develops oral candidiasis (that is not related to antibiotic therapy), the likelihood of his developing a life threatening opportunistic infection or Kaposi's sarcoma in the next few months is substantial.[117] In one series the interval between oral candidiasis and opportunistic infection in this population was 3 months (median) and 1–23 months (range).[117] Similar figures would probably apply to *Candida* proctitis or recurrent vaginal candidiasis in seropositive individuals.[118] *Candida* pharyngitis is usually annoying and may interfere with nutrition, but does not cause life threatening complications. Oral candidiasis is usually persistent or recurrent when patients are not taking antifungal drugs.

Candida is the most frequent cause of esophagitis in HIV-infected patients.[119–120] Herpes simplex, CMV, Kaposi's sarcoma, peptic disease, *Mycobacteria,* and lymphoma can cause esophogeal lesions, but *Candida* is the most common. Symptoms, radiologic appearance on barium swallow, and endoscopic characteristics are typical of those seen with candida esophagitis associated with other immunodeficiencies. Symptoms can be relatively indolent for many weeks or months before the appropriate diagnosis is established. Life-threatening complications such as perforation or hemorrhage are very uncommon. The non-life-threatening characteristics of *Candida* esophagitis and the overwhelming likelihood that esophagitis will be caused by *Candida* in an HIV positive individual encourage many clinicians to institute empiric antifungal therapy.[120] Diagnosis is sought only if there is no response. Endoscopic biopsy is the optimal technique for establishing this diagnosis and ruling out concomitant processes.

Candidemia or *Candida* involvement of organs other than those mentioned above is very uncommon. When candidemia does occur, it is usually related to intravenous or intra-arterial vascular devices.

Oral candidiasis usually responds readily to topical agents such as nystatin or clotrimazole, or to oral ketoconazole. Amphotericin B is occasionally necessary for patients who do not respond to nystatin, clotrimazole, or ketoconazole. Seven to 10 days of 0.6 mg/kg/day usually suffices although even this therapy will fail to clear a few patients. When therapy is stopped, oral candidiasis usually recurs promptly, so chronic topical or oral therapy is usually needed for life. *Candida*

esophagitis is usually treated with ketoconazole or amphotericin B.

MYCOBACTERIA. *Mycobacterium avium-intracellulare* and *M. tuberculosis* occur with great frequency among HIV-infected patients. *M. kansasii, M. fortuitum, M. ulcerans, M. bemophilum,* and other atypical mycobacteria have also been reported to occur. In assessing the clinical importance of mycobacteria in clinical specimens and determining a therapeutic strategy, it is important to assume that the organism in question is clinically important and is amenable to therapy (which should be started), until the laboratory identifies the mycobacterial species and its susceptibilities, at which time the desirability of therapy can be reassessed. *M. avium-intracellulare* occurs with particular frequency among North American patients.[7,121] The organism can be isolated from at least 40% to 60% of patients before they die. *M. avium-intracellulare* infection is usually a disseminated process.[7,121–123] The organism can be cultured from blood, stool, urine, bone marrow, lymph nodes, intestinal wall, bronchoalveolar lavage fluid, or various organ biopsies.[7,121–123] Histopathology of biopsy or autopsy material often shows large clumps of organisms. Inflammatory response may be well established with granulomas, but more often granulomas are not seen and there is minimal or absent inflammatory response. Clearly the organism can be present in impressive quantities at one or more body sites, but it is not always certain what contribution *M. avium-intracellulare* makes in producing clinical symptoms or signs.

Many HIV-infected patients have fever, weight loss, lympadenopathy, and/or diarrhea. In many of these patients no pathogenic viruses, fungi, or protozoa can be identified as the likely causative organisms, but *M. avium–intracellulare* can be isolated from various sites. Whether the *M. avium-intracellulare* is causing the concurrent symptoms and signs is difficult to establish since this *Mycobacterium* can be cultured or seen histopathologically in some asymptomatic individuals, and because there is no effective therapy that could be used to empirically assess whether eradication of the organism alleviated signs and symptoms.[122,124–126] At this juncture it is the presumption of many clinicians that *M. avium-intracellulare* can contribute substantially to the fever, weight loss, inanition, and diarrhea associated with HIV disease. However, the identification of *M. avium-intracellulare* in a clinical specimen should not deter the clinician from searching for other pathogens that are more amenable to therapy.

M. avium-intracellulare isolates from AIDS patients are usually susceptible *in vitro* to clofazimine (88%), cycloserine (95%), and ethionamide (78%).[124] Isolates are usually not susceptible to concentrations of ansamycin likely to be found in the blood although most (92%) are susceptible to higher concentrations.[124] Isolates are rarely susceptible to isoniazid, and only 25% to 35% are susceptible to rifampin or ethambutol. There are isolated reports of clinical and microbiologic responses to regimens containing amikacin or ethambutol, but no regimen has been consistently effective using clinical or microbiologic criteria.

Although other atypical mycobacteria have been documented to cause localized and disseminated infections and disease in HIV-infected patients, these other atypical organisms are relatively uncommon. *Mycobacterium tuberculosis* is a frequent cause of disease in HIV-infected patients, particularly those who come from populations in which *M. tuberculosis* infection is common.[127-130] The failure of *M. tuberculosis* rates in the United States to continue their long standing downward trend in 1985 appears to be related to substantial numbers of cases among HIV-infected drug abusers and Haitians. In one series from New Jersey 24 of 102 drug abusers and 4 of 8 Haitians had tuberculosis in contrast to 0 of 22 homosexuals.[128] In another series from New York City the frequency of tuberculosis was comparable in drug abusers and homosexuals (11% and 7%, respectively) but over half the patients were Black or Hispanic.[127] Haitians, it would appear, have a particular predisposition to tuberculosis: 61% of 45 Haitian patients in Miami had tuberculosis.[121] Tuberculosis appears to be more common than *M. avium-intracellulare* among AIDS patients in Africa.

Tuberculosis can present months or several years prior to other clinical manifestations of HIV infection although it can be a late complication of AIDS as well. About 50% of patients will present with a pulmonary (as opposed to extrapulmonary) manifestation. Upper lobe lesions and cavities which are ordinarily characteristic of adult reactivated disease are much less common among HIV-infected patients than are lower lobe infiltrates that are unilateral or bilateral.[131] Diffuse pulmonary infiltrates are not uncommon. Infiltrates are often associated with hilar, paratracheal, or mediastinal adenopathy which can be a helpful radiologic clue. Extrapulmonary lesions involving bone, kidney, brain, lymph nodes, and virtually any other site have been reported.

Diagnosis of *M. tuberculosis* can be suggested by sputum smear when the morphology of the acid-fast organisms is carefully assessed to distinguish the organisms from atypical mycobacteria. The yield on sputum smears is relatively low, however, compared to culture of sputum or biopsy material.[121,127,128] Bone marrow, lymph nodes, and other extrapulmonary sites that are clinically abnormal are more likely to show histopathologic evidence of acid-fast organisms than is sputum. In contrast to *M. avium-intracellulare* lesions, *M. tuberculosis* lesions often are associated with granulomas including necrotizing granulomas.[121,127,128]

The susceptibility of *M. tuberculosis* in HIV-infected patients has not differed from the susceptibility from non-AIDS patients. Most organisms are susceptible *in vitro* to isoniazid, rifampin, and ethambutol or pyrizinamide. Clinically tuberculosis in this patient population

responds readily to therapy. Three drug therapy with isoniazid, rifampin, and ethambutol is recommended although there are no comparative studies demonstrating that this three drug regimen is more effective than other regimens. There is little information about the optimal duration of therapy, but it seems unwise to some clinicians to discontinue therapy at any point unless drug toxicity precludes antimycobacterial therapy.

Prevention of tuberculosis could presumably be accomplished in HIV-infected patients who were not yet anergic by skin testing for *M. tuberculosis* and instituting isoniazid prophylaxis in positive patients. Whether isoniazid would be effective prophylaxis and whether it should be continued for life remain to be determined.[130]

***SALMONELLA* SPECIES.** Infection with nontyphoidal *Salmonella* species has recently been reported in patients with AIDS, and appears to be a manifestation of the underlying immunodeficiency.[132-135] Infection can occur prior to the diagnosis of AIDS: in one series, 5/8 patients with salmonellosis had infection documented 3 to 11 months before the development of another opportunistic infection.[135] Salmonellosis was diagnosed in 4.2% (3/71) of AIDS patients at one center, and in 6% (8/130) of patients at another.[133,135]

AIDS patients with salmonellosis usually present with nonspecific symptoms: fever, malaise, fatigue, anorexia, cachexia, myalgias, and weight loss.[132-134] Diarrhea that is watery but not bloody or mucoid is seen very commonly, being reported in 7/8 patients in one series.[135] Symptoms may be present for many weeks. An unusual aspect of salmonellosis in AIDS patients is the high incidence of bacteremia. Whereas nontyphoidal *Salmonella* infections in other patients are usually limited to the gastrointestinal tract, and bacteremia occurs only in an estimated 1% to 5% of patients, bacteremia is very common in the setting of AIDS.[132-136] Of 16 patients reported in three studies, 14 presented with bacteremia.[132-134] Stool cultures are usually positive in patients with bacteremia, although in one report stool cultures were positive for *Salmonella* at presentation in only 1 of 8 patients.[135]

Diagnosis of salmonellosis in patients with AIDS is based on culturing the organism from clinical specimens. As noted above, blood and stool cultures are most frequently positive. Occasionally, urine and bronchoscopy cultures will also be positive. At autopsy the organism has been isolated from the lung, liver, heart, bone marrow, kidneys, and brain. The organism most frequently isolated from patients with AIDS is *Salmonella typhimurium:* all 16 patients in three reports were positive for this organism.[132-135] *Salmonella choleraesuis* and a serogroup D *Salmonella enteridites* have also been reported.[134] It is uncertain if the high incidence of *Salmonella typhimurium* isolation is due to a predisposition for infection with this organism in immunocompromised individuals, or because this is the serotype most commonly found to cause human disease.

Most isolates of *Salmonella* cultured from AIDS patients have been sensitive to antibiotic commonly used to treat salmonellosis, including ampicillin, trimethoprim-sulfamethoxazole, and chloramphenicol. Although in nonimmunocompromised patients with *Salmonella* gastroenteritis, antibiotic therapy is usually not necessary, and may prolong the duration of infection, *Salmonella* infections in AIDS patients should be treated, even if these infections are limited to the gastrointestinal tract, because of the risk of bacteremia. Most patients will respond clinically to intravenous ampicillin (6–12 g/day), given for a 2- to 3-week period.[132–135] Occasionally, blood or stool cultures may remain positive during therapy despite treatment with an antibiotic to which the organism is sensitive; symptoms may persist or may improve despite persistent positive culture. In most patients cultures become negative shortly after institution of therapy.

Once therapy is discontinued, there is a very high incidence of relapse, including bacteremia, in AIDS patients with *Salmonella* infection. Among 22 patients described in 4 reports, 16 (73%) developed recurrent positive cultures, usually associated with symptoms.[132–135] Recurrent bacteremia was seen in 13 of these patients. Despite extensive evaluation for the source of persistent infection, including evaluation of the heart, bones, gall bladder, and urinary tract, no site of persistent infection could be documented. Organisms isolated during recurrence usually remained sensitive to the antibiotics which were used for treatment, and patients responded to a second course of therapy. Because of the high incidence of relapse, a suppressive regimen should be given after completion of therapy. Oral ampicillin or amoxacillin given at doses of 1 to 2 g per day have been used, although there is only limited evidence that such regimens are successful. Occasional patients receiving oral therapy have become culture positive.

OTHER BACTERIAL INFECTIONS. A number of other bacterial infections have been documented in patients with AIDS. Since AIDS patients will remain at risk for commonly acquired infections such as pneumonia or sinusitis, it is not always clear if these infections are occurring with greater incidence in patients with AIDS compared to the general population. At one center, 10% of 176 episodes of pneumonia were caused by bacterial pathogens, including *Haemophilus influenzae* and *Streptococcus pneumoniae,* which accounted for 78% of the bacterial pneumonias.[137] Although chest radiographs in these patients would often show lobar infiltrates, in 6 episodes (4 due to *H. influenzae*) diffuse infiltrates were seen. Bacteremia was seen in 4/18 episodes. Specific antimicrobial therapy resulted in a clinical response in 16/18 episodes.

Bacteremia due to organisms other than *Salmonella* species has been reported in two large studies to occur in 10% of patients with AIDS.[137,139] In one study intravenous drug use may have predisposed to infection, but in the other this etiology could not be implicated. Neu-

tropenia was only rarely seen. Although some infections, especially those due to *Staphylococcus epidermis* and gram-negative rods, appeared to be nosocomial in nature, others, especially those due to *S. aureus,* which was seen in 28% of cases, were most often community acquired. Two patients were reported with bacteremia due to *Listeria monocytogenes,* a pathogen frequently seen in other patients with defects in T-cell mediated immunity.[139] Most evaluable patients responded to appropriate antimicrobial therapy.

Although the incidence of venereal diseases such as syphilis and gonorrhea appear to be decreasing in recent years, a trend possibly related to AIDS, two reports suggest that the occurrence of syphilis in HIV-infected patients may have a different natural history from syphilis in other patients.[140,141] Five patients with HIV infections are reported to have developed neurosyphilis manifest as acute syphilitic meningitis (one patient), meningovascular syphilis (three patients), and asymptomatic neurosyphilis (one patient). At least three patients received adequate treatment for primary or secondary syphilis, and appear not to have been reinfected in the interval. Diagnosis was based on examination of cerebrospinal fluid: VDRL test was positive in all, and white blood cell count, protein, and glucose were abnormal in most patients. All patients responded to high dose intravenous penicillin G, although focal defects persisted in the three patients with meningovascular syphilis. These reports suggest that in patients with HIV infection, standard therapy for primary or secondary syphilis may be inadequate, and neurosyphilis, especially meningovascular syphilis, may occur sooner and more frequently than expected. Although firm recommendations cannot be made based on these cases, it would be reasonable to do lumbar puncture on all patients with HIV infection in whom a diagnosis of syphilis is made, and to closely follow patients who receive benzathine penicillin for therapy.

Infections due to *Nocardia asteroides* have rarely been reported in HIV-infected patients, occurring in an estimated 0.3% of AIDS cases.[142] Pulmonary nocardiosis has been seen most commonly; bronchoscopy with bronchoalveolar lavage may be more sensitive than bronchoscopic biopsy in making the diagnosis.[143] Pericarditis, brain abscess, osteomyelitis, and blood stream infection have also been reported.[142] Patients respond to therapy with trimethoprim-sulfamethoxazole, although relapse may be seen following discontinuation of therapy.[142] Because of the high incidence of adverse reactions associated with trimethoprim-sulfamethoxazole therapy in AIDS patients, alternative therapy may be needed. One patient has been reported to have responded to minocycline plus amikacin followed by minocycline plus cycloserine.[143]

A number of other bacterial infections have been reported in patients with AIDS. *Legionella pneumophila* has been reported as a cause of sinusitis in one patient, and has occasionally caused pneumonia.[144] At the National Institute of Health (NIH), this organism has been isolated from pulmonary specimens of a few patients with a concurrent diagnosis of *P. carinii* pneumonia, and has been found isolated from the blood and spleen of one patient.

CYTOMEGALOVIRUS. Cytomegalovirus (CMV) infection is common in most human populations. In the United States, 45% to 80% of the general population is infected in different cities, with higher frequencies among socioeconomically disadvantaged groups. CMV can be transmitted sexually, congenitally, or by blood. Thus, the patient populations with high frequencies of HIV infection are particularly likely to have been infected with CMV. For homosexual males, for example, over 90% are infected. Even asymptomatic, HIV seronegative individuals often shed CMV in their throat and urine.

As HIV-infected patients become progressively immunosuppressed, the likelihood of finding CMV in their blood as well as their urine and throat increases.[145] A major diagnostic problem is determining whether the CMV recognized by culture, histology, or histopathology is causing concurrent symptoms and signs. Many AIDS patients have fever, weight loss, fatigue, lethargy, altered mental status, and other findings at a time when CMV, *Mycobacterium avium-intracellulare,* and Epstein-Barr virus can all be cultivated from various body sites. Conversely, CMV can be isolated from blood, urine, and throat in AIDS patients who are asymptomatic.[145] Thus in many clinical situations the role of CMV for causing disease is unclear. Further diagnostic efforts and therapeutic trials are needed to delineate the effects of CMV on producing disease.

CMV is the most common opportunistic pathogen recognized when AIDS patients come to autopsy.[1-5] In about 30% of AIDS patients CMV is recognized as a major contributor to death. The CMV syndromes of clinical importance that most commonly present in HIV-infected individuals are retinochoroiditis, enteritis, and pneumonitis.[146-149]

CMV is by far the most common cause of retinochoroiditis in HIV-infected patients.[150] Rare cases of retinochoroiditis due to fungi, mycobacteria, and *Toxoplasma* have been seen, but CMV causes well over 95% of cases. Patients with severe depression in T4 lymphocyte number usually complain of floaters, blurred vision, or decreased field of vision. Funduscopic examination reveals findings that are quite distinct from cotton wool spots, which are retinal infarcts that have no etiologic, pathogenetic, or prognostic relationship to CMV disease. Findings of CMV disease include yellow-white exudate, hemorrhage, edema, vessel attenuation, and sheathing. These findings can be confused with other infectious or neoplastic causes of retinal disease, but experienced ophthalmologists are usually confident that these etiologies can be excluded on clinical grounds. The natural history of CMV retinochoroiditis in HIV-infected patients is progression at a variable rate to complete visual loss in the affected eye. Progression may be quite indolent

at certain time points. However, no cases of spontaneous resolution have been reported.

There is no easy and safe way to establish a definitive diagnosis of CMV retinitis. CMV disease is unlikely in a CMV seronegative, blood culture negative patient, but most HIV-infected patients are also CMV seropositive, so serology is not useful. Blood culture results are not available for many weeks even if a reliable laboratory facility is available. Vitreal aspirates or biopsies can be done but there are potential complications, especially retinal detachment when the latter procedure is performed. Since CMV retinochoroiditis has a distinctive clinical appearance and since other etiologies are so uncommon, diagnosis is established usually on the basis of clinical findings.

CMV also causes enteritis.[146,148,151] CMV enteritis may be the initial clinical manifestation of HIV infection or may be a late manifestation after other opportunistic infections and tumors have occurred. Chapter 13 describes in detail the gastrointestinal manifestations of AIDS including the long list of potential etiologies for diarrhea and for esophagitis. CMV is not among the more common causes of diarrhea, but because it is potentially lethal and because it is treatable, it is an important entity to recognize. CMV colitis can manifest as cramps, increase in stool frequency, voluminous watery diarrhea, bloody diarrhea, or rectal discharge. Bowel perforation and substantial gastrointestinal hemorrhage can occur. Colitis is the most common gastrointestinal manifestation of CMV, but esophagitis, proctitis, and small bowel disease also occur.[146-148] The natural history of these entities when untreated are still being defined.

To establish a diagnosis of CMV enteritis, other more common causes of diarrhea, proctitis, or esophagitis must be evaluated as described in Chapter 13. If stool examination is unrevealing of enteric bacterial or protozoan or helminthic pathogens when evaluating diarrhea, colonoscopy with colonic biopsy should be performed. The diagnostic criteria for determining when bowel disease is caused by CMV are not yet clear, but the presence of gross inflammation by visual inspection combined with typical CMV inclusion bodies on histopathology are probably solid bases for instituting therapy. Endoscopic biopsy is also the basis for establishing a diagnosis of CMV esophagitis.

CMV causes pneumonitis in HIV-infected patients. There is considerable debate about the diagnostic criteria for CMV pneumonitis, so that characterizing the clinical manifestations is currently difficult. Many immunosuppressed patients including those who are HIV-infected have various combinations of the following findings: rare CMV inclusion body on biopsy; many CMV inclusion bodies on biopsy; CMV culture positivity of lavage fluid; presence of CMV antigens on lavage cells; positive CMV cytology; minimal to severe mononuclear cell inflammatory response. Which of these findings correlate with CMV being the cause of pulmonary dysfunction is unclear. Some patients with occasional CMV inclusion bodies or CMV culture positive lavage fluid (which may represent oropharyngeal contamination) survive for many months without specific antiviral therapy, while some patients with many CMV inclusion clearly respond to antiCMV therapy or die with extensive CMV pneumonia at autopsy if they are untreated.

CMV has been reported to cause cerebral disease, myelitis, pericarditis, endometritis, glomerulitis, epididymitis, hepatitis, and adrenal necrosis.[148-155] It is not apparent that any of these manifestations are commonly of clinical importance. Neurologic disease caused by CMV is discussed in Chapter 11.

Ganciclovir (DHPG or 1,3-dihydroxy-2-propoxy methyl guanine) has *in vitro* activity against CMV at concentrations that can be achieved clinically. Preliminary results treating retinochoroiditis and enteritis have been encouraging.[146-148,156] For retinochoroiditis, doses of 5 mg/kg intravenously q12h for 14–21 days will usually but not invariably produce resolution of the inflammatory lesions. In the largest series to date, 87% of 60 patients and 77% of 22 patients improved or stabilized.[146,149] Viremia was cleared in 77% to 88% of patients. Discordance is sometimes observed between response of CMV retinochoroiditis and enteritis or pneumonitis.[148] Therapy is usually instituted when lesions are close to the macula or extensive areas of the peripheral retina are involved. Visual acuity often improves as the edema and inflammation subside, but areas of retina that were directly involved by the necrotizing process do not recover but merely scar. After therapy is terminated, retinochoroiditis usually recurs at the original sites within days or several weeks, and thus a maintenance suppressive regimen is necessary for the patient's lifetime. The optimal regimen is not yet known, but 6 mg/kg IV once daily 5 to 7 days per week is often used. Ganciclovir causes bone marrow suppression: neutropenia is often a complication which requires suspension of therapeutic or maintenance regimens, especially when the patient is receiving other marrow suppressive drugs. An oral form of ganciclovir is not currently available.

Ganciclovir has been shown to be effective in the treatment of enteritis in preliminary trials.[147,148] In one cooperative trial, 74% of 31 patients with colitis had clinical improvement including 35% with a complete response. For patients with esophagitis and proctitis, 80% of 5 patients and 75% of 4 patients, respectively, had complete responses.[147] Of 33 patients evaluable for relapse, 40% relapsed at a median time of 9 weeks. All improved with a second course of therapy.

Several cases of CMV pneumonia in HIV-infected patients have been successfully treated, although several treatment failures have also been reported.[148] The role of ganciclovir for the therapy of CMV pneumonia is therefore less well established.

Phosphonoformate has activity against CMV *in vitro* and has undergone some clinical trials.[157] Preliminary trials suggest that it has clinical efficacy but its role in relation to ganciclovir remains to be established.

HERPES SIMPLEX. Herpes simplex is a frequent cause of mucosal and cutaneous disease in HIV-infected patients. Most disease appear to reflect reactivation of latent infection. Manifestations may represent the initial clinical indication of HIV-induced immunosuppression, or they can become apparent and recurrent later in the course of AIDS.

The most common manifestations of Herpes simplex disease in homosexual males with HIV infection is colitis or perirectal ulceration.[10] Chronic genital lesions are also seen occasionally.[158] The perirectal lesions may present as erythema or tenderness and proceed to ulcerate. They can reach many centimeters in diameter and be mistaken for decubitus ulcers or cellulitis. A diagnosis can be readily established by stained lesion smears or by culturing a swab of the lesion. Herpes simplex colitis is usually confined to the rectum and can present with itching, burning, pain, hematochezia, fever, or rectal discharge. Proctoscopy can show mild inflammation or severe mucosal inflammation with considerable friability. Severe pain can be associated with reflex spasm of the anal and urethral sphincters. Diagnosis can be readily established by rectal swab or rectal biopsy.

Patients with rectal or perirectal lesions can infect their fingers with Herpes simplex and then infect other sites. Ulcerated lesions of the finger and lip may be associated with rectal lesions or can occur independently.

A few cases of Herpes simplex encephalitis, meningitis, esophagitis, and pericarditis have been observed in HIV-infected patients, but it is not clear if the frequency or severity of these manifestations are altered by the HIV infection. Disseminated Herpes simplex infection has not been reported as a complication of HIV infection.

Acyclovir administered orally or intravenously is very effective for cutaneous or mucosal Herpes simplex disease in HIV-infected patients. A course of 200 mg orally five times daily or 5 mg/kg IV three times daily for 7 to 10 days is usually enough to cause lesions to resolve. Like other treatable causes of infectious diseases in HIV-infected individuals, Herpes simplex lesions often recur within days or weeks of cessation of therapy and the patient must be maintained on a chronic regimen of oral acyclovir at doses of 200 mg two to five times daily.

HERPES ZOSTER. Herpes zoster is a herpesvirus that is the etiologic agent of chickenpox and dermatomal zoster (shingles). Dermatomal zoster has been noted with a high frequency among members of groups at risk for AIDS, and appears to be related to infection with HIV. In one study, 35/48 (73%) consecutive patients with dermatomal zoster were infected with HIV.[159] Dermatomal zoster appears to be an early marker for the immunosuppression associated with HIV infection. It frequently occurs months to years before other opportunistic infections or tumors develop. In one study zoster was diagnosed approximately 1 year prior to the development of oral thrush and oral hairy leukoplakia, two infections that are highly predictive of the development of AIDS.[160] In that study AIDS occurred in 22% of patients with zoster. It was estimated that within 4 years of diagnosis of dermatomal zoster, nearly 50% of patients will have developed AIDS. It is important to remember, however, that dermatomal zoster can occasionally occur in healthy young HIV seronegative individuals, and is thus not specific for HIV infection.

Herpes zoster has been found to cause both dermatomal and disseminated disease in patients with HIV infection, occurring in 10% and 6%, respectively, of patients with AIDS in one series.[145] Shingles can localize to any dermatome; ophthalmic zoster has been seen frequently and may be associated with an increased incidence of complications such as keratitis and uveitis.[161,162] Painful zoster, severe zoster, and zoster of the head and neck have been associated with development of AIDS.[160] Disseminated zoster may occur either after dermatomal presentation or in the absence of such lesions. It is unknown how often dissemination occurs following localized disease, but the incidence appears to be low. Disseminated zoster in AIDS patients has manifested primarily as cutaneous vesicles, particularly on the hands and feet. One patient with AIDS developed progressive neurologic dysfunction 3 months after an episode of shingles, and was documented at autopsy to have Herpes zoster encephalitis.[163] Herpes zoster has also been cultured from the spinal fluid of a patient with subacute encephalitis, although it is uncertain what role this virus played in disease.[164]

A clinical diagnosis of dermatomal zoster is usually sufficient. Multinucleated giant cells can be seen in scrapings from the vesicles of patients with local or disseminated disease, and the virus can be cultured readily. Histopathologically, intranuclear inclusions can be seen, but this does not distinguish among the herpesviruses.

Patients with disseminated zoster should be treated because painful lesions will often persist without therapy. Intravenous acyclovir at high doses (10 mg/kg 3 times daily) has resulted in prompt resolution of lesions in several patients, although the lesions have usually recurred in the same distribution within a few weeks of stopping therapy. Chronic suppression with oral acyclovir may be necessary in such patients, although the efficacy of such an approach has not been documented. Oral acyclovir is not very effective in treating H. zoster infection, although high doses (800 mg 5 times a day) should be used if oral therapy is attempted. The need for therapy in dermatomal zoster has not been evaluated. However, most patients, especially those who do not have AIDS, will resolve the lesions without therapy. There is no evidence that acyclovir will resolve the lesions more rapidly or result in less severe pain in such patients. Patients with ophthalmic zoster probably should receive therapy with intravenous acyclovir because of the risk of ocular complications. Corticosteroids should be avoided in HIV-infected individuals with zos-

ter because they may produce further immunosuppression.

EPSTEIN–BARR VIRUS. Epstein–Barr virus (EBV) infection can cause fever, lymphadenopathy, and fatigue in immunocompetent or immunosuppressed patients. The virus can be isolated from throat-washings of over 90% of AIDS patients, and one-third of patients have EBV antigens on their circulating lymphocytes.[145] Virtually all AIDS patients have serologic evidence of infection with EBV.[165]

It is not clear what role EBV plays in causing disease in patients with HIV infection. The virus has been found in oral hairy leukoplakia lesions, in conjunction with papillomavirus.[166,167] Oral hairy leukoplakia usually does not cause significant patient discomfort, but may predict the development of AIDS in HIV-infected individuals. EBV has also been associated with lymphoid interstitial pneumonitis in children with AIDS, as well as undifferentiated, Burkitt-like lymphomas in adults and children with HIV infection.[168,169] It is uncertain what role, if any, EBV plays in fevers and lymphadenopathy that are frequently seen in HIV-infected patients. Currently there is no effective therapy for EBV infection, although anecdotal reports have suggested that acyclovir may have a beneficial effect on oral hairy leukoplakia.

FREQUENT CLINICAL SYNDROMES CAUSED BY INFECTIOUS AGENTS

PNEUMONIA. Pulmonary dysfunction is one of the most common diagnostic and therapeutic problems that develops in HIV-infected individuals. The major concern is to determine whether a treatable infectious or neoplastic process is causing the abnormal symptoms, signs, or radiologic findings. Because pneumocystis pneumonia is by far the most common treatable cause of pulmonary dysfunction (Table 12-5) and because pneumocystis pneumonia can be so subtle and indolent in presentation, the initial problems confronting physicians is to determine if lower respiratory dysfunction is really present, and if it is, whether *Pneumocystis* can be demonstrated. If lower respiratory dysfunction is present, but *Pneumocystis* cannot be demonstrated by sputum or bronchoscopic techniques, the next phase of management is to decide if further diagnostic evaluation is merited.

Deciding whether or not lower respiratory tract disease is present is not easy in HIV-infected patients who may have difficulty distinguishing true shortness of breath from weakness, fatigue, myalgia, or the other systemic toxicities of chemotherapeutic agents such as alpha interferon. When patients develop cough, it is not always easy to determine if the cough represents an upper or lower respiratory tract process. Because early institution of appropriate antimicrobial therapy appears to improve survival for pneumocystis pneumonia as well as presumably other pulmonary processes, it is important to educate patients and health care providers to bring these symptoms to medical attention early, before they are severe and prognosis is presumably worse. The chest radiograph is not terribly helpful. Patients with histopathologically florid pneumocystis pneumonia may have normal or minimally abnormal radiographs. *Pneumocystis* can present with nodules, cavities, upper lobe infiltrates, or lobar processes. The presence of pleural effusions may suggest pulmonary Kaposi's sarcoma, especially if thoracentesis shows a bloody effusion. The chest radiograph is also helpful to assess heart size and pulmonary vascularization to help assess whether the pulmonary process is due to congestive heart failure (e.g., AIDS-related cardiomyopathy) rather than pneumonitis. Evaluation of the chest radiograph may cause the clinician to expedite the work up and direct the bronchoscopist, but by itself a normal chest radiography should never be a reason to delay or defer further evaluation.

When HIV-infected patients present with pulmonary manifestations, their immunologic status is a major clue to the likelihood that they have an opportunistic process. HIV-infected patients, regardless of their immunologic status, are subject to community and hospital acquired pathogens such as *Influenza, Mycoplasma, Legionella, Pneumococcus,* and *Hemophilus.* As their immunologic function deteriorates they reach a threshold for susceptibility for opportunistic infection. The precise degree of immunologic dysfunction necessary to produce susceptibility to *M. tuberculosis,* histoplasmosis, and coccidioidomycosis is not clear but patients may develop these processes, as well as Kaposi's sarcoma, lymphoma, and non-specific pneumonitis many months or years before they become susceptible to *Pneumocystis* or cytomegalovirus. These latter two infections rarely if ever develop in patients with T4 lymphocyte counts greater than 250/mm³ (unless circulating lymphocyte counts have been altered by splenectomy or experimental therapies). Thus, the urgency to proceed to sputum evaluation, bronchoscopy, and perhaps open lung biopsy is much greater in patients with less than 250/mm³ T4 cells.

To assess whether the lower respiratory tract as opposed to the upper respiratory tract is infected, a variety of tests have been proposed including determination of diffusion capacity, gallium scanning, DTPA scanning, and computerized tomography. These techniques are all time consuming, costly, and not completely sensitive, so they are becoming less popular. Cases of pneumocystis pneumonia have been documented with normal gallium scans, diffusing capacities, or CT scans.

Since there is no reliable, noninvasive technique to determine if a lower respiratory process is present, diagnostic evaluation should proceed as outlined in Figure 12-1. Sputum can be induced with 3% saline in most patients. When pneumocystis pneumonia is present, sputum can establish the diagnosis in 55% to 90% of patients if the sample is carefully assessed.[20,21] The use-

Table 12-5
Etiology of 232 Episodes of Pneumonitis in 174 AIDS Patients at National Institutes of Health, 1982–87, Determined by Bronchoscopy or Open Lung Biopsy

Etiology	Percent of Episodes
Pneumocystis (N = 94)	40.5
Nonspecific pneumonitis (N = 75)	32.3
CMV (N = 7)	3.0
Mycobacterium avium-intracellulare (N = 4)	1.7
Kaposi's sarcoma (N = 12)	5.2
Bacteria (N = 6)	2.6
Cryptococcus (N = 3)	1.3
Legionella (N = 1)	<1.0
Lymphoma (N = 1)	<1.0
No diagnosis (N = 24)	10.3
Negative lavage only or normal lung	

fulness of induced sputum for diagnosing other pathogenic processes is less clear. If the sputum examination is negative, bronchoscopy with bronchoalveolar lavage and transbronchoscopic biopsy is indicated. Bronchoalveolar lavage has a sensitivity of about 95% for detecting *Pneumocystis.*[19,25] Other pathogenic microorganisms can also be seen, although the efficiency of yield is not as well documented, and the criteria for diagnosing some infections, such as CMV pneumonitis, is uncertain. Transbronchial biopsy may document a few cases of pneumocystis pneumonia that are missed by bronchoalveolar lavage, and can document CMV inclusion bodies, granulomas, nonspecific pneumonitis, and lymphoma. Kaposi's sarcoma cannot be reliably diagnosed by transbronchial biopsy because of the potential to confuse crush artifact and inflammatory cells with Kaposi's sarcoma in small tissue fragments.[170–172] The presence of endobronchial Kaposi's sarcoma is not a reliable indicator that the parenchymal disease is necessarily due to the same process. If no diagnosis is established by bronchoscopy, the decision to proceed to open lung biopsy is determined by the severity and rate of progression of the pulmonary problem, and the institutional likelihood that a treatable process was missed by bronchoscopy. At institutions where there is considerable experience with lavage, where large tissue fragments are obtained by transbronchial biopsy, and where the pathologists and microbiologists are skilled, the likelihood of missing a pathogen may be low enough to minimize the enthusiasm for proceeding to open lung biopsy unless the patient is rapidly deteriorating. Patients with non-specific pneumonitis may spontaneously resolve their symptoms and radiographic abnormalities, thus obviating the need for further evaluation.[173] If the pulmonary disease is severe or deteriorating, open lung biopsy may be appropriate. The most common process missed by bronchoscopic evaluation is Kaposi's sar-

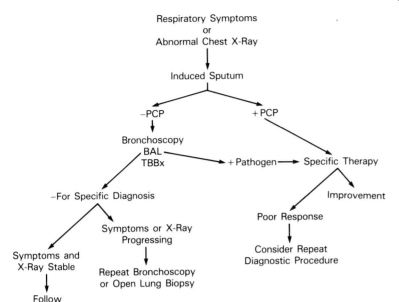

FIG. 12-1. Diagnostic evaluation for infection of the lower respiratory tract.

coma.[170-172] Occasionally a fungal or mycobacterial or CMV pneumonia will be recognized only at open lung biopsy. When Kaposi's sarcoma is documented in the lung, it may be difficult to determine if the Kaposi's sarcoma is extensive enough to cause the pulmonary dysfunction, or whether a second process is also present. A CT scan may be useful to assess this by distinguishing between exudate and tumor. Preliminary evidence suggests that chemotherapy or radiation therapy may palliate patients with pulmonary Kaposi's sarcoma, so this diagnosis is useful to pursue.

Pulmonary dysfunction is a recurrent problem in HIV-infected patients with poor immunologic function. Aggressive prophylaxis against the most common pathogen, *Pneumocystis,* combined with patient education about seeking prompt medical attention, and expeditious diagnostic evaluation should reduce the deleterious impact of pulmonary disease on the quality and duration of patient survival.

FEVER. AIDS patients have many reasons to have temperature elevations that may be related to infection, tumor, or drug therapy. If the AIDS patient has no localizing findings after careful routine examination for the pathogens already discussed, a reasonable evaluation would include:

1. Culture of blood for routine bacteria, fungus, mycobacteria (using lysis-centrifuged or radiometric system), cytomegalovirus
2. Serum cryptococcal antigen
3. Bone marrow aspirate for culture (bacteria, fungus, mycobacteria) and special stains (the latter should be performed even if no granulomas are seen)
4. Stool culture for pathogenic bacteria
5. Stool examination for protozoa and helminths
6. Lumbar puncture
7. Gallium scan
8. Biopsy of clinically abnormal lymph node
9. Culture of urine for mycobacteria, fungus
10. Culture of sputum for mycobacteria, fungus
11. Abdominal CT scan

The cause of fever is often difficult to identify. If the gallium scan shows increased uptake in the lungs or lymph nodes, biopsy procedures may reveal unsuspected *P. carinii* in the former, or fungus, mycobacteria, or Kaposi's sarcoma in the latter. Often such biopsies, directed only by gallium scan, show nonspecific inflammation and thus are not helpful. Cryptococcal infection, mycobacterial infection, or (less often) histoplasmosis or coccidiodomycosis may be identified by cultures of blood, bone marrow, urine, or lymph nodes even when there are no prominent abnormalities other than fever. Culture of stool for *Salmonella* or for other enteric pathogens may reveal a source of fever that was unsuspected from the quantity of stool passed, for example, *Salmonella* or *Shigella.*

As mentioned in previous sections, even if an identified pathogen is treated, the fever may persist, and it becomes difficult to decide if the infective agent in question, such as *C. neoformans* or *Salmonella,* is adequately treated or if another process is responsible for the fever. Similarly, if cytomegalovirus is identified in the blood or EBV is present in circulating leukocytes, it is impossible to be certain that these agents are causing the fever. In some patients there is no apparent new pathogenic organism, and the suspicion may be that Kaposi's sarcoma (particularly extensive visceral disease) is producing fever: in several patients aggressive chemotherapy for the Kaposi's sarcoma has led to shrinkage of tumor and resolution of fever. In other patients HIV may be the cause of fever, but there is no current evidence proving this.

The focus of a fever work-up should be on those causes that are reversible by current therapy: *P. carinii,* fungal processes, *Salmonella,* CMV, and *M. tuberculosis.* Only when effective therapy for EBV, or *M. avium-intracellulare* is available will identification of these organisms be worthwhile from a therapeutic point of view.

CENTRAL NERVOUS SYSTEM DISORDERS. About 10% to 20% of AIDS patients develop an infectious complication in the central nervous system at some point during the course of the disease. Progressive dementia without focal lesions radiologically, anatomically, or clinically is often recognized. HIV can infect the brain and is probably the etiologic agent of subacute encephalitis in many patients, although the role of other as yet unidentified viruses is also commonly discussed.[174] CMV has occasionally been detected in the brain, and may be an agent of encephalitis and myelitis. Herpes zoster has rarely been found to cause encephalitis.

Focal neurologic lesions are also recognized frequently in AIDS patients. Patients may present initially with cognitive disorders, seizures, or focal motor and sensory deficits. If a CT scan shows any contrast-enhancing lesion(s), the differential diagnosis includes toxoplasmosis, lymphoma, or, conceivably, cryptococcoma or tuberculoma. If there are multiple hyodense lesions that do not contrast-enhance, progressive multifocal encephalopthy is the most likely cause. Brain biopsy should be considered although an empiric trial with pyrimethamine and sulfadiazine is often appropriate if the lesion is consistent with toxoplasmosis. If the patient does not respond promptly to therapy, a biopsy becomes more imperative.

Meningitis is also a common complication of AIDS. Aseptic meningitis is often recognized in HIV seropositive patients: HIV may be the causative organism. Cryptococcal meningitis is the most common cause of life threatening meningitis, but tuberculosis, coccidiodomycosis, and lymphoma have also been documented. Some patients present with meningoencephalitis and multiple cranial nerve abnormalities in association with other evidence of disseminated viral processes such as zoster, but the relationship of the zoster to the meningoencephalitis has not been conclusively established.

Neurological abnormalities are discussed in greater detail in Chapter 11.

DIARRHEA. Many AIDS patients complain of frequent bowel movements with or without cramps, tenesmus, mucus or blood. In some patients the symptoms are due to a colitis that can be caused by a multitude of organisms that are included in the term *gay bowel syndrome.* In many patients, however, the stools are frequent, watery, and associated with midepigastric cramps, suggesting a small bowel etiology. In some patients the problem is more annoying than medically important. In other patients, however, the diarrhea can be so voluminous and associated with so much nausea and vomiting that the patient becomes incapacitated by weight loss and inanition.

A comprehensive evaluation including multiple stool examinations for pathogenic bacteria, protozoa, and helminths, upper endoscopy with quantitative bacterial counts and appropriate blind biopsies, and lower endoscopy, may reveal abnormalities. Microorganisms commonly found in homosexual men may be present, such as *G. lamblia, E. histolytica,* or *Salmonella, Shigella,* or *Campylobacter* sp. Other pathogens specific to the immunodeficiency of AIDS, such as *Cryptosporidium,* CMV or *M. avium–intracellulare,* may also be seen. In patients from outside the United States, especially, for example, Haiti, *Cryptosporidium* and *I. belli* are by far the most common pathogens isolated.[75] Most of these infections can be treated, although as with other opportunistic infections in AIDS patients, recurrence of gastrointestinal infections such as CMV colitis or *I. belli* infection, is common following discontinuation of therapy. Even when identified pathogens are eradicated, diarrhea often persists. It is uncertain whether the diarrhea is due to viruses, undetected cryptosporidia, Kaposi's sarcoma of the mucosa, or *M. avium-intracellulare,* all of which can be found at autopsy.

From a practical point of view, pathogenic bacteria, protozoa, and helminths should be sought and treated specifically. If such treatment fails to eradicate the diarrhea, palliative therapy with antidiarrheal agents may be the only alternative left for clinicians. If the patient has extensive Kaposi's sarcoma of the gastrointestinal tract, chemotherapy has in some cases been associated with marked diminution in volume and frequency of diarrhea. Until more information is available about the benefits and toxicities of various chemotherapeutic regimens, diarrhea alone cannot be a reasonable indication for chemotherapy.

Severe diarrhea can be one of the most distressing complications of AIDS. When it is fulminant, the patient's mobility is restricted, family and medical personnel often become reluctant to participate in his care, and the nutritional depletion of the patient magnifies other clinical difficulties.

Gastrointestinal manifestations of HIV infection are discussed more fully in Chapter 13.

REFERENCES

1. Moskowitz L, Hensley GT, Chen JC et al: Immediate causes of death in acquired immunodeficiency syndrome. Arch Path Lab Med 109:735, 1985
2. Niedt GW, Schinella RA: Acquired immunodeficiency syndrome: Clinicopathologic study of 56 patients. Arch Path Lab Med 109:727, 1985
3. Welch K, Finkbeiner W, Alpers C et al: Autopsy findings in the acquired immunodeficiency syndrome. JAMA 252:1152, 1984
4. Hui AN, Koss MN, Meyer PR: Necropsy findings in the acquired immunodeficiency syndrome: A comparison of

premortem diagnosis with postmortem findings. Hum Pathol 15:670, 1984

5. Guarda LA, Luna MA, Smith JL et al: Acquired immunodeficiency syndrome: Postmortem findings. Am J Clin Path 81:549, 1984

6. Kovacs JA, Hiemenz JW, Macher AM et al: *Pneumocystis carinii* pneumonia: A comparison between patients with the acquired immunodeficiency syndrome and patients with other immunodeficiencies. Ann Intern Med 100:663, 1984

7. Green JB, Sidhu GS, Lewin S et al: *Mycobacterium avium-intracellulare:* A cause of disseminated life-threatening infection in homosexuals and drug abusers. Ann Intern Med 97:539, 1982

8. Current WL, Reese NC, Ernst CL et al: Human cryptosporidiosis in immunocompetent and immunodeficient persons. N Engl J Med 308:1252, 1983

9. Levy RM, Bredesen DE, Rosenblum ML: Neurological manifestations of the acquired immunodeficiency syndrome (AIDS): Experience at UCSF and review of the literature. J Neurosurg 62:475, 1985

10. Siegel FP, Lopez C, Hammer G et al: Severe acquired immunodeficiency syndrome in male homosexuals manifested by chronic perianal ulcerative *Herpes simplex* lesions. N Engl J Med 305:1439, 1981

11. Hughes WT, Rivera GK, Schell MJ et al: Successful intermittent chemoprophylaxis for *Pneumocystis carinii* pneumonitis. N Engl J Med 316:1627, 1987

12. Hughes WT: *Pneumocystis carinii* pneumonitis. CRC Press, Boca Raton, FL, 1987

13. Grimes MM, LaPook JD, Bar MH et al: Disseminated *Pneumocystis carinii* infection in a patient with acquired immunodeficiency syndrome. Hum Pathol 18:307, 1987

14. Heyman MR, Rasmussen P: *Pneumocystis carinii* involvement of the bone marrow in acquired immunodeficiency syndrome. Am J Clin Pathol 87:780, 1987

15. Coulman CV, Greene I, Archibald RWR: Cutaneous *Pneumocystis.* Ann Intern Med 106:396, 1987

16. Mason GR, Duane GB, Mena I et al: Accelerated solute clearance in *Pneumocystis* pneumonia. Am Rev Respir Dis 135:864, 1987

17. Coleman DL, Dodek PM, Golden JA et al: Correlation between serial pulmonary function tests and fiberoptic bronchoscopy in patients with *Pneumocystis* pneumonia and the acquired immunodeficiency syndrome. Am Rev Resp Dis 129:491, 1984

18. Tuazon CV, Delaney MD, Simon GL et al: Utility of Gallium-67 scintigraphy and bronchial washings in patients with the acquired immunodeficiency syndrome. Am Rev Respir Dis 132:1087, 1985

19. Ognibene FP, Shelhamer J, Gill V et al: The diagnosis of *Pneumocystis carinii* pneumonia in patients with the acquired immunodeficiency syndrome using subsegmental bronchoalveolar lavage. Am Rev Resp Dis 129:929, 1984

20. Pitchenik AE, Ganjei P, Torres A et al: Sputum examination for the diagnosis of *Pneumocystis carinii* pneumonia in the acquired immunodeficiency syndrome. Am Rev Resp Dis 133:226, 1986

21. Bigby TD, Margolskee D, Curtis JL et al: The usefulness of induced sputum in the diagnosis of *Pneumocystis carinii* pneumonia in patients with the acquired immunodeficiency syndrome. Am Rev Respir Dis 133:515, 1986

22. Kovacs JA, Gill V, Swan JC et al: Prospective evaluation of a monoclonal antibody in the diagnosis of *Pneumocystis carinii* pneumonia. Lancet 2:1, 1986

23. Lau WK, Young LS, Remington JS: *Pneumocystis carinii* pneumonia: Diagnosis by examination of pulmonary secretions. JAMA 236:2399, 1976

24. Caughey G, Wong H, Gamsu G et al: Nonbronchoscopic bronchoalveolar lavage for the diagnosis of *Pneumocystis* pneumonia in the acquired immune deficiency syndrome. Chest 88:659, 1985

25. Stover DE, White DA, Romano PA et al: Diagnosis of pulmonary disease in acquired immune deficiency syndrome (AIDS): role of bronchoscopy and bronchoalveolar lavage. Am Rev Respir Dis 130:659, 1984

26. Wharton MJ, Coleman DL, Wofsey CB et al: Trimethoprim-sulfamethoxazole or pentamidine for *Pneumocystis carinii* pneumonia in the acquired immune deficiency syndrome: A prospective randomized trial. Ann Intern Med 105:37, 1986

27. Haverkos HW: Assessment of therapy for *Pneumocystis carinii* pneumonia: PCP therapy project group. Am J Med 76:501, 1984

28. Brenner M, Ognibene FP, Lack EE et al: Prognostic factors and life expectancy of acquired immune deficiency syndrome patients with *Pneumocystis carinii* pneumonia. Am Rev Resp Dis 139:1199, 1987

29. Murray JF, Garay SM, Hopewell PC et al: Pulmonary complications of the acquired immune deficiency syndrome: An update. Am Rev Respir Dis 135:509, 1987

30. Allegra CJ, Chabner BA, Tuazon CU et al: Trimetrexate, a novel and effective agent for the treatment of *Pneumocystis* pneumonia in patients with acquired immune deficiency syndrome. N Engl J Med 317:978, 1987

31. Wachter RM, Luce JM, Turner J et al: Intensive care of patients with the acquired immune deficiency syndrome: Outcome and changing patterns of utilization. Am Rev Respir Dis 134:891, 1986

32. Gordin FM, Simon GL, Wofsy CB et al: Adverse reactions to trimethoprim-sulfamethoxazole in patients with the acquired immune deficiency syndrome. Ann Intern Med 100:495, 1984

33. Pearson RD, Hewlett EL: Pentamidine for the treatment of *Pneumocystis carinii* and other protozoal diseases. Ann Intern Med 103:782, 1985

34. Mallory DL, Parrillo JE, Baily KR et al: The cardiovascular effects and safety of intravenous and intramuscular pentamidine isethionate. Crit Care Med 15:503, 1987

35. Hughes WT, Smith BL: Efficacy of diaminodiphenylsulfone and other drugs in murine *Pneumocystis carinii* pneumonitis. Antimicrob Agents Chemother 26:436, 1984

36. Mills J, Leoung G, Medina I et al: Dapsone is ineffective therapy for *Pneumocystis* pneumonia in patients with AIDS. Clin Res [Abstr] 34:101A, 1986

37. Leoung GS, Mills J, Hopewell PC et al: Dapsone-trimethoprim for treatment of *Pneumocystis carinii* pneumonia in the acquired immunodeficiency syndrome. Ann Intern Med 105:45, 1986

38. Bernard EM, Pagel L, Schmitt HJ et al: Clinical trials with aerosol pentamidine for prevention of *Pneumocystis carinii* pneumonia. Clin Res 35:468A, 1987

39. Montgomery AB, Luce JM, Turner J et al: Aerosolized pentamidine as sole therapy for *Pneumocystis carinii* pneumonia in patients with acquired immunodeficiency syndrome. Lancet 11:480, 1987

40. Allegra CJ, Kovacs JA, Drake JC et al: Activity of antifolates against *Pneumocystis carinii* dihydrofolate reductase and identification of a potent new agent. J Exp Med 165:926, 1987

41. Golden JA, Sjoerdsma A, Santi DV: *Pneumocystis carinii* pneumonia treated with alpha-difluoromethylornithine: A prospective study among patients with acquired immunodeficiency syndrome. West J Med 141:613, 1984

42. Neibart E, Sacks HS, Hammer G et al: Difluoromethylorinithene (DFMO) in the treatment of *Pneumocystis carinii* pneumonia (PCP). Abstracts of the 26th Interscience Conference on Antimicrobial Agents and Chemotherapy. New Orleans, LA. American Society for Microbiology, Washington, DC, p 224, 1986

43. Paulson YJ, Gilman TM, Boylen OP et al: Eflornithine treatment of *Pneumocystis carinii* pneumonia in twenty patients failing other therapy. Abstracts of the 26th Interscience Conference on Antimicrobial Agents and Chemotherapy. New Orleans, LA. American Society for Microbiology, Washington, DC, p 224, 1986

44. MacFadden DK, Hyland RH, Inouye T et al: Corticosteroids as adjunctive therapy in treatment of *Pneumocystis* pneumonia in patients with acquired immunodeficiency syndrome. Lancet 1:1477, 1987

45. Hughes WT, Kuhn S, Chaudhary S et al: Successful chemoprophylaxis for *Pneumocystis carinii* pneumonitis. N Engl J Med 297:1419, 1977

46. Madoff LC, Scairizzo D, Roberts RB: Fansidar secondary prophylaxis of *Pneumocystis carinii* in AIDS patients. Clin Res 34:524A, 1986

47. Navia BA, Petito CK, Gold JWM et al: Cerebral toxoplasmosis complicating the acquired immune deficiency syndrome: Clinical and neuropathological findings in 27 patients. Ann Neurol 19:224, 1986

48. Wanke C, Tuazon CU, Kovacs A et al: *Toxoplasma* encephalitis in patients with acquired immune deficiency syndrome: diagnosis and response to therapy. Am J Trop Med Hyg 36:509, 1987

49. Wong B, Gold JWM, Brown AE et al: Central-nervous-system toxoplasmosis in homosexual men and parenteral drug abusers. Ann Intern Med 100:36, 1984

50. Frenkel JK: Toxoplasmosis: Parasite life cycle, pathology, and immunology. In Hammond DM (ed): The Coccidia, p 343. Baltimore, University Park Press, 1983

51. Remington JS, Desmonts G: Toxoplasmosis. In Remington JS, Klein JO (eds): Infectious Diseases of the Fetus and Newborn, 2nd ed, p 143. Philadelphia, WB Saunders, 1983

52. Centers for Disease Control: Update: Acquired immunodeficiency syndrome—United States. Morbid Mortal Week Rep 35:542, 1986

53. Derouin F, Beauvais B, Lariviere M: Serologic study of the prevalence of toxoplasmosis in 167 patients with acquired immunodeficiency syndrome (AIDS) or chronic lymphadenopathy syndrome (LAS). Biomed Pharmacother 40:231, 1986

54. Luft BJ, Brooks RG, Conley FK et al: Toxoplasmic encephalitis in patients with acquired immune deficiency syndrome. JAMA 252:913, 1984

55. Weiss A, Margo CE, Ledford DK et al: Toxoplasmic retinochoroiditis as an initial manifestation of the acquired immune deficiency syndrome. J Ophthalmol 101:248, 1986

56. Parke DW, Font RL: Diffuse toxoplasmic retinochoroiditis in a patient with AIDS. Arch Ophthalmol 104:571, 1986

57. Catteral JR, Hofflin JM, Remington JS: Pulmonary toxoplasmosis. Am Rev Respir Dis 133:704, 1986

58. Nistal M, Santana A, Paniaqua R et al: Testicular toxoplasmosis in two men with the acquired immunodeficiency syndrome. Arch Pathol Lab Med 110:744, 1986

59. Luft BJ, Conley F, Remington JS et al: Outbreak of central-nervous-system toxoplasmosis in Western Europe and North America. Lancet 1:781, 1983

60. McCabe RE, Remington JS: *Toxoplasma gondii.* In Mandell RG, Douglas JR, Bennett JE (eds): Principles and Practice of Infectious Disease, 2nd ed, p 1540. New York, John Wiley & Sons, 1985

61. Naot Y, Remington JS: An enzyme-linked immunosorbent assay for the detection of IgM antibodies of *Toxoplasma gondii:* Use for diagnosis of acute acquired infection. J Infect Dis 142:757, 1980

62. Sun T, Greenspan J, Tenenbaum M et al: Diagnosis of cerebral toxoplasmosis using fluorescein-labeled antitoxoplasma monoclonal antibodies. Am J Surg Pathol 10:312, 1986

63. Hofflin JM, Remington JS: Tissue culture isolation of *Toxoplasma* from blood of a patient with AIDS. Arch Intern Med 145:925, 1985

64. Toubol JL, Salmen D, Lancaster F et al: Pneumopathie à *Toxoplasma gondii* chez un patient atteint de syndrome d'immunodepression acquis' mise en evidence du parasite par lavage bronchiolo-alveolaire. Rev Pneumol Clin 42:150, 1986

65. Frenkel JK, Hitchings GH: Relative reversal by vitamins (p-aminobenzoic, folic, and folinic acids) of the effects of sulfadiazine and pyrimethamine on *Toxoplasma,* mouse and man. Antibiot Chemother 7:630, 1957

66. Haverkos W: Assessment of therapy for *toxosplasma* encephalitis. Am J Med 82:907, 1987

67. Allegra CJ, Kovacs JA, Drake JC et al: Potent *in vitro* and *in vivo* antitoxoplasma activity of the lipid-soluble antifolate trimetrexate. J Clin Invest 79:478, 1987

68. Araujo FG, Remington JS: Effect of clindamycin on acute and chronic toxoplasmosis in mice. Antimicrob Agents Chemother 5:647, 1974

69. Garin JP, Eyles DE: Le traitement de la toxoplasmose experimentale de la souris par la spiramycine. Presse Med 66:957, 1958

70. Leport C, Vilde JL, Katlama C et al: Failure of spiramycin to prevent neurotoxoplasmosis in immunosuppressed patients. JAMA 255:2290, 1986

71. Norrby R, Eilard T, Svedhem A et al: Treatment of toxoplasmosis with trimethoprim-sulfamethoxazole. Scand J Infect Dis 7:72–75, 1975

72. Kovacs JA, Allegra CJ, Chabner BA et al: Potent effect of trimetrexate, a lipid-soluble antifolate, on *Toxoplasma gondii.* J Infect Dis 155:1027, 1987

73. Chabner BA: Improved therapy for pneumocystis pneumonia and toxoplasmosis, p 578. In DeVita VT, Jr (moderator): Developmental therapeutics and the acquired immunodeficiency syndrome. Ann Intern Med 106:586, 1987

74. Navin TR, Hardy AM: Cryptosporidiosis in patients with AIDS. J Infect Dis 155:150, 1987

75. DeHovitz JA, Pape JW, Boncy M et al: Clinical manifestations and therapy of *Isospora belli* infection in patients with the acquired immunodeficiency syndrome. N Engl J Med 315:87, 1986

76. Whiteside ME, Barkin JS, May RG et al: Enteric coccidiosis among patients with the acquired immunodeficiency syndrome. Am J Trop Med Hyg 33:1065, 1984

77. Soave R, Danner RL, Honig CL et al: Cryptosporidiosis in homosexual men. Ann Intern Med 100:504, 1984

78. Kazlow PG, Shak K, Benkov KJ et al: Esophageal cryptosporidiosis in a child with acquired immunodeficiency syndrome. Gastroenterology 91:1301, 1986

79. Margulis SJ, Honig CL, Soave R et al: Biliary tract obstruction in the acquired immunodeficiency syndrome. Ann Intern Med 105:207, 1986

80. Blumberg RS, Kelsey R, Perrone T et al: Cytomegalovirus- and Cryptosporidium-associated acalculous gangrenous cholecystitis. Am J Med 76:1118, 1984

81. Ma P, Villanueva TG, Kaufman D, Gillooley JF: Respiratory cryptosporidiosis in the acquired immunodeficiency syndrome. JAMA 252:1298, 1984

82. Brady EM, Margolis ML, Korzeniowski OM: Pulmonary cryptosporidiosis in acquired immunodeficiency syndrome. JAMA 252:89, 1984

83. Ma P, Soave R: Three-step stool examination for cryptosporidiosis in 10 homosexual men with protracted watery diarrhea. J Infect Dis 147:824, 1982

84. Update: treatment of cryptosporidiosis in patients with acquired immunodeficiency syndrome (AIDS). Morbid Mortal Week Rep 33:117, 1984

85. Portnoy D, Whiteside ME, Buckley E et al: Treatment of intestinal cryptosporidiosis with spiramycin. Ann Intern Med 101:202, 1984

86. Restrepo C, Macher AM, Radany EM: Disseminated extraintestinal isosporiasis in a patient with acquired immunodeficiency syndrome. Am J Clin Pathol 87:536, 1987

87. Tietze KJ, Gaska JA, Cosgrove EM: Treatment of *I. belli* enteritis in patients with AIDS. Clin Pharm [letter] 5:191, 1986

88. Wiley CA, Safrin RE, Davis CE et al: Acanthamoeba meningoencephalitis in a patient with AIDS. J Infect Dis 155:130, 1987

89. Kovacs JA, Kovacs AA, Polis M et al: Cryptococcosis in the acquired immunodeficiency syndrome. Ann Intern Med 103:533, 1985

90. Zuger A, Louie E, Holzman RS et al: Cryptococcal disease in patients with the acquired immunodeficiency syndrome. Diagnostic features and outcome of treatment. Ann Intern Med 104:234, 1986

91. Rico MJ, Penneys NS: Cutaneous cryptococcosis resembling molluscum contagiosum in a patient with AIDS. Arch Dermatol 121:901, 1985

92. Borton LK, Wintroub BU: Disseminated cryptococcosis presenting as herpetiform lesions in a homosexual man with acquired immunodeficiency syndrome. J Am Acad Dermatol 10:387, 1984

93. Gal AA, Koss MN, Hawkins J et al: The pathology of pulmonary cryptococcal infections in the acquired immunodeficiency syndrome. Arch Pathol Lab Med 110:502, 1986

94. Ricciardi DD, Sepkowitz DV, Berkowitz LB et al: Cryptococcal arthritis in a patient with acquired immunodeficiency syndrome. Case report and review of the literature. J Rheumatol 13:455, 1986

95. Robinson PG, Sulita MJ, Matthews EK et al: Failure of the Bactec 460 radiometer to detect *Cryptococcus neoformans* fungemia in an AIDS patient. Am J Clin Pathol 87:783, 1987

96. Bottone EJ, Toma M, Johansson BE, Wormser GP: Poorly encapsulated *Cryptococcus neoformans* from patients with AIDS. I: Preliminary observations. AIDS-Res 2:211, 1986

97. Eng RH, Bishburg E, Smith SM et al: Cryptococcal infec-tions in patients with acquired immunodeficiency syndrome. Am J Med 81:19, 1986

98. Stamm AM, Diasio RB, Dismukes WE et al: Toxicity of amphotericin B plus flucytosine in 194 patients with cryptococcal meningitis. Am J Med 83:236, 1987

99. Polsky B, Depman MR, Gold JWM et al: Intraventricular therapy of cryptococcal meningitis via a subcutaneous reservoir. Am J Med 81:24, 1986

100. Diamond RD, Bennett JE: Prognostic factors in cryptococcal meningitis. Ann Intern Med 80:176, 1974

101. Palou-de-Fernanez E, Patino MM et al: Treatment of cryptococcal meningitis in mice with fluconazole. J Antimicrob Chemother 18:261, 1986

102. Wheat LJ, Slama TG, Zekel ML: Histoplasmosis in the acquired immunodeficiency syndrome. Am J Med 78:203, 1985

103. Bonner JR, Alexander WJ, Dismukes ME et al: Disseminated histoplasmosis in patients with the acquired immunodeficiency syndrome. Arch Intern Med 144:2178, 1984

104. Huang CT, McGarry T, Cooper S et al: Disseminated histoplasmosis in the acquired immunodeficiency syndrome. Report of five cases from a nonendemic area. Arch Intern Med 147:1181, 1987

105. Mandell W, Goldberg DM, Neu HC: Histoplasmosis in patients with the acquired immunodeficiency syndrome. Am J Med 81:974, 1986

106. Sathapatayavongs B, Batteiger BE, Wheat LJ et al: Clinical and laboratory features of disseminated histoplasmosis during two large urban outbreaks. Medicine 62:263, 1983

107. Henochowicz S, Sahovic E, Pistole M et al: Histoplasmosis diagnosed on peripheral blood smear from a patient with AIDS. JAMA 253:3148, 1985

108. Paya CV, Roberts GD, Cockerill FR: Laboratory methods for the diagnosis of disseminated histoplasmosis: Clinical importance of the lysis-centrifugation blood culture techniques. Mayo Clin Proc 62:480, 1987

109. Bille J, Stockman L, Roberts GD et al: Evaluation of a lysis-centrifugation system for recovery of yeasts and filamentous fungi from blood. J Clin Microbiol 18:469, 1983

110. Gustafson PR, Henson A: letter: Ketoconazole therapy for AIDS patients with disseminated histoplasmosis. Arch Intern Med 145:2272, 1985

111. Wheat LJ: Ketoconazole therapy for AIDS patients with disseminated histoplasmosis. Arch Intern Med 145:2272, 1985

112. Bronnimann DA, Adam RD, Galgiani JN et al: Coccidioidomycosis in the acquired immunodeficiency syndrome. Ann Intern Med 106:372, 1986

113. Kovacs A, Forthal DN, Kovacs JA et al: Disseminated coccidioidomycosis in a patient with acquired immunodeficiency syndrome. West J Med 140:447, 1984

114. Abrams DI, Robia M, Blumenfeld W et al: letter: Disseminated coccidioidomycosis in AIDS. N Engl J Med 310:986, 1984

115. Ampel NM, Ryan KJ, Carry PJ et al: Fungemia due to *Coccidioides immitis*. An analysis of 16 episodes in 15 patients and a review of the literature. Medicine (Baltimore) 65:312 (Review), 1986

116. Chandrasekar PH, Molinari JA: Oral candidiasis: Forerunner of acquired immunodeficiency syndrome? Oral Surg Oral Med Oral Pathol 60:532, 1985

117. Klein RS, Harris CA, Small CB et al: Oral candidiasis in high risk patients as the initial manifestation of the ac-

quired immunodeficiency syndrome. N Engl J Med 311: 354, 1984

118. Rhoads JL, Wright DC, Redfield RR et al: Chronic vaginal candidiasis in women with human immunodeficiency virus infection. JAMA 257:3105, 1987

119. Holmberg K, Meyer RD: Fungal infections in patients with AIDS and AIDS related complex. Scand J Infect Dis 18:179, 1986

120. Dworkin B, Wormser GP, Rosenthal WS et al: Gastrointestinal manifestations of the acquired immunodeficiency syndrome: A review of 22 cases. Am J Gastroenterol 80: 774, 1985

121. Pitchenik AE, Cole C, Russell BN et al: Tuberculosis, atypical mycobacteriosis, and the acquired immunodeficiency syndrome among Haitians and non-Haitians in South Florida. Ann Intern Med 101:641, 1984

122. Hawkins CC, Gold JWM, Whimbey E et al: *Mycobacterium avium* complex infections in patients with the acquired immunodeficiency syndrome. Ann Intern Med 105:184, 1986

123. Macher AM, Kovacs JA, Gill V et al: Bacteremia due to *Mycobacterium avium-intracellulare* in the acquired immunodeficiency syndrome. Ann Intern Med 99:782, 1983

124. Horsburgh CR, Cohn DL, Roberts RB et al: *Mycobacterium avium-intracellulare* from patients with and without AIDS. Antimicrob Agent Chemother 30:955, 1986

125. O'Brien RJ, Lyle MA, Snider DE: Ansamycin LM-427 in the treatment of *M. avium* complex disease and drug resistant tuberculosis: A preliminary report. Am Rev Respir Dis 131:A223, 1985

126. Masur H, Tuazon C, Gill V et al: Effect of combined clofazimine and ansamycin therapy on *Mycobacterium avium-Mycobacterium intracellulare* bacteremia in patients with AIDS. J Infect Dis 155:127, 1987

127. Louie E, Rice LB, Holaman RS: Tuberculosis in non-Haitian patients with acquired immunodeficiency syndrome. Chest 90:542, 1986

128. Sunderam G, McDonald RJ, Maniatis T et al: Tuberculosis as a manifestation of the acquired immunodeficiency syndrome. JAMA 256:362, 1986

129. Barnes PF, Arvalo C: Six cases of *Mycobacterium tuberculosis* bacteremia. J Infect Dis 156:377, 1987

130. Centers for Disease Control: Diagnosis and Management of mycobacterial infection and disease in persons with human immunodeficiency virus infection. Ann Intern Med 106:254, 1986

131. Pitchenik AE, Rubinson HA: The radiographic appearance of tuberculosis in patients with the acquired immunodeficiency syndrome (AIDS) and pre-AIDS. Am Rev Respir Dis 131:393, 1985

132. Jacobs JL, Gold JWM, Murray MW et al: *Salmonella* infections in patients with the acquired immunodeficiency syndrome. Ann Intern Med 102:86, 1985

133. Smith PD, Macher AM, Bookman MA et al: *Salmonella typhimurium* enteritis and bacteremia in the acquired immunodeficiency syndrome. Ann Intern Med 102:207, 1985

134. Fischl MA, Dickinson GM, Sinave C et al: *Salmonella* bacteremia as manifestation of acquired immunodeficiency syndrome. Arch Intern Med 146:113, 1986

135. Glaser JB, Morton–Kute L, Berger SR et al: Recurrent *Salmonella typhimurium* bacteremia associated with the acquired immunodeficiency syndrome. Ann Intern Med 102:189, 1985

136. Cherubin CE, Neu HC, Imperato PJ et al: Septicemia with nontyphoid *Salmonella*. Medicine 53:365, 1974

137. Polsky B, Gold JW, Whimbey E et al: Bacterial pneumonia in patients with the acquired immunodeficiency syndrome. Ann Intern Med 104:38, 1986

138. Eng RH, Bishburg E, Smith SM et al: Bacteremia and fungemia in patients with acquired immunodeficiency syndrome. Am J Clin Pathol 86:105, 1986

139. Whimbey E, Gold JWM, Polsky B et al: Bacteremia and fungemia in patients with the acquired immunodeficiency syndrome. Ann Intern Med 104:511, 1986

140. Johns DR, Tierney M, Felsenstein D: Alteration in the natural history of neurosyphilis by concurrent infection with the human immunodeficiency virus. N Engl J Med 316:1569, 1987

141. Bery CD, Hooton TM, Collier AC et al: Neurologic relapse after benzathine penicillin therapy for secondary syphilis in a patient with HIV infection. N Engl J Med 316:1587, 1987

142. Holtz HA, Lavery DP, Kapila R: Actinomycetales infection in the acquired immunodeficiency syndrome. Ann Intern Med 102:203, 1985

143. Rodriquez JL, Barrio JL, Pitchenik AE: Pulmonary nocardiosis in the acquired immunodeficiency syndrome. Chest 90:912, 1986

144. Schlanger G, Lutwick LI, Kurzman M et al: Sinusitis caused by *Legionella pneumophila* in a patient with the acquired immunodeficiency syndrome. Am J Med 77:957, 1984

145. Quinnan GV Jr, Masur H, Rook AH et al: Herpesvirus infections in the acquired immune deficiency syndrome. JAMA 252:72, 1984

146. Laskin OL, Cederberg DM, Mills J et al: Ganciclovir for the treatment and suppression of serious infections caused by cytomegalovirus. Am J Med 83:201, 1987

147. Chachoua A, Deterich D, Krasinski K et al: 9-(1,3-dihydroxy-2-propoxymethyl) guanine (Ganciclovir) in the treatment of cytomegalovirus gastrointestinal disease with acquired immunodeficiency syndrome. Ann Intern Med 107:133, 1987

148. Masur H, Lane HC, Palestine A et al: Effect of 9-(1,3-dihydroxy-2-propoxymethyl) guanine on serious cytomegalovirus disease in eight immunosuppressed homosexual men. Ann Intern Med 104:41, 1986

149. Collaborative DHPG Treatment Study Group: Treatment of serious cytomegalovirus infections with 9-(1,3-dihydroxy-2-propoxymethyl) guanine in patients with AIDS and other immunodeficiencies. N Engl J Med 314:801, 1986

150. Palestine AG, Rodrigues MM, Macher AM et al: Ophthalmic involvement in acquired immunodeficiency syndrome. Ophthal 91:1092, 1984

151. Fernandes B, Brunton J, Koven I: Ileal perforation due to cytomegalovirus enteritis. Can J Surg 29:453, 1986

152. Margello S, Cho ES, Nielsen S et al: Cytomegalovirus encephalitis in patients with acquired immunodeficiency syndrome: An autopsy study of 30 cases and a review of the literature. Hum Pathol 18:289, 1987

153. Petito CK, Cho ES, Lemann W et al: Neuropathology of acquired immunodeficiency syndrome (AIDS): An autopsy review. J Neuropathol Exp Neurol 45:635, 1986

154. Anders KH, Guerra WF, Tomigasu V et al: The neuropathology of AIDS. UCLA experience and review. Am J Pathol 124:537, 1986

155. Navia BA, Cho ES, Petito CK et al: The AIDS dementia complex: II. Neuropathology. Ann Neurol 19:525, 1986

156. Palestine AG, Stevens G, Lane HC et al: Treatment of cytomegalovirus retinitis with dihydroxypropoxymethyl guanine. Am J Ophthal 101:95, 1986

157. Oberg B: Antiviral effects of phosphonoformate (PFA, Foscarnet Sodium). Pharmac Ther 19:387, 1983

158. Maier JA, Bergman A, Ross MG: Acquired immunodeficiency syndrome manifested by chronic primary genital herpes. Am J Obstet Gynecol 155:756, 1986

159. Friedman–Kien AE, Lafleur FL, Gendler E et al: *Herpes zoster:* A possible early clinical sign for development of acquired immunodeficiency syndrome in high-risk individuals. J Am Acad Dermatol 14:1023, 1986

160. Melbye M, Grossman RJ, Goedert JJ et al: Risk of AIDS after *herpes zoster.* Lancet 1:728, 1987

161. Sandor EV, Millman A, Croxson TS et al: *Herpes zoster ophthalmicus* in patients at risk for the acquired immunodeficiency syndrome (AIDS). Am J Ophthalmol 101: 153, 1986

162. Cole EL, Meisler DM, Calabrese LH et al: *Herpes zoster ophthalmicus* and acquired immunodeficiency syndrome. Arch Ophthalmol 102:1027, 1984

163. Ryder JW, Croen K, Kleinschmidt–DeMasters BK et al: Progressive enchephalitis three months after resolution of cutaneous zoster in a patient with AIDS. Ann Neurol 19:182, 1986

164. Dix RD, Bredesen DE, Erlich KS et al: Recovery of herpesviruses from cerebrospinal fluid of immunodeficient homosexual men. Ann Neurol 18:611, 1985

165. Rogers MF, Morens OM, Stewart JA et al: National case-control study of Kaposi's sarcoma and *Pneumocystis carinii* pneumonia in homosexual men: Part 2, Laboratory results. Ann Intern Med 99:151, 1983

166. Greenspan JS, Greenspan D, Conant M et al: Oral ''hairy'' leukoplakia in male homosexuals: Evidence of association with both papillomavirus and a herpes-group virus. Lancet 2:831, 1984

167. Greenspan JS, Greenspan D, Lennette ET et al: Replication of Epstein–Barr virus within the epithelial cells of oral ''hairy'' leukoplakia, an AIDS-associated lesion. N Engl J Med 313:1564, 1985

168. Andiman WA, Eastman R, Martin K et al: Opportunistic lymphoproliferations associated with Epstein–Barr viral DNA in infants and children with AIDS. Lancet 2:1390, 1985

169. Peterson JM, Tubbs RR, Savage RA et al: Small noncleaved B cell Burkitt-like lymphoma with chromosome t(8;14) translocation and Epstein–Barr virus nuclear-associated antigen in a homosexual man with acquired immune deficiency syndrome. Am J Med 78:141, 1985

170. Hamm PG, Judson MA, Aranda CP: Diagnosing of pulmonary Kaposi's sarcoma with fiberoptic bronchoscopy and endobronchial biopsy: A report of five cases. Cancer 59:807, 1987

171. Meduri GU, Stover DE, Lee M et al: Pulmonary Kaposi's sarcoma in the acquired immunodeficiency syndrome: Clinical, radiographic, and pathologic manifestations. Am J Med 81:11, 1986

172. Ognibene FP, Steis RG, Macher AM et al: Kaposi's sarcoma causing pulmonary infiltrates and respiratory failure in the acquired immunodeficiency syndrome. Ann Intern Med 102:471, 1985

173. Suffredini A, Ognibene FP, Lack EE: Non specific interstitial pneumonitis: A common cause of pulmonary disease in the acquired immunodeficiency syndrome. Ann Intern Med 107:7, 1987

174. Gabuzda DM, Hirsch MS: Neurological manifestations of infection with human immunodeficiency virus. Ann Intern Med 107:383–391, 1987

Gastrointestinal Complications of AIDS

John G. Bartlett
Barbara Laughon
Thomas C. Quinn

13

Human immunodeficiency virus (HIV) infection and its consequences on the immune defenses may ultimately affect every organ system. The gastrointestinal (GI) tract is one of the most common sites of clinical expression, and all levels from the oral cavity to the anus are frequently involved. Large-scale studies indicate that 30% to 90% of AIDS patients develop chronic diarrhea; these cases are ascribed to a diverse array of superimposed opportunistic infections or opportunistic tumors, or they remain unexplained under the appellation "AIDS enteropathy." Most patients have oral and/or esophageal candidiasis and about one-third develop perirectal lesions. A variety of gastrointestinal conditions that are almost unique to these patients have been unveiled, including visceral Kaposi's sarcoma, oral hairy leukoplakia, Whipple's-like enteropathy due to mycobacteria, chronic cryptosporidiosis and cytomegalovirus colitis. A source of considerable concern is that many of these conditions are difficult to detect and refractory to therapy, although new diagnostic and therapeutic strategies are rapidly being developed. The purpose of this chapter is to review the gastrointestinal manifestations of AIDS.

THE GAY BOWEL SYNDROME

During the past 15 years there has been increasing recognition of sometimes alarmingly high rates of enteric disease among homosexual men. The various syndromes include proctitis, proctocolitis, and enteritis known collectively as the *gay bowel syndrome*. Pathogens encountered in these patients include three groups: (1) commonly recognized enteric pathogens such as *Shigella, Entamoeba histolytica* and *Giardia lamblia;* (2) commonly recognized sexually transmitted pathogens including *Neisseria gonorrhoeae,* herpes simplex virus, *Chlamydia trachomatis,* and *Treponema pallidum,* and (3) occasional enteric pathogens that appear

to be idiosyncratic to this population such as *Campylobacter cinaedi* and *Campylobacter fennelliae.*

The high prevalence of enteric pathogens in gay men presumably reflects promiscuity, specific sexual practices and the high incidence of asymptomatic or untreated infections. There have been numerous reports that describe the frequency of detection of various agents in men who either are asymptomatic or have clinical evidence of intestinal disease. However, most studies are restricted to a relatively small number of organisms, and there is an obvious potential sampling bias since clinics for sexually transmitted diseases are used as the source of subjects in nearly all studies.

The first comprehensive report dealing with a large sample with a comprehensive microbiologic analysis was published by Quinn and colleagues.[1] This was a study of 119 homosexual men with intestinal symptoms and 75 homosexual men without intestinal symptoms studied during the period 1978–81 at a sexually transmitted disease (STD) clinic in Seattle. One or more known rectal or intestinal pathogens were recovered from 80% of symptomatic men compared to 39% for those without symptoms (Table 13-1). Two or more pathogens were recovered from 22% of symptomatic patients, and 4% of those who were asymptomatic. Associated clinical findings were defined as proctitis, proctocolitis, or enteritis. Patients with proctitis had abnormal findings with flexible sigmoidoscopy limited to the distal 15 cm, and nearly all had anorectal symptoms including constipation, rectal discharge, anorectal pain and/or tenesmus. Microbiologic correlations showed that 33 of 41 patients in this category had infections involving *N. gonorrhoeae,* herpes simplex virus, non-lymphogranuloma (LGV) strains of *Chlamydia trachomatis* or *T. pallidum.* The definition of proctocolitis was sigmoidoscopic evidence of inflammation in both the rectum and sigmoid colon that extended beyond 15 cm. The dominant pathogen in the 15 patients with proc-

Table 13-1
Pathogens Recovered in Homosexual Men With and Without Enteric Symptoms

	Seattle Study (1)		Baltimore Study (2)	
	Symptomatic	*Asymptomatic*	*Symptomatic*	*Asymptomatic*
Number of patients	119 (%)	75 (%)	70 (%)	243 (%)
Sexually transmitted pathogens				
N. gonorrhoeae	37 (31)	17 (23)	9 (13)	1 (0.4)
Herpes simplex	23 (19)	3 (4)	13 (19)	6 (2.5)
Chlamydia trachomatis	12 (10)	4 (5)	6 (9)	7 (3)
Treponema pallidum	6 (5)	1 (1)	0	0
Enteric pathogens				
Entamoeba histolytica	20 (29)	6 (25)	3 (4)	3 (1)
Giardia lamblia	10 (14)	1 (4)	7 (10)	5 (2)
Campylobacter sp.	8 (7)	2 (3)	13 (19)	6 (2.6)
Clostridium difficile	3 (3)	1 (1)	3 (4)	0
Shigella	3 (3)	1 (1)	6 (9)	1
Any agent	95 (80)	29 (39)	43 (61)	29 (12)

tocolitis were *Campylobacter jejuni, Shigella flexneri,* LGV strains of *Chlamydia trachomatis, E. histolytica* and *Clostridium difficile.* The definition of enteritis was a normal sigmoidoscopic examination to 25 cm in association with diarrhea, abdominal pain, nausea, and bloating. *G. lamblia* was recovered in 4 of 8 patients in this category.

The Seattle study has subsequently been repeated by our group in Baltimore using similar clinical and microbiologic methods.[2] The major difference was that the Baltimore study (see Table 13-1) was conducted at an infectious disease referral clinic rather than an STD clinic, and the period during which the study took place was October 1984 through December 1985, which post dated the AIDS epidemic with its attendant consequences on sexual practices and HIV infection. The Baltimore study included 243 asymptomatic patients and 68 patients with either diarrhea (35 episodes in 33 patients) or proctitis (35 episodes in 35 patients). In comparing results, the Baltimore study showed a substantially larger proportion of symptomatic patients had diarrhea (enteritis) rather than proctitis. With regard to microbiologic studies, the Baltimore study showed a substantially reduced recovery rate for *N. gonorrhoeae* and *E. histolytica* for both symptomatic and asymptomatic men.

Enteric Pathogens in Patients With AIDS

Diarrhea is a common clinical feature of symptomatic HIV infection. This symptom persisting for at least 1 month in association with unexplained weight loss of 10% of the premorbid weight was previously included in the AIDS-related complex (ARC), sometimes referred to as the *diarrhea–wasting syndrome.* The syndrome, in association with HIV infection, now comprises an "AIDS-defining illness" in both the World Health Organization (WHO) and the recently revised Centers for Disease Control (CDC) definitions.[3,4] The incidence of diarrhea is reported at 30% to 50% among patients in industrialized countries[5–8] and 70% to 90% for AIDS patients in Haiti[9–12] or Africa.[13–20] Incidence of anorectal disease in 340 patients with HIV infection at St. Luke's Roosevelt Hospital Center was 34%, of whom 52 (15%) presented with anorectal symptoms prior to the diagnosis of AIDS or ARC.[21]

Homosexual men comprise the great majority of patients with AIDS in industrialized countries. Data reviewed above (see Table 13-1) indicate a high prevalence of gastrointestinal pathogens in this patient population. Nevertheless, a quite different menu of enteric pathogens is found in patients with AIDS even when the analysis is restricted to homosexual men (Table 13-2). This difference is ascribed to abnormalities in immunologic defenses, the major defects being a quantitative and qualitative defect of CD4 cells combined with polyclonal B-cell activation plus reduced humoral response to newly presented antigens.[21] The major pathogens in homosexual men who are seronegative for HIV infection or asymptomatic seropositive men are the traditionally recognized enteric pathogens and sexually transmitted pathogens (see Table 13-2). By contrast, patients with AIDS often have no defined pathogen or have pathogens that most frequently reflect defective cell-mediated immunity or humoral response.

Most studies of enteric disease in patients with AIDS from industrialized countries are limited in the microbiologic techniques employed, and most show that no likely agent of enteric disease can be detected. The Baltimore study is more comprehensive in that it was designed to detect 20 to 30 types of organisms, including bacteria, fungi, parasites, and viruses.[2] This study included 77 homosexual men with AIDS, 49 with diarrhea

Table 13-2

Enteric Pathogens Encountered in the "Gay Bowel Syndrome" and in Patients with AIDS

Site	AIDS With Diarrhea	Gay Bowel Syndrome
Mouth	*Candida albicans*	*Neisseria gonorrhoeae*
	Herpes simplex	Herpes simplex
		Chlamydia trachomatis
Esophagus	*Candida albicans*	
	Herpes simplex	
	Cytomegalovirus	
Small intestine and colon	*Mycobacterium avium-intra-cellulare*	*Giardia lamblia*
		Entamoeba histolytica
	Salmonella	*Campylobacter*
	Cytomegalovirus	*Shigella*
	Cryptosporidia	*Chlamydia trachomatis*
	Isospora	
Anorectal area	Herpes simplex	Herpes simplex
		Neisseria gonorrhoeae
		Treponema pallidum
		papillomavirus

Table 13-3

Microbiology Studies for Enteric Pathogens in Patients With AIDS (2)

	Diarrhea	No Diarrhea
Number of patients	49 (%)	28 (%)
Pathogens		
Herpes simplex virus	7 (18)*	8 (40)*
Cryptosporidium	7 (16)	0
Chlamydia trachomatis	5 (11)	2 (8)
Campylobacter sp.	5 (11)	2 (8)
Clostridium difficile (toxin)	3 (7)	0
Shigella	2 (5)	0
Giardia lamblia	2 (4)	1 (5)
V. parahemolyticus	2 (4)	0
Isospora belli	1 (2)	0
Any pathogen	28 (55)	11 (39)
Organisms of uncertain clinical significance		
Candida albicans	20 (53)	4 (24)
Cytomegalovirus (rectum)	9 (27)	2 (15)
Blastocystis hominis	7 (15)	3 (16)
Intestinal spirochetes	4 (11)	3 (12)

* Not all specimens were analyzed for all pathogens; % reflects percent of specimens yielding the organism based on the number assessed.

and 28 without diarrhea. The results in this group (Table 13-3) may be compared with results using identical microbiologic techniques in homosexual men without AIDS (see Table 13-1) to illustrate the previously noted differences in pathogens for these two populations. The major difference for patients with AIDS is the relatively high recovery rates for cryptosporidia and cytomegalovirus. Cryptosporidia accounted for 16% of AIDS patients with diarrhea and 1 of 34 episodes of diarrhea in homosexual men without AIDS, and it was never encountered in the absence of diarrhea in 243 homosexual men or in 28 AIDS patients. Herpes simplex virus is not a recognized agent of diarrhea, but was found in 20% to 40% of homosexual men without AIDS with proctitis and in 20% to 40% of AIDS patients. The role of cytomegalovirus (CMV) is somewhat controversial, since this organism is frequently detected either in biopsy specimens or cultures from immunocompromised patients both with and without enteric symptoms. Cytomegalovirus was recovered from 2 of 235 asymptomatic gay men without AIDS, 2 of 13 AIDS patients without diarrhea, and 9 of 34 AIDS patients with diarrhea. Organisms that play no clearly established role in enteric disease due to high prevalence rates in asymptomatic, healthy persons include *Blastocystis hominis,* intestinal spirochetes (*T. hyodysenteriae* and *Brachyspira aalborgi*), and *Candida* species (excluding oral and esophageal candidiasis). *E. histolytica* is also somewhat enigmatic; this well-established enteric pathogen has generally been detected in stools from 10% to 30% of homosexual men,[22-25] but nearly all are asymptomatic carriers.

An overview of the report reviewed indicates that an established pathogen can be recovered in approximately one-half of AIDS patients with diarrhea. Cryptosporidiosis accounted for approximately one-third of patients with positive tests, and a heterogeneous group of pathogens comprise the balance. If cytomegalovirus is accepted as pathogenic when recovered with rectal swab culture, the total yield in symptomatic patients is approximately 75%.

Slim Disease

Serwadda and others[18] reported a "new disease that has recently been recognized in rural Uganda" characterized by weight loss and diarrhea in 1985. There were 71 patients reviewed, the majority of whom were bedridden with intermittent, non-bloody diarrhea, anorexia, marked change in taste and weight losses exceeding 10 kg. Serologic tests for HIV showed 63 of the 71 were positive. The authors noted that the clinical features were similar to the enteropathy associated with AIDS as seen in Zaire, except for the paucity of patients with Kaposi's sarcoma even though this disease is endemic in Uganda. Stool exams were reportedly negative for enteric pathogens including cryptosporidia. Most authorities now recognize slim disease as simply AIDS in which gastrointestinal manifestations represent a dominant clinical feature and the major question concerns the unusually high prevalence of these symptoms in AIDS patients in Africa and Haiti.

AIDS in developing countries appears to be different than that encountered in Europe and the United States in terms of epidemiology, clinical expression and recovery rates for both intestinal and extra-intestinal opportunistic pathogens. In Africa, the disease appears to be far more frequently transmitted by heterosexual rather than homosexual exposure, and there is the obvious difference in prevalence rates for diverse pathogens reflecting unsanitary conditions and the tropical climate. Resources for diagnostic studies are also far more limited, making it difficult to compare microbiologic results in different geographic areas. Studies from Haiti indicate that approximately 50% of AIDS patients had cryptosporidiosis and 15% had isosporosis.[12] These protozoan parasites are the only enteric pathogens that have been detected to account for geographic differences in prevalence rates of GI symptoms.

AIDS Enteropathy

The data reviewed above indicate that a major portion of AIDS patients with diarrhea have no identifiable etiologic agent to account for gastrointestinal symptoms, a condition commonly referred to as *AIDS enteropathy*. Functional studies of the GI tract have been accomplished in patients with this syndrome,[5,26] although it should be acknowledged that these studies were not performed in association with a comprehensive assessment to exclude enteric pathogens that are not readily detected. Within the confines of this limitation, patients with "AIDS enteropathy" appear to have malabsorption characterized by abnormal D-xylose and 14 C-glycerol-tripalmitin absorption tests.[5,26] Small bowel biopsies generally show blunting of villi, epithelial damage, and chronic inflammation of the small intestine; rectal biopsies often demonstrate focal epithelial necrosis in crypts (apoptosis) and intranuclear inclusions that are presumably viral agents, possibly herpes simplex virus or cytomegalovirus.

Electron microscopic studies of gut tissue in patients with AIDS show tubuloreticular structures that are considered ultrastructural markers of considerable interest in AIDS.[27,28] These are irregular, tube-like structures measuring 20 to 30 nm in diameter that are seen in lymphocytes, monocytes, and endothelial cells located in the endoplasmic reticulum, from whence they appear to arise. Tubuloreticular structures are considered nonspecific, but they were encountered in seven of eight patients reviewed by Dobbins and associates and only once (in a patient with Crohn's disease) in over 200 biopsies from patients without AIDS.[27]

Gut Immunity

Immunologic studies have shown the expected findings with respect to lymphocyte subset populations in gut tissue. Immunohistologic staining with monoclonal antibodies show nearly complete depletion of T4 lymphocytes accompanied by an increase in T8 cells in both the small bowel and rectum.[29–31] Ellakany and co-workers[30] reported mean T4:T8 ratios in small bowel

biopsies of 0.1 ± 0.02 for AIDS patients compared to normal values of 2.3 ± 0.2; for rectal biopsies the mean ratio for AIDS patients was 0.2 ± 0.06 compared to 2.6 ± 0.3 for normals. This is not surprising in view of analogous findings with lymphocytes in the peripheral circulation. Rodgers and others[32] confirmed these findings and also showed that the phenotype distribution of gut lymphocytes in healthy homosexual men was normal. This observation supports the concept that the differences in enteric pathogens noted in Table 13-2 may be ascribed to specific sexual practices in otherwise healthy gay men and are due to immune deficits in patients with HIV infection. Weber and colleagues[33] utilized electron microscopy to define the morphology of 86 intestinal and 55 rectal intraepithelial lymphocytes in 11 patients with AIDS for comparison with patients with celiac sprue and healthy persons. The lymphocytes in AIDS patients showed more organelles; they had multiple surface projections and appeared "activated." The authors speculated that these activated lymphocytes could represent cytotoxic effector cells responsible for immune injury. With regard to local expression of humoral defects, Kotler and associates[34] showed depletion of IgA plasma cells and reduced IgA and IgM fluorescene intensity implying reduced cytoplasmic immunoglobulin.

Management

The great majority of AIDS patients with chronic diarrhea have intermittent symptoms with stools that do not show blood or leukocytes, and are associated with the aforementioned absorptive defects, anatomic changes in the small bowel and colon, and electron microscopic studies that reveal the somewhat unique tubuloreticular structures. The severity of diarrhea is highly variable. For most patients it is intermittent, but many have debilitating diarrhea with large volume losses and the attendant consequences of dehydration, electrolyte imbalance, and emaciation. Extensive studies for microbial agents sometimes yield treatable agents, such as *Shigella, Salmonella, Isospora,* and herpes simplex virus, although all of these are prone to recur when treatment is discontinued. Many cases involve untreatable microbial pathogens such as cryptosporidia, *Mycobacterium avium,* and possibly CMV. There remains a relatively large number of patients with no definable enteric pathogen who are classified as having AIDS enteropathy. It is unknown if these represent a primary manifestation of HIV infection. It should be noted parenthetically that stool and bowel tissue have not been subject to analysis for HIV, although this organism has been found in virtually all body fluids in which it has been sought. It is conceivable that some of the GI manifestations of AIDS may reflect HIV infection of the gut *per se* or may be a consequence of immune injury. Alternatively, there may be an as yet undetected opportunistic pathogen or pathophysiologic mechanism such as small bowel overgrowth.

Recommendations for diagnostic studies to detect

microbial agents are summarized in Table 13-4. Use of these tests will depend to a large extent on clinical findings (Table 13-5), diagnostic resources, and idiosyncrasies of methodology for specific laboratories.

Endoscopy is often indicated, although this may pose special concerns for the endoscopist. A survey of chiefs of gastroenterology in U.S. medical centers showed 73% of respondents felt the procedure placed personnel at risk for acquiring HIV infection.[35] Nearly half of institutions used a designated instrument for AIDS patients and 85% employed gas sterilization of equipment. Despite these concerns, the diagnostic yield is high.[36] Contrast studies also show a high yield, and many patients have multiple lesions. A review of 63 barium studies in 44 AIDS patients showed 38 (86%) had at least one abnormal study; 27 of these had multifocal disease, most commonly in the duodenum with an upper GI series and the sigmoid colon with barium enema.[37]

Similarly, abdominal computed tomography (CT) scan provides a high yield.[38] Patients with ARC commonly show retroperitoneal and mesenteric adenopathy, splenomegaly, and perirectal inflammation.[38,39] Large intra-abdominal lymph nodes (over 1.5 cm) specifically suggests *Mycobacterium avium-intracellulare,* Kaposi's sarcoma, or a lymphoma. These distinctions can often be made with fine-needle percutaneous aspiration or CT-guided biopsy.

Recommendations for therapy are summarized in Table 13-6 and reviewed in detail in the following discussions.

Opportunistic Infections

ORAL AND OROESOPHAGEAL CANDIDIASIS. Oral candidiasis or thrush is a common complication in debilitated patients, the immunosuppressed, and persons

---

Table 13-4
Diagnostic Studies for Microbial Agents or Noninfectious Lesions in the Gastrointestinal Tract

Infectious Diseases	Diagnostic Method	Comment
Fungi		
Candida albicans		
Thrush	KOH or Gram's stain of typical lesion to show sheets of yeast forms	Often a presumptive diagnosis based on characteristic white plaques
Esophagitis	Thin barium swallow or endoscopy to show typical esophageal lesion ± biopsy	Often a presumptive diagnosis based on thrush plus dysphagia
Histoplasmosis	Biopsy of oral or intestinal lesion with Giemsa or other appropriate stain and culture on Sabaroud's media	Serology is often supportive, but infrequently definitive
Viral agents		
Herpes simplex virus	Tzanck smear and/or biopsy for smear and culture	Best yield is from lesions at active border
Cytomegalovirus	Culture of rectal swab; biopsy for culture and stain to detect inclusion bodies	Associated pathology and possibly quantitative assessment of inclusion bodies are important in interpretation
Parasites		
Cryptosporidia	Ziehl–Neelson or modified Kinyoun AFB smear of stool or small bowel biopsy	Stool concentration methods necessary when parasite load is low. Monoclonal antibody stains preferred when available
Isospora	As for cryptosporidia, to show typical large oocysts	
Microsporidia	Small bowel biopsy for electron microscopy	Significance of detection unclear
Bacteria		
Salmonella	Stool culture on selective media; blood cultures	
Shigella	Stool culture on selective media; blood cultures	
Campylobacter	Stool culture on selective media	Specialized media and incubation conditions required to detect all species
Mycobacterium	Stool and biopsy for AFB smear and culture	Significance of AFB in stool is often unclear; biopsy for histopathology required for definitive diagnosis
Noninfectious lesions		
Kaposi's sarcoma	Visual appearance in oral cavity or with endoscopy	Biopsies provide a relatively low yield
Oral hairy leukoplakia	Biopsy of tongue	Often suspect in patients with oral lesions that fail to show yeast or fail to respond to antifungal treatment
Lymphoma	Surgery, endoscopy, or percutaneous biopsy	CT scan often shows abdominal lymph node involvement

Table 13-5
Gastrointestinal Manifestations of AIDS: Conditions Associated With Specific Clinical Features

Esophagitis: Candida albicans, herpes simplex virus, cytomegalovirus
Diarrhea without fecal leukocytes (enteritis or enteropathy): Cryptosporidiosis, isosporosis, giardiasis, microsporidia, mycobacteria, cytomegalovirus, lymphoma "AIDS enteropathy"
Diarrhea with fecal leukocytes (colitis): Shigella, Salmonella, *Clostridium difficile, Campylobacter,* cytomegalovirus
Bloody diarrhea: Amebiasis, cytomegalovirus, lymphoma
Steatorrhea: Cytomegalovirus, mycobacteria, cryptosporidiosis, isosporosis, "AIDS enteropathy"
Intestinal perforation: Cytomegalovirus, histoplasmosis, lymphoma
Mesenteric/retroperitoneal adenopathy: Mycobacteria, lymphoma, Kaposi's sarcoma
Proctitis: Herpes simplex, *Chlamydia trachomatis, Neisseria gonorrhoeae, Treponema pallidum,* cytomegalovirus

receiving antibiotic therapy. It is one of the most frequent findings in patients with ARC and carries a relatively poor prognostic sign. Klein and others[40] noted 13 of 22 patients at risk for HIV infection developed AIDS in a median of 3 months following the diagnosis of thrush, compared to none of 20 similar patients without thrush who were followed for 1 year. As expected, the risk was even greater among those who had thrush in association with suppressed T4 levels. The diagnosis is readily established with stains of exudate from typical oral lesions showing sheets of typical yeast and pseudomycelial forms; culture is unnecessary. Patients with oral candidiasis usually respond to traditional therapeutic intervention with clotrimazole troches, nystatin or oral ketoconazole; patients who fail to respond may be treated with a brief, low-dose (0.2–0.5 g) course of amphotericin B. Although these patients generally respond well, they also have a propensity to relapse as soon as therapy is discontinued so that chronic administration of one of these drugs is commonly recommended.

Esophageal candidiasis is also relatively common and represents an AIDS-defining diagnosis. Most patients with established AIDS and thrush have esophageal involvement even when esophageal symptoms are absent.[41] Symptoms, when present, consist of dysphagia with or without retrosternal pain. Oral involvement is usually present, but occasional patients have only esophagitis. Contrast studies of the esophagus show abnormal peristalsis, spasm, and edema with mucosal ulcerations showing a cobblestone appearance.[42] The diagnosis is best established with endoscopy to demonstrate dense plaques of white exudate, that is, "cottage-cheese exudate." Cytologic studies of brushings show yeast and pseudomycelia of *Candida* sp., and biopsies reveal invasion of the mucosa accompanied by an inflammatory response. Tavitian and co-workers[41] noted that 3 of 10 AIDS patients with oral candidiasis had esophageal involvement despite the lack of symptoms suggesting esophageal disease and they further concluded that there was little correlation between the presence of symptoms and the extent of disease seen with endoscopy. The use of endoscopy is often viewed as optional in patients with typical clinical findings. This becomes more important in selected patients who fail to respond to treatment or when this becomes the first AIDS-defining disease. The major differential considerations are esophagitis caused by cytomegalovirus or herpes simplex virus, both of which tend to be more clinically silent.

The treatment of esophageal candidiasis is usually ketoconazole, 200 mg orally twice daily, although some patients respond to oral nystatin (500,000 units swish and swallow 4–6 times daily). Esophagitis is viewed as a more progressive form of candidiasis than thrush since there is invasion beyond the basement membrane. For this reason, the infection is more likely to be refractory to treatment. Severe or refractory cases should be treated with amphotericin B using the low-dose regimen (0.3 mg/kg for 10–15 days). Regardless of the initial treatment, patients should subsequently receive an indefinite course of ketoconazole (200–400 mg/day), nystatin or clotrimazole.

It is uncommon for patients with oral and/or esophageal candidiasis to have *Candida* infections at other anatomic sites. The exception is women with AIDS, who often have *Candida* vaginitis. Lower gastrointestinal involvement with *Candida* invasion of the colon is unusual, as is disseminated candidiasis in these patients. Cultures of the oral cavity and stool often yield *Candida* sp., but this is found in 30% to 60% of healthy individuals without HIV infection. Thus, positive cultures from these sites often reflect the normal flora, and their implication as pathogens must be accompanied by typical clinical findings. With colonic disease there needs to be the demonstration of typical yeast forms invading the mucosa, which is rarely found. When infections occur in the oral cavity, *Candida albicans* is the usual pathogen and any other Candida species must be interpreted with caution.

CYTOMEGALOVIRUS INFECTION. Cytomegalovirus (CMV) infection is found in nearly 90% of AIDS patients at autopsies.[43–45] The sites of involvement are diverse, but may include virtually any level of the gastrointestinal tract including the esophagus, stomach, small bowel, and colon.[46–53] Colonic involvement is most common.[53] It is possible that some of these cases represent new infections, but the majority of AIDS patients have serologic evidence of prior CMV infection and the assumption is that this is a latent infection that has been reactivated in association with immunosuppression. It should be noted that CMV is commonly found in semen, this is now recognized as a sexually transmitted pathogen, prevalence rates in homosexual men according to serologic surveys are high, and rectal intercourse may be a common mode of disease acquisition.[54] Neverthe-

Table 13-6
Treatment of Gastrointestinal Infections Associated With AIDS

Agent	Treatment	Comment
Fungi		
Candida sp.	Clotrimazole: 1 troche 4–5 × daily Nystatin: 500,000–100,000 units swish and swallow tid Ketoconazole: 200 mg po bid	1. Duration is arbitrary: recurrences are common so that chronic suppressive treatment is usually advocated. 2. Patients with documented and/or symptomatic esophagitis should receive ketoconazole. 3. Refractory infections may be treated with amphotericin: 200–500 mg.
Histoplasmosis	Amphotericin B: 2–2.5 g IV	1. Ketoconazole (400–800 mg/day) has been used successfully for disseminated disease, but is not advocated for the compromised host. 2. Relapses common after treatment and may require continuous intermittent treatment.
Virus		
Herpes simplex virus	Acyclovir 200 mg po 5 × daily or 5 mg/kg IV q 8 h × 7–10 days	1. Relapse common: Most patients require chronic suppressive therapy with 200 mg po 3–5 × daily. 2. Occasional patients appear to benefit from topical application of the 5% ointment.
Cytomegalovirus	DHPG: 5 mg/kg IV bid × 2 weeks	1. Relapses are common and may require chronic suppressive treatment.
Parasites		
Cryptosporidiosis	Spiramycin	Efficacy is not established.
Isospora	Trimethoprim-sulfamethoxazole 2 DS po bid × 2 weeks	Relapses are common and may require longer courses or chronic suppressive treatment.
Giardia	Metronidazole: 250 mg tid × 10 days	1. Alternative is quinacrine: 100 mg po tid × 7 days. 2. Treatment of asymptomatic cyst excretors is arbitrary.
Amebiasis	Metronidazole: 750 mg po tid × 5–10 days plus diodoquin: 650 mg po tid × 21 days	Treatment of asymptomatic cyst excretor is arbitrary; preferred drug if treated is Furamide: 500 mg po tid × 10 days.
Microsporidia	None	
Bacteria		
Mycobacterium avium	Rifampin: 600 mg po/day or ansamycin: 150–300 mg po Clofazimine: 100 mg tid po ± amikacin or streptomycin, ethionamide, ethambutal	Efficacy in AIDS patients is not established.
Salmonellosis	Ampicillin: 6 g/day IV × 2–3 weeks, then ampicillin 500 mg tid po for 2–6 mo	1. Alternative for penicillin allergy or ampicillin resistance is trimethoprim sulfamethoxazole: 160 mg trimethoprim bid × 2–3 weeks, then 80 mg bid, or ciprofloxacin 500 mg bid 2. Chronic suppressive treatment required to prevent relapse. 3. Treatment is not advocated for carriers or those with mild gastroenteritis.
Shigella	Tetracycline: 2.5 g po as single dose *or* Trimethoprim-sulfamethoxazole: 160 mg trimethoprim bid × 5 days	1. Ampicillin (but not amoxicillin) may be used if isolate shows in vitro sensitivity. 2. Relapses are common and may require chronic suppressive treatment with tetracycline or doxycycline. 3. Third generation cephalosporins or quinolones may be preferred with septicemia or multiply resistant strains.
Campylobacter	Erythromycin: 250 mg po qid × 5–7 days	Bacteremic patients should receive gentamicin.

less, most patients with CMV infections of the gut have disseminated infections and the means of pathogen acquisition is unclear.

Pathologic findings that may be found in association with CMV infection include esophagitis with esophageal ulcerations, gastritis, enteritis, colitis, or proctitis. The accompanying clinical syndromes include dysphagia and retrosternal pain with esophageal involvement, malabsorption with steatorrhea when there is small bowel involvement, and chronic diarrhea that may be watery, bloody, or associated with excessive mucus when the colon is involved. Most common is diffuse colitis found in association with abdominal pain and watery or bloody diarrhea.[48-51] This may simulate the findings in idiopathic inflammatory bowel disease (IBD);[55] indeed, CMV infection may represent a super-infection in patients without HIV infection who have established IBD accompanied by immunosuppressive treatment. The distinction is important, since further immunosuppressive treatment that is commonly recommended for IBD promotes CMV infection. The point to emphasize is that CMV infection should be excluded in any patient with newly diagnosed IBD whenever the clinical features are atypical, extra-intestinal findings of IBD are absent, the patient is at risk for AIDS, or the patient fails to respond to traditional therapies used for IBD. Patients with CMV infection may also present with a solitary intestinal ulcer, toxic megacolon or, rarely, intestinal perforation.[56-58] Again, confusion may result with IBD or antibiotic-associated colitis. Another source of confusion is an endoscopy finding of violaceous lesions that may resemble Kaposi's sarcoma,[50] the diagnosis being established with a biopsy.

The typical findings with contrast studies are segmental colitis or pancolitis.[53,55,59] Barium enema shows mucosal granularity, thickened folds, spasticity, and superficial erosions. The involvement may be diffuse, segmental, or restricted to the cecum (typhilitis). CT studies may show marked thickening of the colonic wall with mucosal ulcerations. Endoscopy typically shows focal or diffuse inflammatory changes with hemorrhagic plaques and superficial ulcerations. Biopsies of lesions shows CMV vasculitis with hemorrhage and inflammation in the lamina propria; this is accompanied by typical CMV intranuclear inclusions within endothelial cells. Marked involvement of endothelial cells may be associated with vasculitis complicated by ischemic changes and ulcerations. These lesions, when accompanied by typical inclusions, appear to be diagnostic of CMV colitis. The problem is that typical inclusion bodies may also be seen within otherwise normal intestinal mucosa. In this situation, it is not clear that CMV can be implicated in the accompanying pathologic findings at other sites nor with the associated clinical findings. Quantitative assessment may assist in these distinctions. Hinnaut and colleagues[60] calibrated CMV inclusion bodies/mm² tissue and found a direct correlation between counts and grade of inflammation. Response to treatment with 9-(1,3-dihydroxy-2-propoxymethyl) guanine (DHPG)

clearly implicates CMV in some cases even when the organisms appear somewhat remote to the site of documented pathology.[61-63]

There is no FDA-approved treatment for CMV infection of the gastrointestinal tract, but the initial results with DHPG appear promising. Patients with CMV colitis respond by both clinical and pathologic criteria.[53,61-64] Chachoua and others noted clinical improvement in 30 of 41 AIDS patients with CMV infections of the gastrointestinal tract given DHPG in doses of 5 mg/kg twice daily for 2 weeks; 13 had recurrences at a median time of 9 weeks after initiating treatment.[53] A similar experience was reported by the Collaborative DHPG Treatment Study Group.[62] Laskin and associates reported 8 of 12 patients improved with 7.5 mg/kg/day for 2 weeks, but they followed this with a suppressive regimen (three times weekly) to prevent the relapses.[63]

MYCOBACTERIUM AVIUM-INTRACELLULARE. *Mycobacterium avium intracellulare* (MAI) was described in animals over a century ago and was originally recognized as a pathogen in man approximately 30 years ago.[65] This microbe, previously known as battey bacillus, was often considered a dormant organism found in large numbers of healthy persons, with a prevalence rate of about 33% in surveys of over 270,000 military recruits using the intradermal skin test (PPD-B).[66] A review of over 32,000 clinical isolates of mycobacteria reported to the CDC showed that *M. tuberculosis* accounted for 65%, and the next most common species reported was MAI which accounted for nearly 7000, or approximately 25%, of all potentially pathogenic mycobacteria. The highest rates of positive skin tests and the most frequent clinical isolations were from persons residing in the southeastern United States.[67,68] It was further estimated that approximately 30% of the patients with positive cultures actually had disease that could be ascribed to MAI,[69] giving an overall disease incidence of approximately 1/100,000. The great majority of these patients had infection restricted to the lung. Extrapulmonary disease was clearly unusual with only about 30 cases reported prior to the AIDS epidemic, but MAI is now one of the most frequently encountered opportunistic infections in AIDS patients, and represents an AIDS-defining diagnosis.

The source of the organism is usually unclear, but it is believed that man-to-man and animal-to-man transmission is uncommon.[65] Most patients have multiple organ involvement including the lung, lymph nodes, spleen, bone marrow, and gastrointestinal tract.[70-72] The organism may be recovered from any of these sites, and up to one-third of all AIDS patients have MAI recovered from blood cultures.[70,72] Nyberg and co-workers reported that abdominal CT scans in 17 AIDS patients with disseminated MAI showed 14 (82%) had multiple large mesenteric and retroperitoneal lymph nodes.[73]

Patients with gastrointestinal involvement often present with diarrhea, malabsorption, weight loss, and fever. The organism may be detected in the small bowel or colon. With colonic involvement the mucosa may show edema, erythema, and friability. Histologic examination shows typical acid-fast organisms both free and within macrophages of the lamina propria.[74] Pathologic findings with biopsy of the small bowel are often typical of Whipple's disease with foamy macrophages that are distended by vesicles containing periodic acid-Schiff (PAS)-positive material in the lamina propria.[75–77] However, in contrast to the organisms implicated in Whipple's disease, MAI does not cross-react with antibacterial typing sera and is acid-fast. The ultrastructural and pathologic similarities suggest that both of these conditions represent immune deficiencies in which the macrophage has limited capabilities for destroying selected bacteria after phagocytosis. Clinically, both conditions are characterized by fever, malabsorption, and cachexia, but in contrast to Whipple's disease patients, those with AIDS do not have migratory arthritis and they have multiple opportunistic infections with positive HIV serology, anergy, and lymphopenia.

The diagnosis of MAI is based on cultures of stool, recognition of typical organisms with acid-fast stain of stool, and the histology of small-bowel biopsy specimens. With stool specimens, the stain may be performed directly on unprocessed material; stool for culture is processed by the same digestion methods used for sputum. Stacey reported microbiologic studies for acid-fast bacilli (AFB) on 30 stool specimens from 22 AIDS patients.[78] Thirteen specimens from eleven patients yielded MAI in culture, and five showed AFB on Ziehl-Neelsen stain. Only 5 of the 11 had evidence of disseminated infection, raising some questions about the specificity of detecting this organism in stool without biopsy confirmation of mucosal invasion. Kiehn and colleagues[79] reported the Sloan–Kettering Hospital experience, which showed AFB smears of stools were positive in 12 of 17 AIDS patients with disseminated MAI infection, and all 12 specimens grew MAI. The skin test for MAI (PPD-B) is not helpful because of the high prevalence of positive results in healthy controls and the frequency of anergy in patients with AIDS. Similarly, serologic tests for MAI infections to detect antibody specific for this organism with immunofluorescence or other techniques has not proved rewarding.[80]

The treatment of MAI gastrointestinal disease is an enigma. Tetracycline, the traditional agent for Whipple's disease, has no merit. The organism is generally resistant to the usual antimycobacterial agents, and those that are effective *in vitro* do not seem to work *in vivo*. Clofazimine, an FDA approved drug for leprosy, shows good *in vitro* activity.[81] The initial studies in patients with pulmonary infections have been disappointing.[82] However, this may be related to the relatively low levels achieved in pulmonary tissue, suggesting that better results might be expected with extrapulmonary disease since the drug is avidly taken up by epithelium, the bone marrow, and the reticuloendothelial system, where intracellular tissue concentrations are very high. Another relatively new agent is ansamycin, a spiropiperipyl rifampin that shows

considerably better *in vitro* activity against MAI than rifampin.[83] Nevertheless, the clinical experience with clofazimine and/or ansamycin in AIDS patients has been variable.[65]

The current recommendation for disseminated MAI in immunosuppressed adult patients according to a consensus agreement of the American Thoracic Society[84] includes: (1) rifampin (600 mg po/day) if the organism is susceptible to rifampin or ansamycin (150–300 mg orally/day), providing the strain tested is resistant to rifampin and sensitive to ansamycin (these two drugs should not be used simultaneously); (2) clofazimine (100 mg tid orally); (3) ethambutol (25 mg/kg orally per day for 6 weeks followed by 15 mg/kg/day); (4) ethionamide (250 mg po, 2–4 times daily) and (5) streptomycin (15 mg/kg IM daily). Horsberg and others[71] recommend initial treatment with isoniazide (INH), ethambutol, cycloserine, clofazimine, ethionamide, and either rifampin or ansamycin. Furio and Wordell[85] recommend initial treatment with ethambutol, streptomycin, clofazimine, ethionamide, and either rifampin or ansamycin. All of these regimens have extensive potential toxicity and none can be recommended with enthusiasm. Nevertheless, anecdotal cases are reported in which gastrointestinal symptoms ascribed to MAI have responded to antimycobacterial treatment.[86]

HERPES SIMPLEX VIRUS. Herpes simplex virus (HSV) is a common cause of infections of the oral cavity, esophagus and anorectal area in patients with AIDS, and it also represents a common cause of proctitis in homosexual men with or without HIV infection.[87–90] With progressive immunosuppression in the face of HIV infection, the gastrointestinal lesions, particularly those involving the anorectal area, become chronic and progressive. Similar lesions in the oral cavity, esophagus, and perianal region may be seen with other forms of immunosuppression.[91] The usual complaint with perianal involvement is local pain in association with obstipation or constipation; diarrhea cannot be ascribed to this organism since only the most distal level of the GI tract is involved. HSV is notably different from CMV in this regard. The diagnosis is suspected when gross inspection shows single or multiple coalescent perianal ulcerations with a border that is raised and friable with or without vesicles or pustules. The diagnosis is confirmed by Tzanck smear, culture, or biopsy, preferably using specimens from the active border. Esophagitis ascribed to HSV shows the same symptoms and changes with chest radiography as those noted with *Candida* esophagitis. Oral lesions may also be severe and progressive with considerable pain. Treatment of all forms of HSV infection in these patients consists of acyclovir, which is available in topical, oral or intravenous preparations. Patients with severe disease should receive the drug intravenously. The usual oral regimen is 200 mg 5 times daily. Patients with chronic, persistent, or recurrent infections often receive suppressive treatment in the form of oral acyclovir, 200 mg 3–5 times daily.

CRYPTOSPORIDIOSIS. Cryptosporidium shares historical features analogous with two other protozoan parasites, *Pneumocystis carinii* and *Toxoplasma gondii*. These three organisms were originally described in the veterinary literature, were subsequently described as pathogens in humans as zoonotic diseases, and were finally accepted as major pathogens in immunosuppressed hosts in settings where there was usually no clear role of an animal source. Cryptosporidiosis now appears to be a relatively common cause of infectious diarrhea in immunocompetent patients in many settings including sporadic cases, toddlers from day-care centers, travelers, animal handlers, and waterborne epidemics.[93] Homosexual men do not appear to be predisposed to this infection in the absence of HIV infection, but when patients with AIDS have cryptosporidiosis the distribution of cases is somewhat higher among gay men (4.2%) compared to those with other risk categories.[93]

The usual symptoms in immunocompetent patients include nausea, vomiting, low-grade fever, abdominal cramps and watery diarrhea that typically lasts for 1 to 2 weeks. This is a self-limited disease from which immunocompetent patients invariably recover. Most cases are in children, and the incubation period ranges from 1 to 14 days.[92] The clinical pattern is quite different in patients with AIDS. These individuals develop severe, protracted diarrhea accompanied by anorexia, abdominal pain, malabsorption, and marked weight loss. Fever and vomiting are variable.[94-97] Diarrhea may be profound with losses of up to 15 liters daily and a mean of 3.6 liters per day.[96] There is malabsorption of fat and carbohydrate without blood or leukocytes on stool examination. Symptoms may persist for months, resulting in severe weight loss. However, this is variable and symptoms often improve spontaneously. Many patients have remittant symptoms, and rare AIDS patients have spontaneous cures.[98]

The organism is acquired by oral ingestion of oocysts. Sporozoites are released and then colonize and invade the microvilli of the small bowel. Replication is asexual (merogony) with release of merozoites that recycle after release, or sexual (sporogony) with merozoites that differentiate into gametocytes. The sexual cycle results in thin-walled oocysts that autoinfect locally and thick-walled oocysts that are passed.[92,99] Small-bowel biopsies show typical organisms of 2 to 4 μm lining the microvilli in a fashion somewhat analogous to that seen with *G. lamblia*. Histologic changes include partial atrophy and distortion of the villi and a mononuclear infiltration of the lamina propria, primarily in the ileum and jejunum.[100] Oocysts are passed in the stool, where they may be the source of person-to-person transmission and recognized on stool smears in diagnostic testing. Preferred stains are the modified Ziehl–Neelson, modified Kinyoun acid-fast, auramine O fluorescent stains or murine monoclonal antibody stains.[101-105] Stool concentration is recommended in settings where the parasite load is low, especially asymptomatic patients. Methods include Sheather's sugar flotation[101] and the formalin-ethyl acetate (ether) technique.[92] Alternatively,

typical organisms may be detected on the villous border in small bowel biopsies. Serologic tests include an indirect immunofluorescence test and an enzyme-linked immunosorbent assay (ELISA).[106,107] The favored site of infection is the distal small bowel, although any site in the GI tract from esophagus to rectum may be involved. Cryptosporidia also have been occasionally implicated in AIDS patients as a cause of cholecystitis, pancreatitis, or pulmonary infection.[108-112] Occasional asymptomatic carriers with AIDS have been described,[113] but this is unusual.

The prevalence of cryptosporidia among patients with AIDS is highly variable depending on symptoms, geographic location, and diagnostic testing. Data from the CDC indicate that 3.6% of AIDS patients in the United States have cryptosporidiosis;[93] studies from our laboratory show this parasite was detected in stools from 16% of AIDS patients with diarrhea and it was not encountered in the absence of gastrointestinal symptoms (see Table 14-3).[2] Henry and colleagues reported cryptosporidia accounted for 8% of 46 AIDS patients with chronic diarrhea from Zaire.[113] DeHoritz and associates[12] reviewed 110 AIDS patients with chronic diarrhea in Haiti and found cryptosporidia in 76 (57%).

There have been extensive efforts to treat cryptosporidial infections in the immunocompromised host using a variety of antibacterial and antiprotozoal agents, but none have produced a satisfactory result.[96] The possible exception is spiramycin, an antibacterial agent similar to erythromycin that is used extensively in many parts of the world, but available only for investigational use in the United States. One report indicates a good response in the majority of AIDS patients with cryptosporidiosis,[114] but the majority of studies have not shown a satisfactory response. Supportive care in these patients requires attention to fluid and electrolyte disturbances, sometimes requiring enteral or parenteral nutrition support. The role of anti-inflammatory agents, such as indomethacin, bismuth-containing agents and the sugar-electrolyte solutions for oral administration that have been found so successful in managing devastating diarrhea in children have not been adequately explored.

ISOSPORA. *Isospora belli* is another protozoan parasite that invades the microvillus of the small intestine and causes severe protracted diarrhea in patients with AIDS.[116-119] Disseminated isosporosis has been reported in an AIDS patient.[118] The life cycle of the organism,[119] the histologic changes in the small bowel,[116,119,120] and the diagnostic test with stool stains and biopsies[121] are analogous to those ascribed for cryptosporidiosis. The organism is distinguished from cryptosporidium on the basis of its morphology. Modified Kinyoun stains of stool show oval acid-fast oocysts that are much larger (20–30 μm $\times$ 10–20 μm) and contain two sporoblasts. By contrast, oocysts of cryptosporidia are 4 to 6 μm in diameter and contain four sporozoites. As with cryptosporidiosis, *Isospora* infection is AIDS-defining when responsible for diarrhea that persists at least 1 month. It is less common than cryptosporidiosis, but important to recognize since it appears to respond well to treatment with tri-methoprim-sulfamethoxazole. Data from the CDC indicate that only about 0.2% of AIDS cases in the United States involve isosporosis compared to about 3.6% with cryptosporidiosis.[93] A report from Zaire[113] indicates isospora were detected in 19% of AIDS patients with chronic diarrhea and actually exceeded cryptosporidia and all other recognized agents of enteric disease. DeHoritz and co-workers[12] reviewed 110 AIDS patients with chronic diarrhea in Haiti and found 60 (46%) had cryptosporidiosis, 15 (11%) had isosporosis and an additional 5 (4%) had both. The 15 with isosporosis were treated with trimethoprim-sulfamethoxazole for a median of 4 weeks and all responded with resolution of diarrhea within 2 days; 7 patients relapsed and all responded to retreatment.[12]

MICROSPORIDIA. Microsporidia are small protozoan parasites that have been occasionally encountered in patients with AIDS and otherwise unexplained diarrhea. As the name implies, this is a small parasite, and it is not detected with routine microscopic studies or with any diagnostic test on stool. Mature spores measure about $1.5 \times 0.5 \mu$. The preferred diagnostic method is electron microscopy of small bowel biopsies.[27,122,123] The role of this organism as an agent of enteric disease is not clear because of the relatively small number of cases and the lack of any therapeutic agent to evaluate therapeutic response. The true prevalence of this organism is also unclear owing to the rigor and expense required for diagnosis.

SALMONELLA. Salmonellae are relatively common pathogens implicated in four recognized syndromes: the asymptomatic carrier state, the chronic carrier state (defined as positive stool cultures in specimens separated by at least 6 months), gastroenteritis, enteric fever with bacteremia, and extraintestinal sites of infection. Patients with defects in cell-mediated immunity are prone to both more frequent and more serious infections with salmonellae, and so it is with AIDS.[42,124–127] It is estimated that the incidence of salmonellosis is magnified 20-fold over the general population in patients with AIDS.[42] The possibly unique features in this patient population are the predominance of *Salmonella typhimurium,* the lack of a clearly identifiable source of infection for most of the patients, the high rates of bacteremia, and the propensity of the infection to persist or recur despite the use of recommended antimicrobial regimens.

The usual clinical presentation for AIDS patients with salmonellosis is fever and diarrhea that is acute. The putative agent is readily recovered in cultures of stool, and blood cultures are often positive as well. Most authorities do not recommend treatment of *Salmonella* carriers or of patients who simply have gastroenteritis with this organism. However, most AIDS patients have severe disease that clearly merits treatment, and antimicrobial agents are usually recommended for carriers or patients with gastroenteritis who are prone to severe disease that includes the compromised host. The selection of specific agents is based on *in vitro* sensitivity tests of the isolated strain and on precedent, the favored drugs being ampicillin, amoxicillin, or trimethoprim-sulfamethoxazole. The potential role of newer agents such as third-generation cephalosporins or quinolones is under investigation. One of the idiosyncrasies of this infection in AIDS patients concerns the high rate of reactions to trimethoprim-sulfamethoxazole and the propensity of these infections to relapse when therapy has been discontinued. As a consequence, Jacobs and associates[127] recommend long-term suppressive treatment following the initial 2- to 3-week course for acute infection using orally administered amoxicillin. (Amoxicillin is preferred to ampicillin because of the reduced incidence of diarrhea as a side effect and to trimethoprim-sulfamethoxazole owing to the high rate of intolerance to this agent in patients with AIDS).

SHIGELLOSIS. Shigellosis is relatively common in gay men,[128–130] an association that was well recognized prior to the AIDS epidemic. Supporting data are based primarily on reviews of cases showing that 40% to 60% of epidemic[128] sporadic[129,130] cases occur in homosexual men. Shigellosis in patients with AIDS appears to be comparable to the experience with salmonellosis in that there is an unusual propensity for the organism to cause bacteremia and it is also prone to recur following the usual therapeutic regimens.[131,132] Baskin and others[131] report four AIDS patients with *Shigella* bacteremia. This is most unusual in that there are only about 300 reported cases of *Shigella* bacteremia.[133] The only other recognized risk factor for bloodstream invasion by *Shigella* are extreme youth (usually < 1 year) and malnutrition.[133]

CAMPYLOBACTER. *Campylobacter* sp. are a diverse group of microaerophilic, curved gram-negative bacilli that have been recognized enteric pathogens in man since 1947. *C. jejuni* is now recognized as the most commonly identified bacterial agent of diarrheal disease in industrialized countries; studies in symptomatic gay men with diarrhea or proctitis indicate recovery rates of 2% to 6%, suggesting sexual exposure as an occasional mechanism of disease transmission.[134] Other species of *Campylobacter* have a more impressive association with either homosexual exposure or AIDS. *C. cinaedi* and *C. fennelliae* are isolated almost exclusively from gay men, usually in the setting of proctitis or proctocolitis.[135] *C. hyointestinalis* has also been associated with homosexual exposure.[136] All of these species of *Campylobacter* other than *C. jejuni* are relatively infrequent isolates, although the low recovery rates reported may reflect the inadequacy of routine culture methods.

With regard to patients with AIDS, there are anecdotal case reports of two types: One concerns *Campylobacter* sp. encountered almost exclusively in the immunocompromised host, including *C. fetus,* a long recognized pathogen that commonly causes bacteremia in the compromised host,[137,138] and *C. laridis,* a newly recognized and apparently rare agent of bacteremia in the compromised host.[139,140] The second type of case reports concern AIDS patients with unusual *Campylobacter* infections such as *C. cinaedi* bacteremia[141] or refractory diarrhea involving a multiply-resistant strain of *C. jejuni.*[142]

HISTOPLASMOSIS. Histoplasmosis is another infection that is relatively common in immunocompetent hosts, but appears to be more frequent, more severe, and more refractory to therapy in patients with defective cell-mediated immunity including those with AIDS.[143-146] *Histoplasma capsulatum* is a dimorphic fungus in which the form found in the environment is the mycelial phase and the form found at 37°C in infected tissue is the yeast, usually intracellular within macrophages. The organism is distributed worldwide, but is most prevalent in river valley areas in the United States, the endemic area being the region surrounding the Mississippi and Ohio River Valleys. Infection is acquired by inhalation of conidia; the organism replicates in the lung and regional nodes and disseminates hematogenously. Most patients have asymptomatic infections and are detected only by skin tests used in epidemic surveys that reveal up to 90% of persons residing in the endemic area have been infected; some patients develop a self-limited form of pulmonary disease and the disseminated organisms usually remain dormant. Person-to-person transmission does not occur. The favored site for dissemination are the bone marrow, liver, spleen, and oropharynx. The clinical features of disseminated disease reflect these sites with fever, weight loss, pancytopenia, oropharyngeal involvement, and lymphadenopathy. With regard to the gastrointestinal tract, the major site of disseminated disease is the oropharynx with ulcerated lesions that may be associated with pain. Involvement of the small bowel or colon may also occur, but is much less common.[145] The preferred diagnostic methods are the demonstration of typical yeast forms that are usually intracellular within macrophages in biopsy specimens, positive cultures from distant metastatic sites, and serologic tests including the complement fixation (CF) test (with both yeast and mycelial antigens), precipitating antibody detected by immunodiffusion or counterimmunoelectrophoresis (CIE; to detect the H and M bands), and newer, more sensitive tests such as the radioimmunoassay or the enzyme immunoassay). The preferred treatment for disseminated histoplasmosis in the immunocompromised host is amphotericin B usually in a total dose of 2 to 2.5 g. Ketoconazole is active against this organism *in vitro* and is advocated for certain forms of histoplasmosis, but it is not advocated for disseminated disease in the immunosuppressed host.

MALIGNANCIES OF THE GASTROINTESTINAL TRACT

There are numerous tumors of the gastrointestinal tract that are associated with HIV infection. These include Kaposi's sarcoma, non-Hodgkin's lymphoma, cloacogenic carcinoma of the rectum, squamous-cell carcinoma of the rectum and anus, squamous carcinoma of the tongue, and Burkitt's lymphoma.

KAPOSI'S SARCOMA. Kaposi's sarcoma (KS) is a tumor of vascular endothelial cells that typically involves multiple sites, although it is uncertain if these are multiple primary lesions or represent metastatic tumors. This tumor is encountered in 20% to 30% of patients with AIDS; there is an unexplained disproportionate incidence in gay men and an unexplained apparent decrease in the frequency of this tumor in new AIDS cases. Involvement of visceral organs is common, the gastrointestinal tract is one of the most frequent sites for extracutaneous KS lesions, and some reports show that 40% to 50% of patients with KS lesions of the skin have GI involvement.[147-153] The oral cavity is frequently involved, and the lesions are often symmetrical and resemble submucosal hemorrhages.[147,150,151] However, nearly any level of the GI tract may be involved including the pharynx, esophagus, stomach, small bowel, or colon. Friedman performed endoscopy on 50 AIDS patients with KS and found that 10 (20%) had lesions in both the upper and lower tract, 6 had only upper-tract lesions, and 4 (8%) had only colonic lesions. There were no gastrointestinal symptoms ascribed to these lesions, although mortality rates were higher in those with endoscopically detected KS lesions.[148] Most patients with GI lesions also have cutaneous lesions, although visceral lesions occasionally predate cutaneous KS,[152] and one report showed up to 30% of AIDS patients with KS lesions in the GI tract had no skin lesions.[149] Autopsy studies show nodular or diffuse lesions.[154,155]

The usual mechanism of detection beyond visual inspection of the oral cavity is endoscopy. The characteristic endoscopic appearance is a raised, red nodule or nodules measuring several millimeters to 1 to 2 cm in diameter.[147,148,155,156] Larger lesions may show central umbilication. With contrast studies, the KS lesions may appear as nodules with or without a central ulceration.[157] CT scans may be helpful in defining deep tissue plane involvement and extent of nodal disease, especially with upper airway lesions.[157] Most of these lesions are clinically silent, although occasional patients have diarrhea, subacute intestinal obstruction, or protein-losing enteropathy.[158,159] On rare occasions the patient may present with rectal ulcer,[156] patients with pharyngeal involvement may present with dysphagia that is commonly ascribed to other causes,[157] or the clinical features may simulate those of ulcerative colitis.[159] Bleeding is rare and even endoscopic biopsies are not often complicated by bleeding, presumably owing to the location in the submucosa. However, histologic confirmation is difficult to establish with biopsy because of the depth of the lesions. In one study, only 7 of 30 lesions observed by endoscopy were microscopically confirmed.[148]

The mainstay of treatment for cutaneous and accessible mucosal lesions in the oral cavity is radiation using either photon (^{60}Co) or superficial electron beam irradiation. This is generally well tolerated, although irradiation of mucosal lesions is prone to cause mucositis.[161] Complete responses are noted in up to 50% of cases, and pain control is achieved in up to 70%.[161] Chemotherapy with vinca alkaloids (vinblastine, vincristine or etoposide) is also effective in the majority, but is commonly complicated by nausea, anorexia, vomiting, alopecia, paresthesias, and neutropenia.[162-163] Alternative regimens include combination chemotherapy (adriamycin, bleomycin plus vinblastine, vinblastine plus bleomycin, or vinblastine plus methotrexate[164-168] or α-interferon.[169,170] Again, dose-related toxicity is the limiting factor. Data for antiviral therapy with zidovudine in terms of response of KS are sparse. The large collaborative study of this agent in 282 patients with AIDS or ARC clearly showed clinical efficacy for sustaining life and reducing the incidence of opportunistic infection, but there was no convincing evidence of response of KS lesions.[171]

ORAL HAIRY LEUKOPLAKIA. This is a newly recognized disorder that resembles leukoplakia, but shows fibrillar projections that extend outward from the surface of the lesion to account for the name. The gross appearance is raised white thickening on the tongue, usually the lateral border, with a corrugated or hairy surface.[172-174] This may resemble oral candidiasis, and the first clue may be the failure to respond to typical treatment directed against *Candida albicans.* Histologic changes with biopsy resembles leukoplakia except for the absence of a mononuclear infiltrate. The cause of this lesion is unknown, but various studies have implicated papillomaviruses, HSV, CMV, and/or Epstein–Barr virus (EBV). Immunocytochemical staining has demonstrated papillomavirus core antigen in a majority of specimens, but typical viruses were not detected with electronmicroscopy.[172] EBV has been detected by electron microscopy and nucleic acid hybridization using EBV probes.[173]

Oral hairy leukoplakia is not an AIDS-defining diagnosis, but it is seen almost exclusively in the presence of HIV infection and is a relatively poor prognostic sign for the development of AIDS. Serologic studies of 101 patients with this diagnosis in San Francisco showed 100 were positive for HIV. Among 143 patients with oral hairy leukoplakia without AIDS followed prospectively, 43 (30%) developed AIDS. Survival analysis showed the probability of developing AIDS within 16 months was 48% and for 31 months it was 83%.[174] There is no form of treatment with established merit, and given the enigmatic nature of the lesion this is not surprising. Nevertheless, a provocative anecdotal report has shown dramatic resolution with DHPG therapy.[175]

LYMPHOMAS. Lymphomas of the gastrointestinal tract seen in association with AIDS include non-Hodgkin's lymphoma, Burkitt's lymphoma, and occasional cases of small non-cleaved B cell Burkett's-like lymphoma. The majority are high-grade B-cell lymphomas

that are extranodal in origin and respond poorly to chemotherapy.

A review of 119 homosexual males with non-Hodgkins lymphomas showed 68 (57%) of the diseases were high-grade malignant lymphomas, 90% were B-cell types, and 90% had extranodal involvement.[175-181] The third most common site of extranodal lesions is the GI tract, which was involved in up to 20% of patients. Even this may represent underreporting due to insensitive antemortem diagnostic tests. Both contrast studies and endoscopy underestimate true incidence,[182-185] since up to 40% of patients have GI lesions at autopsy.[186-188] Surgery or endoscopy with biopsy is usually required to establish the diagnosis. Any site from the oral cavity to rectum may be involved. In most cases there is a single site within the GI tract so that only about 1% involve two or more anatomic sites within the GI tract, and these usually involve contiguous sites.[189] A patient has been reported with small bowel involvement and two spontaneous perforations.[190] A patient with an HTLV-I associated lymphoma showing continuous involvement from the pharynx to rectum has also been reported.[189] Symptoms reflecting GI lesions are variable depending on the level and extent of involvement, associated opportunistic infections and symptoms ascribed to HIV infection *per se.* Diarrhea, when present, is usually secretory without steatorrhea, perhaps reflecting preservation of the villous architecture.[189] The prognosis is grim even with complete removal of localized small bowel lesions (stage Ie or IIe).[191]

REFERENCES

1. Quinn TC, Stamm WE, Goodell SE et al: The polymicrobial origin of intestinal infections in homosexual men. N Engl J Med 309:576, 1983
2. Laughon BE, Druckman DA, Vernon A et al: Prevalence of enteric pathogens in homosexual men with and without AIDS. Gastroenterology (in preparation)
3. Centers for Disease Control: Revision of the CDC surveillance case definition for Acquired Immunodeficiency Syndrome. Morbid Mortal Week Rep 36:3S, 1987
4. World Health Organization: Acquired immunodeficiency syndrome (AIDS). WHO/CDC case definition of AIDS. Week Epidemiol Rev 61:69, 1986
5. Kotler DP, Gaetz HP, Lange M et al: Enteropathy associated with the acquired immunodeficiency syndrome. Ann Intern Med 101:421, 1984
6. Archer DL, Glinsmann WH: Enteric infections and other co-factors in AIDS. Immunol Today 6:292, 1985
7. Santangelo WC, Krejs GJ: Gastrointestinal manifestations of the acquired immunodeficiency syndrome. Am J Med Sci 292(5):328, 1986
8. Dworkin B, Wormser GP, Rosenthal WS et al: Diarrhea and malabsorption associated with the acquired immunodeficiency syndrome (AIDS). Am J Gastroenterol 80(10):774, 1985
9. Pape JW, Liaudaud B, Thomas F et al: Characteristics of the acquired immune deficiency syndrome in Haitians. N Engl J Med 309:945, 1983

10. Pape JEW, Liautaud B, Thomas F et al: The acquired immunodeficiency syndrome in Haiti. Ann Intern Med 103: 674, 1985

11. Malebranche R, Arnoux E, Grerin JM et al: Acquired immunodeficiency syndrome with severe gastrointestinal manifestations in Haiti. Lancet 2:873, 1985

12. DeHovitz JA, Pape JW, Boncy M et al: Clinical manifestations and therapy of *Isospora belli* infection in patients with the acquired immunodeficiency syndrome. N Engl J Med 315:87, 1986

13. Clumeck N, Sonnet J, Taelman H et al: Acquired immune deficiency syndrome in African patients. N Engl J Med 310:492, 1984

14. Biggar RJ, Bouvet E, Ebbesen P et al: Clinical features of AIDS in Europe. Eur J Cancer Clin Oncol 20:165, 1984

15. Glauser MP, Francioli P: Clinical and epidemiological survey of acquired immune deficiency syndrome in Europe. Eur J Clin Microbiol 3L:55, 1984

16. Piot P, Quinn TC, Taelman H et al: Acquired immunodeficiency syndrome in a heterosexual population in Zaire. Lancet 2:65, 1984

17. Van de Perre P, Rouvroy D, Lepage P et al: Acquired immunodeficiency syndrome in Rwanda. Lancet 2:62, 1984

18. Serwadda E, Mugewrwa RD, Sewankambo NK et al: Slim disease: A new disease in Uganda and its association with HTLV-III infection. Lancet 2:849, 1985

19. Murquart K-H, Muller HA, Sailer J, Moser R: Slim disease (AIDS). Lancet 2:1186, 1985

20. Kamradt T, Niese D, Vogel F: Slim disease (AIDS). Lancet 2:1425, 1985

21. Wexner SE, Smithy WB, Milsom JW et al: The surgical management of anorectal diseases in AIDS and pre-AIDS patients. Dis Colon Rectum 29(11):719, 1986

22. Seligmann M, Pinching AJ, Rosen FS et al: Immunology of human immunodeficiency virus infection and the acquired immunodeficiency syndrome. Ann Intern Med 107:234, 1987

23. Phillips SC, Mildvan D, Wiliam DC et al: Sexual transmission of enteric protozoa and helminths in a venereal-disease-clinic population. N Engl J Med 305:603, 1981

24. William DC, Shookhoff HB, Felman YM et al: High rates of enteric protozoal infections in selected homosexual men attending a venereal disease clinic. Sex Trans Dis 5:155, 1978

25. Kean BH, William DC, Luminais SK: Epidemic of amoebiasis and giardiasis in a biased population. Br J Vener Dis 55:375, 1979

26. Gillin JS, Shike M, Alcock N et al: Malabsorption and mucosal abnormalities of the small intestine in the acquired immunodeficiency syndrome. Ann Intern Med 102:619, 1985

27. Dobbins WO III, Weinstein WM: Electron microscopy of the intestine and rectum in acquired immunodeficiency syndrome. Gastroenterology 88:738, 1985

28. Sidhu GS, Stahl RE, El Sadr W et al: Ultrastructural markers of AIDS. Lancet 1:990, 1983

29. Budhraja M, Levendoglu H, Kooka F et al: Duodenal mucosal T cell subpopulation and bacterial cultures in acquired immune deficiency syndrome. Am J Gastroenterol 82(5):427, 1987

30. Ellakany S, Whiteside TL, Schade RR et al: Analysis of intestinal lymphocyte subpopulations in patients with acquired immunodeficiency syndrome (AIDS) and AIDS-related complex. Am J Clin Pathol 87(3):356, 1987

31. Weber JR Jr, Dobbins WO III: The intestinal and rectal epithelial lymphocyte in AIDS. An electron-microscopic study. Am J Surg Pathol 10(9):627, 1986

32. Rodgers VD, Fassett R, Kagnoff MF: Abnormalities in intestinal mucosal T cells in homosexual populations including those with the lymphadenopathy syndrome and acquired immunodeficiency syndrome. Gastroenterology 90(3):552, 1986

33. Weber JR Jr, Dobbins WO III: The intestinal and rectal epithelial lymphocyte in AIDS. An electron-microscopic study. Am J Surg Pathol 10(9):627, 1986

34. Kotler DP, Scholes JV, Tierney AR: Intestinal plasma cell alterations in acquired immunodeficiency syndrome. Dig Dis Sci 32(2):129, 1987

35. Raufman JP, Straus EW: Gastrointestinal endoscopy in patients with acquired immune deficiency syndrome: an evaluation of current practices. Gastrointest Endoscop 33(2):76, 1987

36. Rotterdam H, Sommers SC: Alimentary tract biopsy lesions in the acquired immune deficiency syndrome. Pathology 17(2):181, 1985.

37. Wall SD, Ominsky S, Altman DF et al: Multifocal abnormalities of the gastrointestinal tract in AIDS. Am J Roentgenol 146(1):1, 1986

38. Jeffrey RB Jr, Nyberg DA, Bottles K et al: Abdominal CT in acquired immunodeficiency syndrome. Am J Roengenol 146(1):7, 1986

39. Albin J, Lewis E, Eftekhari F et al: Computed tomography of rectal and perirectal disease in AIDS patients. Gastrointest Radiol 12(1):67, 1987

40. Klein RS, Harris CA, Small CB et al: Oral candidiasis in high risk patients as the initial manifestation of the acquired immunodeficiency syndrome. N Engl J Med 311: 354, 1984

41. Tavitian A, Raufman J–P, Rosenthal LE: Oral candidiasis as a marker for esophageal candidiasis in the acquired immunodeficiency syndrome. Ann Intern Med 104:54, 1986

42. Bodey GP, Fainstein V, Guerrant R: Infections of the gastrointestinal tract in the immunocompromised patient. Ann Rev Med 37:271, 1986

43. Gottlieb MS, Groopman JE, Weinstein WM et al: The acquired immunodeficiency syndrome. Ann Intern Med 99: 208, 1983

44. Fauci AS, Macher AM, Longo DL et al: Acquired immunodeficiency syndrome: Epidemiologic, clinical, immunologic and therapeutic consideration. Ann Intern Med 100:92, 1984

45. Welch K, Finkbeiner W, and Alpers CE: Autopsy findings in the acquired immunodeficiency syndrome. JAMA 252: 1152, 1984

46. Bathazar EJ, Megibow AJ, Hulnick DH: Cytomegalovirus esophagitis and quantities in AIDS. Am J Radiol 144:1201, 1985

47. Lang DJ, Kummer JF, Hartley DP: Cytomegalovirus in semen: Persistence and demonstration in extracellular fluids. N Engl J Med 291:121, 1974

48. Knapp AB, Horst DA, Eliopoulos G et al: Widespread cytomegalovirus gastroenterocolitis in a patient with AIDS. Gastroenterology 85:1399, 1983

49. Gertier SL, Pressman J, Price P et al: Gastrointestinal cytomegalovirus infection in a homosexual man with severe acquired immunodeficiency syndrome. Gastroenterology 85:1403, 1983

50. Meiselman MS, Cello JP, Margaretten W: Cytomegalovirus colitis: Report of the clinical, endoscopic, and pathologic

findings in two patients with the acquired immune deficiency syndrome. Gastroenterology 88:171, 1985

51. Levinson W, Bennetts RW: Cytomegalovirus colitis in acquired immunodeficiency syndrome: A chronic disease with varying manifestations. Am J Gastroenterol 80:445, 1985

52. Rotterdam H, Sommers SC: Alimentary tract biopsy lesions in the acquired immune deficiency syndrome. Pathology 17:181, 1985

53. Chachoua A, Dieterich D, Krasinski K et al: 9-(1,3-dihydroxy-2-propoxymethyl) guanine (Ganciclovir) in the treatment of cytomegalovirus gastrointestinal disease with the acquired immunodeficiency syndrome. Ann Intern Med 107:133, 1987

54. Collier AC, Meyers JD, Corey L et al: Cytomegalovirus infection in homosexual men. Am J Med 82:593, 1987

55. Frager DH, Frager JD, Wolf EL et al: Cytomegalovirus colitis in acquired immune deficiency syndrome: Radiologic spectrum. Gastrointest Radiol 11:241, 1986

56. Frank D, Raicht FF: Intestinal perforation associated with cytomegalovirus infection in patients with acquired immune deficiency syndrome. Am J Gastroenterol 79:201, 1984

57. Freedman PG, Weiner BC, Balthazar EJ: Cytomegalovirus esophagogastritis in a patient with acquired immunodeficiency syndrome. Am J Gastroenterol 80:434, 1985

58. Kram HB, Hino ST, Cohen RE et al: Spontaneous colonic perforation secondary to cytomegalovirus in a patient with acquired immune deficiency syndrome. Crit Care Med 12:469, 1984

59. Balthazar EJ, Megibow AJ, Fazzini E et al: Cytomegalovirus colitis in AIDS: radiographic findings in 11 patients. Radiology 155:585, 1985

60. Hinnant KL, Rotterdam HZ, Bell ET et al: Cytomegalovirus infection of the alimentary tract: A clinicopathological correlation. Am J Gastroenterol 81(10):944, 1986

61. Bach MC, Bagwell SP, Knapp NP et al: 9-(1,3 dihydroxy-2-propoxymethyl) guanine for cytomegalovirus infection in patients with the acquired immunodeficiency syndrome. Ann Intern Med 103:381, 1985

62. Collaborative DHPG Treatment Study Group: Treatment of serious cytomegalovirus infections with 9-(1,3 dihydroxy-2-propoxymethyl) guanine in patients with AIDS and other immunodeficiencies. N Engl J Med 314:801, 1986

63. Laskin OL, Cederberg DM, Mills J et al: Ganciclovir for the treatment and suppression of serious infections caused by cytomegalovirus. Am J Med 83:201, 1987

64. Masur H, Lane HC, Palestine A et al: Effect of 9-(1,3 dihydroxy-2-propoxymethyl) guanine on serious cytomegalovirus disease in eight immunosuppressed homosexual men. Ann Intern Med 104:41, 1986

65. Colaizzi PA: Disease due to *Mycobacterium avium-intracellulare.* Chest 87:139S, 1985

66. Edwards LB, Acquaviva FA, Livesay VT et al: An atlas of sensitivity to tuberculin, PPD-B, and histoplasmin in the United States. Am Rev Respir Dis 99:1, 1969

67. Good RC: Isolation of nontuberculous mycobacteria in the United States, 1979. J Infect Dis 142:779, 1980

68. Good RC, Snider DE: Isolation of nontuberculous mycobacteria in the United States, 1980. J Infect Dis 142:779, 1982

69. Fogan L: PPD antigens and the diagnosis of mycobacterial diseases: a study of atypical mycobacterial disease in Oklahoma. Arch Intern Med 124:49, 1969

70. Hawkins CC, Gold JWM, Whimbey E et al: *Mycobacterium avium* complex infections in patients with the acquired immunodeficiency syndrome. Ann Intern Med 105:184, 1986

71. Horsburgh CR Jr, Mason UG III, Farhi DC et al: Disseminated infection with *Mycobacterium avium-intracellulare:* A report of 13 cases and review of the literature. Medicine 64:36, 1985

72. Kiehn TE, Edwards FF, Brannon P et al: Infections caused by *Mycobacterium avium* complex in immunocompromised patients: Diagnosis by blood culture and fecal examination, antimicrobial and seroagglutination characteristics. J Clin Microbiol 21:168, 1985

73. Nyberg DA, Federle MP, Jeffrey RB et al: Abdominal CT findings of disseminated Mycobacterium avium-intracellulare in AIDS. Am J Roentgenol 145:297, 1985

74. Damsker B: *Mycobacterium avium-Mycobacterium intracellulare* from the intestinal tracts of patients with the acquired immunodeficiency syndrome: Concepts regarding acquisition and pathogenesis. J Infect Dis 151:179, 1985

75. Roth RI, Owen RL, Keren DF: AIDS with *Mycobacterium avium-intracelluare* lesions resembling those of Whipple's disease. N Engl J Med 309:1324, 1983

76. Ston RL, Grumminger RP: AIDS with *Mycobacterium avium-intracelluare* lesions resembling those of Whipple's disease. N Engl J Med 309:1323, 1983

77. Gillin JS, Urmacher C, West R et al: Disseminated *Mycobacterium avium-intracelluare* infection in acquired infection in acquired immunodeficiency syndrome mimicking Whipple's disease. Gastroenterology 85:1187, 1983

78. Stacey AR: Isolation of Mycobacterium avium-intracellulare-scrofulaceum complex from faeces of patients with AIDS. Brit Med J 293:119A, 1986

79. Kiehn TE, Edwards FF, Brannon P et al: Infections caused by *Mycobacterium avium* complex in immunocompromised patients: Diagnosis by blood culture and fecal examination, antimicrobial susceptibility tests, and morphological and seroagglutination characteristics. J Clin Microbiol 21:168, 1985

80. Winter SM, Bernard EM, Gold JWN et al: Humoral response to disseminated infection by *Mycobacterium avium-intracellulare* in acquired immunodeficiency syndrome and hairy cell leukemia. J Infect Dis 151:523, 1985

81. Gangadharam PR, Pratt PF, Damale PB et al: Dynamic aspects of the activity of clofazimine against *Mycobacterium intracellulare.* Tubercle 62:201, 1981

82. Gribetz AR et al: Solitary pulmonary nodules due to nontuberculous mycobacterial infection. Am J Med 70:39, 1981

83. Woodley CL, Kilburn JO: *In vitro* susceptibility of *Mycobacterium avium* complex and *Mycobacterium tuberculosis* strains to a spiro-piperidyl rifampin. Am Rev Respir Dis 126:586, 1982

84. Iseman MD, Corpe RF, O'Brien RJ et al: Disease due to *Mycobacterium avium-intracellulare.* Chest 87:139S, 1985

85. Furio MM, Wordell CJ: Treatment of infectious complications of acquired immunodeficiency syndrome. Clin Pharmacol 4:539, 1985

86. Schneebaum CW, Novick DM, Chabon AB et al: Terminal ileitis associated with Mycobacterium avium-intracellulare infection in a homosexual man with acquired immune deficiency syndrome. Gastroenterology 92:1127, 1987

87. Siegal FP, Lopez C, Hammer GS et al: Severe acquired immunodeficiency in male homosexuals, manifested by chronic perianal ulcerative herpes simplex lesions. N Engl J Med 305:1439, 1981

88. Goodell SE, Quinn TC, Mkrtichian E et al: Herpes simplex virus proctitis in homosexual men: Clinical, sigmoidoscopic and histopathologic features. N Engl J Med 308:868, 1983

89. Quinnan GV, Masur H, Rock AH: Herpesvirus infections in the acquired immune deficiency syndrome. JAMA 252:72, 1984

90. Goldmeir D: Proctitis and herpes simplex virus in homosexual men. Brit J Vener Dis 56:111, 1980

91. Kalb RE, Grossman ME: Chronic perianal herpes simplex in immunocompromised hosts. Am J Med 80:486, 1986

92. Janoff EN, Reller LB: *Cryptosporidium* species, a protean protozoan. J Clin Microbiol 25:967, 1987

93. Navin TR, Hardy AM: Cryptosporidiosis in patients with AIDS. J Infect Dis 155:150, 1987

94. Whiteside ME, Barkin JS, May RG et al: Enteric cocciodiosis among patients with the acquired immunodeficiency syndrome. Am J Trop Hyg 33:1065, 1984

95. Pittik SD, Fainstein V, Garza D et al: Human cryptosporidiosis: A spectrum of disease. Report of six cases and review of literature. Arch Intern Med 143:2269, 1983

96. Communicable Disease Center: Cryptosporidiosis: Assessment of chemotherapy of males with acquired immune deficiency syndrome (AIDS). Morbid Mortal Week Rep MMWR 31:589, 1982

97. Portnoy D, Whiteside ME, Buckley E III et al: Treatment of intestinal cryptosporidiosis with spiramycin. Ann Intern Med 101:202, 1984

98. Soave R, Danner RL, Honig CL et al: Cryptosporidiosis in homosexual men. Ann Intern Med 100:504, 1984

99. Bird RG, Smith MD: Cryptosporidiosis in man: Parasite life cycle and fine structural pathology. Am J Pathol 132:217, 1980

100. Lefkowitch JH, Krumholz S, Feng–Chen KL et al: Cryptosporidiosis of the human small intestine a light and electron microscopic study. Hum Pathol 15:746, 1984

101. Ma P, Soave R: Three-step stool examination for cryptosporidiosis in 10 homosexual men with protracted watery diarrhea. J Infect Dis 147:824, 1983

102. Dupont HL: Cryptosporidiosis and the healthy host. N Engl J Med 312:1319, 1985

103. Garcia LS, Brewer TC, Bruckner DA: Fluorescence detection of *Cryptosporidium* oocysts in human fecal specimens by using monoclonal antibodies. J Clin Microbiol 25:119, 1987

104. Garcia LS, Bruckner DA, Brewer TC, Shimizu RY: Techniques for the recovery and identification of *Cryptosporidium* oocysts from stool specimens. J Clin Microbiol 18:185, 1983

105. Payne P, Lancaster LA, Heinzman M et al: Identification of *Cryptosporidium* in patients with acquired immunodeficiency syndrome. N Engl J Med 309:613, 1984

106. Campbell PN, Current WL: Demonstration of serum antibodies to cryptosporidium in normal immunodeficient humans with confirmed infections. J Clin Microbiol 18:165, 1983

107. Ungar BLP, Soave R, Fayer R et al: Enzyme immunoassay detection of immunoglobulin M and G antibodies to cryptosporidium in immunocompetent and immunocompromised persons. J Infect Dis 153:570, 1986

108. Blumberg RS, Kelsey P, Perrone T et al: Cytomegalovirus and cryptospordium associated acalculous gangrene cholecystitis. Am J Med 76:1118, 1984

109. Pitlik SD, Fainstein V, Rios A et al: Cryptosporidial cholecystitis. N Engl J Med 308:967, 1983

110. Forgacs P, Tarshis A, Ma P et al: Intestinal and bronchial cryptosporidiosis in an immunodeficient homosexual man. Ann Intern Med 99:793, 1983

111. Ma P, Villanueva TG, Kaufman D et al: Respiratory cryptosporidiosis in the acquired immune deficiency syndrome. JAMA 252:1298, 1984

112. Zar F, Geisler PJ, Brown VA: Asymptomatic carriage of Cryptosporidium in the stool of a patient with the acquired immunodeficiency syndrome. J Infect Dis 151:195, 1985

113. Henry MC, De Clercq D, Lokombe B et al: Parsitological observations in chronic diarrhoea in suspected AIDS adult patients in Kinshasa (Zaire). Trans R Soc Trop Med Hyg 80(2):309, 1986

115. Portnoy D, Whiteside ME, Buckley E et al: Treatment of intestinal cryptosporidiosis with spiramycin. Ann Intern Med 101:202, 1984

116. Shein R, Gelb A: *Isospora belli* in a patient with acquired immunodeficiency syndrome. J Clin Gastroenterol 6:525, 1984

117. Forthal DN, Guest SS: *Isospora belli* enteritis in three homosexual men. Am J Trop Med Hyg 33:1060, 1984

118. Restrepo C, Macher AM, Radany EH: Disseminated extraintestinal isosporiasis in a patient with acquired immune deficiency syndrome. Am J Clin Pathol 87:536, 1987

119. Henderson HE, Gillespie GW, Kaplan P: The human isospora. Am J Hyg 78:302, 1963

120. Brandborg LL, Goldberg SD, Breidenboch WC: Human coccidiosis: A possible cause of malabsorption. The life cycle in small bowel mucosal biopsies as a diagnostic feature. N Engl J Med 283:1306, 1970

121. Ng E, Markell EK, Fleming RL et al: Demonstration of *Isospora belli* by acid fast stain in a patient with acquired immune deficiency syndrome. J Clin Microbiol 20:384, 1984

122. Modigliani R, Bories C, LeCharpentier T et al: Diarrhea and malabsorption in acquired immune deficiency syndrome: A study of four cases with special emphasis on opportunistic protozoan infections. Gut 26:179, 1985

123. Desportes I, Le Charpentier Y, Galian A et al: Occurrence of a new microsporidian: Enterocytozoan bieneusi n.g., sp., in the enterocytes of a human patient with AIDS. J Protozool 32:250, 1985

124. Smith PD, Macher AM, Bookman MA et al: *Salmonella typhimurium* enteritis and bacteremia in the acquired immunodeficiency syndrome. Ann Intern Med 102:207, 1985

125. Nudelman RB, Mathur-Wagh V, Yancovitz SR et al: Salmonella bacteremia associated with the acquired immunodeficiency syndrome (AIDS). Arch Intern Med 145:1968, 1985

126. Glasser JB, Morton–Kute L, Berger SR et al: A recurrent salmonella typhimurium bactermia associated with the acquired immunodeficiency syndrome. Ann Intern Med 102:189, 1985

127. Jacobs JL, Gold JWM, Murray HW et al: Salmonella infections in patients with the acquired immunodeficiency syndrome. Ann Intern Med 102:186, 1985

128. Dritz SK, Back AF: Shigella enteritis venereally transmitted. N Engl J Med 291:1194, 1974

129. Bader M, Pedersen AHB, Williams R: Venereal transmis-

sion of shigellosis in Seattle—King County. Sex Transm Dis 4:89, 1977

130. Brusin LM, Genvert G, Topf–Olstein B et al: Shigellosis: Another sexually transmitted disease?. Brit J Vener Dis 52:348, 1976

131. Baskin DH, Lax JD, Barenberg D: Shigella bacteremia in patients with the acquired immune deficiency syndrome. Am J Gastroenterol 82:338, 1987

132. Glupczynski Y, Hansen W, Jonas C et al: Shigella flexneri bacteremia in a patient with acquired immune deficiency syndrome. Acta Clin Belg 40:388, 1985

133. Struelens MJ, Patte D, Kabir I et al: Shigella septicemia: Prevalence, presentation, risk factors and outcome. J Infect Dis 152:784, 1985

134. Quinn TC, Goodell SE, Fennell C et al: Infections with *Campylobacter jejuni* and *Campylobacter*-like organisms in homosexual men. Ann Intern Med 101:187, 1984

135. Totten PA, Fennell CL, Tenover FC et al: *Campylobacter cinaedi* (sp. nov.) and *Campylobacter fennelliae* (sp. nov.): Two new *Campylobacter* species associated with enteric disease in homosexual men. J Infect Dis 151:131, 1985

136. Edmonds P, Patton CM, Griffin PM et al: *Campylobacter hyointestinalis* associated with human gastrointestinal disease in the United States. J Clin Microbiol 25:685, 1987

137. Riley LW, Finch MJ: Results of the first year of national surveillance of Campylobacter infections in the United States. J Infect Dis 151:956, 1985

138. Guerrant RL, Lahita RG, Winn WC Jr et al: Campylobacteriosis in man: Pathogenic mechanisms and review of 91 bloodstream infections. Am J Med 65:584, 1978

139. Nachamkin I, Stowell C, Skalina D et al: *Campylobacter laridis* causing bacteremia in an immunosuppressed patient. Ann Intern Med 101:55, 1984

140. Tauxe RV, Patton CM, Edmonds P et al: Illness associated with *Campylobacter laridis,* a newly recognized *Campylobacter* species. J Clin Microbiol 21:222, 1985

141. Cimolai N, Gill MJ, Jones A et al: "Campylobacter cinaedi" bacteremia: Case report and laboratory findings. J Clin Microbiol 25:942, 1987

142. Dworkin B, Wormser GP, Abdoo RA et al: Persistence of multiply antibiotic-resistant *Campylobacter jejuni* in a patient with the acquired immune deficiency syndrome. Am J Med 80:965, 1986

143. Haggerty CM, Britton MC, Dorman JM et al: Gastrointestinal histoplasmosis in suspected acquired immunodeficiency syndrome. West J Med 143:244, 1985

144. Taylor MD, Baddour LM, Alexander JR: Disseminated histoplasmosis associated with the acquired immune deficiency syndrome. Am J Med 77:579, 1984

145. Haggerty CM, Britton MC, Dorman JM, Marzoni FA Jr: Gastrointestinal histoplasmosis in suspected acquired immunodeficiency syndrome. AJR 145:297, 1985

146. Cohn JB: The acquired immunodeficiency syndrome: B-cell lymphoma, histoplasmosis and ethics and economics. Ann Intern Med 104:447, 1986

147. Lozada F, Silverman J, Miglioratti CA et al: Oral manifestations of tumors and opportunistic infection in AIDS: Findings in 53 homosexual men with Kaposi's sarcoma. Oral Surg 56:491, 1983

148. Friedman S, Wright T et al: Kaposi's sarcoma and the gastrointestinal tract: The San Francisco experience. Gastroenterology 84:1160, 1983

149. Lemlich G, Schwam L, Lebwohl M: Kaposi's sarcoma and acquired immunodeficiency syndrome. Postmortem

findings in twenty-four cases. J Am Acad Dermatol 16: 319, 1987

150. Gnepp DR, Chandler W, Hyams V: Primary Kaposi's sarcoma of the head and neck. Ann Intern Med 100:107, 1984

151. Patow CA, Steis R, Longo DL et al: Kaposi's sarcoma of the head and neck in acquired immune deficiency syndrome. Otolaryngol Head Neck Surg 92:255, 1984

152. Gottlieb MS, Moderator: The acquired immune deficiency syndrome. Ann Intern Med 99:208, 1983

153. Saltz RK, Kurtz RC, Lightdale CJ et al: Gastrointestinal involvement in Kaposi's sarcoma. Gastroenterology 82: 1168, 1982

154. Stern JO, Dieterich M, Faust L et al: Disseminated Kaposi's sarcoma: Involvement of the GI tract in homosexual men. Gastroenterology 82:1185, 1982

155. Friedman–Kien AE, Laubenstein LJ, Rubinstein P et al: Disseminated Kaposi's sarcoma in homosexual men. Ann Intern Med 96:693, 1982

156. Endean ED, Ross CW, Strodel WE: Kaposi's sarcoma appearing as a rectal ulcer. Surgery 101:767, 1987

157. Emery CD, Wall SD, Federle MP et al: Pharyngeal Kaposi's sarcoma in patients with AIDS. Am J Roentgenol 147: 919, 1986

158. Rose HS, Balthazar EJ, Megibow AJ et al: Alimentary tract involvement in Kaposi's sarcoma: Radiographic and endoscopic findings in 25 homosexual men. Am J Roentgenol 139:661, 1982

159. Laine L, Politoske EJ, Gill P: Protein-losing enteropathy in acquired immunodeficiency syndrome due to intestinal Kaposi's sarcoma. Arch Intern Med 147:1174, 1987

160. Weber JN, Carmichael DJ, Boylston A et al: Kaposi's sarcoma of the bowel—presenting as apparent ulcerative colitis. Gut 26:295, 1985

161. Cooper JS, Fried PR: Defining the role of radiation therapy in the management of epidemic Kaposi's sarcoma. Int J Radiat Oncol Biol Phys 13:35, 1987

162. Lewis B et al: Single agent and combination chemotherapy of Kaposi's sarcoma in acquired immune deficiency syndrome, abstracted. Proc Am Soc Clin Oncol 2:59, 1983

163. Mintzer DM et al: Treatment of Kaposi's sarcoma and thrombocytopenia with vincristine in patients with the acquired immunodeficiency syndrome. Ann Intern Med 102:200, 1985

164. Laubenstein LJ et al: Treatment of epidemic Kaposi's sarcoma with VP-16 (etoposide) or a combination of doxorubicin, bleomycin, and vinblastine. J Clin Oncol 2:1115, 1984

165. Kapkin L et al: Treatment of Kaposi's sarcoma in acquired immunodeficiency syndrome with an alternating vincristine-vinblastine regimen. Cancer Treat Rep 70:1121, 1986

166. Laubenstein LJ et al: Treatment of epidemic Kaposi's sarcoma with VP-16 (etoposide) and a combination of doxorubicin, bleomycin and vinblastine (ABV), abstracted. Proc Am Soc Clin Oncol 2:228, 1983

167. Wernz J et al: Chemotherapy and assessment of response in epidemic Kaposi's sarcoma with bleomycin/velban, abstracted. Proc Am Soc Clin Oncol 5.4, 1986

168. Gelmann EP, Longo D, Lane HC et al: Combination chemotherapy of disseminated Kaposi's sarcoma in patients with the acquired immune deficiency syndrome. Am J Med 82:456, 1987

169. Krown SE, Real FX, Cunningham–Rundles S et al: Preliminary observations on the effect of recombinant leu-

kocyte A interferon in homosexual men with Kaposi's sarcoma. N Engl J Med 308:671, 1983

170. Groopman JE, Gottlieb MS, Goodman J et al: Recombinant alpha-2 interferon for Kaposi's sarcoma associated with the acquired immunodeficiency syndrome. Ann Intern Med 100:671, 1984

171. Fischl MA, Richman DD, Grieco MH et al: The efficacy of azidothymidine (AZT) in the treatment of patients with AIDS and AIDS-related complex. N Engl J Med 317:185, 1987

172. Greenspan D, Convant M, Silverman S Jr et al: Oral "hairy" leucoplakia in male homosexuals: Evidence of association with both papillomavirus and A herpes-group virus. Lancet 831, October 13, 1984

173. Greenspan JS, Greenspan D, Lennette ET: Replication of Epstein-Barr virus within the epithelial cells of oral "hairy" leukoplakia, an AIDS-associated lesion. N Engl J Med 313:1564, 1985

174. Greenspan D, Greenspan JS, Hearst NG et al: Relation of oral hairy leukoplakia to infection with the human immunodeficiency virus and the risk of developing AIDS. J Infect Dis 155:475, 1987

175. Newman C, Polk BF: Resolution of oral hairy leukoplakia during therapy with 9-(1,3 dihydroxy-2-propoxymethyl) guanine (DHPH). Ann Intern Med 107:348, 1987

176. Lowenthal DA, Safai B, Koziner B: Malignant neoplasia in AIDS. Infect Surg 413, July 1987

177. Brynes RK, Chan CW, Spira TJ et al: Value of lymph node biopsy in unexplained lymphadenopathy in homosexual men. JAMA 250:1313, 1983

178. Ziegler JL, Beckstead JA, Volberding PA et al: Non-Hodgkin's lymphoma in 90 homosexual men: relation to generalized lymphadenopathy and the acquired immunodeficiency syndrome. N Engl J Med 311:565, 1984

179. Levine AM, Meyer PR, Begandy MK et al: Development of B-cell lymphoma in homosexual men: Clinical and immunologic findings. Ann Intern Med 100:7, 1984

180. Gill PS, Levine AM, Meyer PR et al: Primary central nervous system lymphoma in homosexual men: Clinical, immunologic and pathologic features. Am J Med 78:742, 1985

181. Kalter SP, Riggs SA, Cabanillas F et al: Aggressive non-Hodgkin's lymphomas in immunocompromised homosexual males. Blood 66:655, 1985

182. Brady LW, Asbell SO: Malignant lymphoma of the gastrointestinal tract. Radiology 137:291, 1980

183. Crowley KS, Don G, Gibson GE et al: Primary gastrointestinal tract lymphoma A clinicopathologic study of 28 cases. Aust NZ J Med 12:135, 1982

184. Loehr WJ, Mujahed Z, Zahn FD, Gray GF, Thorbjarnarson B: Primary lymphoma of the gastrointestinal tract: A review of 100 cases. Ann Surg 170:232, 1969

185. Sandler RS: Primary gastric lymphoma: A review. Am J Gastroenterol 79:21, 1984

186. Rosenberg SA, Diamond HD, Jaslowitz B et al: Lymphosarcoma: A review of 1269 cases. Medicine 40:31, 1961

187. Herrmann R, Panahon AM, Barcos MP et al: Gastrointestinal involvement in non-Hodgkin's lymphoma. Cancer 46:215, 1980

188. Sherlock P: The gastrointestinal manifestations and complications of malignant lymphoma. Schweiz Med Wochenschr 110:1031, 1980

189. Cappell MS, Chow J: HTLV-1-associated lymphoma involving the entire alimentary tract and presenting with an acquired immune deficiency. Am J Med 82:649, 1987

190. Collier PE: Small bowel lymphoma associated with AIDS. J Surg Oncol 32:131, 1986

191. Steinberg JJ, Bridges N, Feiner HD et al: Small intestinal lymphoma in three patients with acquired immune deficiency syndrome. Am J Gastroenterol 80:21, 1985

Kaposi's Sarcoma in AIDS: Diagnosis and Treatment

Robert L. Krigel
Alvin E. Friedman-Kien

14

The acquired immunodeficiency syndrome (AIDS) was first recognized in New York and California in early 1981 as a combined epidemic of *Pneumocystis carinii* pneumonia and Kaposi's sarcoma (KS) in young men of homosexual or bisexual orientation. As of September 1987 the Centers for Disease Control (CDC) had reported over 40,000 patients with AIDS in the United States and over 55,000 worldwide, with new cases continuing to present at an increasing rate. The true incidence of the disease is probably much higher than the statistics indicate. The disease has become a world health problem with cases being reported from more than 123 countries. The etiology of this alarming disease appears to be a family of T-cell lymphotropic retroviruses, known as the human immunodeficiency virus (HIV, see Chapter 2). Various epidemiologic cofactors may also be involved in predisposing certain individuals in groups known to be at high risk to develop AIDS. The underlying immunologic deficiency that characterizes AIDS is an acquired profound disorder of cell-mediated immune functions. This immunologic deficiency predisposes the host to a variety of opportunistic infections (OIs) and unusual neoplasms, especially the previously uncommon tumor KS.[1-6]

Kaposi's sarcoma was first described in 1872 by the Austro-Hungarian dermatologist, Moritz Kaposi, in an article entitled "Idiopathic Multiple Pigmented Sarcoma of the Skin."[7,8] From that time until the recent epidemic, classic KS remained a rare and unusual tumor. While most of the cases seen in Europe and North America have occurred in elderly men of Italian or Eastern European Jewish ancestry, the neoplasm has also been reported to occur in several other distinct populations as well: young black African adult males and prepubescent children, renal allograft recipients, and other patients receiving immunosuppressive therapy.[9-14] The recent epidemic of a disseminated, fulminant form of KS was first observed among young homosexual men in large urban centers in the United States. This new form of KS shall be referred to as epidemic KS in light of its association with AIDS and to distinguish it from the classic, African, and transplant-related varieties of the neoplasm. Although the histopathology of the different stages of the Kaposi's tumor is essentially identical in all of these groups, the clinical manifestations and course of the disease differ remarkably.[15]

ETIOLOGY

The most current hypotheses regarding the etiology of AIDS suggest that the underlying immune disfunction is caused by a virus. The putative agent appears to behave similarly to the hepatitis B virus (HBV) in its manner of transmission, that is, by intimate sexual contact or through exposure to blood or blood products. Currently, the human retrovirus HIV-1 (formerly known as human T-cell leukemia virus [HTLV-III] and/or the lymphadenopathy-associated virus [LAV]) is considered the most likely cause of AIDS. Although HIV is now known to infect other host cells such as macrophages, Langerhans cells, and cells of the central nervous system, the virus seems to have a particular tropism for infecting the host's T-helper lymphocytes or their precursors, thus leading to their destruction and an irreversible state of severe cell-mediated immune deficiency. The victim thus becomes susceptible to a wide range of uncommon opportunistic infections or the development of KS and other lymphoreticular neoplasms. In 1987, the populations identified to be at high risk for contracting AIDS included sexually active homosexual men, female and male intravenous drug users, hemophiliacs who had received lyophilized Factor VIII clotting concentrates, recipients of HIV-infected blood transfusion, the sexual partners of those listed above, and infants born to HIV-infected mothers. However, HIV infection appears to be spreading to the general heterosexual population in these areas as well. Apparently, AIDS has also been found to be epidemic in equatorial Africa, where both men and women have been reported to have this disease in large numbers. Most of these groups found to be at high risk for AIDS have histories of repeated infections with multiple organisms or intravenous antigenic protein exposure, which may overwhelm and overload the host's immune system in such a way as to serve as cofactors in rendering certain individuals more vulnerable to HIV infection, resulting in the irreversible immune dysregulation that is characteristic of AIDS.[16-25]

Serologic testing has consistently shown that patients with epidemic KS have markedly elevated serum antibody levels to more than one virus, including Epstein–Barr virus (EBV) and cytomegalovirus (CMV), as well as to hepatitis A virus, hepatitis B virus and herpes simplex virus types 1 and 2.[26,27] The possible role of recurrent or latent CMV infection in the etiology of AIDS and particularly epidemic KS has been under investigation since the onset of the epidemic. It has been reported that over 94% of homosexual men studied at a venereal disease clinic had antibodies to CMV as compared to 54% of heterosexual male controls. Moreover, approximately 19% of the homosexual patients had CMV isolated from their urine.[28] CMV has also been isolated from blood, semen, gastrointestinal tract, central nervous system, and lungs of patients with AIDS. Based on limited studies, CMV has, for many years, been thought to be associated with the African form of KS. Elevated CMV serum antibody titers have been demonstrated in some of these patients, and part of the CMV genome has been reported to be incorporated into the DNA of the KS tumor specimens examined from patients with the classic, African, and epidemic types of KS. However, there have been conflicting results in associating CMV with both the epidemic and the classic varieties of KS. Recent studies have demonstrated a relatively low antibody titer to CMV in North American cases of classic KS when compared to patients with the epidemic variety, and the lack of any conclusive evidence of infection with the CMV genomes in classic, African, or epidemic KS tissue as determined by in situ hybridization. In addition, no difference has been established for the association of CMV in AIDS patients with epidemic KS as compared to AIDS patients with OIs.[29,30] Whether CMV plays a significant role as a cofactor in the etiology of AIDS in general and KS in particular or simply represents yet another opportunistic infection or reactivation of a latent infection once the patient becomes immunocompromised has yet to be determined.[31-33]

The possible role of predisposing genetic factors in the development of KS has been suggested by the prevalence of the classic form of KS in men of eastern European and Mediterranean backgrounds. Early in the recognition of the AIDS epidemic, a large comparative study of the major histocompatibility antigens among heterosexual patients in New York City with classic KS and homosexuals with epidemic KS demonstrated that both populations had a significantly higher incidence of the HLA DR5 antigen (43%) as compared to a control population of healthy, heterosexual white men (23%).[26] As the AIDS epidemic progressed and the HLA typing of increasing numbers of patients with epidemic KS was studied, the percentage of patients with HLA DR5 was found to be diminished. This observation suggested that in the beginning of the epidemic persons within the homosexual population at risk for AIDS who carried the HLA DR5 allele were possibly more susceptible to the development of KS. However, the high incidence of HLA DR5 among the patients studied with classic KS has continued to be present at a statistically significant level; most of these patients have been of Italian or Jewish extraction. Thirty-nine percent of Eastern European, Ashkanazic Jews in Israel carry the HLA DR5 allele, and its incidence in American Jews of various backgrounds is 32%. The incidence of HLA DR5 in black African patients with KS is 40%. In American blacks, the incidence is approximately 30%. Thus, KS has been seen most prominently in populations with a relatively high occurrence of the HLA DR5 antigen.[34-37]

Recent observations on epidemic KS have led to the hypothesis that this tumor is not a metastasizing neoplasm, but rather a multicentric tumor arising from local hyperplasia of a cell of endothelial origin.[38,39] Immunohistochemical studies have suggested that the cell of origin of KS is from vascular endothelium. Immunoperoxidase techniques have demonstrated in the cellular components of KS tumor the presence in situ of the Factor VIII related antigen and the HLA DR antigen, both of which are histochemical markers characteristic of endothelial tissue.[40,41] It has been suggested that the profound depression of cell-mediated immunity in patients with AIDS when combined with a growth factor specific for endothelial cells permits the uncontrolled de novo development of the multifocal, mucocutaneous and visceral lesions typically observed with epidemic KS. The marked predilection for the continuous development of multiple lesions on the skin observed in KS is unlike the distribution pattern of metastatic lesions seen in other malignancies except for melanomas. Thus, rather than label KS a metastasizing malignancy, we have referred to it as an "opportunistic neoplasm" similar to the opportunistic infections that are prone to develop in the severely immunocompromised host.[42,43]

THE DIAGNOSIS OF KAPOSI'S SARCOMA

Patients with classic KS usually present with asymptomatic brownish-red to purple or blue-colored patches, plaques or nodular skin lesions most frequently located on the lower extremities, especially the ankles and soles (Color Figs. 14-1 through 14-6). Initially, the disease may be limited to a single or a few discrete macular or papular lesions that range in size from a few millimeters to several centimeters in diameter. Lesions tend to increase in size slowly, often coalescing with time into large plaques and nodules. Occasionally, individual lesions may regress spontaneously.[44]

Although the lesions appear to be highly vascular, they rarely bleed excessively when cut or traumatized. New lesions are slow to develop, and often tend to occur near an original tumor site; they can appear at any time on any part of the body surface, including the arms, upper legs, face, and trunk. Lesions that persist for long periods often become hyperpigmented, especially in darker complexioned individuals. With time untreated tumors often increase in size, becoming fungated and ulcerated. In patients with long-standing classic KS, chronic venous stasis and lymphedema of the involved lower extremities frequently develop as a complication of the disease.[45,46]

Epidemic KS is characterized by the sudden and often widespread occurrence of lesions at the onset of the disease involving the skin, oral mucosa, lymph nodes and visceral organs. The gastrointestinal tract, lung, liver, and spleen may also be involved, although the spectrum of clinical manifestations and lesion morphology of epidemic KS are much more varied than those seen in the classic type of the disease (see Color Figs. 14-7 through 14-30). The earliest faint, flat, macular lesions (patch stage) may be so unobtrusive as to be totally overlooked. The early flat lesions may be mistaken for pityriasis rosea, purpura, pigmented nevi, early melanomas or vascular lesions such as flat hemangiomas and venous lakes, progressive pigmented purpuric eruptions (such as Schamberg's disease or purpura of Gougerot–Blum), or secondary syphilis. The mucocutaneous KS lesions are usually asymptomatic, may be single or multiple, and sometimes appear simultaneously or sequentially (see Color Figs. 14-11 through 14-13). New lesions usually continue to appear throughout the course of the disease. They may be found in localized clusters and can be widely disseminated (see Color Figs. 14-14, 14-16, 14-18). As the lesions become more numerous, they tend to occur in a bilateral symmetrical distribution along the lines of skin cleavage (Langer's lines) (see Color Figs. 14-9, 14-17, 14-25). Unlike classic KS, the lesions of epidemic KS are often elongated, fusiform, or oval in shape (see Color Figs. 14-14, 14-16, 14-17, 14-19). As these tumors evolve, the flat lesions rapidly become elevated, developing into papules or plaques (plaque stage) (see Color Figs. 14-15 to 14-17, 14-25). When numerous, these raised lesions can resemble the generalized eruptions of secondary syphilis, lichen planus, sarcoidosis, eruptive xanthomas, widespread congenital hemangiomas, urticaria pigmentosa, multiple intradermal, junctional or dysplastic nevi, chronic inflammatory reactions to insect bites, papular urticaria, dermatofibromas, pyogenic granulomas, glomus tumors, cutaneous lymphomas, basal cell carcinomas, cutaneous metastases of internal tumors, and angiosarcomas of the head and neck. Eventually, the plaque stage lesions may enlarge, coalesce and become elevated nodules (nodular stage) (see Color Figs. 14-22, 14-23, and 14-25 through 14-30). The lesions may appear any place on

the skin of the face, trunk, or extremities, but particularly common skin sites include the occipital region behind the ears and the earlobes themselves (Color Fig. 14-21). Deep red to blue macular, plaque, and nodular oropharyngeal lesions are seen in the hard and soft palates, gingival and buccal mucosa, and pharynx, including the tonsils. In the epidemic form of KS multiple lesions are frequently detected by upper endoscopy and colonoscopy along the alimentary tract from the esophagus, throughout the gastrointestinal tract, including the rectum and anus. KS has rarely been reported in the central nervous system, and lesions in the testicles are extremely uncommon.[47-49]

HISTOPATHOLOGIC CLASSIFICATION

The characteristic histopathology of all types of KS is similar regardless of the differences in clinical behavior seen in the various populations involved. The chronologic, progressive clinical sequence from the early faint-pink to bluish macular lesions to larger red to purple indurated plaques and subsequently into dark red to brown or blue tumor nodules is paralleled in the histopathologic changes as well. Like the clinical appearance of the early macular lesions, the histopathology of the earliest patch-stage skin lesions of KS can be difficult to diagnose because of the subtlety of the changes. These changes include, in the upper portion of the dermis, a slight increase in the number of bizarre-shaped, dilated, vascular spaces lined with thin endothelial cells which tend to be contiguous with pre-existing vessels (Color Figs. 14-31, 14-32). In the dermis, there is a sparse superficial and deep perivascular mononuclear cell infiltrate composed of lymphocytes and plasma cells. Histologically, plaque lesions of KS are characterized by an increased number of jagged, irregular, endothelial-lined vascular spaces. A dense, mononuclear, inflammatory cell infiltrate composed of plasma cells and lymphocytes is present throughout the dermis, and there is an increased number of grouped spindle-shaped cells located between collagen bundles. Characteristically, a few extravasated erythrocytes are often found interspersed in the intercellular spaces between the spindle cells (Color Figs. 14-33, 14-34).

Microscopic examination of the more advanced nodular lesions reveals very few, thin, endothelial-lined, vascular slits surrounded and compressed by dense, interweaving bundles or fascicles of spindle-shaped cells (Color Figs. 14-35, 14-36). Some erythrocytes can be seen within the exceedingly fine vascular clefts. At this stage, the inflammatory cells are absent, but a few extravasated erythrocytes and hemosiderin-laden macrophages are seen throughout the interstices between the spindle cells. The mononuclear cell infiltrate consisting of lymphocytes and plasma cells seen in the patch- and plaque-stage lesions is absent in the nodular lesions. Nuclear and cytologic atypia, and a few cells in mitosis are occasionally seen. Both the spindle-shaped cells and the thin endothelial cells lining the abnormally shaped vascular spaces stain for Factor VIII using indirect immunoperoxidase techniques, suggesting the endothelial cell origin for both cell types that comprise this neoplasm.

Histopathologically involved lymph nodes contain multiple small foci of KS tumors located in the capsular and sinusoid regions of the nodes associated with generalized lymphoid hyperplasia, atypical of metastatic tumor invasion. Similarly, the disseminated KS tumor lesions occurring in visceral organs are found in close association with and appear to arise from pre-existing organ vessels in the connective tissue structure.[50,51]

NON AIDS-RELATED KAPOSI'S SARCOMA

Classic Kaposi's Sarcoma

Although considered a rare disease, several hundred cases of classic KS have been reported in the literature since its first description over 100 years ago. The vast majority of such cases occur in males with a ratio of approximately 10 to 15 males to one female. In North Americans and Europeans the usual age is between 50 and 70. Occasionally, cases have been seen in patients below the age of 30, although such cases are very rare. The classic variety of KS has rarely been seen in siblings or in other members of the same family. However, the high incidence and association of this tumor within particular ethnic groups has contributed to the suspicion that there may be a genetic predisposition to the disease.[52-55]

The tumors usually present with one or more asymptomatic red, purple, or brown patch, plaque, or nodular skin lesions (see Color Figs. 14-1 through 14-6). The disease is often limited to a single or multiple lesions that most often appear either simultaneously or gradually in tandem sequence in clusters which are usually localized to one or both lower extremities, especially involving the ankle and soles.

The disease most commonly runs a relatively benign, indolent course for 10 to 15 years or more with slow enlargement of the original tumors and the gradual development of additional lesions. Most patients eventually die from causes unrelated to KS. Although new cutaneous lesions may appear throughout the course of the disease, and on any part of the body, they commonly tend to occur close to the original tumor site on the lower extremities. The oral mucosa and conjunctiva have occasionally been found to be sites for tumor growth during the protracted course of the classic form of the disease. In rare cases, spontaneous regression of one or more individual lesions has been observed. Skin lesions that persist for prolonged periods often become hyperpigmented. Untreated tumors increase in size, coalesce, and often become fungating and eventually ulcerated. Although it is uncommon, local invasion of underlying subcutaneous tissue and bone may occur in

lesions of several years' duration. With time, chronic venous stasis and lymphedema of the involved lower extremity frequently complicate the clinical course of the disease. In long-standing cases, discrete systemic lesions eventually develop along the gastrointestinal tract, in lymph nodes, and in other organs. These visceral lesions are generally asymptomatic and are most often discovered only at autopsy.

Up to one-third of the patients with classic KS develop a second primary malignancy, most often a lymphoproliferative disorder, such as non-Hodgkin's lymphoma. These second malignancies may either antedate or follow the appearance of KS during the indolent course of the disease. This observation has further suggested the role of common constitutional factors in predisposing certain individuals to the development of particular neoplasms.[56-58]

Local treatment of skin lesions with irradiation, surgical excision or electrocauterization and curettage is generally effective. In more advanced cases with disseminated cutaneous and visceral tumor involvement, local therapeutic modalities are impractical. In such cases, systemic chemotherapy has achieved relatively good control of the lesions and effective short-term palliation.

African Kaposi's Sarcoma

In 1950 new interest in this rare tumor arose with the report of 43 cases of KS in Bantu tribesmen of South Africa. Shortly thereafter, it was recognized that KS is a relatively common neoplasm in native populations in equatorial Africa. At the First International Symposium on Kaposi's Sarcoma held in Kampala in 1961, it was reported that this disease comprised approximately 9% of all cancers seen in Ugandan males, whereas the incidence of KS among the white and Asian populations living in these same regions was comparable to the low incidence of classic KS in Europe. The geographic distribution of KS in equatorial Africa appears to overlap the same regions where Burkitt's lymphoma, a tumor closely associated with EBV, is endemic. However, KS appears to be more prevalent in this endemic region at higher altitudes than where Burkitt's lymphoma is seen.[10,59-61]

Typical African KS is seen as either an indolent neoplasm reminiscent of the classic disease seen in Europe and North America or as a uniquely "florid," aggressive disease. Three distinct clinical types have been identified, as shown in Table 14-1. There is an indolent variety characterized by cutaneous plaque and nodular lesions. This relatively benign type is similar in behavior to the classic type of KS in its clinical pattern and is associated with a long survival. The more aggressive forms of KS observed in young, black Africans include the florid, infiltrative, and generalized lymphadenopathic types which progress rapidly and, if not treated appropriately, may kill the patient within 1 year. The florid, aggressive

Table 14-1
Classification of Endemic African Kaposi's Sarcoma

Clinical Type	Behavior	Age Group (yrs)	Bone Involvement	Lymph Node Involvement	Predominant Skin Tumor
Nodular	Indolent	>25	Rare	Rare	Nodules, plaques
Florid	Locally aggressive	>25	Often	Rare	Fungating (exophytic)
Infiltrative	Locally aggressive	>25	Always	Rare	Diffuse infiltration
Lymphadenopathic	Disseminated aggressive	<25	Rare	Always	Nodules (very rare)

(Adapted from Taylor JF, Templeton AL, Vogel CL et al: Kaposi's Sarcoma in Uganda: A clinicopathological study. Int J Cancer 8:122, 1971)

lesions grow into fungating and exophytic tumors and often invade the subcutaneous and surrounding tissue including the underlying bone. In Africa both the indolent and locally more aggressive forms of KS occur with a male:female ratio comparable to that observed for the classic KS tumor seen in North America and Europe. In general, however, the patients in Africa are significantly younger than their European counterparts. Both the localized and aggressive forms of KS occur most commonly in young adults between the ages of 25 and 40. A unique lymphadenopathic form of KS is seen in Africa, primarily in prepubescent children and occasionally in very young adolescent adults (male:female ratio 3:1). It presents with a diffuse lymphadenopathy, usually without cutaneous manifestations. In these cases the generalized lymph node disease is frequently associated with visceral organ involvement. The prognosis is very poor, with a 100% fatality rate within 3 years.[62]

Many treatment trials with various chemotherapeutic agents have been carried out in the African varieties of KS. The locally aggressive tumors of the florid, infiltrative type are very responsive to combinations of chemotherapy. However, at 3 years follow-up, 36% of this group had died with disease and only 14% were disease free. The children with the lymphoadenopathic, generalized form of the disease have an extremely poor prognosis and run a more fulminant and rapidly fatal course despite rigorous treatment with systemic chemotherapy.[43]

The AIDS epidemic is now recognized as a growing problem throughout Central Africa.[63-65] In one recent series, 34% of the inpatients at a hospital in Kinshasa, Zaire were serologically positive for HIV.[65] Since AIDS is occurring in the same area in which African KS is endemic, there has been considerable confusion regarding the relationship between African AIDS and the endemic form of KS. There are several important differences between AIDS in Africa and AIDS seen in the Western world. African AIDS afflicts equal numbers of men and women. Most of the men are heterosexuals with multiple sex partners, and many of the women are prostitutes. Homosexuality and intravenous drug use are apparently rare in this setting. However, there are con-

flicting data on how such behavior has influenced the pattern of KS in Africa. Because both KS and HIV are endemic to the region, the occurrence of the tumor and the virus infection together in an individual in Africa is becoming an increasing likelihood. In Zambia and Uganda, for instance, there has been a marked increase in an aggressive form of KS clinically similar to the KS seen in Western AIDS patients; these patients are HIV antibody–positive.[66,67] However, it is clear that there are cases of the endemic forms of African KS occurring similar to those recognized prior to the AIDS epidemic, which are unrelated to HIV infection.[68-70]

Renal Transplant–Associated Kaposi's Sarcoma

In 1969 the first case of KS in association with a renal transplant was described. Since that time a number of renal allograft recipients receiving prednisone and azathioprine were found to develop KS shortly after the onset of immunosuppressive therapy. The incidence of KS in renal transplants has been estimated at between 150 and 200 times the expected incidence of this tumor in the general population. The average time to develop KS after transplantation is about 16 months. Although the tumor in these iatrogenically immunosuppressed patients often remains localized to the skin, widespread dissemination with mucocutaneous or visceral organ involvement is common. In this group of immunosuppressed patients, the tumor appears with a male:female ratio of approximately 2.3:1. The degree of depression of cellular immunity has been found to correlate with the extent of KS. In some cases, the KS tumors have regressed as a result of reduction or changes in immunosuppressive therapy.[13,71-74]

The course of the neoplasm ranges from localized skin lesions to a more progressive and widespread form resembling the aggressive, lymphadenopathic disease pattern seen in black African children and homosexual men with AIDS. Approximately 30% of these transplant patients die with generalized KS. A number of other iatrogenically immunosuppressed patients die from opportunistic infections or from complications related to their organ transplants, such as chronic renal failure.

Radiotherapy, when used, has been generally effective in patients with KS lesions localized to the skin or the oral cavity. Clinical management of renal transplant patients who develop KS is difficult and requires a delicate balance between the risk of death from generalized KS and the risk of death from renal rejection and the complications of renal failure that may occur if the immunosuppressive therapy is stopped.[75]

There are also reports of KS developing after the use of immunosuppressive agents in the treatment of a variety of autoimmune diseases. These include systemic lupus erythematosus, rheumatoid arthritis, pemphigus vulgaris or pemphigoid, temporal arteritis, and hemolytic anemia.[76-79]

EPIDEMIC KAPOSI'S SARCOMA

In the 18 months prior to the spring of 1981, 21 cases of a previously undescribed fulminant and disseminated form of KS in young homosexual or bisexual men were identified in New York City and California. The sudden and rapidly increasing occurrence of this neoplasm heralded the recognition of the epidemic of a new devastating disease now known as AIDS. Simultaneously and independently, five cases of a rare opportunistic infection, *Pneumocystis carinii* pneumonia, were also observed in young, previously healthy homosexual men in Los Angeles.[80] Epidemiologically, these patients with *P. carinii* pneumonia were similar in sexual preference, the use of a variety of recreational drugs, and a high incidence of past histories of sexually transmitted diseases to the homosexual men with KS.[5] The simultaneous recognition of the concurrent epidemics led to the realization that these clinical entities were in fact different manifestations of a common underlying disease characterized by a profound and irreversible disorder of cell-mediated immunity.

Incidence

Although AIDS continues to be most prevalent in homosexual or bisexual men (65% of the total reported cases), the disease has also occurred in other populations. Specifically, these groups include both male and female intravenous drug users (16% of the total), and individuals who are both intravenous drug users and homosexual men (8% of the total). The remaining 11% include people of Haitian origin (2% of the total) and hemophiliacs who have received factor VIII clotting concentrates (1% of the total). AIDS has also been reported in women who have been sexual partners of men with AIDS (2% of the total), men and women whose diagnosis of AIDS is suspected of being related to blood transfusions (2% of the total), and children whose parents either had or were at risk for AIDS (1% of the total). The remaining 3% of the cases of AIDS have occurred in persons who did not fit into any of the described high-risk groups. Approximately 26% of all AIDS cases in the United States are from New York City, 23% from California, and 6% to 7% each from Florida, Texas, and New Jersey, accounting for 68% of all adult AIDS patients.[6,81]

Approximately 96% of all male cases of epidemic KS in the United States have been diagnosed in homosexuals or bisexuals. The cases have occurred in men as young as 19 and as old as 64 with a mean age of 37.7. Approximately 26% of all homosexual males with AIDS present with or will eventually develop KS during the course of their illness, whereas 77% present with *P. carinii* pneumonia or other opportunistic infections. By comparison, only about 3% of all heterosexual intravenous drug users with AIDS and about 9% of Haitian AIDS patients develop epidemic KS. To date, 1% of the hemophiliac patients with AIDS who received lyophilized clotting factor concentrates have developed KS. Similarly, KS has been observed in 3% of the AIDS cases associated with blood transfusions, in 3% of the women in the United States who had AIDS, and in 3% of the pediatric AIDS patients. Epidemic KS has also been reported in Haiti, western Europe, and Central Africa.[6,81-86]

The proportion of AIDS patients with KS has steadily decreased since the epidemic was first identified in 1981. Twenty-five percent of AIDS patients in 1982 had KS as their presenting AIDS diagnosis. By August 1987 the cumulative proportion of AIDS patients with KS had diminished to approximately 20%.[81] Selik and co-workers have recently analyzed this trend.[87] The frequency of epidemic KS in white homosexual men who were not intravenous drug users was almost twice as great in the five states with the most AIDS cases (28% in New York, California, Florida, Texas, and New Jersey) as in the 35 states with fewer than 310 cases per state (15%). In the District of Columbia, Puerto Rico, and the ten states with an intermediate frequency of AIDS, the proportion of AIDS patients with KS was 22%. This geographic difference parallels the decreasing proportion of AIDS patients identified within the early epicenters such as New York City (43% before 1983, 26% in 1986). As AIDS has spread to other areas, the incidence of epidemic KS has decreased. However, even controlling for geographic trends, the incidence of KS has decreased. There is no obvious explanation for this change in incidence except the suggestion that there has been a decline in exposure to cofactors necessary to cause KS.

Epidemiology

Table 14-2 summarizes some of the epidemiologic features of epidemic KS. Most of the patients with epidemic KS have past histories of multiple, often recurrent, sexually transmitted diseases including syphilis, gonorrhea, genital *herpes simplex,* anogenital warts (*condylomata*

Table 14-2
*Epidemiology and Immunology in Patients
with Epidemic Kaposi's Sarcoma*

Homosexual or bisexual orientation
Occasional IV drug use or Haitian origin
Use of recreational drugs
Multiple sexually transmitted diseases
Enteric parasitic diseases
Antibodies to the EBV, CMV, HAV, HBV, and HIV
Genetic predisposition (HLA DR-5)?
Alterations in Immunity:
  Cell-Mediated Immunity
    1. Cutaneous anergy
    2. Absolute deficiency of T-helper lymphocytes
    3. Inversion of normal T-helper:T-suppressor lymphocyte
       ratio
    4. Diminished lymphocyte response to mitogen stimulation
  Humoral Immunity
    1. Polyclonal hyperglobulinemia ⎫
    2. Antibodies to ⎬ Cross-reacting
       T-lymphocytes ⎪
    3. Antibodies to semen ⎭
    4. Acid-labile α-interferon in serum (similar to lupus
       erythematosus)
    5. Elevated circulating immune complexes
    6. Immune complex–mediated thrombocytopenic purpura
    7. Inability to mount *de novo* antibody response

acuminata), *molluscum contagiosum, lymphogranuloma venereum* and non-gonococcal urethritis. Most had had a variety of systemic viral illnesses, including hepatitis A and B. More than 80% of the initial patients with epidemic KS had medical histories that included intestinal parasitic infections, especially amebiasis and giardiasis, both of which are now considered sexually transmitted diseases among urban homosexual men and are treated with different medications, including metronidazole, a known potential carcinogen in laboratory animals. In addition to a history of sexually transmitted diseases, the use of amyl nitrite (an inhalant recreational drug) has been shown in one study to be correlated with the development of KS in homosexual men.[88,89]

It has been suggested that sexual promiscuity and certain sexual practices involving exposure to fecal matter (e.g., anal lingus, anal intercourse, and fist fornication) have been common in AIDS patients. In fact, it has been demonstrated that homosexual men with AIDS-related KS when compared to a group of "healthy" homosexual controls gave sexual histories which included a much higher rate of passive (receptive) anal–genital intercourse associated with the rectal deposition of the sexual partner's semen. This suggests that exposure of the rectal mucosa to semen during anal–genital intercourse increases the risk for the development of AIDS and epidemic KS. It has been recommended that the use of condoms during rectal sex may offer at least partial protection against this risk.[90–92]

Clinical Features

A comparison of epidemic KS with the classic, African, and renal-transplant associated variants of KS is shown in Table 14-3. Frequently, epidemic KS is characterized by multifocal, widespread lesions at the onset of illness. These lesions may involve the skin, oral mucosa, lymph nodes, and visceral organs such as the gastrointestinal tract, lung, liver, and spleen. Most AIDS patients who present with the mucocutaneous lesions of KS often feel healthy and are usually free of systemic symptoms as compared to those AIDS patients who first develop an opportunistic infection. However, in addition to KS lesions, systemic manifestations may be present simultaneously or even precede the appearance of the tumor lesions by several months and include persistent or intermittent fever, weight loss, diarrhea, malaise, and fatigue. Impetigo, vague psoriasiform or pruritic, eczematous skin eruptions, superficial fungal infections of the skin and nails, oral or esophageal candidiasis (thrush) may occur. Persistent, progressive viral disease such as anogenital herpes simplex infections as well as severe herpes zoster infections (often with systemic dissemination) and CMV enteritis, encephalopathy, and retinitis are also common complications observed in patients with AIDS and epidemic KS.[1,2]

The sites of disease at presentation of epidemic KS are much more varied than that seen in the other types of this neoplasm and are summarized in Table 14-4. In an early report on the clinical manifestations of the disease, 49 patients were described. Eight percent had no skin involvement whatsoever, 27% had localized or fewer than five skin lesions, and 63% had innumerable skin lesions widely distributed over the skin surface area. One patient had a single, locally aggressive exophytic lesion. Sixty-one percent of the patients had generalized lymphadenopathy at the time of the first examination. Four of these patients who had generalized lymphadenopathy in the absence of skin lesions or detectable visceral organ involvement at the time of presentation were found to have biopsy-proven KS localized to the lymph nodes. In 45% of the patients studied, KS lesions were found in one or more sites along the gastrointestinal tract. Twenty-nine percent of the patients had either unexplained fever or weight loss when first seen. Thus, while most patients present with skin disease, uncommonly KS involvement of lymph nodes or the gastrointestinal tract may precede the appearance of the cutaneous lesions.[93]

Eventually, almost all patients with epidemic KS developed progressive disease. Progression often proceeds in an orderly fashion from a few localized or widespread mucocutaneous lesions to more numerous and generalized skin disease with lymph node involvement and gastrointestinal tract disease. Pleuropulmonary KS involvement is an ominous sign usually occurring terminally in those patients who die of KS.[94–96] A recent report of 112 patients with epidemic KS diagnosed prior to 1983 and followed for a minimum of 15 months found

Table 14-3
Comparison of Kaposi's Sarcoma Variants

Type	Population	Clinical Characteristics	Course
Classic	Older men (age 50–80) of Jewish and Italian heritage	Usually confined to lower extremities often with venous statis and lymphedema; late widespread cutaneous and visceral involvement; male:female 10–15:1	Indolent; survival 10–15 years; 37% associated with other malignancies
African	Young adult (age 25–40) black men in Central Africa	Localized modular lesions (57%); large, aggressive exophytic tumors or invasive to underlying bone (38%); male:female 13:1	Indolent if nodular; otherwise slowly progressive and fatal within 5–8 years
	Children (age 2–13)	Generalized lymphadenopathy, (5%), rarely involving the skin; male:female 3:1	Rapidly progressive; fatal within 2–3 years
Renal transplant	Iatrogenically immunosuppressed patients; usually Jewish and Mediterranean heritage	May be localized to skin or widespread with systemic involvement; male:female 2.3:1	Can be indolent or rapidly progressive; may regress when immunosuppressive therapy is discontinued; fatal in 30%
Epidemic	AIDS patients; Primarily homosexual men; few Haitians, intravenous drug users, and Africans	Disseminated mucocutaneous lesions often involving lymph nodes and visceral organs, especially gastrointestinal tract and lungs	Fulminant; less than 20% survival at 2 years if associated with opportunistic infections

Table 14-4
Sites of Disease and Systemic Signs at Presentation in 49 Patients with Epidemic Kaposi's Sarcoma

Manifestation	No. of Patients (% of total group)
Skin Lesions	
None	4 (8)
Localized	13 (27)
Generalized	31 (63)
Locally aggressive	1 (2)
Lymph Node Involvement	
None	19 (39)
Localized	—
Generalized	30 (61)
Splenomegaly	5 (10)
Visceral Involvement	
Bone	1 (2)
Hepatomegaly	5 (10)
Lung	5 (10)
Gastrointestinal tract	22 (45)
Systemic Signs*	
Fever and weight loss	9 (18)
Fever only	4 (8)
Weight loss only	1 (2)
Total	14 (29)

* Unexplained fever >100°F (orally) and ≥10% weight loss.

that 65 (58%) had died. Of these 65 only 10 (15%) had died without a history of an opportunistic infection. And of these, two (20%) died of progressive non-Hodgkin's lymphoma, whereas only eight died directly from KS. In fact, as shown in Figure 14-1, patients with epidemic KS who never developed an opportunistic infection are predicted to have an 80% survival at 28 months from diagnosis as compared to a less than 20% survival in those who have had an opportunistic infection at some time during the course of their illness.[97-99] A recent autopsy series of patients with AIDS included 18 cases with epidemic KS. Ten (56%) patients had disseminated KS that contributed significantly to morbidity and mortality. Nine (50%) had lung involvement and 3 (17%) had KS in the adrenal glands.[100]

Laboratory Abnormalities

Leukopenia (especially lymphopenia) and mild anemia are common findings in those patients who present with epidemic KS as their only manifestation of AIDS.[101,102] Less frequently, immune thrombocytopenic purpura (ITP) occurs as a further complication of the syndrome. This has recently been demonstrated to be due to immune complexes rather than antiplatelet antibodies, as in the case of autoimmune thrombocytopenic purpura.[103-105] In general, liver chemistries are normal unless there is an associated opportunistic infection.

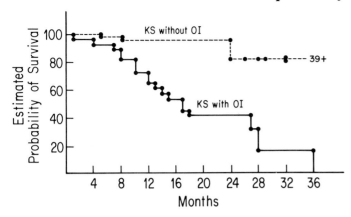

FIG. 14-1. Survival in Kaposi's sarcoma with and without opportunistic infection.

HIV has been isolated in cultured lymphocytes of patients with AIDS, and antibodies to HIV have been detected in up to 90% of these patients.[106,107] The characteristic underlying immunologic disorder is a profound deficiency of cell-mediated immunity. As shown in Table 14-2, the vast majority of patients with epidemic KS display cutaneous anergy, have a marked reduction in the absolute number of helper T-lymphocytes, and have an inversion of the ratio of T-helper to T-suppressor lymphocytes. Their lymphocytes show a markedly diminished *in vitro* response to mitogenic stimulation. While the B-cell mediated humoral arm of the patient's immune system appears to be hyperfunctional as evidenced by polyclonal hypergammaglobulinemia and high levels of circulating immune complexes, in fact, AIDS patients have been shown to be unable to mount antibody responses when exposed to new antigens.[108–110]

It has been reported that there is a significant correlation in epidemic KS patients between the absolute numbers of T-helper and T-suppressor cells and between the number of T-helper lymphocytes and the numbers of granulocytes and erythrocytes. Thus, the immunologic alterations are only part of the multiple disturbances seen in this disease. Moreover, autoantibodies to T-lymphocytes have been demonstrated in homosexual AIDS patients which cross-react with autoantibodies to semen, thereby suggesting a possible role for the exposure to allogeneic semen as a cofactor in the development of epidemic KS. Other immunologic abnormalities characteristic of AIDS covered in detail elsewhere in this text include elevated levels of β_2 microglobulins, the presence of an acid-labile α-interferon in serum, depressed natural-killer cell activity, elevated thymosin α_1 levels, and impaired interleukin-2 production by peripheral blood lymphocytes in response to antigens.[111–117]

Staging

To account for the variation in disease presentation and facilitate following the progression of disease and response to therapy, a staging classification (Table 14-5)

Table 14-5
Staging System of Kaposi's Sarcoma

Stage I	cutaneous, locally indolent (classic)
Stage II	cutaneous, locally aggressive or without regional lymph nodes (African locally agressive)
Stage III	generalized cutaneous and/or lymph node involvement (African lymphadenopathic and epidemic)
Stage IV	visceral (epidemic)

Subtypes
  A. No systemic signs or symptoms
  B. Systemic signs: 10% weight loss or fever greater than 100°F orally, unrelated to an identifiable source of infection lasting more than 2 weeks.

has been proposed that is inclusive of all of the clinical variants of KS.[93] Stage I represents the classic KS seen most commonly in elderly male patients of Mediterranean or Middle Eastern origin. Stage II represents the typical African KS when locally invasive. Stages III and IV stratify the disseminated and systemic KS observed in AIDS patients and in African children with generalized lymphadenopathic disease. Each stage is further subtyped according to the absence of systemic symptoms (A) or the presence of systemic symptoms (B). These B symptoms include fever unrelated to an identifiable source of infection, night sweats, weight loss greater than or equal to 10% of normal body weight, and unexplained diarrhea.

With this staging system approximately 10% to 15% of patients with epidemic KS have stage I disease, 20% to 25% will be stage III-A, and another 20% to 25% will be Stage IV-A. Approximately 20% to 25% will have B symptoms (one-half each in Stages III-B and IV-B), and an additional 15% to 20% will have a prior or coexistent OI (defined as an OI diagnosed within 3 months of the diagnosis of epidemic KS). Actuarial survivals are shown in Fig. 14-2. Stage I patients were alive up to 2 years after diagnosis, although most had progressive disease. Patients with generalized tumor lesions without B symptoms (Stages III-A and IV-A) have an estimated

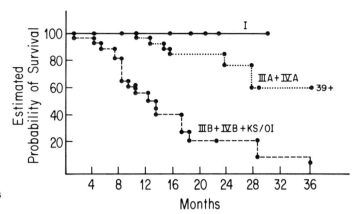

FIG. 14-2. Survival in patients with epidemic Kaposi's sarcoma as a function of stage.

survival of 60% at 28 months. Patients with palate or gastrointestinal KS involvement do somewhat worse than those without alimentary tract lesions. Patients with disseminated disease with symptoms (stages III-B and IV-B) have a median survival of 15 months, and those who have a prior or coexistent opportunistic infection have a median survival of only 7 months.[99,118,119]

However, there is no universally accepted classification for epidemic Kaposi's sarcoma. Other staging schemes have been proposed that incorporate laboratory parameters as well as clinical features. Several studies have demonstrated the importance of both the absolute number of T-helper lymphocytes and the T-helper to T-suppressor ratio, as shown in Table 14-6.[120,121] The presence of acid-labile α-interferon in the patient's serum has been described as an indicator of poor prognosis.[122] Others have also identified as prognostic factors the hematocrit and number of systemic symptoms.[123] Thus, there are distinct clinical as well as laboratory prognostic factors with epidemic KS, as summarized in Table 14-7.

TREATMENT

The natural course of disease progression within each of the different types of KS is highly variable. It has therefore been difficult to evaluate the efficacy of systemic treatment with a variety of chemotherapeutic agents. In fact, it has never been demonstrated that either local or systemic treatment of classic KS alters the ultimate course of the disease. Treatment may, however, result in a disappearance or reduction in size of specific skin lesions and thereby alleviate the discomfort associated with the chronic edema and ulcerations that often accompany multiple skin tumors seen on the lower extremeties, in control of symptoms associated with mucosal or visceral lesions, and rarely also in promoting the healing of locally invasive bone lesions. There are no data, however, to show that treatment improves survival.[124] Despite some temporary effects on the existing tumors, none of the current systemic agents under in-

Table 14-6
Impact of T-Cell Subsets on Survival in Epidemic KS

	Prognostic Groups		
	Good	Intermediate	Poor
T-helper lymphocytes/ml (survival at 12 months)	>300 (85%)	300–100 (intermediate)	<100 (35%)
T-helper to T-suppressor ratio (survival at 12 months)	>0.5 (>95%)	0.5–0.2 (intermediate)	<0.2 (25%)

(Adapted from Taylor J, Afrasiabi R, Fahey JL et al: Prognostically significant classification of immune changes in AIDS with Kaposi's sarcoma. Blood 67: 666, 1986)

Table 14-7
Prognostic Factors in Epidemic Kaposi's Sarcoma

1. Extent of disease	1. Hematocrit
2. Visceral involvement	2. Absolute number of T-helper lymphocytes
3. Systemic symptoms	3. T-lymphocyte helper–suppressor cell ratio
4. Prior or coexistent opportunistic infection	4. Acid-labile α-interferon

vestigation in the treatment of epidemic KS has been found to alter the development of new lesions, to increase survival, or to consistently improve the underlying immune deficiency.

Local Modalities: Surgery and Radiation

Small localized lesions of KS may be satisfactorily treated by electrodessication and curettage or by surgical excision. However, KS tumors are generally very responsive to local radiation therapy, and excellent palliation has been obtained with doses not much higher than 2000 cGy (rad). While most of this experience has been obtained in the cutaneous lesions of classic KS, the early skin and oral lesions of epidemic KS seem to be equally radiosensitive. Radiation has infrequently been employed for the treatment of the rare, but sometimes painful bone lesions of KS or localized visceral disease. Long-standing tumor lesions and extensive confluent areas of KS have been found to be less radiosensitive. In the presence of moderate to severe edema, complications are frequently encountered. Localized skin recurrences may also be effectively treated with electron-beam therapy. Thus, with these techniques, successful control of at least the localized mucocutaneous lesions can be achieved in most patients with either classic or epidemic KS.[125-131]

Chemotherapy

Therapeutic strategies have varied greatly with the different forms of KS. This has been especially true in epidemic KS where the already profoundly depressed immunologic status of the host has limited the therapeutic efficacy of systemic chemotherapy. Historically, the most commonly used chemotherapeutic agent has been vinblastine. Reports on the treatment of classic KS have consistently shown a 90% to 95% response rate with vinblastine, although response durations rarely exceeded 1 year, and a beneficial effect on survival has never been documented. In a group of unselected patients with epidemic KS, weekly administration of vinblastine was found to have only a 26% objective response rate. However, in patients with early-stage disease, vinblastine has been reported to have a 50% to 75% response rate as compared to a 20% or less response rate in patients with more advanced epidemic KS.[132-136]

Experience with other chemotherapeutic agents has been obtained in African KS. At the Uganda Cancer Institute in the early 1970s, trials of bleomycin, BCNU (carmustine), ICRF-159 (rozaxone), actinomycin D, and dacarbazine (DTIC) as single agents and combinations of actinomycin D and vincristine with or without dacarbazine documented the chemoresponsiveness of KS. The response rates with these agents were impressive, varying from 38% to 89% for single agents and 100% for the combinations.[137-141] Whether such results are applicable to epidemic KS is uncertain. The antitumor efficacy of these drugs and combinations was established on relatively short-term observations of tumor regression, and duration of response and survival are unknown.

The first systemic chemotherapy studies in epidemic KS began in 1981 with the recognition of AIDS as a new disease. Treatment of the initial patients consisted of vinblastine and bleomycin, which provided only a transient improvement. Long-lasting responses were observed in two patients treated with a combination of doxorubicin (Adriamycin), bleomycin, vinblastine, and dacarbazine (ABVD).[4] The combination of actinomycin D and dacarbazine was used as second-line therapy and found to be poorly tolerated as well as ineffective. These preliminary observations led to the formulation of treatment strategies using combinations of doxorubicin, bleomycin, and either vinblastine or vincristine in patients with visceral involvement, systemic symptoms, or a history of prior treatment failure. Etoposide (VP-16), both as a single agent and in combinations, has been utilized because of its relatively good subjective tolerance, known antitumor activity against other neoplasms, and a presumed lack of cross resistance to the combination drug regimens described above.[142-148] These treatment results are shown in Table 14-8. The wide variation in response rates reflects patient selection rather than a significant difference in chemosensitivities. In general, single-agent therapy has been used in early-stage disease and the combinations in more advanced disease. When single-agent therapy has been used in patients with more advanced disease, response rates have been significantly lower.

Biologic Response Modifiers

The search for and use of potential immune modulators was prompted by the observation of a higher than expected incidence of opportunistic infection following treatment of patients with epidemic KS with combination chemotherapy. Among the biologic response mod-

Table 14-8
Systemic Treatments of Epidemic Kaposi's Sarcoma

	Response Rate (%)	*Reference*
Chemotherapy		
vinblastine (VBL)	26	135
etoposide (VP-16)	76	142
vincristine (VCR)	61	143
bleomycin (Bleo)	77	144
VCR + VBL	45	145
Bleo + VBL	62	144
VBL + methotrexate	77	146
doxorubicin + Bleo + VBL or VCR (ABV)	66–86	142, 147, 148
Biologic Response Modifiers		
α-interferons		
α-2a	38	149, 153
α-2b	40	150
α-N1	10–67	151, 152
+ VP-16	21	154
+ VBL	29–60	155, 156
+ VCR	15	157
γ-interferon	0	159
interleukin-2	0–6	160, 161

ifiers tested, the α-interferons have been most widely studied in the treatment of patients with epidemic KS. In general, there has been a 40% major response rate with both recombinant and nonrecombinant α-interferons. In these studies, high-dose therapy was found to be much more effective than low-dose therapy. In general, the treatments were well tolerated with side-effects consisting of a flu-like syndrome with fever, headache, and malaise. Objective toxicity was minimal, consisting primarily of myelosuppression and reversible changes in the serum transaminase levels. No consistent or sustained changes were seen in the patient's deficient immunologic status during or after treatment; there was no change in the carrier state of HIV, nor did this therapy prevent opportunistic infections. In these reports the responses differed significantly according to the prognostic factors of extent of disease, prior opportunistic infection, prior treatment with chemotherapy, and the presence of circulating acid-labile α-interferon.[149-153] Several studies have combined α-interferon with chemotherapy (see Table 14-8). Overall, these trials have shown no benefit in the combinations as compared to the single-agent activities. In fact, there was a higher incidence of constitutional and hematologic toxicities.[154-157]

Other biologic response modifiers are currently being studied in an attempt to reverse the underlying immune deficiency. γ-(immune) interferon is produced by T-lymphocytes and promotes macrophage antibody-dependent, cell-mediated cytotoxicity. T-lymphocytes have deficient production of this lymphokine in AIDS patients. When γ-interferon is added *in vitro,* there is an increase in the cytotoxic activity of mononuclear phagocytes.[158] However, in one clinical treatment study employing a partially purified γ-interferon preparation, no objective tumor responses were seen in seven patients with epidemic KS.[159] Treatment studies have also been performed with recombinant Interleukin-2 (IL-2). Patients with AIDS are deficient in the production of IL-2, and it is thought that IL-2 may reconstitute some aspects of the immune system deficient in patients with AIDS. In a recent study, nonrecombinant IL-2 derived from the Jurkat human T-cell tumor cell line was administered to 10 cancer patients, including 5 who had epidemic KS. No therapeutic responses were seen.[160] In a second study using recombinant IL-2, only 3 responses were seen in 55 patients with epidemic KS.[161] Thus, neither γ-interferon nor IL-2 is active in this setting.

Current Recommendations

There are several problems with treating epidemic KS. First, chemotherapy may actually worsen the underlying immune deficiency as evidenced by the increased incidence of opportunistic infections following aggressive combination chemotherapy. Second, although this possibility has led to experimental treatment studies utilizing immunotherapy in AIDS, these immunomodulators are relatively new agents with potential long-term effects that are still unknown. Third, immunomodulators, even if they improve the immunologic deficiency, may not have an effect on the KS tumor. The clinical response of the KS tumor in AIDS patients to the various treatments tested to date, whether chemotherapy agents or interferons, appears to be a function of the stage of the disease (Table 14-9). This variation in response is consistent with the theory that a tumor develops resistance with increasing duration and extent of disease. The optimal duration of treatment is still unknown. In general, a complete response is difficult to achieve, and maintenance therapy is necessary to effect an improvement in long-term survival. Current recommendations for the treatment of epidemic KS are shown in Table 14-10. Patients with localized disease are treated with local modalities only: surgical excision, electrocautery and curettage, or radiation therapy. Patients with disseminated disease without B symptoms are candidates for treatment with potential immunomodulators or single-agent chemotherapy. Patients with disseminated, aggressive, extensive visceral involvement or with B symptoms are treated with combination chemotherapy.[162]

Table 14-9
Impact of Prognostic Factors on Response to Systemic Agents

	Response Rate (%)	
Regimen	Early Stage/ No Symptoms	B Symptoms/ Prior OI or Prior Treatment
Etoposide		
Vinblastine	86	20
ABV	75	10–20
Recombinant α-interferons	92 60–88	80 5–30

Table 14-10
Treatment of Kaposi's Sarcoma

Extent of Disease	Preferred Treatment*
Localized	Surgical excision or radiation therapy
Indolent disseminated cutaneous and/or lymphadenopathic	Immunotherapy and/or single-agent chemotherapy
Aggressive, disseminated or with systemic B symptoms	Combination chemotherapy

* Patients should be treated with protocol therapies whenever possible.

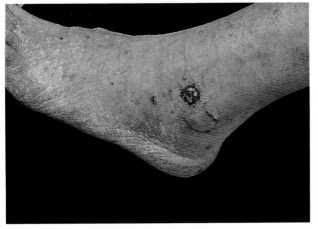

COLOR PLATE 14-1.

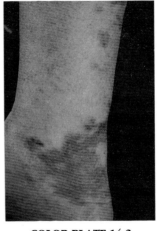

COLOR PLATE 14-2.

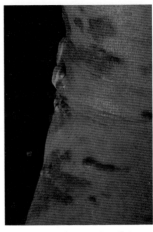

COLOR PLATE 14-3.

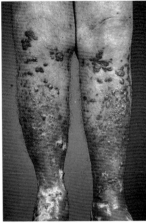

COLOR PLATE 14-4.

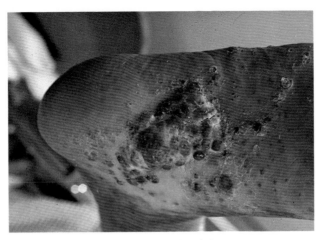

COLOR PLATE 14-5.

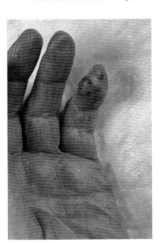

COLOR PLATE 14-6.

COLOR PLATE 14-1.   Classic Kaposi's sarcoma. There is a purplish 1.5 cm tumor nodule located on the lateral ankle region of the foot in this 70-year-old Italian man. Numerous small, violet-to-blue papules surrounded the larger tumor.

COLOR PLATE 14-2.   Classic Kaposi's sarcoma. There is a large hyperpigmented confluent plaque stage lesion located on the ankle region of the lower extremity. Numerous small bluish and brown nodules are present within the area of the hyperpigmented plaque. A few faint pink macular tumor lesions are seen further up the leg.

COLOR PLATE 14-3.   Classic Kaposi's sarcoma. There are several asymptomatic brown and violet discrete and confluent thick plaques located along the lower extremity just above the ankle. There are several pink-to-red nodules interspersed among the plaques. Chronic edema is frequently associated with long-standing cases of the classic form of Kaposi's sarcoma involving the lower extremities.

COLOR PLATE 14-4.   Classic Kaposi's sarcoma. This patient, a 72-year-old Eastern European Jewish male had Kaposi's sarcoma of 12 years' duration. There is bilateral involvement of his lower extremities with slowly progressive appearance of deep violet and brown plaque and nodular tumor lesions extending up both legs. The disease is associated with painful chronic lymphedema of the feet-ankle regions, and there are several large ulcerations.

COLOR PLATE 14-5.   Classic Kaposi's sarcoma. An untreated large multiloculated tumor mass located on the sole of the foot is surrounded by multiple small satellite reddish-to-purple papules. Such lesions respond well to local radiation therapy.

COLOR PLATE 14-6.   Classic Kaposi's sarcoma. There is a red-to-violet nodular lesion present on the tip of the fifth finger of this patient with classic Kaposi's sarcoma. The patient's disease (localized to his lower extremities) had run an indolent course for 8 years prior to the appearance of this distant solitary lesion.

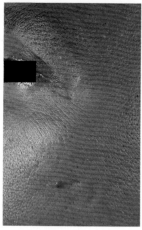

COLOR PLATE 14-7.

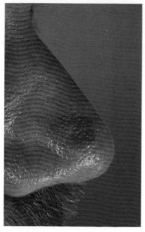

COLOR PLATE 14-8.

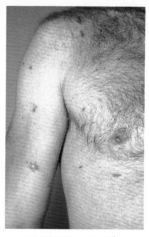

COLOR PLATE 14-9.

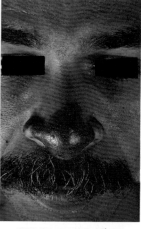

COLOR PLATE 14-10.

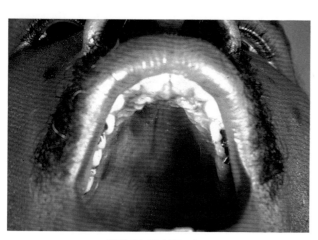

COLOR PLATE 14-11.

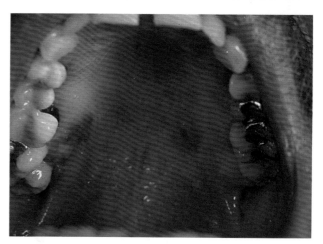

COLOR PLATE 14-12.

COLOR PLATE 14-7. Epidemic Kaposi's sarcoma. A 5 mm, reddish, solitary papular tumor that appeared suddenly on the cheek of this 33-year-old healthy intravenous drug user proved to be AIDS-associated Kaposi's sarcoma. This was the only lesion present at the time of diagnosis.

COLOR PLATE 14-8. Epidemic Kaposi's sarcoma. Patch stage. This totally asymptomatic flat violaceous macule spontaneously appeared on the nose. Several similar patch stage skin lesions had developed at distant sites on the patient's body at about the same time. No systemic symptoms were associated with the appearance of these lesions.

COLOR PLATE 14-9. Epidemic Kaposi's sarcoma. Widely disseminated multiple pink and red, round and elongated lesions appeared over the arm and trunk of this 23-year-old homosexual male, who was otherwise totally asymptomatic. The diagnosis of Kaposi's sarcoma was confirmed by biopsy.

COLOR PLATE 14-10. Epidemic Kaposi's sarcoma. There is a large, confluent, hyperpigmented patch stage lesion of Kaposi's sarcoma located on the nose of this black patient with AIDS. There were similar dark brown macular lesions located on other parts of his body. In black skin, the lesions of Kaposi's sarcoma rapidly become hyperpigmented.

COLOR PLATE 14-11. Epidemic Kaposi's sarcoma. Deep blue to brown flat tumor lesions are seen on the hard palate of this black patient. Note the numerous hyperpigmented plaques also present on the cheeks of this patient as well.

COLOR PLATE 14-12. Epidemic Kaposi's sarcoma. Note the red-to-purple papules located on the hard palate; there is a cluster of tumor lesions near the gingival margin. Lesions commonly develop on the oral mucosa in patients with AIDS-associated Kaposi's sarcoma.

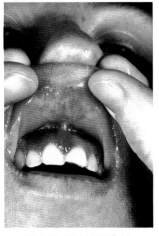

COLOR PLATE 14-13.

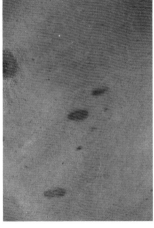

COLOR PLATE 14-14.

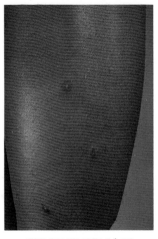

COLOR PLATE 14-15.

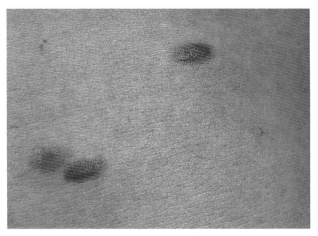

COLOR PLATE 14-16.

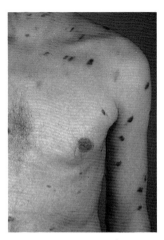

COLOR PLATE 14-17.

COLOR PLATE 14-13. Epidemic Kaposi's sarcoma. There are numerous hemorrhagic-looking, deep red lesions distributed all over the gingiva and some diffuse small flat lesions present on the inner mucosal surface of the upper lip.

COLOR PLATE 14-14. Epidemic Kaposi's sarcoma. The elongated, pinkish-brown macules and early plaque stage lesions located on the chest are typical of this tumor seen in patients with AIDS. Some of the lesions are slightly hyperpigmented.

COLOR PLATE 14-15. Epidemic Kaposi's sarcoma. Multiple, hyperpigmented, deep brownish-purple papular and plaque lesions on the thigh in a black AIDS patient.

COLOR PLATE 14-16. Epidemic Kaposi's sarcoma. In fair-skinned individuals, the infiltrated plaque stage lesions may retain a pinkish-red color without hyperpigmentation. The ovoid shape of the lesions is a common feature of AIDS-associated Kaposi's sarcoma.

COLOR PLATE 14-17. Epidemic Kaposi's sarcoma. With time, an increasing number of patch, plaque, and eventually nodular lesions may continue to appear throughout the course of the disease. The symmetrical distribution of lesions along the lines of skin cleavage (Langer's lines) is typical of AIDS-associated Kaposi's sarcoma.

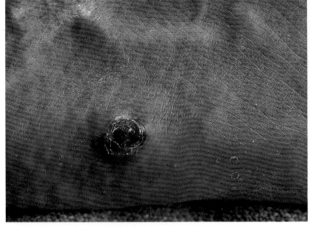

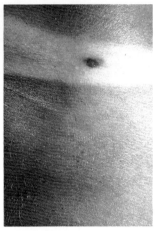

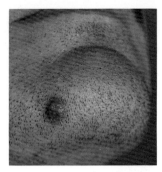

COLOR PLATE 14-20.

COLOR PLATE 14-18.

COLOR PLATE 14-19.

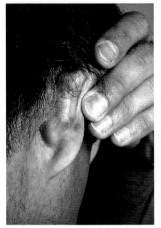

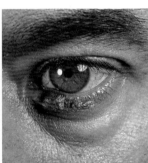

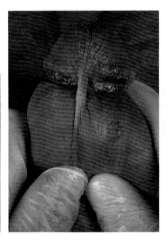

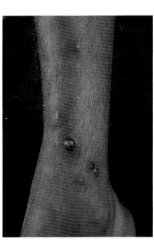

COLOR PLATE 14-21.   **COLOR PLATE 14-22.**   **COLOR PLATE 14-23.**   **COLOR PLATE 14-24.**

COLOR PLATE 14-18.   Epidemic Kaposi's sarcoma. This patient presented with only a single nodular lesion located on the lateral aspect of the sole of his foot. The lesion was totally asymptomatic. Thereafter, the patient rapidly developed multiple and widely disseminated patch, plaque, and nodular lesions over his entire body.

COLOR PLATE 14-19.   Epidemic Kaposi's sarcoma. This 49-year-old bisexual male developed a few hyperpigmented nodular lesions on his trunk that persisted for several months prior to his seeking medical attention. This patient, who was German, travelled frequently to Haiti for winter vacations. He was one of the first cases of AIDS recognized from the Federal Republic of Germany.

COLOR PLATE 14-20.   Epidemic Kaposi's sarcoma. This isolated, pink nodular tumor is located on the chin. A few other patch and plaque stage lesions were widely distributed over the patient's trunk and extremities.

COLOR PLATE 14-21.   Epidemic Kaposi's sarcoma. Nodular lesion on the skin of the dorsum of the ears and the occipital region behind the earlobes are a particularly frequent site for lesions of AIDS-associated Kaposi's sarcoma.

COLOR PLATE 14-22.   Epidemic Kaposi's sarcoma. Although uncommon, lesions can also develop on the eyelids. In this case there is a blue-violet nodular lesion on the margin of the lower eyelid.

COLOR PLATE 14-23.   Epidemic Kaposi's sarcoma. This patient presented with multiple papular and nodular lesions surrounding the corona of the penis. No other mucocutaneous lesions were present. Initially, it was suspected that these lesions represented condylomata acuminata; however, a biopsy proved the lesions to be Kaposi's sarcoma.

COLOR PLATE 14-24.   Epidemic Kaposi's sarcoma. There are several pink to violaceous translucent nodular lesions present on the lower extremities in this individual. Additional plaque and patch stage lesions continued to appear throughout the course of his disease. Several of these developed into nodules.

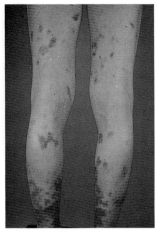

COLOR PLATE 14-25.

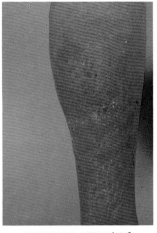

COLOR PLATE 14-26.

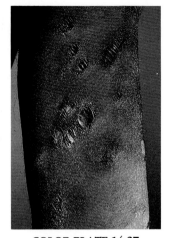

COLOR PLATE 14-27.

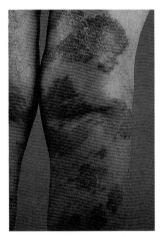

COLOR PLATE 14-28.

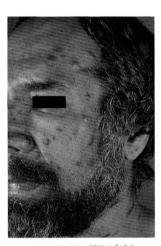

COLOR PLATE 14-29.

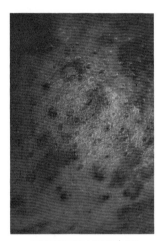

COLOR PLATE 14-30.

COLOR PLATE 14-25. Epidemic Kaposi's sarcoma. Throughout the course of the disease, increasing numbers of lesions continue to appear, although lesions often remain as flat plaques rather than develop into nodules. In this patient, lesions rapidly increased in number and were widely disseminated with confluency of neighboring lesions occurring in certain areas. The symmetry of the eruption is quite typical of the epidemic form of Kaposi's sarcoma.

COLOR PLATE 14-26. Epidemic Kaposi's sarcoma. This patient had the disease for 2 years. The lesions, which initially appeared on the lower extremity as discrete plaques, rapidly increased in number and became confluent. The appearance of the disease in this AIDS-associated case is remarkably similar to that seen in patients with the classic form of Kaposi's sarcoma.

COLOR PLATE 14-27. Epidemic Kaposi's sarcoma. This black patient with AIDS rapidly developed progressive cutaneous lesions involving his entire body with extensive visceral involvement within 2 years of onset.

COLOR PLATE 14-28. Epidemic Kaposi's sarcoma. Large, confluent, hyperpigmented, violet-colored, infiltrated plaque lesions developed over most of this patient's body. This patient's disease ran a fulminant course within 1 year after onset, complicated by several opportunistic infections. He developed visceral lesions of Kaposi's sarcoma involving lungs, lymph nodes, spleen, and liver.

COLOR PLATE 14-29. Epidemic Kaposi's sarcoma. This patient had nodular and papular lesions located over most of his body within 2 years. There was a marked edema of the face associated with extensive tumor involvement of the lymph nodes in the head and neck region.

COLOR PLATE 14-30. Epidemic Kaposi's sarcoma. The disseminated deep violet lesions seen in this patient were observed at the terminal stage of his illness, which had been present for only 2 years. The clinical behavior of Kaposi's sarcoma in patients with AIDS may vary enormously.

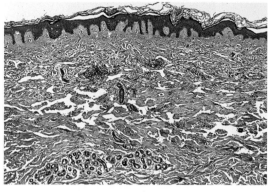

COLOR PLATE 14-31.

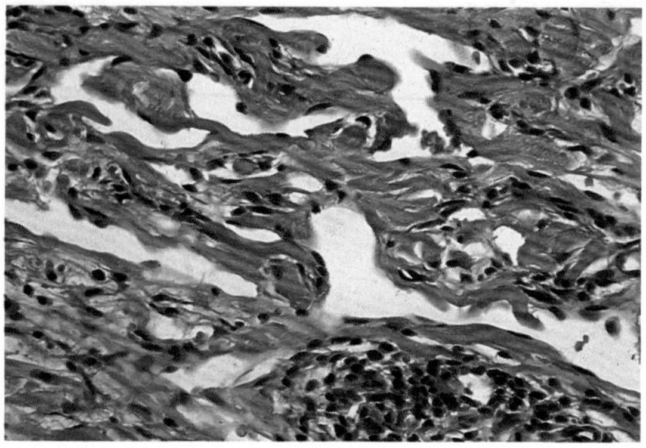

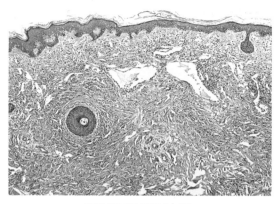

COLOR PLATE 14-32.

COLOR PLATE 14-33.

COLOR PLATE 14-31.   Patch stage lesion, low-power magnification. Numerous jagged, bizarre-shaped, endothelial-lined vascular spaces are seen within the dermis. A sparse superficial and deep perivascular mononuclear inflammatory cell infiltrate is present throughout the dermis (×32).

COLOR PLATE 14-32.   Patch stage lesion, high-power magnification. The sparse superficial and deep perivascular mononuclear cell infiltrate found in the dermis is composed of lymphocytes and plasma cells, surrounding multiple, irregularly shaped vascular slits lined with what appeared to be thin but normal-looking endothelial cells (×250).

COLOR PLATE 14-33.   Plaque stage lesions, low-power magnification. There are multiple jagged-shaped, dilated endothelial-lined vascular spaces within the dermis surrounded by an increased mononuclear infiltrate consisting of lymphocytes and plasma cells, much denser than that seen in the earlier patch stage lesions (×35).

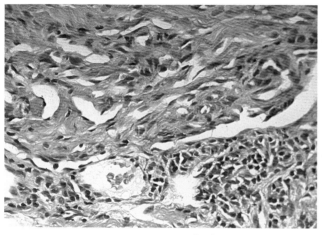

COLOR PLATE 14-34.

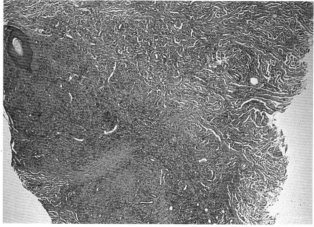

COLOR PLATE 14-35.

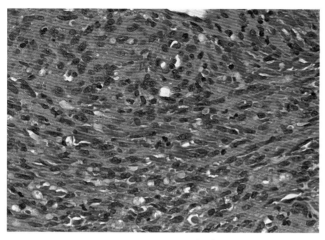

COLOR PLATE 14-36.

COLOR PLATE 14-34.   Plaque stage lesion, high-power magnification. The mononuclear cell infiltrate seen in plaque stage lesions is more pronounced than that in patch stage lesions. A large number of spindle-shaped cells between collagen bundles surround irregularly-shaped dilated endothelial-lined vessels. The combination of bizarre-shaped vascular spaces and the presence of spindle cells between collagen bundles is typical of plaque stage Kaposi's sarcoma lesions (×272).

COLOR PLATE 14-35.   Nodular stage lesion, low-power magnification. The mononuclear cell infiltrate is almost totally absent. There are, however, fine vascular slits compressed and surrounded by thick bundles or fascicles of spindle cells. This pattern is diagnostic of the nodular stage of Kaposi's sarcoma lesions (×25).

COLOR PLATE 14-36.   Nodular stage lesions, high-power magnification. Swirling fascicles of spindle cells surround thin endothelial-lined spaces. The mononuclear infiltrate found in patch and plaque lesions is absent. Some extravasated red blood cells are seen between the spindle cells. The characteristic cell types, diagnostic of the plaque and nodular stages of Kaposi's sarcoma lesions, are the endothelial cells lining the vascular slits and spindle cells. Both are believed to be of endothelial origin, since both stain for Factor VIII and for DR antigens by immunoperoxidase techniques (×310).

FUTURE CONSIDERATIONS

The impact of available treatments on survival among patients with epidemic KS has not been demonstrated. Therefore, currently treatment should be considered palliative. Early stages of the disease may not need systemic treatment, whereas advanced disease requires treatments with demonstrated antitumor activity. A complete response is difficult to achieve, and if obtained, maintenance therapy may be necessary. Although it is clear that epidemic KS is responsive to a number of chemotherapeutic drugs and interferons, the impact of such tumor control on host survival is uncertain. The overall prognosis for patients with AIDS-associated KS appears more related to the immunosuppression and on-going HIV infection than to the neoplastic proliferation. The development of potential methods to promote immune restoration are playing a prominent role in current therapeutic strategies for patients with epidemic KS.[163] Major efforts to develop specific antiviral (anti-HIV) agents and treatment modalities as well as vaccines are under investigation all over the world. However, to date none of these experimental immunorestorative or antiviral treatments has shown any significant antineoplastic activity upon epidemic KS.[164,165] Ultimately, the ideal treatment for the AIDS patient with KS may be a combination of antiviral therapy, immunotherapy, and chemotherapy.

REFERENCES

1. Friedman–Kien AE, Laubenstein L, Marmor M et al: Kaposi's sarcoma and pneumocystis pneumonia among homosexual men–New York and California. Morbid Mortal Week Rept 30:250, 1981
2. Friedman–Kien AE: Disseminated Kaposi-like sarcoma syndrome in young homosexual men. J Am Acad Dermatol 5:468, 1981
3. Gottleib MS, Schroff R, Schanker HM et al: *Pneumocystis carinii* pneumonia and mucosal candidiasis in previously healthy homosexual men: Evidence of a new acquired cellular immunodeficiency. N Engl J Med 305:1425, 1981
4. Hymes K, Cheung T, Greene JB et al: Kaposi's sarcoma in homosexual men. Lancet 2:598, 1981
5. Centers for Disease Control Task Force on Kaposi's Sarcoma and Opportunistic Infections: Epidemiological aspects of the current outbreak of Kaposi's sarcoma and opportunistic infections. N Engl J Med 306:248, 1982
6. CDC Update: acquired immunodeficiency syndrome (AIDS)—United States. Morbid Mortal Week Rept 33:337, 1984
7. Kaposi M: Idiopathiches multiples pigment sarcom der Haut. Arch Dermatol Syphil 4:465, 1872
8. Classics in oncology: Kaposi M: Idiopathic multiple pigmented sarcoma of the skin. Cancer 32:342, 1982
9. Safai B, Good RA: Kaposi's sarcoma: A review and recent developments. Cancer 31:3, 1981
10. Oettle AG: Geographical and racial differences in the frequency of Kaposi's sarcoma as evidence of environmental or genetic causes. Acta Unio Int Contra Carcum 18:330, 1962
11. Davies JNP, Loethe F: Kaposi's sarcoma in African children. Acta Unio Int Contra Carcum 18:394, 1962
12. Olweny CLM, Kaddumukasa AA, Atine I et al: Childhood Kaposi's sarcoma: Clinical features and therapy. Br J Cancer 33:555, 1976
13. Harwood AR, Osoba D, Hofstader SL et al: Kaposi's sarcoma in recipients of renal transplants. Am J Med 67:759, 1979
14. Penn I: Kaposi's sarcoma in organ transplant recipients. Transplantation 27:8, 1979
15. Gottlieb GJ, Ackerman AB: Kaposi's sarcoma: An extensively disseminated form in young homosexual men. Hum Pathol 13:10, 1982
16. Barré–Sinoussi F, Chermann JC, Rey F et al: Isolation of a T-lymphotropic retrovirus from a patient at risk for acquired immune deficiency syndrome (AIDS). Science 220(4599):868, 1983
17. Gelmann EP, Popovic M, Lomonico A et al: Evidence for HTLV infection in two patients with AIDS. In Friedman–Kien AE, Laubenstein LJ (Eds): AIDS: The Epidemic of Kaposi's Sarcoma and Opportunistic Infections, p 127. New York, Masson, 1984
18. Gelmann EP, Popovic M, Blayney D et al: Proviral DNA of a retrovirus, human T-cell leukemia virus, in two patients with AIDS. Science 220:862, 1983
19. Gallo RC, Sarin PS, Gelmann EP et al: Isolation of human T-Cell leukemia virus in acquired immune deficiency syndrome (AIDS). Science 220:865, 1983
20. Brun–Vezinet F, Barré–Sinoussi F, Salmot AG et al: Detection of IgG antibodies to lymphadenopathy-associated virus in patients with AIDS or lymphadenopathy syndrome. Lancet 1:1253, 1984
21. Popovic M, Sarngadharan MG, Read E et al: Detection, isolation and continuous production of cytopathic retroviruses (HTLV-III) from patients with AIDS and pre-AIDS. Science 224:497, 1984
22. Gallo R, Salahuddin SZ, Popovic M et al: Frequent detection and isolation of cytopathic retrovirus (HTLV-III) from patients with AIDS and at risk for AIDS. Science 224:500, 1984
23. Schupbach J, Popovic M, Gilden RV et al: Serological analysis of a subgroup of human T-lymphotropic retroviruses (HTLV-III) associated with AIDS. Science 224:503, 1984
24. Sarngadharan MG, Popovic M, Bruch L et al: Antibodies reactive with human T-lymphotropic retroviruses (HTLV-III) in the serum of patients with AIDS. Science 224:506, 1984
25. Levy JA, Hoffman AD et al: Isolation of lymphocytopathic retroviruses from San Francisco patients with AIDS. Science 225:840, 1984
26. Friedman-Kien AE, Laubenstein L, Rubinstein P et al: Disseminated Kaposi's sarcoma in homosexual men. Ann Intern Med 96(1):693, 1982
27. Marmor M, Friedman–Kien AE, Zolla–Pazner S et al: Kaposi's sarcoma in homosexual men: A seroepidemiologic case-control study. Ann Intern Med 100:809, June 1984
28. Drew WL, Mintz L, Miner RC et al: Prevalence of cytomegalovirus infection in homosexual men. J Infect Dis 143:188, 1981
29. Ambinder RF, Newman C, Hayward GS et al: Lack of association of cytomegalovirus with endemic African Kaposi's sarcoma. J Infect Dis 156:193, 1987
30. Polk BF, Fox R, Brookmeyer R et al: Predictors of the acquired immunodeficiency syndrome developing in a

cohort of seropositive homosexual men. N Engl J Med 316:61, 1987

31. Fenoglio CM, McDougall JK: The relationship of cyto-megalovirus to Kaposi's sarcoma. In Friedman–Kien AE, Laubenstein LJ (Eds): AIDS: The Epidemic of Kaposi's Sarcoma and Opportunistic Infections, p 329. New York, Masson, 1984

32. Giraldo G, Beth E, Huang E–S: Kaposi's sarcoma and its relationship to human cytomegalovirus (CMV). III. CMV DNA and CMV early antigens in Kaposi's sarcoma. Int J Cancer 26:23, 1980

33. Drew WL, Conant MA, Miner RC et al: Cytomegalovirus and Kaposi's sarcoma in young homosexual men. Lancet 2:125, 1982

34. Rubinstein P, Walker ME, Mollen N et al: Immunogenetic aspects of epidemic Kaposi's sarcoma (EKS) in homo-sexual men. In Ma P, Armstrong R (Eds): AIDS and In-fections of Homosexual Men. New York, New York Med-ical Books, 1983

35. Rubinstein P, Walker M, Mollen D et al: Immunogenetic aspects of epidemic Kaposi's sarcoma in homosexual men. In Friedman–Kien AE, Laubenstein LJ (Eds): AIDS: The Epidemic of Kaposi's Sarcoma and Opportunistic In-fections, p 139. New York, Masson, 1984

36. Baur MR, Danilova JA: Population analysis of HLA-A,B,C,Dr and other genetic markers. Histocompatibility Testing 955:93, 1980

37. Melbye M, Kestens L, Biggar RJ et al: HLA studies of en-demic African Kaposi's sarcoma patients and matched controls: No association with HLA-DR5. Int J Cancer 39:182, 1987

38. Costa J, Rabson AS: Generalized Kaposi's sarcoma is not a neoplasm. Lancet 1:58, 1983

39. Friedman–Kien AE: Kaposi's Sarcoma: An Opportunistic Neoplasm. J Invest Dermatol 82:446, 1984

40. Modlin RL, Hofman FM, Kempf RA et al: Kaposi's sarcoma in homosexual men: An immunohistochemical study. J Am Acad Dermatol 8:620, 1983

41. Guarda LG, Silva EG, Ordonex NG et al: Factor VIII in Kaposi's sarcoma. Clin Pathol 76:197, 1981

42. Levy JL, Ziegler JL: Hypothesis: Acquired immunodefi-ciency syndrome is an opportunistic infection and Ka-posi's sarcoma results from secondary immune stimula-tion. Lancet 2:78, 1983

43. Ziegler JL, Templeton AC, Vogel CL: Kaposi's sarcoma: A comparison of classical, endemic, and epidemic forms. Semin Oncol 11:47, 1984

44. Templeton AC: Kaposi's sarcoma. In Andrade R, Cumport SL, Popkin GL et al (Eds): Cancer of the Skin: Biology, Diagnosis, and Management. Philadelphia, WB Saunders, 1976

45. Cox FH, Helwig EB: Kaposi's sarcoma. Cancer 12:289, 1959

46. Rothman S: Remarks on sex, age, and racial distribution of Kaposi's sarcoma and on possible pathogenic factors. Acta Unio Int Contra Carcum 18:326, 1962

47. Epstein E: Kaposi's sarcoma and para-psoriasis en plaque in brothers. JAMA 219:1477, 1972

48. Rothman S: Some clinical aspects of Kaposi's sarcoma in the European and North American population. Acta Unio Int Contra Carcum 18:364, 1962

49. Friedman–Kien AE, Ostreicher R: Overview of classical and epidemic Kaposi's sarcoma. In Friedman–Kien AE, Laubenstein LJ (Eds): AIDS: The Epidemic of Kaposi's Sarcoma and Opportunistic Infections, p 23. New York, Masson, 1984

50. Gottlieb GJ, Ragaz A, Vogel JV et al: A preliminary com-munication on extremely disseminated Kaposi's sarcoma in young homosexual men. Am J Dermatopathol 3:111, 1981

51. Gottlieb GJ, Ackerman AB: Kaposi's sarcoma: An exten-sively disseminated form in young homosexual men. Hum Pathol 13:10, 1982

52. Reynolds WA, Winkelmann RK, Soule EH: Kaposi's sar-coma: A clinicopathological study with particular refer-ence to its relationship to the reticuloendothelial system. Medicine 44:419, 1965

53. Rothman S: Some clinical aspects of Kaposi's sarcoma in the European and North American population. Acta Unio Int Contra Cancer 18:364, 1962

54. Davis J: Kaposi's sarcoma. Present concept of clinical cause and treatment. NY State J Med 68:2067, 1968

55. DiGiovanna JJ, Safai B: Kaposi's sarcoma: Retrospective study of 90 cases with particular emphasis on the familial occurrence, ethnic background and prevalence of other diseases. Am J Med 71:779, 1981

56. Safai B, Mike V, Giraldo G et al: Association of Kaposi's sarcoma with secondary primary malignancies. Possible etiopathogenic implications. Cancer 45:1472, 1980

57. Greenstein RH, Conston AS: Co-existent Hodgkin's dis-ease and Kaposi's sarcoma: A report of a case with unusual features. Am J Med Sci 218:384, 1949

58. Ulbright TM, Santa Cruz DJ: Kaposi's sarcoma: Relation-ship with hematologic, lymphoid, and thymic neoplasia. Cancer 47:963, 1981

59. Olweny CLM: Epidemiology and clinical features of Ka-posi's sarcoma in tropical Africa. In Friedman–Kien AE, Laubenstein LJ (Eds): AIDS: The Epidemic of Kaposi's Sarcoma and Opportunistic Infections, p 35. New York, Masson, 1984

60. Taylor JF, Templeton AC, Vogel CL et al: Kaposi's sarcoma in Uganda: A clinicopathological study. Int J Cancer 8:122, 1971

61. Loethe R, Jurray JF: Kaposi's sarcoma: Autopsy findings in the African. Acta Unio Int Contra Carcum 18:429, 1962

62. Templeton AC, Bhana D: Prognosis in Kaposi's Sarcoma. J Nat Cancer Inst 55:1301, 1975

63. Biggar RJ: The AIDS problem in Africa. Lancet 1:79, 1986

64. Denis F, Barin F, Gershy–Damet G et al: Prevalence of human T-lymphotropic retroviruses type III (HIV) and type IV in Ivory Coast. Lancet 1:408, 1987

65. Colebunders R, Mann JM, Francis H et al: Evaluation of a clinical case-definition of acquired immunodeficiency syndrome in Africa. Lancet 1:492, 1987

66. Bayley AC, Downing RG, Cheingsong–Popov R et al: HTLV-III distinguishes atypical and endemic Kaposi's sarcoma in Africa. Lancet 1:359, 1985

67. Bayley AC. Aggressive Kaposi's sarcoma in Zambia, 1983. Lancet 1:1318, 1984

68. Biggar RJ, Melbye M, Kestens L et al: Kaposi's sarcoma in Zaire is not associated with HTLV-III infection. N Engl J Med 311:1051, 1984

69. Downing RG, Elgin RP, Bayley AC: African Kaposi's sar-coma and AIDS. Lancet 1:478, 1984

70. Kestens L, Melbye M, Biggar RJ et al: Endemic African Kaposi's sarcoma is not associated with immunodefi-ciency. Int J Cancer 36:49, 1985

71. Stribling J, Wertzner S, Smith GV: Kaposi's sarcoma in renal allograft recipients. Cancer 42:442, 1978
72. Myers BD et al: Kaposi's sarcoma in kidney transplant recipients. Arch Intern Med 133:307, 1974
73. Penn I: Kaposi's sarcoma in organ transplant recipients. Transplantation 27:8, 1979
74. Myers BD, Kessler E, Levi D et al: Kaposi's sarcoma in kidney transplant recipients. Arch Intern Med 133:307, 1974
75. Harwood AR: Kaposi's sarcoma in renal transplant patients. In Friedman–Kien AE, Laubenstein LJ (Eds): AIDS: The Epidemic of Kaposi's Sarcoma and Opportunistic Infections, p 41. New York, Masson, 1984
76. Klepp O, Dahl O, Stenwig JT: Association of Kaposi's sarcoma and prior immunosuppressive therapy. Cancer 42:2626, 1978
77. Gange RW, Wilson–Jones E: Kaposi's sarcoma and immunosuppressive therapy: An appraisal. Clin Exp Dermatol 3:135, 1978
78. Klein MB, Periera FA, Kantor I: Kaposi's sarcoma and complicating systemic lupus erythematosus treated with immunosuppression. Arch Dermatol 110:602, 1974
79. Leung F, Fam AG, Osoba D: Kaposi's sarcoma complicating corticosteroid therapy for temporal arthritis. Am J Med 71:320, 1981
80. Centers for Disease Control. Pneumocystis pneumonia. Los Angeles. Morbid Mortal Week Rept. 30:250, 1981
81. Morgan M: personal communication, 1987
82. Drotman DP, Curran JW: AIDS: An epidemiologic overview. In Friedman–Kien AE, Laubenstein LJ (Eds): AIDS: The Epidemic of Kaposi's Sarcoma and Opportunistic Infections, p 279. New York, Masson, 1984
83. Masur H, Michelis MA, Wormser GP et al: Opportunistic infection in previously healthy women: Initial manifestations of a community-acquired cellular immunodeficiency. Ann Intern Med 97:533, 1982
84. Pitchenik AE, Fischl MA, Dickinson GM et al: Opportunistic infections and Kaposi's sarcoma among Haitians: Evidence of a new acquired immunodeficiency state. Ann Intern Med 98:277, 1983
85. Brunet JB, Bouvet E, Chaperon J et al: Acquired immunodeficiency syndrome in France. Lancet 1:700, 1983
86. Clumeck N, Mascart Lemone F, de Maugeuge J et al: Acquired immune deficiency syndrome in black Africans. Lancet 4:642, 1983
87. Selik RM, Starcher ET, Curran JW: Opportunistic diseases reported in AIDS patients: Frequencies, associations, and trends. AIDS 1:175, 1987
88. Marmor M, Friedman–Kien AE, Laubenstein L et al: Risk factors for Kaposi's sarcoma in homosexual men. Lancet 1:1083, 1982
89. Jaffe HW, Choi K, Thomas PA et al: National case-control study of Kaposi's sarcoma and *Pneumocystis carinii* pneumonia in homosexual men: Part I. Epidemiologic results. Ann Intern Med 99:145, 1983
90. Marmor M: Epidemic Kaposi's sarcoma and sexual practices, among male homosexuals. In Friedman–Kien AE, Laubenstein LJ (Eds): AIDS: The Epidemic of Kaposi's Sarcoma and Opportunistic Infections, p 291. New York, Masson, 1984
91. Darrow WW, Jaffe HW, Curran JW: Letter: Passive anal intercourse as a risk factor for AIDS in homosexual men. Lancet 2:160, 1983
92. Marmor M, Friedman–Kien AE, Zolla-Pazner S et al: Kaposi's sarcoma in homosexual men: A serioepidemiologic case-control study. Ann Intern Med 100:809, 1984
93. Krigel R, Laubenstein LJ, Muggia F: Kaposi's sarcoma: A new staging classification. Canc Treat Rep 67:531, 1983
94. Hamm PG, Judson MA, Aranda CP. Diagnosis of pulmonary Kaposi's sarcoma with fiberoptic bronchoscopy and endobronchial biopsy. Cancer 59:807, 1987
95. Meduri GU, Stover DE, Lee M et al: Pulmonary Kaposi's sarcoma in the acquired immune deficiency syndrome. Am J Med 81:11, 1986
96. Ognibene FP, Steis RG, Macher AM et al: Kaposi's sarcoma causing pulmonary infiltrates and respiratory failure in the acquired immunodeficiency syndrome. Ann Intern Med 102:471, 1985
97. Krigel RL: The treatment and natural history of epidemic Kaposi's sarcoma. In Selikoff IJ, Tierstein AS, and Hirschman SZ (Eds): Annals of the New York Academy of Sciences. New York, New York Academy of Sciences, 1984
98. Krigel R: Prognostic factors in Kaposi's sarcoma. In Friedman–Kien AE, Laubenstein LJ (Eds): Epidemic Kaposi's Sarcoma and Opportunistic Infections in Homosexual Men. New York, Masson, 1984
99. Krigel RL: Kaposi's sarcoma. In Carter S, Issel B (Eds): Etoposide: Current Status and New Developments. New York, Academic Press, 1984
100. Welch K, Finkbeiner W, Alpers CE et al: Autopsy findings in the acquired immune deficiency syndrome. JAMA 252:1152, 1984
101. Rogers MF, Morens DM, Stewart JA et al: National case-control study of Kaposi's sarcoma and *Pneumocystis carinii* pneumonia in homosexual men: Part 2. Laboratory results. Ann Intern Med 99:151, 1983
102. Abrams DI, Chinn EK, Lewis BJ et al: Hematologic manifestations in homosexual men with Kaposi's sarcoma. Am J Clin Pathol 81(1):13, 1984
103. Morris L, Distenfeld A, Amorosi E et al: Autoimmune thrombocytopenic purpura in homosexual men. Ann Intern Med 96:714, 1982
104. Walsh CM, Nardi MA, Karpatkin S: On the mechanism of thrombocytopenic purpura in sexually active homosexual men. N Engl J Med 311:635, 1984
105. Walsh CM, Krigel R, Lennette E et al: Prognosis, response to therapy and anti-AIDS associated retrovirus antibody in homosexual patients with thrombocytopenia. Ann Intern Med 103:542, 1985
106. Siegal FP: Immune function and dysfunction in AIDS. Semin Oncol 11:29, 1984
107. Fauci AS, Macher AM, Longo DL et al: Acquired Immunodeficiency Syndrome: Epidemiologic, Clinical, Immunologic, and Therapeutic Considerations. Ann Intern Med 100:92, 1984
108. Friedman-Kien AE, and Ostreicher R: Overview of classical and epidemic Kaposi's sarcoma. In Friedman–Kien AE, Laubenstein LJ (Eds): AIDS: The Epidemic of Kaposi's Sarcoma and Opportunistic Infections, p 23. New York, Masson, 1984
109. Ammann AJ, Abrams D, Conant M et al: Acquired immune dysfunction in homosexual men: Immunologic profiles. Clin Immunol Immunopathol 27:315, 1983
110. Lane HC, Masur H, Edgar LC et al: Abnormalities of B-cell activation in patients with the acquired immunodeficiency syndrome. N Engl J Med 309:453, 1983
111. Stahl RE, Friedman-Kien A, Dubin R et al: Immunologic

abnormalities in homosexual men: Relationship to Kaposi's sarcoma. Am J Med 73:171, 1982

112. Zolla–Pazner S, William D, El-Sadr W et al: Elevated serum beta-2 microglobulin as a surrogate marker for the acquired immune deficiency syndrome. JAMA 251:2951, 1984

113. DeStefano E, Friedman RM, Friedman–Kien AE et al: Acid-labile human leukocyte interferon in homosexual men with Kaposi's sarcoma and lymphadenopathy. J Infect Dis 146:451, 1982

114. Rook AH, Masur H, Lane JC et al: Interleukin-2 enhances the depressed natural killer and cytomegalovirus-specific cytotoxic activities of lymphocytes from patients with the acquired immune deficiency syndrome. J Clin Invest 72: 398, 1983

115. Hersh EM, Reuben JM, Rios A et al: Elevated serum thymosin alpha 1 levels associated with evidence of immune dysregulation in male homosexuals with a history of infectious diseases or Kaposi's sarcoma. N Engl J Med 308: 45, 1983

116. Biggar RJ, Taylor PH, Goldstein AL et al: Thymosin alpha 1 levels and helper/suppressor ratios in homosexual men. N Engl J Med 309:49, 1983

117. Shearer GM: Allogenic leukocytes as a possible factor in induction of AIDS in homosexual men. N Engl J Med 308(4):223, 1983

118. Krigel RL, Laubenstein LJ, Friedman–Kien AE et al: Kaposi's sarcoma: Evaluation of a new staging classification [Abstr]. Proc Am Soc Clin Oncol 3:61, 1984

119. Krigel R, Ostreicher R, LaFleur F et al: Epidemic Kaposi's sarcoma: identification of a subset of patients with a good prognosis [Abstr]. Proc Am Soc Clin Oncol 4:4, 1985

120. Safai B, Johnson KG, Myskowski PL et al: The natural history of Kaposi's sarcoma in the acquired immunodeficiency syndrome. Ann Intern Med 103:744, 1985

121. Taylor J, Afrasiabi R, Fahey JL et al: Prognostically significant classification of immune changes in AIDS with Kaposi's sarcoma. Blood 67:666, 1986

122. Vadhan–Raj S, Wong G, Gnecco C et al: Immunological variables as predictors of prognosis in patients with Kaposi's sarcoma and the acquired immunodeficiency syndrome. Cancer Res 46:417, 1986

123. Volberding P, Kaslow K, Bille M et al: Prognostic factors in staging Kaposi's sarcoma in the acquired immune deficiency syndrome [Abstr]. Proc Am Soc Clin Onc 3:51, 1984

124. Muggia FM: Treatment of classical Kaposi's sarcoma: A new look. In Friedman–Kien AE, Laubenstein LJ (Eds): AIDS: The Epidemic of Kaposi's Sarcoma and Opportunistic Infections, p 57. New York, Masson, 1984

125. Holecek MJ, Jarwood AR: Radiotherapy and Kaposi's sarcoma. Cancer 41:1733, 1978

126. Harwood AR: Extended field radiotherapy of Kaposi's sarcoma. Arch Dermatol 117:203, 1981

127. Lo TC, Salzman FC, Smedel MJ et al: Radiotherapy of Kaposi's sarcoma. Int J Radiol Oncol 4[Suppl 12]:98, 1978

128. Nisce LZ, Safai B, Poussin–Rosillo H: Once weekly total and subtotal skin electron beam therapy of Kaposi's sarcoma. Cancer 47:640, 1981

129. Cooper JS, Fried PR, Laubenstein LJ: Initial observations of the effect of radiotherapy on epidemic Kaposi's sarcoma. JAMA 252:934, 1984

130. Nobler MP, Leddy ME, Huh SH: The impact of palliative irradiation on the management of patients with acquired immune deficiency syndrome. J Clin Oncol 107, 1987

131. Hill DR: The role of radiotherapy for epidemic Kaposi's sarcoma. Semin Oncol 14[Suppl 3]:19, 1987

132. Scott WP, Voight JA: Kaposi's sarcoma management with vincaleucoblastine. Cancer 19:557, 1966

133. Tucker SB, Winkelmann RK: Treatment of Kaposi's sarcoma with vinblastine. Arch Dermatol 112:958, 1976

134. Salan AJ, Greenwald ES, Silvay O: Long term complete remission of Kaposi's sarcoma with vinblastine therapy. Cancer 47:637, 1981

135. Volberding PA, Abrams DI, Conant M et al: Vinblastine therapy for Kaposi's sarcoma in the acquired immunodeficiency syndrome. Ann Intern Med 103:335, 1985

136. Laubenstein LJ: Staging and treatment of Kaposi's sarcoma in patients with AIDS. In Friedman–Kien AE, Laubenstein LJ (Eds): AIDS: The Epidemic of Kaposi's Sarcoma and Opportunistic Infections, p 51. New York, Masson, 1984

137. Vogel CL, Clements D, Wanume AK et al: Phase II clinical trials of 1, 3-BIS (2-chloreoghyl-1-nitrosuourea, BCNU, NSC 4099621) and bleomycin (NSC 125066) in Kaposi's sarcoma. Cancer Chemo Rep (Part I) 57:325, 1973

138. Olweny CLM, Masaba JP, Sikyewunda W et al: Treatment of Kaposi's sarcoma with ICRF-159 (NSC 129943). Cancer Chemo Rep 60:111, 1976

139. Vogel CL, Templeton CJ, Templeton AC et al: Treatment of Kaposi's sarcoma with actinomycin-D and cyclophosphamide: Results of a randomized clinical trial. Int J Cancer 8:136, 1971

140. Vogel DL, Primakc A, Owor R et al: Effective treatment of Kaposi's sarcoma with 5-(3, 3-dimethyl-1-triazeno) imidazole-4-carboxamide (DTIC, NSC 45388). Cancer Chemo Rep (Part 1) 57:65, 1973

141. Olweny CLM, Toya T, Katangole–Mbiddie E et al: Treatment of Kaposi's sarcoma by a combination of actinomycin-D, vincristine and imidazole carboxamide. Results of a randomized clinical trial. Int J Cancer 14:649, 1974

142. Laubenstein LJ, Krigel RL, Hymes KB et al: Treatment of epidemic Kaposi's sarcoma with VP-16 (etoposide) or a combination of doxorubicin, bleomycin, and vinblastine. J Clin Oncol 2:1115, 1984

143. Mintzer DM, Real FX, Jovino L et al: Treatment of Kaposi's sarcoma and thrombocytopenia with vincristine in patients with the acquired immunodeficiency syndrome. Ann Intern Med 102:200, 1985

144. Wernz J, Laubenstein L, Hymes K et al: Chemotherapy and assessment of response in epidemic Kaposi's sarcoma with bleomycin/Velban [Abstr]. Proc Am Soc Clin Oncol 5:4, 1986

145. Kaplan L, Abrams D, Volberding P: Treatment of Kaposi's sarcoma in acquired immunodeficiency syndrome with an alternating vincristine–vinblastine regimen. Cancer Treat Rep 70:1121, 1986

146. Minor DR, Brayer T: Velban and methotrexate combination chemotherapy for epidemic Kaposi's sarcoma [Abstr]. Proc Am Soc Clin Oncol 5:1, 1986

147. Gill P, Deyton L, Rarick M et al: Results of a prospective trial of adriamycin, bleomycin, and vincristine in the treatment of epidemic Kaposi's sarcoma [Abstr]. Proc Am Soc Clin Oncol 6:5, 1987

148. Gelmann EP, Longo D, Lane HC et al: Combination chemotherapy of disseminated Kaposi's sarcoma in patients with the acquired immune deficiency syndrome. Am J Med 82:456, 1987

149. Krown SE, Real FX, Cunningham–Rundles S et al: Preliminary observations on the effect of recombinant leu-

kocyte A interferon in homosexual men with Kaposi's sarcoma. N Engl J Med 308:1071, 1983

150. Groopman JE, Gottlieb MS, Goodman J et al: Recombinant alpha-2 interferon therapy for Kaposi's sarcoma associated with the acquired immunodeficiency syndrome. Ann Intern Med 100:671, 1984

151. Rios A, Mansell PWA, Newell GR et al: Treatment of acquired immunodeficiency syndrome–related Kaposi's sarcoma with lymphoblastoid interferon. J Clin Oncol 3: 506, 1985

152. Gelman EP, Preble OT, Steis R et al: Human lymphoblastoid interferon treatment of Kaposi's sarcoma in the acquired immune deficiency syndrome. Am J Med 78: 737, 1985

153. Real FX, Oettgen HF, Krown SE: Kaposi's sarcoma and the acquired immunodeficiency syndrome: Treatment with high and low doses of recombinant leukocyte A interferon. J Clin Oncol 4:544, 1986

154. Lonberg M, Odajnyk C, Krigel R et al: Sequential and simultaneous alpha 2 interferon and VP16 in epidemic Kaposi's sarcoma [Abstr]. Proc Am Soc Clin Oncol 4:2, 1985

155. Rios A, Mansell P, Newell G et al: The use of lymphoblastoid interferon and vinblastine in the treatment of acquired immunodeficiency syndrome related Kaposi's sarcoma [Abstr]. Proc Am Soc Clin Oncol 4:6, 1985

156. Krown SE, Real FX, Lester T et al: Interferon alfa-2a ± vinblastine in AIDS-related Kaposi's sarcoma: A prospective randomized trial [Abstr]. Proc Am Soc Clin Oncol 5:6, 1986

157. Fischl M, Lucas S, Richman S et al: Phase II study of Wellferon and vincristine in AIDS related Kaposi's sarcoma [Abstr]. Proc Am Soc Clin Oncol 6:2, 1987

158. Murray HW, Rubin BY, Masur H et al: Impaired cell-mediated immune responses in the acquired immune deficiency syndrome: Patients with opportunistic infection fail to secrete activating lymphokine and gamma interferon. N Engl J Med 310:883, 1984

159. Krigel RL, Odajnyk C, Laubenstein L et al: Therapeutic trial of gamma interferon in patients with epidemic Kaposi's sarcoma. J Biol Respir Modif 4:358, 1985

160. Lotze M, Robb R, Frana L et al: Systemic administration of interleukin-2 in patients with cancer and AIDS: Initial results of a phase I trial [Abstr]. Proc Am Soc Clin Oncol 3:51, 1984

161. Volberding P, Moody DJ, Beardslee D et al: Therapy of acquired immune deficiency syndrome with recombinant interleukin-2. AIDS Res Hum Retroviruses 3:115, 1987

162. Krigel RL, Friedman–Kien AE: Kaposi's sarcoma. In Prevost TT, Farmer ER (Eds). Current Therapy in Dermatology. New York, Decker, 1985

163. Groopman JE, Mitsuyasu RT, DeLeo MJ et al: Effect of recombinant human granulocyte–macrophage colony-stimulating factor on myelopoiesis in the acquired immunodeficiency syndrome. N Engl J Med 317:593, 1987

164. Broder S, Yarchoan R, Collins JM et al: Effects of suramin on HTLV-III/LAV infection presenting as Kaposi's sarcoma or AIDS-related complex: Clinical pharmacology and suppression of virus replication in vivo. Lancet 2: 627, 1985

165. Fischl MA, Richman DD, Grieco MH et al: The efficacy of azidothymidine (AZT) in the treatment of patients with AIDS and AIDS-related complex. N Engl J Med 317:185, 1987

Reactive and Neoplastic Lymphoproliferative Disorders and Other Miscellaneous Cancers Associated with HIV Infection

Alexandra M. Levine

15

REACTIVE LYMPHOPROLIFERATIVE DISORDERS: PERSISTENT, GENERALIZED LYMPHADENOPATHY

Early in the AIDS epidemic, it became apparent that individuals at risk for AIDS were also at risk for the development of generalized lymphadenopathy of a reactive nature. The term *persistent, generalized lymphadenopathy* or *PGL* was used by the Centers for Disease Control (CDC) to characterize this disorder, described as generalized lymphadenopathy involving at least two or more extra-inguinal sites, of three months' duration or longer, in the absence of any known specific cause of adenopathy. Microscopically, the involved nodes were consistent with a reactive hyperplastic process.[1]

Histologic Features

Although many of the histologic characteristics of PGL could be considered nonspecific, certain morphologic features were noteworthy and have been described in great detail.[2-8] These features can best be summarized as consisting of a florid, hyperplastic B-lymphoid response, with marked follicular hyperplasia, frequently comprising over 75% to 80% of the cross-sectional area of the node, while compressing the interfollicular tissue. In cases that are not as extreme, prominent interfollicular components have also been described, with vascular proliferation and increase in perisinus and plasma cells. Aside from their prominence, peculiar alterations of these follicles include disruption of the follicular dendritic network, presence of naked follicular centers without the typical mantle zones, infiltration of follicles by mantle cells and islets of lymphocytes, and disruption of the follicles by lymphocytes or hemorrhage.

Immunophenotypically, the nodes in PGL were also distinct from the expected pattern in reactive hyperplasia, with decreased paracortical CD4$^+$ lymphocytes, increased CD-8$^+$ cells in follicles and paracortical areas, and increased numbers of activated lymphocytes.[9-10]

As the illness progressed, Fernandez and colleagues and other researchers described a gradual change in lymph node histology, with development of decreased follicle size, involution and atrophy of follicles, and the eventual evolution to a picture of lymphocyte depletion.[6,11]

Importance of Initial Lymph Node Biopsy

Although this assertion was somewhat controversial at the outset, Levine and co-workers have demonstrated that the diagnosis of PGL cannot be made with real accuracy in the absence of lymph node biopsy.[12,13] Thus, in a study of the natural history of PGL among homosexual men, which required confirmatory lymph node biopsy for accrual, 6 of the first 40 potential PGL study cases were found to have conditions other than PGL at the time of node biopsy. Two of these cases were found to have node-based Kaposi's sarcoma in the absence of cutaneous involvement, two individuals had malignant lymphoma, one patient had *Mycobacterium* tuberculosis, and the sixth had histoplasmosis. In evaluating all clinical and laboratory data obtained prior to the time of actual node biopsy, the group of patients who were subsequently proved by biopsy to have PGL could not be distinguished from those who had these other conditions. The clinical finding of generalized lymphadenopathy in a patient with HIV infection, then, does not prove the diagnosis of PGL.[12]

Aside from substantiating the precise underlying

diagnosis, lymph node biopsy may be valuable in terms of individual patient prognosis. Thus, the histologic development of progressive follicular involution and then lymphocyte depletion may be associated with clinical deterioration and the subsequent development of frank AIDS.[6,11]

Clinical Characteristics of Disease

Several large cohorts of patients with PGL have been described.[14-21] Sixty-three homosexual men with biopsy-proven PGL have been followed at University of Southern California since 1982, with a mean follow-up of 1.5 years (9–>62 months; 76.1 person years).[20,21] The mean age of the PGL cases was 32.4 years (range 19–59). The study population was composed of 46 Caucasians (72.6%), 8 Blacks (12.9%), and 9 Hispanics (14.5%). All patients were homosexual or bisexual males; two cases also gave a history of intravenous drug abuse.

The initial symptom complex in these patients may best be classified as a typical viral-like illness, with significant myalgias noted in 67%, fatigue and malaise requiring change in work habits or life-style in 39%, headache in 23%, diarrhea in 35%, and systemic B symptoms, consisting of fever, drenching night sweats, and/or unexplained weight loss in 35%. Interestingly, when followed over time, approximately 40% of patients experienced fluctuation of these symptoms. Thus, in characterizing the total percentage of patients who eventually developed one or all of these complaints, 47% have noted systemic B symptoms at some time during the follow-up interval, 36% have had headache, 60% have had noteworthy fatigue, 46% have had diarrhea, and 41% have had nonspecific cough. The new onset of fever, then, in a patient with PGL does not necessarily imply that a change in underlying disease process has occurred and may simply reflect the expected fluctuations in symptomatology over time.

By definition, patients with PGL must have generalized lymphadenopathy. In our study group, very unusual sites for reactive lymphadenopathy were recorded, with definite fluctuation in lymph node size during the follow-up interval. Thus, in the course of illness, 100% had cervical adenopathy at some time, 98% had enlarged axillary nodes, 93% had enlarged inguinal nodes, and 38% had supraclavicular adenopathy, whereas lymph node enlargement in the infraclavicular area was noted in 20%, in the epitrochlear area in 20%, and in popliteal nodes in 5%; 21% were found to have splenomegaly at some time.

Retroviral Characteristics of Disease

At study entry, 62 of 63 PGL cases (98%) were found to have antibody to HIV, determined by the ELISA method, and confirmed by Western blot. During the follow-up period, all cases were found to be HIV seropositive. Interestingly, 80% of cases (33 of 41) were found to be live-virus positive by analysis of reverse transcriptase levels from cultured peripheral blood lymphocytes at the same time that antibody against HIV was present.[22]

Immunologic Characteristics of Disease

A profound abnormality in B-cell function has been described in AIDS and in PGL.[23-25] Thus, high spontaneous IgG production has been documented, with paradoxic suppression of IgG synthesis after stimulation with pokeweed mitogen (PWM).[24]

Abnormalities in T-lymphocyte subsets have also been described, and although similar in a general sense to those changes noted in AIDS, the degree of abnormality in PGL is less extreme, indicating that a spectrum of immunologic dysfunction exists among HIV-infected individuals. Early in PGL, a specific decrease in $CD4^+CDw29^+$, or helper–inducer cells, has been documented, whereas, over time, a decrease in $CD4^+$ suppressor–inducers also occurs. An increase in cytotoxic T cells ($CD8^+CD11b^-$) is apparent throughout the course of illness, whereas activated T cells ($CD2^+Ta1^+$) and circulating B-lymphocytes are reduced compared to HIV seronegative homosexual controls.[26,27]

Aside from abnormalities in B- and T-lymphocytes, various other makers of immune dysfunction have been described in PGL, including an increase in serum β-2 microglobulin levels, which may reflect changes in disease activity over time.[28]

Relationship to AIDS in General and to AIDS–Lymphoma

At the outset of the AIDS epidemic there was some question concerning the eventual outcome of patients with PGL. Most of the early patients had remained stable over time, and the question remained unanswered.[18]

With further follow-up, it has become apparent that some patients with PGL will develop AIDS. The precise rates of development of AIDS among cohorts of PGL cases have ranged from approximately 1% to 6% per person per year.[14-21,29-31]

In our own PGL series, 7 of 63 PGL patients have AIDS, with a median follow-up interval of 1.5 years (9–>62 months). Four of these cases were eventually diagnosed with *Pneumocystis carinii* pneumonia, whereas three additional cases developed AIDS-related lymphoma, representing a rate of conversion from PGL to AIDS of approximately 9% per person per year. The development of AIDS among this cohort occurred as events which were scattered throughout the period of follow-up, with no plateau apparent.[20,21] This would imply that, given time, potentially all PGL patients would eventually develop AIDS.

In an attempt to predict which PGL patients may remain relatively stable over the short term, and which are likely to develop progressive illness more rapidly, an 11-factor multifactorial analysis was performed. Interestingly, the factors that could predict development of AIDS, as characterized by opportunistic infection (OI) and those that could predict AIDS as defined by B-cell lymphoma were distinct. Thus, the development of AIDS-OI could be predicted by the finding of decreased T4 cells at study entry (p < 0.001), decreased T4:T8 ratio (p < 0.001), and increasing IgA levels over time (p = 0.005). Conversely, the development of AIDS-related lymphoma among our PGL cohort could be predicted by the presence of anemia at study entry (p < 0.001), and increasing levels of IgG (p = 0.0036).[20,21]

The development of B-cell lymphoma in our PGL patients was not particularly surprising, given the extreme degree of polyclonal B-cell activation that has been noted in PGL in the setting of HIV-induced immune dysfunction.[32] Pelicci and others have described the presence of monoclonal and oligoclonal immunoglobulin light-chain gene rearrangement in as many as 20% of PGL nodal biopsy specimens,[33] and we have documented the same finding in our own cohort. In the setting of on-going B-cell proliferation, development of specific chromosomal translocations may provide the opportunity for selective growth advantage, leading eventually to a monoclonal B-cell proliferation. In fact, three of our initial 63 PGL patients have now developed lymphoma, representing a specific rate of conversion of approximately 3% per person per year. Based upon the expected incidence rates of lymphoma in the United States, from the age-adjusted Third National Cancer Survey,[34] the relative risk of lymphoma in patients with PGL is over 850 times the expected rate. With ever-increasing numbers of HIV-infected individuals who may eventually develop PGL, it is expected that increasing numbers of patients with AIDS-related lymphoma will continue to be diagnosed.

MALIGNANT LYMPHOMA ASSOCIATED WITH AIDS

Incidence Rates of Lymphoma in Never-Married Men

Lymphoma was not considered part of the spectrum of AIDS until June 1985, when the case-definition criteria were expanded to include individuals who have high-grade B-cell lymphomas with positive serology and/or virology to HIV.[35] Although several series of homosexual men with lymphoma had been published before that time,[36–43] the relation between these cases and prior HIV infection was not documented until 1985,[44] and it was at that time, as well, that population-based epidemiologic data began to indicate a statistical increase in lymphomas, occurring specifically among "never-married men."[45]

Using data from the Cancer Surveillance Program (CSP), a population-based cancer registry in Los Angeles County,[46] it is apparent, as shown in Figure 15-1, that a sizable increase in lymphomas has occurred in never-married males, beginning in 1980 and continuing to the present time.[47] No such increase has been identified among ever-married males, or in married or never-married females. Although the never-married male category is obviously not synonymous with homosexual male, no such specific data is available through the CSP registry, and it is assumed that a majority of homosexual men at risk for AIDS would fall within the never-married category.

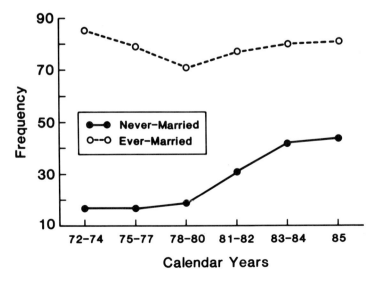

FIG. 15-1. Numbers of cases of lymphoma diagnosed among never-married and ever-married males aged 18 to 24 in Los Angeles County from 1972 to 1985, using data from the Cancer Surveillance Program, a population-based cancer registry.

Although the overall incidence of lymphoma has increased among never-married males, it is specifically the high-grade B-cell types of disease that have shown the most significant increases when the years 1972–1980 are compared to 1980–1985 (Table 15-1). Thus, the categories of Burkitt's lymphoma, immunoblastic sarcoma, and "undifferentiated lymphoma, not otherwise specified" have increased both in number and in proportion among never-married men in Los Angeles County since 1980.[45,47]

Epidemiologic Features

Although AIDS-related lymphomas have been reported in intravenous drug abusers and in hemophiliacs, the majority of reported cases to date have occurred in homosexual men.[48]

High-grade lymphoma may be the first manifestation of AIDS. However, a sizable number of these cases have had opportunistic infections or Kaposi's sarcoma (KS), which would have resulted in an AIDS diagnosis prior to the development of lymphoma. Thus, Ziegler and colleagues reported that 42 of 90 (47%) patients with AIDS-lymphoma had AIDS prior to the time of initial diagnosis of lymphoma, with OI occurring in 25%, KS in 11%, and both OI and KS in 10%.[37] Unusual cases have been reported, including the simultaneous occurrence of *Pneumocystis carinii* pneumonia, systemic cytomegalovirus infection, KS, and immunoblastic lymphoma, all present within one nodal biopsy in a homosexual male.[49]

Aside from prior diagnosis of AIDS, many patients with AIDS-related lymphoma have had prior diagnosis of AIDS-related complex (ARC), with persistent, generalized lymphadenopathy the most prominent of these pre-existing conditions, as demonstrated by Levine and co-workers,[21,32] and by Ziegler and others, who described a history of generalized lymphadenopathy in 33 of 77 (43%) lymphoma cases, diagnosed antemortem.[37]

Pathologic Spectrum of Disease

As indicated by the cancer registry data, the vast majority of patients with AIDS-related lymphoma have had B-cell tumors of high-grade pathologic type.[35] These would include small non-cleaved lymphoma, either Burkitt's or Burkitt's-like (previously termed undifferentiated lymphoma), and immunoblastic lymphoma (also called immunoblastic sarcoma).[50-51] Thus, in the series reported by Ziegler and others 62% had high-grade disease,[37] whereas in the series of Levine and co-workers approximately 81% have had high-grade B-cell lymphomas.[44] This pathologic spectrum of lymphomatous disease is most unusual, when compared to previous series of spontaneous lymphomas. Thus, in a review of 425 cases of lymphoma diagnosed at the University of Southern California, and published in 1978, the incidence of B-immunoblastic sarcoma was only 3.5%, while small non-cleaved lymphoma was present in 6.8% of the group.[50] Likewise, in a series of 1175 patients with lymphoma reported by the Working Formulation on Lymphoma classification 7.9% of the group were diagnosed as having immunoblastic lymphoma, while 5% had small non-cleaved disease.[51]

Although the majority of patients with AIDS-related lymphoma have had high-grade B-cell disease, it is also apparent that almost all series have noted the presence of intermediate-grade lymphoma in some patients.[37,43] This area is somewhat problematic, because of the known difficulties in consistency and reproducibility in the field of lymphoma pathology.[52] It is highly probable that a case diagnosed as a small non-cleaved "high-

Table 15-1
Changes in Number and Histologic Pattern of Non-Hodgkin's Lymphoma in Married and Never-Married Men Ages 18–54 in Los Angeles County: Pre-1980 versus 1980–1985

| | | Never-Married Males | | | | Ever-Married Males | | | |
| | | 1972–1980 (n = 138) | | Post–1980 (n = 197) | | 1972–1980 (n = 636) | | Post–1980 (n = 428) | |
Histology	*ICD-O*	n	%	n	%	n	%	n	%
Lymphoma:NOS	9591	0	0	12	6	8	1	15	3
Undifferentiated, NOS	9600	3	2	18	9	5	1	17	4
Immunoblastic sarcoma	9612	4	3	23	12	11	3	30	7
Burkitt's lymphoma	9750	1	1	20	10	5	1	3	1
	Total	8	6	73	37	29	5	65	15

grade" lymphoma in some centers might be considered a large non-cleaved "intermediate-grade" lymphoma in others. Thus, it is possible that some of the reported intermediate-grade cases may reflect the subjectivity inherent in lymphoma diagnosis. However, it is also probable that some cases of intermediate-grade lymphoma do exist within the spectrum of AIDS-related disease. Furthermore, as described by Kalter,[43] it is possible that patients with intermediate-grade disease may fare better than those with high-grade histology, although this has not been confirmed.

It is now apparent, as well, that the spectrum of pathologic types of disease associated with HIV infection is somewhat wider than originally appreciated. Thus, in Ziegler's series, 7% had low-grade lymphomas, whereas 5 of 27 (19%) patients described by Levine and co-workers had low-grade disease, including small cleaved lymphoma, and plasmacytoid–lymphocytic lymphoma.[37,44] Interestingly, of the three patients with biopsy-proven PGL followed serially by Levine and colleagues who subsequently developed lymphoma, two of these developed high-grade immunoblastic lymphomas, whereas the third developed low-grade, plasmacytoid–lymphocytic lymphoma. This would imply that the spectrum of B-cell lymphoma that may occur in association with HIV infection may be quite broad, even though epidemiologic data to prove such an association is still lacking. Other lymphoproliferative malignancies that have been reported in association with HIV infection include multiple myeloma[53,54] and B-cell acute lymphocytic leukemia (L-3, or Burkitt's leukemia.[55]) Of real interest is that essentially all of these processes have been similar with respect to the B-cell nature of disease. Although there have been occasional reports of T-lymphoblastic lymphoma occurring in homosexual men, this disorder is expected to occur in young men,[56,57] and the finding of an occasional patient with lymphoblastic lymphoma, who happens to be young and homosexual would not be particularly noteworthy.

AIDS-Related Primary Central Nervous System Lymphoma

Lymphoma primary to the central nervous system has been considered a diagnostic criterion for AIDS from the onset of the epidemic. The development of primary central nervous system (P-CNS) lymphoma in association with severe HIV-induced immunocompromise would not be surprising, since CNS lymphoma has previously been well described in individuals with congenital or acquired immune deficiency diseases.[58–61] Thus, individuals with IgA deficiency, or Wiskott–Aldrich syndrome, or those who have undergone organ transplantation with subsequent administration of immunosupressive agents are at increased risk for the development of P-CNS lymphoma, which normally occurs very rarely (0.2%–1% of all lymphomas) in patients with no such underlying immunologic defect.[62–64]

The most common presenting features in patients with P-CNS lymphoma include headache, cranial nerve palsies, seizure disorder, or hemiparesis.[42,65,66] However, another common initial symptom complex may include altered mental status or personality change. Thus, although most such patients present with symptoms or signs that would mandate a careful CNS work-up, it is most important to realize that many of these individuals may first seek medical attention because of rather subtle changes in personality. The development of apathy, for example, has been the only initial manifestation of disease in some of our patients with P-CNS lymphoma.[65]

Radiographic analysis of patients with P-CNS lymphoma has also proved problematic at times. Most patients demonstrate definite space-occupying lesions with contrast enhancement on computed tomographic (CT) scanning. The majority of lesions are isodense or hyperdense prior to administration of contrast media, with varying degrees of surrounding edema and mass effect.[65] With double-dose delay (DDD) contrast studies, most lesions appear as homogeneous or heterogeneous contrast-enhancing masses. Interestingly, several investigators have reported the finding of ring-enhancing mass lesions, very similar to the lesions described in CNS toxoplasmosis, in patients who later proved to have P-CNS lymphoma.[66,67] Thus, although ring-enhancing lesions are seen most commonly in CNS infections associated with AIDS, P-CNS lymphoma can also present in this manner. In comparing results of imaging techniques in space-occupying lesions within the brain in patients with AIDS, Gill and colleagues noted several features that were characteristic of P-CNS lymphoma.[67] These lymphomas usually appeared as single lesions, always larger than 3 cm. In a comparison of the CT scan findings in brain of 16 patients with cerebral toxoplasmosis versus 7 with P-CNS lymphoma, multiple lesions were demonstrated in 13 patients with toxoplasmosis, with a total of 50 lesions noted in this group. The median number of such lesions was 2.5 (range 1–7). In the seven patients with P-CNS lymphoma, six had solitary lesions, whereas the seventh had two demonstrable masses. Aside from the greater likelihood of multiple lesions in toxoplasmosis as opposed to P-CNS lymphoma, the size of the individual lesions was also distinct between the groups. Thus, the average lesion size in toxoplasmosis was 1.5 cm (range 1–4 cm), whereas that of lymphomas was 4.5 cm (range 3–5 cm). These differences were highly significant (p < 0.001). While DDD-CT scanning techniques may be somewhat problematic in some cases, the combined radiologic criteria of size, multiplicity, and pre- and postcontrast appearance may be useful in differentiating these two pathologic processes. It would appear reasonable to assume that a patient with multiple, small, ring-enhancing lesions on DDD-CT scan does, in fact, have cerebral toxoplasmosis and may be treated empirically. However, while the diagnosis of P-CNS lymphoma can be strongly suggested by DDD-CT scan results, a definitive diagnosis by brain biopsy would appear warranted. This is especially true since multiple neuropathologic processes may be coexistant in a given patient.[67]

The specific sites of P-CNS lymphoma within the brain may be quite various, including disease that has been described in the basal ganglia, parietal, frontal, or frontoparietal lobes, cerebellum, and pons.[42,65-67]

No prospective therapeutic trial of patients with AIDS-related P-CNS lymphoma has yet been accomplished. However, Formenti and associates have recently reviewed the experience with whole brain radiotherapy, administered to eight patients with AIDS-related P-CNS lymphoma who were diagnosed at University of Southern California (USC).[68] After receiving a total dose of 2200 to 5000 cGy, over 2 to 4 weeks, four cases demonstrated complete resolution of the intracranial mass lesion, a fifth attained partial response, and the remainder experienced either no response, or disease progression. Interestingly, one of the patients who experienced a pathologically and radiographically proven complete remission failed to improve clinically. He died of progressive neurologic dysfunction; at autopsy, there was no evidence of lymphoma, although both toxoplasma and cytomegalovirus encephalitis were present. This case illustrates the importance of careful assessment of the brain, with biopsy in patients who do not respond as expected to a given therapeutic intervention; it is very possible in such a circumstance that the patient may have more than one on-going neuropathologic process.

In Formenti's series, although complete remission was attained in four of eight patients, only two individuals survived more than a year, and both had received 5000 cGy, resulting in complete remission. The median survival of the entire group was only 3.5 months (range 2–>16 months). Two of the complete remissions subsequently died of multiple opportunistic infections, one remains alive at this time, and the fourth relapsed within the brain at 14 months, and died 2 months later. Thus, of all eight patients, one patient remains alive and well beyond 1 year, two of the clinical remissions died of opportunistic infections, one was lost to follow-up, and the remaining four died with active CNS lymphoma. It is thus apparent that patients with AIDS-related P-CNS lymphoma may respond to radiation treatment. However, response duration is usually quite short, and survival is influenced by refractory or recurrent disease or by systemic opportunistic infection. Alternative treatment approaches, with the use of immunomodulators and/or antiretroviral agents, may be necessary.

Systemic AIDS-Related Lymphoma: Clinical Characteristics

The vast majority of patients with AIDS-related lymphoma first present with systemic B symptoms, including fever, drenching night sweats, and/or weight loss. All published series have been consistent in this regard.[36-44,54,69] Currently, 68 patients with AIDS-related lymphoma have been diagnosed at USC. Of these, 49 (72%) have presented with B symptoms. The issue of fever in a patient with HIV infection and associated lymphoma may be problematic, since these individuals are also prone to multiple opportunistic infections, which may be relatively occult. It would seem prudent, therefore, to evaluate such a patient carefully for the possibility of occult *Mycobacterium avium-intracellulare* (MAI), or other such infectious processes before arbitrarily attributing the presence of fever or night sweats to the underlying lymphomatous disease.

Aside from the frequency of systemic symptoms at presentation, another common feature in patients with AIDS-related lymphoma is the frequency of initial disease in extranodal sites.[36-44,54,69] In the USC experience, 43 of 68 patients (63%) have presented with stage IV disease, while another 14 (21%) with stage IE involving a single extranodal site. Thus, 84% first presented with extranodal disease. This is distinct from other series of "spontaneous" lymphoma, in which the majority of patients present with disease in nodal sites alone. Thus, in Jone's series of 405 patients, 61% presented with stage I, II, or III disease, whereas 1% had stage IE, and 38% had disseminated stage IV involvement at the time of initial presentation.[70]

The sites of initial lymphomatous disease are extremely varied, as demonstrated in Table 15-2. Furthermore, it is common for patients to present with more than one extranodal site of involvement. In the USC experience, 12 patients (18%) presented with P-CNS lymphoma, whereas an additional 10 (15%) had CNS

Table 15-2

Stage of Disease and Sites of Involvement in 68 Patients with AIDS-Related Lymphoma

	Number of Patients	*% of Patients*
Stage		
I	3	4
IE	14	21
II	1	1
III	7	10
IV	43	63
Site		
CNS	22	32
GI	18	26
BM	17	25
Liver	8	12
Kidney	6	9
Lung	6	9
Heart	4	6
Adrenal	4	6
Bone	3	4
Skin	3	4
Bladder	2	3
Pancreas	1	1

lymphoma in addition to other sites of systemic lymphomatous disease. It is interesting that patients with P-CNS lymphoma present with mass lesions within the brain, as described above, whereas patients with systemic lymphoma only rarely present with CNS mass lesions, demonstrating leptomeningeal disease instead. Of importance is that this lymphomatous meningitis may be entirely asymptomatic, indicating that all patients with AIDS-related lymphoma should be evaluated by lumbar puncture as part of the routine staging evaluation. Numbness of the jaw has been another unusual presentation of meningeal disease in our experience and is now a clue to us that CNS involvement must be considered. The importance of CNS involvement in the patient with systemic AIDS-related lymphoma has also been emphasized by our autopsy experience.[71] Of 12 patients with systemic AIDS-related lymphoma who were eventually taken to autopsy, 8 (66%) were found to have CNS disease, which had only been suspected in 3 (25%) antemortum. In these 8 cases, 2 had mass lesions within brain, whereas the remainder had diffuse infiltration of leptomeninges.

Aside from CNS, the next most common site of extranodal disease in our experience has been the gastrointestinal (GI) tract, which showed involvement in 18 (26%). These patients often present with a history of abdominal pain or mass, and with recent onset of GI bleeding. All areas of the GI tract may be involved, and several patients have demonstrated radiographic evidence of lymphomatous disease along the entire length of the GI tract, from esophagus to anus, which has subsequently been documented pathologically at the time of autopsy. Isolated involvement of the stomach, small bowel, or colon may also occur, and lymphomatous disease within the rectum has been found in eight of our current series of patients (12%). The patient with rectal lymphoma may present with pain upon defecation, rectal bleeding, or mucoid rectal discharge. Two patients in our series have had lymphomatous disease isolated to the rectum alone.[72]

The bone marrow is another common site of lymphomatous involvement, showing involvement in 17 (25%) of our current series. Of note, two patients presented with Burkitt's leukemia;[55] one 33 year old presented with the prolymphocytic variant of chronic lymphocytic leukemia, and two young men presented with leukemic stages of low-grade disease, including small cleaved lymphoma in one, and plasmacytoid-lymphocytic lymphoma in the other.[44] Varying degrees of marrow infiltration were observed in the total patient group, with varying degrees of peripheral cytopenias. In some patients with bone marrow involvement, normal hemograms were observed.

As shown in Table 15-2, extremely unusual sites of initial lymphomatous disease were observed in our patients, including involvement of the heart in four. All patients with involvement of the myocardium also had multiple other sites of lymphomatous disease. Several of these patients presented with a history of chest pain, which was indistinguishable from that of an acute myocardial infarction, with electrocardiographic findings consistent with this diagnosis. The most sensitive radiologic technique in detecting space occupying lesions within the heart was found to be two-dimensional echocardiography.[73]

Virologic Characteristics

The initial inclusion of lymphoma within the spectrum of AIDS was somewhat difficult at the outset prior to the clear recognition that these cases were increasing epidemiologically, and prior to the identification of HIV as the etiologic organism in AIDS. In 1985, Levine and others demonstrated that 13 of 15 (87%) homosexual patients with high-grade, B-cell lymphoma, diagnosed at USC in the 1980s had either positive serology or virology to HIV. In a control group of 11 patients who had been diagnosed with the same types of high-grade lymphoma in the same time interval, but who did not belong to known groups at risk for AIDS, only one individual has antibodies to HIV (p < 0.001). It was thus apparent that there was an association between prior infection with HIV and subsequent development of high-grade B-cell lymphoma, in populations at risk for AIDS.[44] The revision of the case definition of AIDS made by the CDC in 1985 specifically requires that the individual in question must have some evidence of HIV infection, either presence of antibody, or presence of live HIV virus, in order for inclusion within the AIDS designation.[35] It is thus currently understood that patients with AIDS-related lymphoma must have evidence of prior infection with HIV.

Aside from HIV, several reports have recently documented the presence of coexistant infection with HTLV-I in some patients with AIDS-related lymphoma.[32,48] Although endemic in southwest Japan and the West Indies,[74,75] cases of adult T-cell leukemia/lymphoma, caused by HTLV-I, have also been reported in the United States. HTLV-I, as a potential coinfecting virus in the AIDS-related lymphomas, is an interesting area of further study, since Mann and colleagues have recently described B-cell chronic lymphocytic leukemia in two West Indian patients, who had circulating antibodies to HTLV-I.[76] The B-CLL cells secreted immunoglobulin M (IgM), with preferential reactivity against the p24 protein, or the large envelope protein (gp 61) of HTLV-I. It was concluded that HTLV-I played an indirect role in the development of B-CLL, serving as the source for initial antigenic stimulation of B-cells, and also as a source of altered T-cell regulation, leading eventually to malignancy.[76] Recent studies in intravenous drug abusers from the United States have indicated the presence of anti-HTLV-I antibodies in approximately 50% of black drug abusers in New Orleans, and 30% of black drug abusers from New Jersey.[77] It is thus apparent that HTLV-I has entered the population in this country, and that further work related to HTLV-I as a possible coinfecting virus in patients with AIDS-related lymphoma would be warranted.

Yet another potential coinfecting virus in patients with AIDS-related lymphoma is the human B-lymphoma virus (HBLV). This DNA virus, distinct from Epstein–Barr virus (EBV), has been isolated from six individuals, two of whom also had antibodies to HIV. One of the HIV-positive patients had AIDS-associated lymphoma, and the second had reactive dermatopathic lymphadenopathy.[78] It is thus clear that further study of HBLV as a potential cofactor in the lymphomas seen in AIDS would be of interest.

Aside from the viruses discussed above, it is clear that most patients with AIDS, and those with AIDS-related lymphoma have also been infected with EBV.[48,79,80] The majority of patients have had serologic profiles consistent with a normal response to prior infection, although some have had antibody profiles suggestive of immune compromise or viral reactivation.[80] The presence of EBV DNA has been confirmed by Southern blot analysis of AIDS-lymphoma tissues, and the presence of c-myc oncogene rearrangement or translocation has been demonstrated by Pelicci and co-workers in 9 of 10 AIDS–lymphoma cases.[33] Still, the precise relationship between EBV and the subsequent development of AIDS-associated lymphoma has yet to be defined.

Therapeutic Considerations

At this time, the therapy of choice in AIDS-related lymphoma is unknown. The specific problems faced by the clinician are numerous. First, these patients usually have high-grade disease that would mandate the use of intensive, multiagent chemotherapy. However, because of the underlying HIV-induced immunosuppression, the use of multiagent chemotherapy may lead to even greater risk of immune compromise and opportunistic infection. Thus, in 20 patients from USC who eventually underwent autopsy, 13 were found to have one or multiple opportunistic infections, and an additional 3 had systemic bacterial infections that had been unsuspected antemortem.[71] The incidence of bacterial infection was higher in individuals who had received chemotherapy. The second therapeutic problem encountered by these patients is the issue of CNS involvement, either at diagnosis or at the time of relapse.[65,66,71] As discussed, in the USC series CNS disease was present in 22 patients at diagnosis and occurred in an additional 7 patients at the time of relapse. Thus, 29 of 68 (43%) of cases had documented CNS involvement at some time during the course of illness. Of note, in our autopsy series, 8 in 12 (66%) patients with systemic lymphoma were found to have involvement of the brain, which had been suspected clinically in only 3. There was no relationship between prior bone marrow involvement and the subsequent likelihood of CNS disease at the time of autopsy.[71] We therefore believe the incidence of lymphomatous disease within the brain is much higher than

clinically suspected or diagnosed. A third problem encountered by the clinician is underlying bone marrow compromise secondary to HIV infection.[81] In chemotherapy the importance of appropriate dose and dose-interval as determinants of tumor response is recognized[82]; when bone marrow reserve is inadequate, it may be extremely difficult to administer the optimal chemotherapy necessary for long-term, disease-free survival.

With these issues in mind, it is not particularly surprising that the median survival of patients with AIDS-related lymphoma has been less than 1 year in most reported series. Various chemotherapeutic regimens have been employed without significant success. Kalter and associates[43] noted a complete remission in 6 of 8 cases after the use of one of five different regimens commonly employed in the 1970s. Long-term follow-up on these cases is not available. Since many of these patients had intermediate-grade disease, the authors concluded that intermediate histologic types may offer a survival advantage. In our experience, complete remission status may be achieved quite rapidly, with impressive tumor lysis observed after administration of relatively small doses of chemotherapy. The real problem is not attainment of complete remission, but rather relapse of disease, either systemically or in the CNS, despite the continuation of therapy. In a prospective series performed at USC, 13 patients received the M-BACOD regimen,[83] resulting in complete remission in 54%. However, only four of the seven responders remained alive beyond 1 year (31% of the treated group). Subsequently, a second trial of very intensive chemotherapy was begun consisting of multiple agents, including high-dose cytosine arabinoside, administered on the first day of therapy in an attempt to prevent CNS relapse. Complete remission was obtained in 3 of 9 treated patients (33%), and only one of these remains alive and disease free beyond 1 year. The regimen was extremely toxic, resulting in opportunistic infections in seven patients and mandating an early termination of the trial.[84] At the current time, a multicenter prospective trial is in progress using relatively low doses of commonly employed agents, in addition to azidothymidine (AZT), in an attempt to restore immune function and prevent relapse, while hopefully preventing the development of opportunistic infections. Results of this trial are awaited with interest.

Pathogenesis of Disease

The development of lymphoma in patients with congenital, acquired or iatrogenic immune deficiency states has been well described;[58–61] these lymphomas are most commonly of B-lymphoid derivation and of high-grade pathologic type. The development of lymphoma in persons with HIV infection would be fully consistent with these prior reports.

The precise cause of the lymphomas seen in AIDS, however, has yet to be defined. Although initially entertained as a possibility, the HIV infection *per se* does not appear to be the direct oncogenic event. It is possible that HIV, along with other coinfecting viruses such as HTLV-I[76] or HBLV,[78] may be causative, but this remains speculative. The role of EBV in the setting of HIV-induced immune compromise remains an intriguing possibility, especially in light of the X-linked lymphoproliferative disorder described by Purtilo.[85,86] In this disorder, affected individuals are immunocompromised relative to EBV, and when infected by this organism may develop high-grade B-cell lymphomas that may be indistinguishable from those seen in AIDS. The intense reactive B-cell response seen in PGL, and in AIDS in general, may certainly be a predisposing factor in the development of B-cell lymphomas. This intense B-cell response, secondary to HIV *per se,* or to EBV in the setting of immune compromise, or to other, undefined factors could lead eventually to chromosomal translocations (8;14 or 8;22),[87–90] *c-myc* rearrangement,[33] and the eventual selection of multiple (oligoclonal) and then single (monoclonal) B-cell clones with growth advantage and the potential for malignant transformation.

HODGKIN'S DISEASE IN HIV-INFECTED INDIVIDUALS

Although there has been no increase in the diagnosis of Hodgkin's disease (HD) among HIV-infected patients or among populations at risk for AIDS, several case reports and small series of such patients have been published.[91–97] It is apparent that the patient with underlying HIV-induced immunosuppression who then develops HD may not do as well as would normally be expected. Thus, these patients often present with systemic B symptoms and with widely disseminated disease, with involvement of bone marrow, skin, and/or lung, sometimes without mediastinal or hilar adenopathy. Additionally, several unusual cases have been reported, including that of a 31-year-old homosexual male with biopsy-confirmed KS and HD, both present within the same lymph node.[96] Furthermore Coonley and others reported a 33-year-old homosexual male who was found to have HD involving a posterior rectal mass, with associated pelvic lymphadenopathy.[97] These cases are most unusual, and would warrant further explanation.

It is also apparent that an HIV-infected patient with disseminated HD may not be able to tolerate the chemotherapeutic regimens that may be curative in usual settings. Thus, the development of significant bone marrow compromise due to both HIV and chemotherapy may limit the potential to deliver the optimal drug doses in the time intervals required for cure.[82] Furthermore, the development of multiple opportunistic infections in these patients may further delay the appropriate administration of chemotherapy while predisposing to early demise due to the infections *per se.*

Although HD is not associated epidemiologically with AIDS, it is thus apparent that special consideration must be given to overcome the difficulties inherent in administering chemotherapeutic regimens to persons who are already immunocompromised. Clearly, alternative therapeutic measures may be required.

OTHER MALIGNANCIES IN HIV-INFECTED INDIVIDUALS

Although epidmiologic data linking HIV infection with development of other solid tumors does not yet exist, numerous case reports of such an association are most worrisome. The transplantation model may be useful in this regard. Thus, patients who have undergone organ transplantation, with subsequent use of long-term immunosuppressive agents to prevent graft rejection are at definite increased risk for development of various malignancies. These include basal cell carcinoma of the skin (3-fold relative risk [RR]), squamous cell carcinoma of the skin (4–21-fold RR), lip cancers (29-fold RR), lymphomas (28–49-fold RR), carcinoma of the uterine cervix (14-fold RR), and KS (400–500-fold RR); furthermore, as reported recently by Penn, these patients are also at risk (100-fold RR) for the development of carcinoma of the vulva and anus.[98] It has been postulated that the factors responsible for these malignancies include an underlying state of immunodeficiency, such that normal mechanisms of immune surveillance are inoperative, with the additional presence of on-going infection by various oncogenic viruses. In the example of organ transplantation, the immunosuppression is iatrogenic. The potential oncogenic viruses that have been described in these patients include papillomavirus, which has been associated with condyloma acuminatum, as well as anogenital carcinomas,[99–102] and herpes simplex virus type II (HSV-II), which has been implicated in the pathogenesis of carcinoma of the uterine cervix.[103]

Although KS and high-grade lymphoma have already been linked epidemiologically with AIDS, the other cancers that have been noted in organ transplant recipients have not yet increased statistically in association with the HIV epidemic. It is conceivable that such associations may not be documented in future years. However, when one considers that the risk of anogenital cancer in transplant recipients increases much later than the development of KS or lymphoma,[98] occurring an average of 88 months from transplantation (range 9–125 months), it becomes apparent that major increases in the numbers of these cases among HIV-infected persons may only be a matter of time.

Anal Cancer

As discussed, the incidence of carcinomas of the vulva and anus is 100 times greater in renal transplant recipients than in the general population.[98] At least 29% of these patients have had prior condyloma acuminatum of the anogenital region, or known papilloma virus in association with the subsequent carcinoma. A history of prior infection with HSV-II has also been documented in some of these patients.[98]

In patients at risk for AIDS, various case reports have described the coexistance of HIV infection, with development of carcinoma in situ, or invasive carcinoma of the anus.[101,102,104–106] Dahling and colleagues used national cancer registry data and reported that 33.6% of men with squamous cell carcinoma of the anus between 1974 and 1979 had never been married, versus 7.8% "never-married" status in patients who developed colon cancer, suggesting the possibility that homosexual behavior, with receptive anal intercourse, anal warts, fissures, fistulae, and/or abcesses may be a risk factor for development of anal carcinoma.[107]

Gal and co-workers studied all cases of squamous cell carcinoma of the anus or rectum, diagnosed at Los Angeles County-USC Medical Center between 1981 and 1985, and found that seven in ten such cases occurred in homosexual men. Carcinoma tissues from these seven, plus another from a homosexual male diagnosed elsewhere, were studied by immunoperoxidase technique for the presence of papillomavirus antigens, which were found in five of eight cases (63%), suggesting the possibility that this virus, in a setting of HIV-induced immunosuppression, may be etiologic in anal cancer, either alone or with other coinfecting oncogenic viruses.[101] Likewise, Croxson and associates have described anal condylomata acuminata in seven homosexual men, all associated with presence of human papillomavirus within the condyloma or adjacent anal mucosa. Biopsy of these anal warts revealed carcinoma in situ in all seven, indicating the importance of excision and evaluation of all such chronic condylomata in HIV-infected individuals, and also indicating that the incidence of anal carcinoma in homosexual men may be increasing.[102] Two additional cases were noted in an addendum, with all nine patients diagnosed within an 18-month period in one medical center.

Miscellaneous Carcinomas

An extremely unusual case of widely metastatic basal cell carcinoma of the skin has been reported by Sitz and others in a 21-year-old HIV-infected homosexual male.[108] Although such an occurrence was first reported as early as 1894, fewer than 200 cases of metastatic disease have since been reported in the English literature. Since the relative risk of basal cell carcinoma is three times higher in organ transplant recipients than in normal individuals,[109] the possibility of a relationship between this tumor and underlying immunodeficiency must be considered.

A case of squamous cell carcinoma of the tongue occurring in the homosexual partner of an AIDS patient has been described,[110] and several additional such cases have been reported.[111]

Single case reports of adenosquamous carcinoma of the lung[112] and adenocarcinoma of the colon and of pancreas[54] have been described in HIV-infected individuals; the significance of these reports is unclear.

Testicular carcinoma has also been described recently occurring in young homosexual men.[54,113] Testicular cancer is the most common type of cancer in white males between the ages of 20 and 34 years, and the incidence of this cancer has doubled in the United States between 1937 and 1971.[113] The precise cause of this increase is currently not understood, and its relationship, if any, to homosexual behavior, or to HIV infection, remains speculative.

It is thus apparent that many unusual cancers may be seen in HIV-infected patients. Although no epidemiologic link between these cancers and AIDS yet exists, it is certainly possible that anogenital carcinomas, squamous cell carcinomas of the tongue, and other such tumors may be increasing in patients at risk for AIDS. Careful attention to these cases may result in a better understanding of their relationship to AIDS *per se,* as well as providing additional information regarding the potential etiology of cancer in man.

REFERENCES

1. Centers for Disease Control: Persistent, generalized lymphadenopathy among homosexual males. Morbid Mortal Week Rept. 31:249, 1982
2. Meyer PR, Yanagihara ET, Parker JW et al: A distinctive follicular hyperplasia in the acquired immunodeficiency syndrome (AIDS) and the AIDS-related complex: A prelymphomatous state for B-cell lymphoma? Hematol Oncol 2:319, 1984
3. Levy N, Boone D, Hechinger M et al: Cytofluorographic analysis of lymph nodes from patients with the persistent generalized lymphadenopathy (PGL) syndrome. Diag Immunol 3:15, 1985
4. Brynes RK, Chan WC, Spira TJ et al: Value of lymph node biopsy in unexplained lymphadenopathy in homosexual men. JAMA 250:1313, 1983
5. Burns BF, Wood GS, Dorfman RF: The varied histopathology of lymphadenopathy in the homosexual male. Am J Surg Pathol 9:287, 1985
6. Fernandez R, Mouradian J, Metroka C et al: Letter. The prognostic value of histopathology in persistent generalized lymphadenopathy in homosexual men. N Engl J Med 309:185, 1983
7. Ewing EP, Chandler FW, Spira TJ et al: Primary lymph node pathology in AIDS-related lymphadenopathy. Arch Pathol Lab Med 109:977, 1985
8. Ioachim HL, Lerner CW, Tapper ML: The lymphoid lesions associated with the acquired immunodeficiency syndrome. Am J Surg Pathol 7:543, 1983
9. Wood GS, Garcia CF, Dorfman RF, et al: The immunohistology of follicle lysis in lymph node biopsies from homosexual men. Blood 66:1092, 1985
10. Turner RR, Meyer PR, Taylor CR et al: Immunohistology of persistent generalized lymphadenopathy. Evidence for progressive lymph node abnormalities in some patients. Am J Clin Pathol 88:10, 1987

11. Turner RR, Levine AM, Gill PS et al: Progressive histopathologic abnormalities in the persistent generalized lymphadenopathy syndrome. Am J Surg Pathol 1987 (In Preparation)

12. Levine AM, Meyer PR, Gill PS et al: Results of initial lymph node biopsy in homosexual men with generalized lymphadenopathy. J Clin Oncol 4:165, 1986

13. Abrams DI: AIDS-related lymphadenopathy: The role of biopsy. J Clin Oncol 4:126, 1986

14. Mathur–Wagh U, Enlow RW, Spigland I et al: Longitudinal study of persistent generalized lymphadenopathy in homosexual men: Relation to the acquired immunodeficiency syndrome. Lancet 1:1033, 1984

15. Mathur–Wagh U, Mildvan D, Senie RT: Follow-up at $4\frac{1}{2}$ years on homosexual men with generalized lymphadenopathy. N Engl J Med 313:1542–3, 1985 (letter)

16. Gold JWM, Weikel CS, Godbold J et al: Unexplained persistent lymphadenopathy in homosexual men and the acquired immune deficiency syndrome. Medicine 64:203, 1985

17. Fishbein DB, Kaplan JE, Spira TJ et al: Unexplained lymphadenopathy in homosexual men: A longitudinal study. JAMA 254:930, 1985

18. Abrams DI, Lewis BJ, Beckstead JF et al: Persistent diffuse lymphadenopathy in homosexual men: Endpoint or prodrome? Ann Intern Med 100:801, 1984

19. Abrams D, Mess T, Volberding P: Lymphadenopathy: Endpoint or prodrome? Update of a 36-month prospective study. International Conference on AIDS-Associated Syndromes, Irvine, CA, 1984

20. Levine AM, Gill PS, Rasheed S, et al: Natural history of human immunodeficiency virus (HIV) infection among a cohort of homosexual men. Proc ASCO 6:3, 1987

21. Levine AM, Krailo M, Gill PS et al: Natural history of biopsy-proven persistent, generalized lymphadenopathy (PGL) and human immunodeficiency virus (HIV) infection among a cohort of homosexual men from Los Angeles (Submitted)

22. Rasheed S, Norman GL, Gill PS et al: Virus-neutralizing activity, serologic heterogeneity and retrovirus isolation from homosexual men in the Los Angeles area. Virology 150:1, 1986

23. Lane HC, Masur H, Edgar LC et al: Abnormalities of B-cell activation and immunoregulation in patients with the acquired immunodeficiency syndrome. N Engl J Med 309:453, 1983

24. Burkes RL, Abo W, Levine AM et al: Characterization of immunologic function in homosexual men with persistent, generalized lymphadenopathy and acquired immune deficiency syndrome. Cancer 59:731, 1987

25. Yarchoan R, Redfield RR, Broder S: Mechanisms of B cell activation in patients with acquired immunodefiency syndrome and related disorders. J Clin Invest 78:439, 1986

26. De Martini RM, Turner RR, Formenti SC et al: Peripheral blood mononuclear cell abnormalities and their relationship to clinical course in homosexual men with HIV infection. Diagnostic and Clin Immunol 5:194, 1988

27. Seligmann M, Pinching AJ, Rosen FS et al: Immunology of human immunodeficiency virus infection and the acquired immunodeficiency syndrome: An update. Ann Intern Med 107:234, 1987

28. Burkes RL, Sherrod AE, Stewart ML et al: Serum beta-2 microblobulin levels in homosexual men with AIDS and with persistent, generalized lymphadenopathy. Cancer 57:2190, 1986

29. Francis DP, Jaffe HW, Fultz PN et al: The natural history of infection with the lymphadenopathy-associated virus human T-lymphotropic virus type III. Ann Intern Med 103:719, 1985

30. Goedert JJ, Biggar RF, Weiss SH et al: Three year incidence of AIDS in five cohorts of HTLV-III infected risk group members. Science 235:992, 1986

31. Mann JM, Bila K, Colebunders RL et al: Natural history of human immunodeficiency virus infection in Zaire. Lancet 2:707, 1986

32. Levine AM, Gill PS, Krailo M et al: Natural history of persistent, generalized lymphadenopathy (PGL) in gay men: Risk of lymphoma and factors associated with development of lymphoma. Blood 68:130a, 1986

33. Pelicci P, Knowles DM, Arlin ZA et al: Multiple monoclonal B cell expansions and c-myc oncogene rearrangements in acquired immune deficiency syndrome-related lymphoproliferative disorders: Implications for lymphomagenesis. J Exp Med 164:2049, 1986

34. National Cancer Institute: Third National Cancer Survey: Incidence Data. National Cancer Institute Monograph 41. DHEW Publ No (NIH) 75-787. US Department of Health, Education and Welfare, 1975

35. Centers for Disease Control: Revision of the case definition of acquired immunodeficiency syndrome for national reporting—United States. Ann Intern Med 103:402, 1985

36. Levine AM, Meyer PR, Begandy MK et al: Development of B-cell lymphoma in homosexual men: Clinical and Immunologic Findings. Ann Intern Med 100:7, 1984

37. Ziegler JL, Beckstead JA, Volberding PA et al: Non-Hodgkin's lymphoma in 90 homosexual men: Relationship to generalized lymphadenopathy and acquired immunodeficiency syndrome (AIDS). N Engl Med 311:565, 1984

38. Levine AM, Burkes FL, Walker M et al: Development of B-cell lymphoma in two monogamous homosexual men. Arch Intern Med 145:479, 1985

39. Doll DC, List AF: Letter: Burkitt's lymphoma in homosexuals. Lancet 1:1026, 1982

40. Centers for Disease Control: Diffuse, undifferentiated non-Hodgkin's lymphoma among homosexual males—United States. Morbid Mortal Week Rept 31:277, 1982

41. Ziegler JS, Drew WL, Miner RC et al: Outbreak of Burkitt-like lymphoma in homosexual men. Lancet 1:631, 1982

42. Snider WD, Simpson DM, Aronyk KE et al: Letter: Primary lymphoma of the nervous system associated with acquired immunodeficiency syndrome. N Engl J Med 308:45, 1983

43. Kalter SP, Riggs SA, Cabanillas F et al: Aggressive non-Hodgkin's lymphomas in immunocompromised homosexual males. Blood 66:655–659, 1985

44. Levine AM, Gill PS, Meyer PR et al: Retrovirus and malignant lymphoma in homosexual men. JAMA 254:1921, 1985

45. Ross RK, Dworsky RL, Paganini–Hill A et al: Non-Hodgkin's lymphomas in never married men in Los Angeles. Brit J Cancer 52:785, 1985

46. Hisserich JC, Martin SP, Henderson BE: An areawide cancer reporting network. Publ Health Rept 90:15, 1975

47. Ross R, Levine AM, Mack T: Increasing incidence of lymphoma among never married males in Los Angeles: Update. (Submitted)

48. Levine AM, Gill PS, Rasheed S: AIDS related B-cell lymphoma. In Broder S (Ed): AIDS, p 233, New York, Marcel Dekker, 1986

49. Burkes RL, Gal AA, Stewart ML et al: Simultaneous oc-

currence of pneumocystis cartini pneumonia, cytomegalovirus infection, Kaposi's sarcoma, and B-cell immunoblastic sarcoma in a homosexual male. JAMA 253:3425, 1985

50. Lukes RJ, Parker JW, Taylor CR et al: Immunologic approach to non-Hodgkin's lymphomas and related leukemias. Analysis of the results of multiparameter studies of 425 cases. Semin Hematol 15:322, 1978

51. Non-Hodgkin's lymphoma pathologic classification project: National Cancer Institute sponsored study of classifications of non-Hodgkin's lymphomas: Summary and description of a working formulation for clinical usage. Cancer 49:2112, 1982

52. NCI Non-Hodgkin's Lymphoma Classification Project Writing Committee: Classification of non-Hodgkin's lymphomas: Reproducibility of major classification systems. Cancer 55:91, 1985

53. Vandermolen LA, Fehir KM, Rice L: Multiple myeloma in a homosexual man with chronic lymphadenopathy. Arch Intern Med 145:745, 1986

54. Kaplan MH, Susin M, Pahwa SG et al: Neoplastic complications of HTLV-III infection: Lymphomas and solid tumors. Am J Med 82:389, 1987

55. Gill PS, Meyer PR, Pavlova Z et al: B-cell acute lymphocytic leukemia in adults: Clinical, morphologic and immunologic findings. J Clin Oncol 4:737, 1986

56. Lukes RJ, Collins RD: Immunologic characterization of human malignant lymphomas. Cancer 34:1488, 1974

57. Rosen PG, Feinstein DI, Pattengal PF et al: Convoluted lymphocytic lymphomas in adults: A clinicopathologic entity. Ann Intern Med 89:319, 1978

58. Frizzera G, Rosai J, Dehner LP et al: Lymphoreticular disorders in primary immunodeficiency: New findings based on an up to date histologic classification of 35 cases. Cancer 46:692, 1980

59. Good AE, Russo RH, Schnitzer B et al: Intracranial histiocytic lymphoma with rheumatoid arthritis. J Rheumatol 5:75, 1978

60. Cleary ML, Warnke R, Sklar J: Monoclonality of lymphoproliferative lesions in cardiac-transplant recipients: Clonal analysis based on immunoglobulin-gene rearrangements. N Engl J Med 1984; 310:477

61. Schneck SA, Penn I: De-novo brain tumors in renal-transplant recipients. Lancet 1:922, 1971

62. Henry JM, Heffner RR Jr, Dillard SF et al: Primary malignant lymphomas of the central nervous system. Cancer 34:1293, 1974

63. Burstein SD, Kernohan JW, Uihelein A: Neoplasms of the reticuloendothelial system of the brain. Cancer 16:289, 1963

64. Levitt LJ, Dawdson DM, Rosenthal DS et al: CNS involvement in Non-Hodgkin's lymphomas. Cancer 45:545, 1980

65. Gill PS, Levine AM, Meyer PR et al: Primary Central Nervous System Lymphoma in Homosexual Men. Clinical, Immunologic, and Pathologic Features. Am J Med 78:742, 1985

66. So YT, Beckstead JH, Davis RL: Primary central nervous system lymphoma in acquired immune deficiency syndrome: A clinical and pathological study. Ann Neurol 20:566, 1986

67. Gill PS, Graham RA, Boswell W et al: A comparison of imaging, clinical and pathologic aspects of space occupying lesions within the brain in patients with acquired immune deficiency syndrome. Am J Physiol Imaging 1:134, 1986

68. Formenti SC, Gill PS, Lean E et al: Primary central nervous system lymphoma in AIDS: Results of radiation therapy. (Submitted)

69. Mernick M, Malamud S, Haubenstock A et al: Non-Hodgkin's lymphoma in AIDS: Report of 11 cases and literature review. Mt Sinai J Med 53:664, 1986

70. Jones SE, Fuks Z, Bullm M et al: Non-hodgkin's lymphomas. IV. Clinicopathologic correlation of 405 cases. Cancer 31:806, 1973

71. Loureiro C, Gill PS, Levine AM et al: Autopsy findings in AIDS-related lymphoma. (Submitted)

72. Burkes RL, Meyer PR, Gill PS et al: Primary rectal lymphoma in homosexual men. Arch Intern Med 146:913, 1986

73. Gill PS, Chandraratna P, Meyer PR et al: Malignant lymphoma: Cardiac involvement at initial presentation. J Clin Oncol 5:216, 1987

74. Hinuma Y, Komoda H, Chosa T et al: Antibodies to adult T cell leukemia associated antigen (ATLA) in sera from patients with ATL and controls in Japan: A nationwide seroepidemiologic study. Int J Cancer 29:631, 1982

75. Catovsky D, O'Brian C, Lampert I: Diagnostic features of adult T-cell lymphoma/leukemia (ATLL). Lancet 1:639, 1982

76. Mann DL, DeSantis P, Mark G et al: HTLV-I associated B-cell CLL: Indirect role for retrovirus in leukemogenesis. Science 236:1103, 1987

77. Weiss SH, Sazinger WC, Ginzburg HM et al: Human T-cell lymphotropic virus type I (HTLV-I and HIV prevalences among US drug abusers. Proc ASCO 6:4, 1987

78. Salahuddin SZ, Ablashi DV, Markham PD et al: Isolation of a new virus, HBLV, in patients with lymphoproliferative disorders. Science 234:596, 1986

79. Peterson JM, Tubbs RR, Savage RA et al: Small noncleaved B-cell Burkitt-like lymphoma with chromosome t (8;14) translocation and Epstein Barr virus nuclear-associated antigen in a homosexual man with acquired immune deficiency syndrome. Am J Med 78:141, 1985

80. Birx DL, Redfield RR, Tosato G: Defective regulation of Epstein Barr infection in patients with acquired immunodeficiency syndrome (AIDS) or AIDS-related disorders. N Engl J Med 314:874, 1986

81. Spivak JL, Bender BS, Zuinn TC: Hematologic abnormalities in the acquired immune deficiency syndrome. Am J Med 77:224, 1984

82. Frei E III, Canellos GP: Dose: A critical factor in cancer chemotherapy. Am J Med 69:585, 1980

83. Skarin AT, Canellos GP, Rosenthal DS et al: Improved prognosis of diffuse histiocytic and undifferentiated lymphoma by use of high dose methotrexate alternating with standard agents (M-BACOD). J Clin Oncol 1:91, 1983

84. Gill PS, Levine AM, Krailo M et al: AIDS-related malignant lymphoma: Results of prospective treatment trials. J Clin Oncol 5:1322, 1987

85. Purtilo DT: Immune deficiency predisposing to Epstein-Barr virus induced lymphoproliferative diseases. The X-linked lymphoproliferative syndrome as a model. Adv Cancer Res 34:279, 1981

86. Purtilo DT: Epstein–Barr virus induced oncogenesis in immune deficient individuals. Lancet 1:300, 1980

87. Klein G: Specific chromosomal translocations and the genesis of B-cell derived tumors in mice and men. Cell 32:311, 1983

88. Wang PG, Lee EC, Sieverts H et al: Burkitt's lymphoma in AIDS: Cytogenetic study. Blood 63:190, 1984

89. Chaganti RSK, Jhanwar SC, Koziner B et al: Specific translocations characterize Burkitt's like lymphoma of homosexual men with the acquired immunodeficiency syndrome. Blood 61:1265, 1983

90. Magrath I, Erikson J, Whang-Peng J et al: Synthesis of kappa light chains by cell lines containing an 8;22 chromosomal translocation derived from a male homosexual with Burkitt's lymphoma. Science 222:1094, 1983

91. Scheib RG, Siegel RS: Letter: Atypical Hodgkin's disease and the acquired immunodeficiency syndrome. Ann Intern Med 102:554, 1985

92. Schoeppel SL, Hoppe RT, Dorfman FT et al: Hodgkin's disease in homosexual men with generalized lymphadenopathy. Ann Intern Med 102:68, 1985

93. Robert NJ, Schneiderman H: Letter: Hodgkin's disease and the acquired immunodeficiency syndrome. Ann Intern Med 101:142, 1984

94. Subar M, Chamulak G, Dall-Favera R et al: Clinical and pathologic characteristics of AIDS associated Hodgkin's disease [abstr]. Blood 68:135a, 1986

95. Schoeppel S, Hoppe R, Abrams D et al: Hodgkin's disease in homosexual men: The San Francisco bay area experience [abstr]. Proc ASCO 5:3, 1986

96. Mitusuyasu RT, Colman MF, Sun NCJ: Simultaneous occurrence of Hodgkin's disease and Kaposi's sarcoma in a patient with the acquired immune deficiency syndrome. Am J Med 80:954, 1986

97. Coonley CJ, Straus DJ, Flippa D et al: Hodgkin's disease presenting with rectal symptoms in a homosexual male. A case report and review of the literature. Cancer Invest 2:279, 1984

98. Penn I: Cancers of the anogenital region in renal transplant recipients. Cancer 58:611, 1986

99. Jenson AB, Lim LY, Lancaster WD: Role of papilloma virus in proliferative squamous lesions. Surv Synth Pathol Res 4:8, 1985

100. Zur Hausen H: Human papillomaviruses and their possible role in squamous cell carcinomas. Curr Top Microbiol Immunol 78:1, 1977

101. Gal AA, Meyer PR, Taylor CR: Papillomavirus antigens in anorectal condyloma and carcinoma in homosexual men. JAMA 257:337, 1987

102. Croxson T, Chabon AB, Rorat E et al: Intraepithelial carcinoma of the anus in homosexual men. Dis Colon Rectum 27:325, 1984

103. Fenoglio CM: Viruses in the pathogenesis of cervical neoplasia: An update. Hum Pathol 13:785, 1982

104. Li FP, Osborn D, Cronin CM: Anorectal squamous carcinoma in two homosexual men. Lancet 2:391, 1982

105. Cooper HS, Patchefsky AS, Marks G: Cloacogenic carcinoma of the anorectum in homosexual men: An observation of four cases. Dis Colon Rectum 22:557, 1979

106. Leach RD, Ellis H: Carcinoma of the rectum in male homosexuals. J R Soc Med 74:490, 1981

107. Daling JR, Weiss NS, Klopfenstein LL et al: Correlates of homosexual behavior and the incidence of anal cancer. JAMA 247:1988, 1982

108. Sitz KV, Keppen M, Johnson DF: Metastatic basal cell carcinoma in acquired immunodeficiency syndrome-related complex. JAMA 257:340, 1987

109. Hoxtell EO, Mandel JS, Murray SS et al: Incidence of skin carcinoma after renal transplantation. Arch Dermatol 113:436, 1977

110. Conant MC, Volberding P, Fletcher V et al: Squamous cell carcinoma in sexual partner of Kaposi's sarcoma patient. Lancet 1:286, 1982

111. Lozada F, Silverman S Jr, Conant M: New outbreak of oral tumors, malignancies and infectious disease strikes young male homosexuals. Calif Dent Assoc J 10:39, 1982

112. Irwin LE, Begandy MK, Moore TM: Adenosquamous carcinoma of the lung and the acquired immunodeficiency syndrome. Ann Intern Med 100:158, 1984

113. Logothetis CJ, Newell GY, Samuels ML: Testicular cancer in homosexual men with cellular immune deficiency: Report of two cases. J Urol 133:484, 1985

Pharmacologic Treatment of HIV Infection

Robert Yarchoan
Samuel Broder

16

Acquired immunodeficiency syndrome (AIDS) was recognized as a new clinical entity in the summer of 1981.[1-3] By 1984, a newly discovered pathogenic human retrovirus, human immunodeficiency virus (HIV), had been shown to be the etiologic agent causing AIDS.[4-6] This virus is also called human T-cell immunodeficiency virus type III (HTLV-III),[4,5] lymphadenopathy associated virus (LAV),[6] and AIDS-related virus (ARV).[7] The following year, 1985, a nucleoside analog, 3'-azido-2',3'-dideoxythymidine (AZT) was found to be an effective inhibitor of HIV replication in the laboratory[8] and was given to the first patient.[9] Over the next $1\frac{1}{2}$ years, AZT was found to induce immunologic and clinical improvements in patients with severe HIV infection[9] and to improve the survival of certain patients with AIDS.[10,11] In March 1987, 6 years after the recognition of AIDS as a new clinical entity, and slightly more than 2 years after the first laboratory observation that AZT had activity against HIV, AZT was approved by the U.S. Food and Drug Administration for use in patients with severe HIV infection.

This rapid drug development, unprecedented in the modern era, was in part possible because of a number of pioneering efforts in the fields of nucleoside biochemistry, cell biology, and retrovirology, some of which antedated the recognition of AIDS as a clinical illness. It involved an intense collaboration between at least one government agency, a private sector pharmaceutical corporation, and 12 medical centers around the United States. In this chapter, we will discuss the rationale for antiviral therapy in patients with HIV infection, the specific development of AZT, and finally, several additional agents that are being considered as possible therapeutic modalities in this disorder. The reader is also referred to Chapter 5, which summarizes the life cycle of HIV and outlines possible new therapeutic strategies that might emerge based on a knowledge of this life cycle.

RATIONALE FOR THE USE OF ANTIVIRAL DRUGS FOR THE TREATMENT OF AIDS

Before discussing the specific development of AZT, it is perhaps worthwhile to discuss briefly the rationale for the use of an antiviral approach in HIV infection. In this regard, it should perhaps be mentioned that the validity of this approach could ultimately be proved only by the finding of an antiretroviral drug that could improve the morbidity and mortality of patients with AIDS; before the development AZT, no antiviral drug had been shown to affect significantly the course of an established retroviral infection in humans or an animal model, and there was some skepticism in the scientific community that any antiretroviral drug could affect the course of patients with established AIDS.

The rationale for the use of antiretroviral therapy in patients with AIDS is based on a number of premises concerning this disease:

That active replication of HIV is important in the pathogenesis and maintenance of the disease state

That at any one point in time, most helper T cells (or other relevant cells) are not infected with HIV

That infected cells die in a relatively short period of time

That it is possible to stop the replication of HIV and thus to block the spread of the virus

That the damaged organs have at least some regenerative potential

277

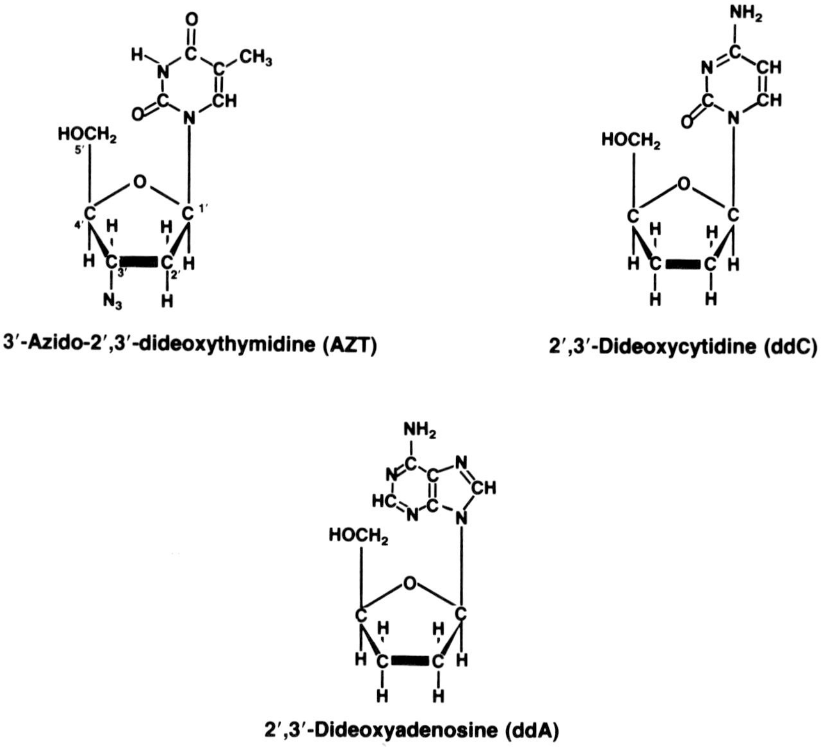

3'-Azido-2',3'-dideoxythymidine (AZT)

2',3'-Dideoxycytidine (ddC)

2',3'-Dideoxyadenosine (ddA)

FIG. 16-1. Structure of three dideoxy-nucleosides with activity against HIV. Certain unsaturated (2',3'-didehydro) analogs are also active.

As for the hallmark helper–inducer (T4[+] or CD4[+]) T cells, these premises are for the most part true. Even in a patient with established AIDS, the vast majority of helper T cells at any given time appear to be free of virus;[12] Most die in a short period of time after being infected.[5] And finally, the lymphoid system has a well-known capacity for regeneration (which provides the basis for bone marrow transplantation).

However, there is increasing evidence that for other cell types (and even in the case of certain T cells), these premises may not strictly be true. It has been shown, for example, that monocytoid cells and Epstein–Barr virus (EBV)–infected B cells can be infected with HIV and may remain infected (and produce virus) for a long period of time without dying.[13,14] In addition, some T cells may become latently infected with HIV, not producing virus or being killed until they are antigenically stimulated some time later.[15–17] Perhaps more importantly, it has been shown that the brain, an organ with limited regenerative potential at best, is an important site of replication of HIV[18–20] and that dementia can be an important consequence of HIV infection.[21] Finally, it has been shown that CD4[+] T cells can be killed upon contact with HIV-producing cells without the T cells themselves being infected.[22,23] As demonstrated by the clinical results obtained with AZT, an antiviral strategy can be efficacious even though these premises may not be strictly true in all cases. The instances where these premises do not apply, however, may account in part

for the observation that AZT can only partially and temporarily reverse the defects in advanced AIDS, and they should be considered in developing future therapeutic strategies.

IN VITRO ACTIVITY OF DIDEOXYNUCLEOSIDE ANALOGS AGAINST HIV

Mitsuya and Broder reported that a number of nucleoside analogs in which the 3'-hydroxy group is replaced with another chemical moiety (Fig. 16-1) are potent *in vitro* inhibitors of HIV infection.[8,24,25] These compounds are phosphorylated to a 5'-triphosphate form by mammalian enzymes,[26] and as 5'-triphosphates, act at the level of HIV DNA polymerase (reverse transcriptase) to prevent viral replication.[26–28] In each case, because of the 3'-substitution, the nucleosides cannot form subsequent 3'-diester linkages once they are added to a growing chain of viral DNA; they can thus act as chain terminators to prevent subsequent elongation of the DNA chain (Fig. 16-2).[25–28] One such compound, 3'-azido-2',3'-dideoxythymidine (AZT), was found by Mitsuya and colleagues to effectively inhibit HIV replication (even under conditions of a high multiplicity of infection of virus) at concentrations of 5 μM (Table 16-1).[8] Toxicity was not observed in T cells until concentrations of 50 μM were attained. As will be discussed in detail, AZT was subsequently shown to reduce the morbidity and

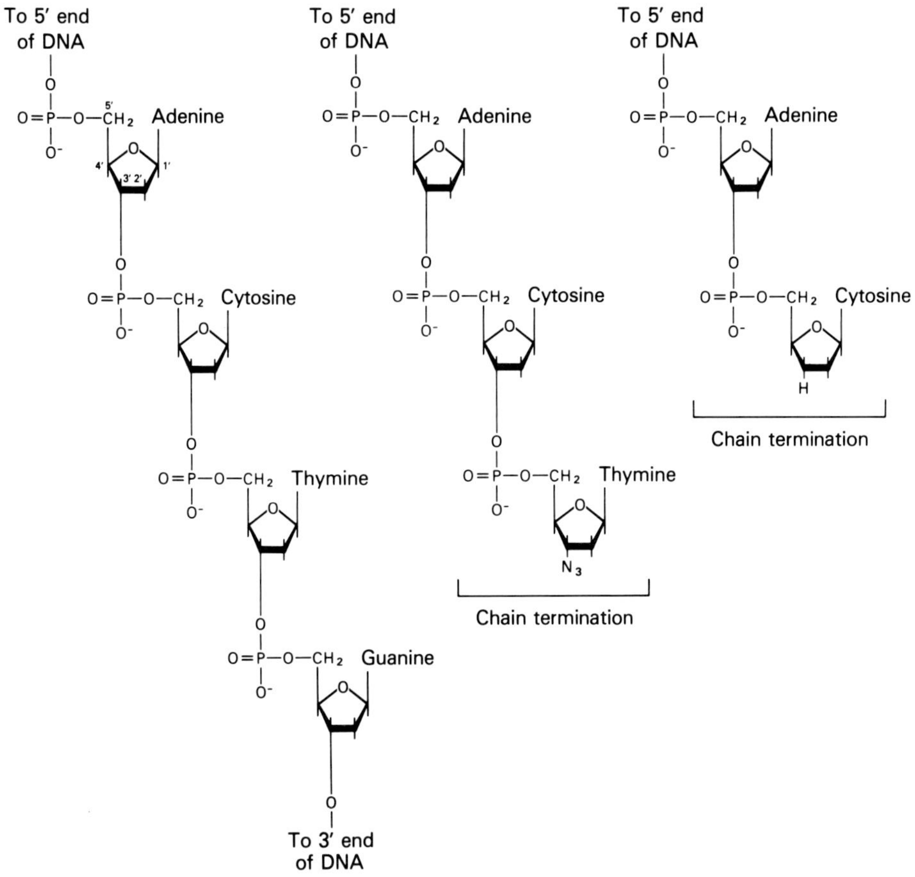

FIG. 16-2. Chain termination, one postulated mechanism of the action of dideoxynucleoside triphosphates. Shown at left is a normal DNA chain. When AZT-5'-triphosphate (*center*) or 2',3'-dideoxycytidine-5'-triphosphate (*right*) are incorporated into the growing 3' end of a DNA chain, it is not possible to form subsequent 5'→3' phosphodiester linkages, and chain termination occurs. (Yarchoan R, Broder S: Progress in the development of antiviral therapy for the acquired immunodeficiency syndrome and related disorders: A progress report. N Engl J Med 316: 557, 1987)

increase the survival of patients with AIDS and is now approved for use in this condition.

Mechanism of Action of Dideoxynucleosides

Although there are several unresolved issues concerning the mechanism of action of these compounds in inhibiting the replication of HIV, it appears that they are successively phosphorylated in a target cell to yield 2',3'-dideoxynucleoside-5'-triphosphates (Fig. 16-3). In this form, they become analogs of the 2'-deoxynucleoside-5'-triphosphates that are the natural substrates for HIV DNA polymerase (reverse transcriptase) and for cellular DNA polymerases.

There are two demonstrable mechanisms by which these 5'-triphosphates can inhibit reverse transcriptase, and the relative contribution of these two mechanisms is at present unclear. The first mechanism is chain termination. As was mentioned above, because of the 3'-alteration of these compounds, once they are incorporated into DNA, subsequent 5'→3' diester linkages cannot be formed (see Fig. 16-2). Indeed, at concentrations that are attainable in human cells, 2',3'-dideoxynucleo-

tide analogs have been shown to serve as substrates for HIV reverse transcriptase, resulting in chain termination after the addition of a single dideoxynucleotide residue.[28]

The other mechanism of action of these drugs is as a competitive inhibitor of the normal nucleoside-5'-triphosphate for HIV reverse transcriptase. In the case of AZT, for example, HIV has a K_m of 2.8 μM for 2'-deoxythymidine-5'-triphosphate (the normal nucleotide analog), while the K_i for AZT-5'-triphosphate is 0.04 μM.[26] In contrast to this low K_i value for viral reverse transcriptase, the K_i of AZT-5'-triphosphate against mammalian DNA polymerase α is 230 μM, and the K_i against mammalian DNA polymerase β is 70 μM.[26] A similar preferential utilization of AZT-5'-triphosphate as compared to 2'-deoxythymidine-5'-triphosphate has been found for avian myeloblastosis virus reverse transcriptase.[36] Thus, reverse transcriptase selectively utilizes AZT-5'-triphosphate, whereas DNA polymerase α and β do not; this preferential utilization (either as a competitive inhibitor or for incorporation and subsequent chain termination) is believed to be the basis for the ability of this compound to exert an antiviral effect at certain concentrations without cellular toxicity. It should be

Table 16-1
Partial Listing of Dideoxynucleosides with In Vitro *Activity Against HIV*

Compound Name	Effective in Vitro Anti-HIV Concentration*	Clinical Status	Reference(s)
3'-azido-2',3'-dideoxythymidine	1–5 μM	Prescription drug	8
2',3'-dideoxycytidine	0.5 μM	Phase I trials	24
2',3'-dideoxyadenosine	10 μM	Phase I trials	24
2',3'-dideoxyinosine	10 μM	Same as 2',3'-dideoxyadenosine	24
2',3'-dideoxyguanosine	10 μM	Preclinical	24
2',3'-dideoxythymidine	200 μM	Preclinical; no current plans for development	24
5-fluoro-2',3'-dideoxycytidine	0.5 μM	Preclinical	29
2',3'-dideoxycytidinene (didehydro analog)	0.2–0.3 μM	Preclinical	30, 31
2',3'-dideoxythymidinene (didehydro analog)	1–3 μM	Preclinical	31, 32
3'-azido-2',3'-dideoxyadenosine	10 μM	Preclinical	33
3'-azido-2',3'-dideoxyuridine	0.2 μM	Preclinical	34
3'-fluoro-2',3'-dideoxythymidine	4–20 μM	Preclinical	35

* Extreme caution must be used in comparing the effective antiviral concentrations of these compounds, as they have been tested in different laboratories using different assays, different multiplicities of infection, and different endpoints for antiviral effect.

noted, however, that, like reverse transcriptase, DNA polymerase γ (found in mitochondria) is sensitive to the effects of dideoxynucleoside-5'-triphosphates,[27] and this may contribute to the toxicity of these compounds.

A similar preferential utilization by reverse transcriptase has been found for other dideoxynucleoside-5'-triphosphates, including ddC, ddA, 2',3'-dideoxythymidine, and 2',3'-dideoxyguanosine.[27,37] Interestingly, the K_is of these compounds against the normal nucleoside-5'-triphosphate for HIV or avain myeloblastosis virus are all roughly similar, suggesting that the differences in activity of these compounds in cell cultures is not due to differing affinities of their triphosphates for reverse transcriptase. Instead, it appears that the different activities are the result of differential phosphorylation of these compounds and differences in the pool sizes of the competing normal nucleoside-triphosphates.[37]

Anabolic Phosphorylation of Dideoxynucleosides

As noted above, dideoxynucleosides must undergo anabolic phosphorylation by mammalian enzymes to an active 5'-triphosphate moiety. In the case of AZT, for example, upon entry into a cell, the drug is phosphorylated by thymidine kinase to form AZT-5'-monophosphate (AZT-MP). AZT-MP, in turn is phosphorylated by dTMP kinase (thymidylate kinase) to form AZT-5'-di-

phosphate (AZT-DP), which is subsequently phosphorylated to AZT-5'-triphosphate (AZT-TP) (see Fig. 16-3).[26] The relative efficiency of phosphorylation is an important determinant of the activity of these drugs *in vitro*. AZT, for example, is an excellent substrate for human thymidine kinase (K_m = 3.0 μM)[26] and is effective at concentrations of 5 μM. However, substitution of the 3' position with a hydrogen yields 2',3'-dideoxythymidine, which is poorly phosphorylated and is a rather poor agent against HIV *in vitro* (see Table 16-1).[24]

For many deoxynucleoside analogs, the rate-limiting step in phosphorylation is the initial addition of a phosphate group to form the 5'-monophosphate. AZT is somewhat unusual in that regard in that the rate-limiting step appears to be the phosphorylation of AZT-MP (see Figure 16-3).[26] Cells exposed to AZT develop large pools of AZT-MP, but relatively small pools of AZT-TP, and AZT is phosphorylated very slowly by dTMP kinase (relative maximum velocity only 0.3% as compared to dTMP; K_m = 8.6 μM).[26] Because of this interaction of AZT-MP with dTMP-kinase, it also may act as a substrate inhibitor for the phosphorylation of dTMP by this enzyme (see Figure 16-3), and cells exposed to AZT may have high levels of dTMP and decreased levels of dTTP.[26]

Other dideoxynucleosides with *in vitro* activity against HIV have also been found to be phosphorylated to a triphosphate form in human cells. In the case of 2',3'-dideoxycytidine (ddC), for example, an OKT4+ T cell line produced 0.5 pmole ddC-triphosphate per million cells after exposure to 1 μM of ddC for 24 hours.[38]

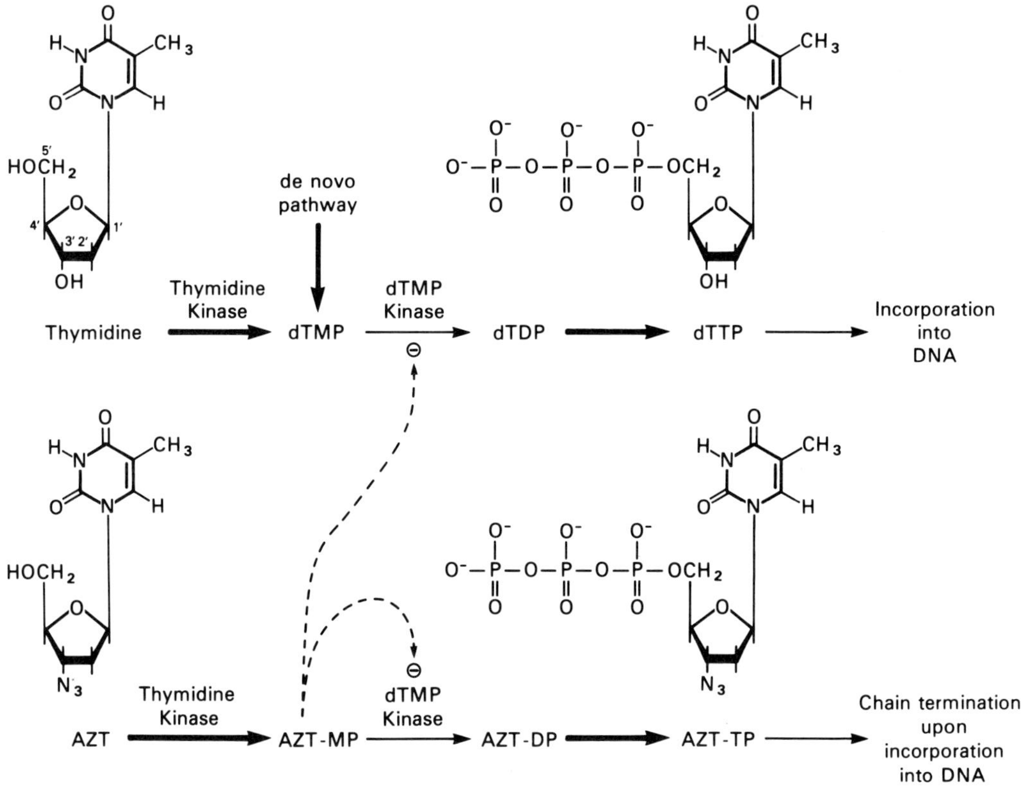

FIG. 16-3. Intracellular metabolism of AZT and thymidine. Abbreviations used: dTMP, thymidine-5'-monophosphate; dTDP, thymidine-5'-diphosphate; dTTP, thymidine-5'-triphosphate; AZT-MP, AZT-5'-monophosphate; AZT-DP, AZT-5'-diphosphate; AZT-TP, AZT-5'-triphosphate. (Yarchoan R, Broder S: Progress in the development of antiviral therapy for the acquired immunodeficiency syndrome and related disorders: A progress report. New Engl J Med 316:557, 1987)

This efficient phosphorylation (plus the relative small pool size of the competing normal analog, deoxycytidine-5'-triphosphate) most likely contributes to its potent *in vitro* activity in human T cells against HIV. Interestingly, this rather efficient phosphorylation occurs even though ddC is a relatively poor substrate for human cytoplasmic and mitochondrial deoxycytidine kinase (K_ms 180 and 120 μM, respectively).[39] 2',3'-dideoxyadenosine (ddA) is also efficiently phosphorylated by human cells.[40] Thus, each dideoxynucleoside that has been found to provide a protective effect against HIV *in vitro* can be demonstrated to be well phosphorylated in the relevant target cell lines, supporting the hypothesis that the triphosphates are the active forms of these drugs.

Since these drugs must undergo intracellular metabolism in the relevant target cells, and since the enzymes responsible for this anabolic phosphorylation may vary among different cell types, the question must be asked whether other cells (besides T-lymphocytes) that are targets for HIV infection can phosphorylate these drugs and be protected against infection. In the case of EBV-infected B cells and monocytoid cell lines, it appears that protection against HIV infection can be afforded by each of the drugs tested: AZT, ddC, and ddA.[41] Resting monocytes (another important target for HIV infection) may have different activities of deoxynucleoside kinases than monocytoid cell lines, however, and the activity of these drugs in monocytes is presently under investigation.

CLINICAL ACTIVITY OF AZT IN PATIENTS WITH AIDS AND RELATED DISORDERS

Initial Clinical Studies in Patient with AIDS or ARC

The activity of AZT against HIV *in vitro* was demonstrated at the National Cancer Institute in February 1985.[8] Several months later, our group in collaboration with investigators at Duke University Medical Center, the

University of Miami, and the Wellcome Research Laboratories, began a phase I trial of AZT in patients with AIDS and related disorders.[9] The purpose of this trial was to investigate the toxicity and pharmacokinetics of AZT and to gain information on whether it might have some clinical, immunologic, or virologic activity in patients with severe HIV infection. This was an escalating-dose trial, in which each patient received 2 weeks of intravenous dosing followed by 4 weeks of oral dosing at twice the intravenous dose. After this initial period, many of the patients continued to receive oral dosing (in some cases after a period during which they did not receive drug).[9,42]

Pharmacokinetic analysis revealed that AZT was well absorbed when given orally (bioavailability approximately 60%).[9,43] Also, it was found that levels that inhibited HIV replication *in vitro* could be achieved in patients. The half-life of AZT was found to be approximately 1 hour, with most of the drug being cleared by hepatic glucuronidation (to an inactive metabolite) and renal tubular secretion.[9,43,44] Finally, AZT was found to have excellent penetration across the blood–brain barrier; levels in the cerebrospinal fluid (CSF) 3 to 4 hours after a dose of AZT were an average of 55% of plasma levels obtained simultaneously.[9,43,45]

In subsequent studies, it was found that at least one drug that is known to inhibit hepatic glucuronidation, probenecid, can substantially increase the half-life of AZT.[44] It is quite possible that other glucuronidation inhibitors such as acetaminophen, morphine, or sulfonamides will be found to have similar clinically relevant effects. Indeed, any factor that affects hepatic blood flow or liver function could affect AZT metabolism and thus change its toxicity (and efficacy) profiles.

In the phase I trial of AZT, it was found that patients who received intermediate doses of AZT (oral doses of 15–30 mg/kg/day) had partial restoration of their immune function over a 6-week period of time, specifically twofold increases in the number of CD4+ (helper–inducer) T cells and restoration of delayed-type cutaneous hypersensitivity reactions in 6 of 16 previously anergic persons.[9] In addition, patients had an average 2.2 kg weight gain during the initial 6 weeks on AZT. Finally, some of the patients had other evidence of clinical improvement, particularly cessations of chronic fevers and in two patients clearing of chronic fungal nailplate infections without systemic antifungal therapy.

The ability to detect HIV in mitogen-stimulated cultures of peripheral blood mononuclear cells[46] was assessed in this phase I study. There was a suggestion that it was harder to culture HIV from patients receiving the highest doses of AZT;[9] however, this was an inconsistent finding, and patients who experienced immunologic improvement frequently continued to have detectable virus by this technique. The detection of HIV in mitogen-stimulated cultures involves the activation of cells that may be latently infected, and it is perhaps not surprising that such a system would fail to detect an antiviral effect. We subsequently have examined serum

collected from some of these patients for HIV p24 antibody, measured by an enzyme-linked immunosorbent assay (developed by Abbott Laboratories, Abbott, IL), and found that there was a consistent decline in the p24 antigen.* Interestingly, even some patients receiving the lowest dose of AZT (1 mg/kg IV q8h) had declines in their serum p24 antigen. Thus, this phase I study suggested that AZT could induce clinical, immunologic, and virologic benefits in patients with severe HIV infection.

The principal toxicity associated with AZT administration was found to be bone marrow suppression.[9,11] This was observed more often in patients with AIDS than those with ARC and appeared to be particularly troublesome in patients with *Mycobacterium avium* or cytomegalovirus infections.† Anemia and leukopenia (including decreases in the number of CD4+ T cells) were most frequently observed. These toxicities consistently developed in patients receiving oral doses (or intravenous equivalents) of 90 mg/kg/day after 4 to 6 weeks, and also developed in some patients receiving lower doses (25–30 mg/kg/day) for 8 weeks or longer.[9,47] Another observation in this study was that while patients receiving intermediate doses of AZT had sustained increases in their CD4+ cells for at least up to a 6-week period of time, those receiving higher doses (25–30 mg/kg/day) frequently had only transient increases lasting 2 weeks. This observation suggested that the late falls in CD4+ cells in these patients was at least in part a manifestation of AZT toxicity.[9,48] Finally, thrombocytopenia was observed less frequently, and indeed, some patients had brief increases in their platelet counts upon being administered AZT.[9] However, some patients who were continued on AZT for longer than 6 months eventually developed thrombocytopenia, suggesting that this may be a late manifestation of drug toxicity in some patients.

Many of the patients who initially developed bone marrow suppression on the higher doses of AZT were found subsequently to tolerate lower doses (6–15 mg/kg/day orally); however, we do not know if the lower doses confer a clinical benefit. Increases in the red blood cell mean corpuscular volume (reflecting megaloblastic changes) were found to often predate frank bone marrow toxicity. As mentioned above, because AZT-MP acts as a substrate inhibitor for dTMP-kinase (see Fig. 16-3), cells exposed to AZT *in vitro* frequently have a decline in their intracellular thymidine-triphosphate pools,[26] and it is likely that this drug-induced deficiency contributes to the megaloblastic changes and marrow toxicity.

Vitamin B_{12} and folic acid are involved in the synthesis of dTMP by the *de novo* pathway (see Fig. 16-3), and deficiencies of these vitamins are associated with megaloblastic anemias. Thus, it might be predicted that

---

* Yarchoan R, Allain JP, Broder S: Unpublished data.

† Yarchoan R, Broder S: Unpublished data.

patients who have underlying reductions in the production of thymidine triphosphate would be more susceptible to the toxic effects of AZT, and indeed, this has been found to be true.[9,48] Thus, patients receiving AZT should be screened for these vitamin deficiencies and replacement therapy initiated if low or even low-normal levels are found. Parenthetically, it should be noted that patients with AIDS develop vitamin deficiencies, and specifically vitamin B_{12} deficiency, with a higher incidence than the general population.

Other toxicities associated with AZT administration include headaches (found in approximately half the patients),[9,11] nausea and vomiting,[11,45] seizures (reported in one near-terminal patient),[49] myalgias,[11] and confusion (occurring in three patients who were receiving 90 mg/kg/day of AZT or who were receiving other medicines).[9,47] Some of these symptoms, particularly the headaches, nausea, and myalgias, appear to be most prominent during the first several weeks of therapy, and subsequently become less severe. The maximal tolerated dose over a 6-week period of time was found to be 90 mg/kg/day orally; however, as mentioned above, over an 8- to 16-week period of time, lower doses (25 to 30 mg/kg/day orally) are associated with bone marrow toxicity in almost half the patients with AIDS.[11,42] In general, ARC patients or patients with KS and relatively intact immune function tolerate AZT better than patients with AIDS who have had opportunistic infections, and most patients who develop bone marrow toxicity can subsequently tolerate lower doses of the drug (6–15 mg/kg/day orally);[48] however, while some patients on these lower doses were found to have increases in the number of $CD4^+$ cells[9] and decreases in serum p24 antigen in the phase I study, we reemphasize that it is a topic of ongoing research whether such lower doses will confer a significant clinical benefit.

As noted above, patients in our phase I study were continued on the drug after the initial 6-week period (in some cases following a 1- to 3-month period without drug), and some patients have tolerated 10 to 25 mg/kg/day of AZT for up to 28 months.* Many of the patients with AIDS were noted to have late decreases in their $CD4^+$ cells after 12 to 20 weeks of therapy.[60] In contrast, some ARC patients (or patients with Kaposi's sarcoma [KS] and minimal immunologic dysfunction) have had sustained increases in their $CD4^+$ T cells. We stress, however, that in absolute numbers, certain $CD4^+$ T-cell increases were rather modest; nevertheless, it now appears clear that even modest increments of $CD4^+$ T-cell counts can confer significant survival benefits to patients with AIDS.

Eighteen patients with AIDS or severe ARC from the initial phase I study of AZT have been followed at the National Cancer Institute; this group comprises 6 patients with AIDS who had had Pneumocystis carinii pneumonia (PCP) prior to entry, 2 patients who had both PCP and KS, 6 with KS, and 4 with ARC. (This

group includes 12 of the 19 patients reported in the original report[9] and 6 additional patients who initially received a higher dose of AZT). Of these 18 patients, 9 are still alive 19 to 25 months after their initial entry into the protocol. Some of those patients have had second or third episodes of PCP; however, it is our clinical impression that these episodes were frequently mild and that the patients overall have done better over a 2-year period of time than one would have expected in the absence of therapy. However, the results do suggest that AZT clearly has limitations in advanced AIDS; half of the patients have now died and a number of the patients who are presently alive have low numbers of circulating $CD4^+$ (helper–inducer) T cells.

To specifically address the question of whether AZT indeed increased the survival of patients with AIDS or ARC, a phase II multicenter placebo-controlled trial was initiated in February 1986.* 282 patients were entered into this study including 160 with AIDS who had had their first episode of PCP within 120 days of entry and 122 with ARC (with either weight loss or oral candidiasis). Each patient received either 250 mg of AZT every 4 hours around the clock or placebo.

By September 1986, 20 deaths had occurred in this trial, 1 in a patient randomized to AZT and 19 in patients on placebo ($p < 0.001$).[10,11] Because of the dramatic difference in the mortality between these two groups, an independent data safety monitoring board at that time elected to prematurely terminate the study and to give AZT to all the patients who had been on placebo.[10] Starting in September 1986, under the mechanism of a Treatment IND, AZT was made widely available to AIDS patients who had PCP and who fulfilled certain other criteria, and on March 20, 1987, the Food and Drug Administration approved AZT for use in patients with symptomatic HIV infection (AIDS and advanced ARC) who have a history of cytologically confirmed PCP or an absolute CD4 lymphocyte count of less than 200/mm^3 in the peripheral blood before therapy is begun.

This trial also confirmed that patients receiving AZT had increases in their weight and immune function, and demonstrated that they had a decreased incidence of opportunistic infections. Overall, the patients receiving AZT had a 0.5 kg increase in their mean body weight, while the placebo recipients lost 0.1 kg ($p < 0.05$).[10] In addition, by week 4 of the study, the AIDS patients receiving AZT had a mean 86/mm^3 increase in their absolute $CD4^+$ cell count, while those receiving placebo had an 8/mm^3 decrease ($p < 0.0001$). In addition, a

---

* Yarchoan R, Broder S: Unpublished data.

* Principal investigators who participated in this trial were D. Durack, Duke University Medical Center, NC; M. Fischl, University of Miami, FL; M. Gottlieb, University of California Medical Center, CA; M. Grieco, St. Luke's–Roosevelt Hospital, NY; J. Groopman, New England Deaconess Hospital, MA; G. Jackson, University of Illinois, IL; O. Laskin, Cornell Medical College, NY; J. Leedom, LAC–USC Medical Center, CA; D. Mildvan, Beth Israel Medical Center, NY; D. Richman, University of California San Diego Medical Center, CA; R. Schooley, Massachusetts General Hospital, MA; and P. Volberding, University of California San Francisco, CA.

higher proportion of the AIDS patients who received AZT and who were anergic at entry developed positive delayed-type hypersensitivity reactions to at least one recall antigen during the study. Similar increases in CD4+ cells and improvement in skin test reactivity were seen in the ARC patients. There was evidence from this study, however, that these effects were only transient. By week 20, the CD4+ count in the AIDS patients who received AZT had returned to baseline and was only slightly higher than that of the patients taking placebo. There was a suggestion that the ARC patients in this study had somewhat more sustained increases in their CD4+ T cells; however, even in this patient population, by week 24, there was not a statistically significant difference between the treated and untreated groups.

In regard to virologic assessment, there were no differences overall between the AZT and placebo-treated patients in the ability to isolate HIV in mitogen-stimulated cultures of peripheral blood mononuclear cells.[10] However, in the patients in whom the circulating HIV p24 (core) protein was examined, there were statistically significant decreases from entry at weeks 4, 8, and 12.[10,50] Thus, as assessed by the circulating p24 antigen that could be detected in an immunologic assay, AZT induced a decrease in the viral load in treated patients.

Fewer opportunistic infections developed in the patients receiving AZT in this phase II study than in those receiving placebo; 24 patients in the AZT group developed opportunistic infections as compared to 45 patients in the placebo group.[10] Interestingly, differ-

ences between these groups did not appear until week 6 of the study, suggesting that the protection from opportunistic infections in the patients receiving AZT followed their improvement in immune function and was not the result of a direct effect of the AZT on the organisms causing the opportunistic infections.

At the termination of this trial in September 1986, all the study participants were given the opportunity to receive AZT (although in some cases there was a delay of several weeks before this was effected). Among the original placebo recipients (including those who later received AZT for less than 3 weeks and were therefore unlikely to benefit from it), the mortality 36 weeks after entry was 39.3%. In contrast, among the original AZT recipients, the mortality at 36 weeks was only 6.2% (Fig. 16-4), and even after 52 weeks, only 10.3% of the original AZT recipients had died.[10] Therefore, patients receiving AZT had a better survival than untreated patients (e.g., those on placebo) for at least 1 year. The total increase in survival afforded by AZT therapy is at present unknown, and as the placebo arm of the phase II study has been terminated, it will most likely never be demonstrated in a placebo-controlled study. However, it may be possible to estimate the increase by continuing to follow the patients on the phase I and phase II studies.

It should perhaps be mentioned at this point that two patients on our phase I trial of AZT developed B-cell lymphomas; one, a severely immunosuppressed ARC patient, developed a large-cell lymphoma of the esophagus after 12 months on drug, and the second, a

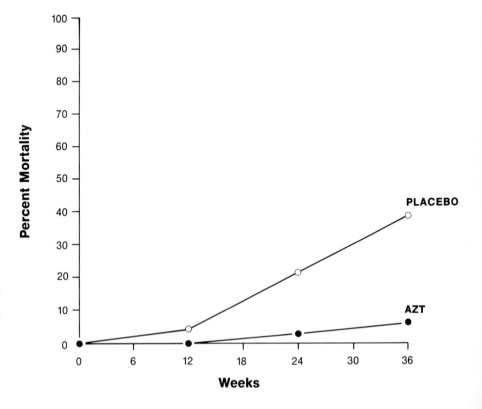

FIG. 16-4. Survival of patients in the randomized multicenter phase II study of AZT.[10] Placebo patients who at the termination of the study were switched to AZT are still scored as placebo patients if they received 3 weeks or less of AZT prior to their death, as it is unlikely that they would have derived clinical benefit from this short a time of therapy. (Data of M. Fischl, D.D. Richman, D. Barry, and the AZT Collaborative Working Group)

patient who had had PCP prior to entry, developed a large-cell lymphoma in the lung after 22 months of AZT.* High-grade B-cell lymphomas have been observed to develop with increased frequency in patients with HIV infection in the absence of antiviral therapy,[51] and it has been speculated that an increased frequency of EBV-infected B cells, B-cell activation induced by HIV, or a failure of T-cell immunologic surveillance might contribute to the development of these lymphomas.[52-55] Lymphoid tumors are a well-known complication of a variety of congenital immunodeficiencies such as Wiskott–Aldrich syndrome or ataxia telangiectasia, and as we have developed expertise in controlling their infections and the patients have lived longer, such tumors have been seen more often.[56] It is possible that as AIDS patients live longer as a result of effective antiviral therapy, we will observe an increased incidence of lymphomas. At this point, however, this remains a theoretical possibility, and it should be stressed that overall, AZT therapy results in decreased morbidity and mortality in patients with severe HIV infection.

Effect of AZT on Kaposi's Sarcoma

In the phase I study of AZT, 9 patients had KS. During the first 6 weeks of therapy, none of those patients had regressions of their KS, and some of the patients had detectable increases in their lesions.[9,42] Six of those 9 patients were continued on AZT for longer than 6 weeks. Of these 6 patients, one had a complete response in his KS starting at week 8, and another three patients had partial responses starting between weeks 6 and 14.[47,57] These partial responses, however, were only temporary, and the patients eventually developed new lesions while on AZT. In a subsequent small-scale trial in which patients with KS were randomized to receive either KS or placebo, there was also a suggestion that the patients receiving AZT had less progression or in some cases minor regressions of their KS lesions.[58] Thus, the initial clinical experience with AZT in patients with KS suggests that occasional patients may have an initial increase in their KS upon being given AZT and also that some temporary tumor regression may later be observed in certain patients; these effects are in general not dramatic. It is possible, however, that a subset of patients who may have a higher chance of having KS responses to AZT will be defined.

The mechanism by which AZT exerts its antineoplastic effect on those patients who respond is unclear: possibilities include an antitumor effect as a result of improved immunologic function,[59] a direct antitumor effect of the drug (AZT was originally synthesized as a possible antitumor agent[60]), or as a result of decreased production of a tumorigenic lymphokine by HIV-infected cells. It should perhaps be stressed that although KS is a hallmark manifestation of HIV infection, the pathogenesis of this tumor is poorly understood. In addition, once KS develops, HIV may not be required for its continued growth. Salahuddin and colleagues have recently developed cloned cell lines from KS lesions that have characteristics of lymphatic endothelial cells and that induce KS-like lesions when injected into nude mice.[61] These lines grow in response to conditioned medium from cell lines transformed with another retrovirus (HTLV-II); however, the lines themselves do not contain any detectable viruses. Through experiments such as these, it may be possible to better understand the pathogenesis of KS, to predict how antiviral therapy may (or not) be expected to affect the disorder, and finally, to target specific therapy for those patients in whom the KS itself becomes a major clinical problem.

Effect of AZT on HIV-Induced Neurologic Dysfunction

In contrast to the minimal effects on Kaposi's sarcoma, we have observed that patients with HIV-induced neurologic dysfunction can have substantial clinical improvement upon being administered AZT.[45,62] Indeed, in some patients the neurologic improvements represent the most notable feature of AZT administration.

Since the initial observation in 1985 that the brain was an important site of HIV replication,[18] it has been increasingly recognized that neurologic dysfunction (including dementia, peripheral neuropathy, and myelopathy) is associated with HIV infection.[19-21] In one recent study, half of patients studied with HIV-related lymphadenopathy syndrome had abnormalities on psychometric testing,[63] and it is possible that as we become better able to treat the opportunistic infections in AIDS, neurologic disorders in this disease will become clinically more prominent. In general, HIV-related dementia portends a poor prognosis, and in one recent study, such patients were found to have a median survival of 4.2 months.[21] Some scientists have assumed that HIV-induced neurologic deficits would be irreversible.

The pathogenesis of the neurologic dysfunction in HIV infection is at present not well understood, and it is uncertain which cell types in the nervous system are targets for infection. A recent study of the neuropathology of patients dying of AIDS-associated dementia indicated that abnormalities are most prominent in the white matter; these included inflammatory changes, vacuolation, and microglial nodules.[64] In regard to the affected cells, several studies reported this year have suggested that the target cells for infection with HIV are macrophages.[14,65,66] A particularly intriguing result observed by Gartner and co-workers was that virus isolated from macrophages of affected patients was more efficient at infecting macrophages than virus obtained from T cells.[14,65] Such variants of HIV might be particularly important in causing central nervous system disease. Two other studies reported this year have shown widespread evidence of expression of CD4-like proteins in the brain and have suggested that these may be the

---

* Yarchoan R, Broder S: Unpublished data.

receptors for the virus in the central nervous system.[67,68] Finally, it is possible that some neurologic symptoms may be caused by neuroactive lymphokines released from virally infected cells, by host defense cells responding to retroviral invasion, or by viral proteins that can mimic neuropeptides. In this regard, it is of particular interest that a neuroactive protein called "neuroleukin" was reported to have substantial sequence homology with HIV envelope protein[69] and, like HIV, has been found to activate B cells *in vitro*;[69] it is possible that HIV envelope glycoprotein acts as a competitive inhibitor for neuroleukin and thus starves nerve cells of factor.

As noted above, AZT has been found to have excellent penetration across the blood–brain barrier; levels in the CSF 4 hours after a dose have been found to average 50% to 60% of simultaneous plasma levels.[9,43,45] We have recently described the effects of AZT administration in seven patients with HIV-associated neurologic disease (three with dementia, two with peripheral neuropathy, one with dementia and peripheral neuropathy, and one with a T10 transverse myelitis).[45,57,62] No demonstrable response was noted in the patient with the T10 transverse myelitis, and one patient with a severe neuropathy had only minimal improvement. The other five patients had substantial improvements in their dementia and/or neuropathy over a 3 to 30 week period of AZT administration as assessed by neurologic examination, nerve conduction studies, and/or psychometric testing. Three patients had a positron emission scan (a measure of brain glucose metabolism) done at the onset of therapy and 8 weeks later. In one case, the initial scan was normal, while in two others the initial scan showed an abnormal heterogeneous pattern of cortical glucose metabolism. In each of these two cases where the initial scan was abnormal, subsequent scans done during therapy showed a more normal homogeneous pattern.[57,62] In one patient, the dose of AZT had to be stopped after 6 months because of neutropenia; the dementia subsequently worsened and the patient died of complications of the dementia.[45] These results suggest that AZT can at least transiently induce improvements in some patients with HIV-associated neurologic disease and as a corollary suggest that HIV-induced dementia has a reversible component. This should be an area of further research in the next few years. We are intrigued by the rapidity with which certain patients may experience improvements of dementia. We have seen responses as early as 3 weeks, and perhaps this favors an HIV-induced neurotoxin (or inhibition of an essential neuroactive substance) as the cause of the disordered central nervous system in certain patients.

Current Recommendations and Issues for Future Research

Overall, these studies with AZT have indicated that, although it is not a cure for AIDS, the drug can induce immunologic improvements, increase survival, and reverse certain neurologic abnormalities in patients with AIDS and related diseases. In some patients, the improvement in the quality of life is substantial.

AZT is now approved by the Food and Drug Administration for adult patients with HIV infection who have had Pneumocystis carinii pneumonia or who have less than 200 T4 cells/mm^3 (Retrovir, package insert). The recommended starting dose is 200 mg orally every 4 hours. Patients who develop significant anemia (hemoglobin < 7.5 g/dl) or neutropenia (<750 neutrophils/mm^3) may require dose interruption until some evidence of marrow recovery is obtained; they can then be started on a lower dose. For patients with less severe bone marrow suppression, physicians may want to reduce the dose without first interrupting therapy.

Based on our experience using AZT, we would recommend that physicians using this drug check the serum folic acid and vitamin B_{12} levels and consider replacement therapy with these vitamins (including vitamin B_{12} injections) if the patients have low or even low-normal vitamin levels. Care should be exercised if drugs that affect hepatic glucuronidation (e.g., acetaminophen, probenecid, morphine derivatives, or nonsteriodal inflammatory drugs) are used or if drugs that are by themselves cytotoxic are used concomitantly. In any case, because of the propensity of AZT to cause bone marrow toxicity, blood counts should be obtained at least every 2 weeks if possible.

AZT has been shown to cross the placenta of animals, and in a murine model, administration to pregnant animals has been found to partially protect fetal mice from maternofetal retroviral transmission.[70] Although AZT has not been found to be teratogenic in studies in pregnant rats (Retrovir, package insert), it is not known whether it will cause fetal damage when administered to pregnant women, and it should be given to a pregnant woman only if clearly needed, and perhaps only in a research setting.

It should be stressed that because of the very rapid development of AZT, less is known about this agent than most other drugs approved for prescription use. It is not known, for example, if lower doses of AZT (<200 mg q4h) will also reduce morbidity and mortality in patients, or whether in patients who develop anemia it is better to continue high doses of AZT and provide transfusion support or to reduce the dose of the drug. It is possible in this regard that different subpopulations of patients will have to be treated differently; in patients with HIV-induced dementia, for example, one might tend to be more aggressive in administering higher doses of AZT in the face of toxicity. Another unresolved issue is whether administration of AZT early in the course of HIV infection will prevent or substantially delay the development of AIDS; studies are presently underway to address this point. The use of AZT in combination with other drugs is another important area for future work; this will be discussed further below. Finally, the use of AZT in children and infants with HIV infection is another area being explored. Dr. Philip A. Pizzo in the pediatric branch of the National Cancer Institute is presently conducting a phase I trial of AZT in children with AIDS, and other such trials are also on-going. It is hoped that through these efforts, we can learn how to use this drug optimally.

OTHER DIDEOXYNUCLEOSIDES

2′,3′-Dideoxycytidine

The results with AZT demonstrated that an antiretroviral drug could reduce the morbidity and mortality in patients with AIDS. While important in its own right, the development of AZT has also provided an impetus for the clinical development of other agents with antiretroviral activity. As noted above, 2′,3′-dideoxycytidine (ddC) was found by Mitsuya and Broder to have potent activity against HIV,[24] with complete protection being afforded with 0.5 μM ddC, even under conditions of a high multiplicity of infection.

Additional studies with ddC demonstrated several other properties that might be desirable in a potential therapeutic agent for HIV infection. It was found to be relatively resistant to cytidine deaminase (a major catabolic enzyme for cytidine analogs),[38] it was well absorbed when given to animals, it was found to have straightforward pharmacokinetic clearance by the kidney in animals, and it induced comparatively few side effects in laboratory animals.[71]

Based on these results, we have initiated a phase I study of ddC at the National Cancer Institute. The results of this trial are at present preliminary, but several conclusions can be drawn. ddC appears to be well absorbed when given orally in humans, and levels that are antiviral *in vitro* can be attained in patients.* We have not seen megaloblastic bone marrow suppression (the dose-limiting toxicity for AZT). However, other toxicities, including a "rash symptom-complex" and a painful peripheral neuropathy, have been observed. The rash-symptom complex, including a rash on exposed surfaces, fevers, arthralgias, and mouths sores, was an early toxicity; it usually developed after about 2 weeks of therapy but then subsided 2 weeks later, even with continued ddC administration. Peripheral neuropathy developed in a number of patients as a late toxicity, usually after 9 or more weeks of therapy.†

In terms of antiviral activity, nearly all of the patients on the higher doses of the drug (0.03 mg/kg q4h or greater) had a rapid decline in their detectable serum p24 antigen (as measured by the Abbott assay).‡ However, in some patients, this parameter returned to baseline after a number of weeks on therapy. Some patients also had evidence of immunologic improvement, including rises in their number of helper–inducer (CD4$^+$)

---

* Klecker R, Collins JM, Yarchoan R et al: Unpublished data.

† Yarchoan R, Broder S: Unpublished data.

‡ Yarchoan R, Allain JP, Broder S: Unpublished data.

T cells and improvement in *in vitro* antigen-driven proliferative responses.§ Thus, preliminary results from this phase I study indicate that ddC has evidence of antiviral activity but is also associated with toxicities, and additional studies will be needed to determine whether it has a clinical role in the therapy of AIDS, either as a single agent or in combination with other drugs. One particularly intriguing result in this regard is that patients can tolerate higher cumulative doses of ddC if the drug is given in an alternating regimen with AZT; indeed, patients have tolerated such a regimen for more than 40 weeks.†

2′,3′-Dideoxyadenosine/2′,3′,-Dideoxyinosine

Another dideoxynucleoside with potent *in vitro* activity against HIV is 2′,3′-dideoxyadenosine (ddA).[24] This compound is effectively phosphorylated in human T cells to an active triphosphate moiety.[40] In human serum, ddA is rapidly deaminated by adenosine deaminase to form 2′,3′-dideoxyinosine (ddI); however, as noted in Table 16-1, ddI also has *in vitro* activity against HIV. (Within human cells, ddI can be metabolized to form ddA-5′-triphosphate.) A phase I clinical trial of ddA/ddI (administered as the ddA form) has recently been initiated at the National Cancer Institute.

OTHER RETROVIRAL AGENTS

In addition to the aforementioned dideoxynucleosides, a number of other agents have been shown to have some anti-HIV activity in certain *in vitro* systems. A partial list of these agents is given in Table 16-2.

Reverse Transcriptase Inhibitors

Several of these compounds, including suramin,[72] HPA 23,[73] phosphonoformate,[74,75] and rifabutine[76] are believed to act by interfering with the function of HIV reverse transcriptase, although one should bear in mind that more than one mechanism might apply.

Suramin was described by De Clercq in 1979 as being a profound inhibitor of the reverse transcriptase of certain avian and murine retroviruses,[77] and was the first agent published as having *in vitro* activity against HIV.[72] Initial clinical trials of suramin in patients with ARC and AIDS, using one fixed regimen, showed a suggestive antiviral effect (as measured by culture technology).[78] However, patients did not have clinical or immunologic improvement, and substantial toxicity was observed. It is worth exploring other regimens or methods of administration that might potentiate the therapeutic index of this drug. At present, suramin is being studied as an experimental anticancer agent.

Phosphonoformate and rifabutine are two other

---

§ Yarchoan R, Perno CF, Broder S: Unpublished data.

Table 16-2
Some Other Agents Being Studied for Anti-HIV Activity

Name	Concentration with in Vitro *Antiretroviral* Activity	Comments
AL 721	100 µg/ml (50% inhibition)	Clinical trials underway
Alpha IFN	4–1024 U/ml (partial)	Clinical activity against KS
Dextran sulfate	10 µg/ml	Preclinical
GM-CSF	3 U/ml (partial)	Clinical trials underway
HPA 23	Activity reported	Causes thrombocytopenia; no evidence of efficacy
Peptide T	1 nM	Clinical trials underway
Phosphonoformate	132–680 µM	Clinical trials underway
Ribavirin	100 µg/ml (partial)	Clinical trials underway
Rifabutine	10–100 µg/ml	Clinical trials underway
Suramin	25 µg/ml	No evidence of clinical or immunologic improvement in patients using one fixed regimen; adrenal cortical damage is one side effect

substances that are believed to interfere with reverse transcriptase activity and that have been shown to have activity against HIV *in vitro*.[74–76] Neither substance requires anabolic phosphorylation to an active form, and they might therefore be useful for protecting certain target cells that lack appropriate kinases for dideoxynucleosides. In addition to inhibiting HIV, phosphonoformate (also called foscarnet) has been shown to be an inhibitor of the DNA polymerase of certain human herpesviruses[79] and was once administered to immunocompromised patients with cytomegalovirus.[74] Clinical trials are presently underway in patients with HIV infection.

In the mid-1970s, Ting and co-workers showed that certain rifamycin analogs were inhibitors of reverse transcriptase.[80] Rifabutine, one such analog with *in vitro* activity against *Mycobacterium avium* has more recently been shown to inhibit HIV replication by 90% to 99% at concentrations of 0.1 to 0.5 µg/ml, concentrations that are attainable in patients.[76] This drug thus has the potential advantage that it might inhibit both HIV and an opportunistic pathogen frequently found in these patients. Results of initial clinical studies of activity against HIV should be forthcoming shortly.

Other Agents Being Studied for Anti-HIV Activity

A number of other compounds are presently being investigated as potential antiviral drugs; these appear to work at sites other than reverse transcriptase. In several cases, the mechanism of activity is not known (see Table 16-2). Two of these, the lipid substance AL 721 and an octapeptide called *peptide T,* are believed to inhibit the binding of HIV to target cells.[68,81]

AL 721 is basically a dietary agent composed of neutral glycerides, phosphatidylcholine, and phosphatidylethanolamine in a 7:2:1 ratio.[81] It is postulated that this phospholipid mixture could distort the outer lipid layer of the virus or possibly its cell-receptor attachment site. In very short-term cultures, it has been shown to have partial activity against HIV *in vitro*.[81] However, much remains to be learned about whether this phospholipid complex can effectively suppress HIV replication. It is expected to have very little toxicity in patients since the ingredients are components in the biosynthesis of phospholipids in the body.

Another substance presently entering clinical trials as a potential anti-HIV agent is peptide T. This peptide is a sequence in the envelope glycoprotein (gp120) of HIV that has been reported to block the binding of the virus to target cells and to inhibit *in vitro* vial replication.[68] This point is a matter of active discussion since many laboratories are unable to demonstrate potent suppression of HIV under similar conditions.[82] Because of the possibility that this substance might, like gp120, bind to the CD4 protein, which acts as the receptor for HIV, concerns have been raised that it might be immunosuppressive if administered to patients. A small study in four patients, however, did not find any toxicity associated with peptide T administration.[83]

Another biologic agent, α-interferon, is believed to act by inhibiting the budding of HIV from infected cells. In their original description of HIV (then called HTLV-III), Popovic and colleagues demonstrated that antibodies against α-interferon increased viral production by infected cells.[5] Subsequently, it has been shown that exogenous α-interferon added to cell cultures could partially inhibit virus production.[84,85] Interestingly, α-interferon was tested clinically in patients with KS even before it was known that a retrovirus caused AIDS; in several trials, it was shown to induce partial or, in some cases, complete responses in a subset of patients with KS.[86–88]

Several other agents whose site of action is unknown have been shown to inhibit HIV *in vitro;* these include ribavirin,[89] dextran sulfate,[90] and granulocyte-macrophage colony stimulating factor (GM-CSF).[91,92] Ribavirin is a guanosine analog that has activity against several RNA viruses *in vitro*[93] and has recently been shown to have partial activity against HIV.[89] One proposed mechanism of action for ribavirin in its activity against other viruses is interference with the capping of virus-specific RNA by inhibition of messenger RNA guanylyl transferase activity.[93] It is possible that a similar mechanism might account for its activity against HIV. Initial clinical trials of ribavirin in patients with HIV infection have shown that, while high doses can be associated with difficulty concentrating and anemia, lower doses can often be tolerated. Initial small studies to evaluate its efficacy have yielded inconclusive or negative results,[94] and additional studies are planned. Dextran sulfate (MW 7000–8000) was originally developed as an anticoagulant and has been used clinically in Japan for a number of years as an antilipemic agent. It was recently shown to inhibit HIV replication at concentrations of 10 μg/ml,[90] and plans are underway to evaluate it clinically. Its mechanism of action is uncertain.

Finally, mention should be made of GM-CSF, a glycoprotein that acts as a potent stimulator for hematopoetic precursor cells. It has recently been reported that GM-CSF has some activity against HIV in U937, a monocytoid cell line, at concentrations of 30 U/ml or greater.[91] In addition, unlike AZT and some other drugs being considered, GM-CSF does not have marrow-suppressive properties, but instead would be expected to enhance bone marrow function. Thus, even if it has only limited antiviral activity, GM-CSF might be useful in combination with other agents. Indeed, it has recently been reported that it has synergistic activity when tested with AZT (see Table 16-3).[92]

STUDIES OF AGENTS TESTED IN COMBINATION WITH AZT

An area of recent interest in the development of therapeutic strategies against HIV is the use of two or more agents that might have either synergistic activity or additive activity with nonoverlapping toxicities. Such combination therapy has yielded dramatic results in the area of antitumor chemotherapy.[95] In addition, it has proved useful in the long-term treatment of certain chronic infectious diseases (e.g., *Mycobacterium* infections) in which drug resistance is a problem.

As an initial step in the development of such therapies, several agents have recently been tested for their activity against HIV in combination with AZT; a partial listing of the results of such studies is shown in Table 16-3. As can be seen, a number of such agents have been shown to be synergistic (or at least additive) when tested in at least one system; a notable exception is ribavirin which antagonizes the action of AZT probably by interfering with its phosphorylation.[99]

At least two of these drug combinations, AZT plus acyclovir, and AZT plus α-interferon, are at this time being evaluated in pilot studies in patients with HIV infection. Like AZT, acyclovir is a nucleoside analog that can be phosphorylated to a triphosphate form and is believed to act by chain termination. It was originally developed for use against herpesvirus infections and is now approved for this use.[93] Acyclovir has little toxicity when administered to patients and in particular does not cause bone marrow suppression, most likely because normal cells cannot phosphorylate this drug. While it has little activity against HIV as a single agent, it can substantially enhance the *in vitro* anti-HIV activity of AZT.[24,33] We are presently studying a small group of patients to determine whether acyclovir can be given with AZT over a period of several months without causing unacceptable toxicity.

Another agent that has been shown to be synergistic with AZT *in vitro* is a mismatched double-stranded RNA [poly(I):poly(C$_{12}$,U)], also called ampligen.[97] This agent is believed to act primarily as an immunostimulator and is reported to enhance interferon production and macrophage function.[100] Ampligen was recently studied in a phase I trial in 10 patients with AIDS or ARC, and an improvement in delayed hypersensitivity skin test reactions was observed.[100] Based on these preliminary results, additional clinical studies of ampligen are now planned.

Although the focus of this chapter is on the antiviral therapy of HIV infection, it is perhaps at this point

Table 16-3
In Vitro *Effect of Some Drugs Tested in Combination with AZT*

Drug Combination	Reported Anti-HIV Effect	Reference
AZT + Acyclovir	Synergistic	24, 33
AZT + α-IFN	Synergistic	96
AZT + Ampligen	Potentiates activity of AZT	97
AZT + ddC	Potentiates activity of AZT	*
AZT + Dextran Sulfate	Synergistic	98
AZT + GM-CSF	Synergistic in monocytoid line	92
AZT + Ribavirin	Antagonizes activity of AZT	99

* Mitsuya and Broder, unpublished data.

worthwhile to mention that yet another therapeutic strategy being considered in the treatment of AIDS is the combination of antiviral therapy with some strategy to boost the patient's immune system. In addition to ampligen, some other approaches being considered for the immunostimulation (or immunoreconstitution) of AIDS patients include bone marrow transplantation (being studied by Fauci and others in combination with antiviral therapy), thymus transplantation,[101,102] or interleukin-2.[103]

ACTIVITY OF ANTIRETROVIRAL DRUGS ON VIRUSES OTHER THAN HIV

Many of the drugs being considered as antiretroviral agents against HIV also have activity against other retroviruses.[27,36,70,104] In particular, there is considerable homology in the reverse transcriptase of a number of retroviruses, and agents that act at this step (including dideoxynucleosides) can have a wide range of activity as long as the target cell phosphorylates them.[104] For example, AZT and ddC both exert a profound antiviral effect on a variety of viruses including caprine arthritis encephalitis virus, equine infectious anemia virus, and amphomorphic murine leukemia virus in appropriate target cells. In the case of amphomorphic murine leukemia virus, little activity is found with ddC when the virus is grown in the NIH 3T3 cell line (a murine cell line that does not effectively phosphorylate ddC); however, effective viral inhibition is obtained when the same virus is grown in human cells.[104]

Several of these drugs have recently also been shown to inhibit another pathogenic human retrovirus, human T-cell lymphotropic virus type I (HTLV-I),[105,106] a virus that causes an aggressive leukemia-lymphoma in some infected persons. It is doubtful whether an antiviral drug will directly affect the transformed leukemia cells in such patients. However, HTLV-I-infection has also been shown to cause T-cell immunodeficiency,[107,108,109] and it is possible that AZT or related drugs might improve this manifestation of HTLV-I infection. In addition, HTLV-I has been associated with a group of related neurologic syndromes variously called tropical spastic papaparesis[110] and HTLV-I–associated myelopathy;[111] it is possible that a clinical benefit will be derived in such patients by blocking their viral replication. Also, several viruses related to HIV have recently been described in Africa, and at least one of these (called HIV-2 or LAV-2) has been associated with an AIDS-like illness.[112,113] Finally, there is recent evidence that certain cases of multiple sclerosis might be caused by a retrovirus related to HTLV-I and HIV.[114] The first retrovirus, HTLV-I, was discovered only 7 years ago, and it is likely that in the near future additional human retroviruses will be discovered and found to play a role in the pathogenesis of a variety of illnesses. It is thus possible that drugs now being developed for the treatment of AIDS will in the future have a role in clinical (or veterinary) medicine to treat illnesses not presently known to be caused by retroviruses.

SUMMARY

In the short period of time since AIDS was recognized as a new clinical entity, the virus responsible for causing this disease (HIV) has been identified, several agents have been found to block the replication of the virus *in vitro,* and at least one such agent, AZT, has been shown to reduce the morbidity and mortality of patients with AIDS. The demonstration that one dideoxynucleoside analog has clinical efficacy in some patients with AIDS and that even the neurologic dysfunction caused by the disease may be at least partially reversible in some cases has removed some of the uncertainty about the rationale for an antiretroviral intervention in established AIDS. It may also help to dispel the prevailing sense of hopelessness about the disease.

While AZT is important clinically as a drug in its own right, it may even be more important as an impetus for additional efforts to develop antiretroviral strategies for the treatment of AIDS. It is estimated that over 1.5 million persons in the United States are presently infected with HIV, and many of these will be expected to develop AIDS over the next 10 years. These statistics add a sense of urgency to the development of effective therapies in this disorder, and with the start that has been made, we are confident that scientists and clinicians can rise to meet this challenge.

REFERENCES

1. Gottlieb MS, Schroff R, Schanker HM et al: *Pneumocystis carinii* pneumonia and mucosal candidiasis in previously healthy homosexual men: Evidence of a new acquired cellular immunodeficiency. N Engl J Med 305:1425, 1981
2. Masur H, Michelis MA, Greene JB et al: An outbreak of community-acquired *Pneumocystis carinii* pneumonia: Initial manifestations of cellular immune dysfunction. N Engl J Med 305:1431, 1981
3. Siegal FP, Lopez C, Hammer GS et al: Severe acquired immunodeficiency is male homosexuals, manifested by chronic perianal herpes simplex lesions. N Engl J Med 305:1439, 1981
4. Gallo RC, Salahuddin AZ, Popovic M et al: Frequent detection and isolation of pathogenic retroviruses (HTLV-III) from patients with AIDS and at risk for AIDS. Science 224:500, 1984
5. Popovic M, Sarngadharan MG, Reed E et al: Detection, isolation, and continuous production of cytopathic retrovirus (HTLV-III) from patients with AIDS and pre-AIDS. Science 224:497, 1984
6. Barré–Sinoussi F, Chermann JC, Rey F et al: Isolation of a T cell lymphotropic virus from a patient at risk for the acquired immunodeficiency syndrome (AIDS). Science 220:868, 1983
7. Levy JA, Hoffman AD, Kramer SM et al: Isolation of lymphocytopathic retroviruses from San Francisco patients with AIDS. Science 225:840, 1984

8. Mitsuya H, Weinhold KJ, Furman PA et al: 3'-azido-3'-deoxythymidine (BW A509U): An antiviral agent that inhibits the infectivity and cytopathic effect of human T-lymphotropic virus type III/lymphadenopathy-associated virus *in vitro*. Proc Natl Acad Sci USA 82:7096, 1985

9. Yarchoan R, Klecker RW, Weinhold KJ et al: Administration of 3'-azido-3'-deoxythymidine, and inhibitor of HTLV-III/LAV replication, to patients with AIDS or AIDS-related complex. Lancet 1:575, 1986

10. Fischl MA, Richman DD, Grieco MH et al: The efficacy of azidothymidine (AZT) in the treatment of patients with AIDS and AIDS-related complex. A double-blind, placebo-controlled trial. N Engl J Med 317:185, 1987

11. Richman DD, Fischl MA, Grieco MH et al: The toxicity of azidothymidine (AZT) in the treatment of patients with AIDS and AIDS-related complex. N Engl J Med 317:192, 1987

12. Shaw GM, Hahn BH, Arya SK et al: Molecular characterization of human T-cell leukemia (lymphotropic) virus type III in the acquired immune deficiency syndrome. Science 226:1165, 1984

13. Montagnier L, Gruest J, Chamaret S et al: Adaptation of lymphadenopathy associated virus (LAV) to replication in EBV-transformed B lymphoblastoid cell lines. Science 225:63, 1984

14. Gartner S, Markovits P, Markovitz DM et al: The role of mononuclear phagocytes in HTLV-III/LAV infection. Science 233:215, 1986

15. Hoxie JA, Haggarty BS, Rackowski JL et al: Persistent noncytopathic infection of normal human T lymphocytes with AIDS-associated retrovirus. Science 229:1400, 1985

16. Folks T, Powell DM, Lightfoote MM et al: Induction of HTLV-III/LAV from a non-virus producing T cell line: Implications for latency. Science 231:600, 1986

17. Zagury D, Bernard J, Leonard R et al: Long-term cultures of HTLV-III-infected T cells: A model of cytopathology of T-cell depletion in AIDS. Science 231:850, 1986

18. Shaw GM, Harper ME, Hahn BH et al: HTLV-III infection in brains of children and adults with AIDS encephalopathy. Science 277:177, 1985

19. Ho DD, Rota TR, Schooley RT et al: Isolation of HTLV-III from cerebrospinal fluid and neural tissues of patients with neurologic syndromes related to the acquired immunodeficiency syndrome. N Engl J Med 313:1493, 1985

20. Resnick L, diMarzo–Veronese F, Schüpbach J et al: Intra-blood–brain-barrier synthesis of HTLV-III-specific IgG in patients with neurologic symptoms associated with AIDS or AIDS-related complex. N Engl J Med 313:1498, 1985

21. Navia BA, Jordan BD, Price RW: The AIDS dementia complex. I. Clinical features. Ann Neurol 19:517, 1986

22. Lifson JD, Reyes G, McGrath MS et al: AIDS retrovirus induced cytopathology: Giant cell formation and involvement of CD4 antigen. Science 232:1123, 1986

23. Lifson JD, Feinberg MB, Reyes GR et al: Induction of CD4-dependent cell fusion by the HTLV-III/LAV envelope glycoprotein. Nature 323:725, 1986

24. Mitsuya H, Broder S: Inhibition of the *in vitro* infectivity and cytopathic effect of human T-lymphotropic virus type III/lymphadenopathy-associated virus (HTLV-III/LAV) by 2',3'-dideoxynucleosides. Proc Natl Acad Sci USA 83:1911, 1986

25. Mitsuya H, Broder S: Strategies for antiviral therapy in AIDS. Nature 325:773, 1987

26. Furman PA, Fyfe JA, St. Clair MH et al: Phosphorylation of 3'-azido-3'-deoxythymidine and selective interaction of the 5'-triphosphate with human immunodeficiency virus reverse transcriptase. Proc Natl Acad Sci USA 83:8333, 1986

27. Waqar MA, Evans MJ, Manly KF et al: Effects of 2',3'-dideoxynucleosides on mammalian cells and viruses. J Cell Physiol 121:402, 1984

28. Mitsuya H, Jarrett RF, Matsukura M et al: Long-term inhibition of human T-lymphotropic virus type III/lymphadenopathy-associated virus (human immunodeficiency virus) DNA synthesis and RNA expression in T cells protected by 2',3'-dideoxynucleosides *in vitro*. Proc Natl Acad Sci USA 84:2033, 1987

29. Kim C–H, Marquez VE, Broder S et al: Potential anti-AIDS drugs. 2',3'-dideoxycytidine analogues. J Medicinal Chem 30:862, 1987

30. Balzarini J, Pauwels R, Herdewijn P et al: Potent and selective activity of 2',3'-dideoxycytidinene, the 2',3'-unsaturated derivative of 2',3'-dideoxycytidine. Biochem Biophys Res Comm 140:735, 1986

31. Hamamoto Y, Nakashima H, Matsui T et al: Inhibitory effect of 2',3'-didehydro-2',3'-dideoxynucleosides of infectivity, cytopathic effects, and replication of human immunodeficiency virus. Antimicrob Ag Chemother 31:907, 1987

32. Balzarini J, Kang G–J, Dalal M et al: The anti-HTLV-III (anti-HIV) and cytotoxic activity of 2',3'-didehydro-2',3'-dideoxyribonucleosides: A comparison with their parental 2',3'-dideoxynucleosides. Mol Pharmacol 32:162, 1987

33. Mitsuya H, Matsukura M, Broder S: Rapid *in vitro* systems for assessing activity of agents against HTLV-III/LAV. In Broder S (ed): AIDS: Modern concepts and therapeutic challenges. p 303. New York, Marcel Dekker, 1987

34. Schinazi RF, Chu C–K, Ahn M–K et al: Selective *in vitro* inhibition of human immunodeficiency virus (HIV) replication by 3'-azido-2',3'-dideoxyuridine (CS-87). J Clin Biochem 11D[Suppl]:74, 1987

35. Herdewijn P, Balzarini J, De Clercq E et al: 3'-substituted 2',3'-dideoxynucleoside analogues as potential anti-HIV (HTLV-III/LAV) agents. J Medicinal Chem 30:1270, 1987

36. Eriksson B, Vrang L, Bazin H et al: Different patterns of inhibition of avian myeloblastosis virus reverse transcriptase activity by 3'-azido-3'-deoxythymidine 5'-triphosphate and its *threo* isomer. Antimicrob Ag Chemother 31:600, 1987

37. Hao Z, Dalal M, Cooney DA et al: A comparison of 2',3'-dideoxynucleoside-5'-triphosphates as inhibitors of retroviral reverse transcriptases. Proc Am Assoc Cancer Res 28:323, 1987

38. Cooney DA, Dalal M, Mitsuya H et al: Initial studies on the cellular pharmacology of 2',3'-dideoxycytidine, an inhibitor of HTLV-III infectivity. Biochem Pharmacol 35:2065, 1986

39. Starnes MC, Cheng Y–C: Cellular metabolism of 2',3'-dideoxycytidine, a compound active against human immunodeficiency virus *in vitro*. J Biol Chem 262:988, 1987

40. Cooney DA, Ahluwalia G, Mitsuya H et al: Initial studies on the cellular pharmacology of 2',3'-dideoxyadenosine, an inhibitor of HTLV-III infectivity. Biochem Pharmacol 36·1765, 1987

41. Perno C–F, Yarchoan R, Tosato G et al: Activity of dideoxynucleosides against HTLV-III/LAV *in vitro* in different human cells. Abstracts of the III International Conference on AIDS, June 1–5, 1987, Washington DC, p 165

42. Yarchoan R, Broder S: Strategies for the pharmacological intervention against HTLV-III/LAV. In Broder S (ed):

AIDS: Modern Concepts and Therapeutic Challenges, p 335. New York, Marcel Dekker, 1987

43. Klecker RW, Collins JM, Yarchoan R et al: Plasma and cerebrospinal fluid pharmacokinetics of 3'-azido-3'-deoxythymidine: A novel pyrimidine analog with potential application for the treatment of AIDS and related disorders. Clin Pharmacol Ther 41:407, 1987

44. de Miranda P, Good SS, Blom MR et al: The effect of probenecid on the pharmacokinetic disposition of azidothymidine (AZT). International Conference on Acquired Immunodeficiency Syndrome (AIDS), Paris, June 23–25, 1986 (Abstr)

45. Yarchoan R, Berg G, Brouwers P et al: Response of human-immunodeficiency-virus–associated neurological disease to 3'-azido-3'-deoxythymidine. Lancet 1:132, 1987

46. Markham PD, Salahuddin SZ, Popovic M et al: Advances in the isolation of HTLV-III from patients with AIDS and AIDS-related complex and from donors at risk. Cancer Res 45:4588S, 1985

47. Yarchoan R, Broder S: Progress in the development of antiviral therapy for HTLV-III-associated diseases. In DeVita VT, Hellman S, Rosenberg SA (eds): Important Advances in Oncology 1987, p 293. Philadelphia, JB Lippincott, 1987

48. Yarchoan R, Broder S: Development of antiretroviral therapy for the acquired immunodeficiency syndrome and related disorders: A progress report. N Engl J Med 316: 557, 1987

49. Hagler DN, Frame PT: Azidothymidine neurotoxicity. Lancet 2:1392, 1986

50. Chaisson RE, Allain J–P, Leuther M et al: Significant changes in HIV antigen level in the serum of patients treated with azidothymidine. N Engl J Med 315:1610, 1986

51. Ziegler JL, Beckstead JA, Volberding PA et al: Non-Hodgkin's lymphoma in 90 homosexual men. Relation to generalized lymphadenopathy and the acquired immunodeficiency syndrome. N Engl J Med 311:565, 1984

52. Birx DL, Redfield RR, Tosato G: Defective regulation of Epstein–Barr virus infection in patients with acquired immunodeficiency syndrome (AIDS) or AIDS-related disorders. N Engl J Med 314:874, 1986

53. Yarchoan R, Redfield RR, Broder S: Mechanisms of B cell activation in patients with acquired immunodeficiency syndrome and related disorders: Contribution of antibody-producing B cells, of Epstein–Barr virus–infected B cells, and of immunoglobulin production induced by human T cell lymphotropic virus, type III/lymphadenopathy-associated virus. J Clin Invest 78:439, 1986

54. Pahwa S, Pahwa R, Saxinger C et al: Influence of the human T-lymphotropic virus/lymphadenopathy–associated virus on the functions of human lymphocytes: Evidence for immunosuppressive effects and polyclonal B-cell activation by banded virus preparations. Proc Natl Acad Sci USA 82:8198, 1985

55. Schnittman SM, Lane HC, Higgins SE et al: Direct polyclonal activation of human B lymphocytes by the acquired immune deficiency syndrome virus. Science 233:1084, 1986

56. Waldmann TA, Misiti JM, Nelson DL et al: Ataxia-telangiectasia: A multisystem disease with immunodeficiency, impaired organ maturation, x-ray hypersensitivity, and a high incidence of neoplasia. Ann Intern Med 99:367, 1983

57. Yarchoan R, Broder S: Preliminary results on the use of dideoxynucleosides in the therapy of AIDS. In Chanock RM, Lerner RA, Brown F et al (eds): Vaccine 87. Cold Spring Harbor, NY Cold Spring Harbor Press (In preparation)

58. Walker R, Lane HC, Masur H et al: Therapy of AIDS patients with early Kaposi's sarcoma with 3'-azido-3'-deoxythymidine. Abstracts of the III International Conference on AIDS, June 1987, Washington, DC, p 58

59. Safai B, Johnson KG, Myskowski PL et al: The natural history of Kaposi's sarcoma in the acquired immunodeficiency syndrome. Ann Intern Med 103:744, 1985

60. Horwitz JP, Chua J, Noel M: Nucleosides. V. The monomesylates of 1-(2'-deoxy-beta-D-lyxofuranosyl)thymidine. J Organ Chem 29:2076, 1964

61. Salahuddin Z, Nakamura S, Biberfeld P et al: Development of clonal lines from Kaposi's sarcoma (KS) lesion (AIDS-KS) and their biological properties. Abstracts of the III International Conference on AIDS, June 1987, Washington, DC, p 111

62. Yarchoan R, Thomas RV, Fischl MA et al: Treatment of human immunodeficiency virus–associated neurological disease with 3'-azido-2',3'-dideoxythymidine. In D Bolognesi (ed): Human Retroviruses, Cancer, and AIDS: Approach to Prevention and Therapy. UCLA Symposia on Molecular and Cellular Biology, New Series, Vol 71. New York, Alan Liss, 1987

63. Janssen RS, Saykin A, Kaplan J et al: Neurologic and neuropsychological complications of lymphadenopathy syndrome. Abstracts of the III International Conference on AIDS, June 1987, Washington, DC, p 55

64. Navia BA, Cho E–S, Petito CK et al: The AIDS dementia complex. II. Neuropathology. Ann Neurol 19:525, 1986

65. Gartner S, Markovits P, Markovitz DM et al: Virus isolation from and identification of HTLV-III/LAV-producing cells in brain tissue from a patient with AIDS. JAMA 256:2365, 1986

66. Koenig S, Gendelman HE, Orenstien JM et al: Detection of AIDS virus in macrophages in brain tissue from AIDS patients with encephalopathy. Science 233:1089, 1986

67. Maddon PJ, Dalgleish AG, McDougal JS et al: The T4 gene encodes the AIDS virus receptor and is expressed in the immune system and the brain. Cell 47:333, 1986

68. Pert CB, Hill JM, Ruff MR et al: Octapeptides deduced from the neuropeptide receptor-like pattern of antigen T4 in brain potently inhibit human immunodeficiency virus receptor binding and T-cell infectivity. Proc Natl Acad Sci USA 83:9254, 1986

69. Gurney ME, Heinrich SP, Lee MR et al: Molecular cloning and expression of neuroleukin, a neurotrophic factor for spinal and sensory neurons. Science 234:566, 1986

70. Sharpe AH, Jaenisch R, Ruprecht RM: Retroviruses and mouse embryos: A rapid model for neurovirulence and transplacental antiviral therapy. Science 236:1671, 1987

71. Kelly JA, Litterst CL, Roth JS et al: The disposition and metabolism of 2',3'-dideoxycytidine, an *in vitro* inhibitor of HTLV-III infectivity, in mice and monkeys. Drug Metab Dispos 15:595, 1987

72. Mitsuya H, Popovic M, Yarchoan R et al: Suramin protection of T cells in vitro against infectivity and cytopathic effect of HTLV-III. Science 226:172, 1984

73. Chermann JC, Sinoussi F, Jasmin C: Inhibition of RNA-dependent DNA polymerase of murine oncornaviruses by 5-tungsto-2-antimoniate. Biochem Biophys Res Comm 65:1229, 1975

74. Sandstrom EG, Kaplan JC, Byington RE et al: Inhibition of human T-cell lymphotropic virus type III in vitro by phosphonoformate. Lancet 1:1480, 1985

75. Sarin PS, Taguchi Y, Sun D et al: Inhibition of HTLV-III/LAV replication by foscarnet. Biochem Pharmacol 34: 4075, 1985

76. Anand R, Moore J, Feorino P et al: Rifabitine inhibits HTLV-III. Lancet 1:97, 1986

77. De Clercq E: Suramin: A potent inhibitor of the reverse transcriptase of RNA tumor viruses. Cancer Lett 8:9, 1979

78. Broder S, Yarchoan R, Collins JM et al: Effects of suramin on HTLV-III/LAV infection presenting as Kaposi's sarcoma or AIDS-related complex: Clinical pharmacology and suppression of virus replication in vitro. Lancet 1: 627, 1985

79. Helgstrand E, Eriksson B, Johansson NG et al: Trisodium phosphonoformate: A new antiviral compound. Science 201:819, 1978

80. Ting RC, Yang SS, Gallo RC: Reverse transcriptase, RNA tumour virus transformation, and derivatives of rifamycin SV. Nat New Biol 236:163, 1972

81. Sarin PS, Gallo RC, Scheer DI et al: Effects of a novel compound (AL 721) on HTLV-III infectivity in vitro. N Engl J Med 313:1289, 1985

82. Barnes DM: Debate over potential AIDS drug. Science 237:128, 1987

83. Wetterberg L, Alexius B, Sääf J et al: Peptide T in treatment of AIDS. Lancet 1:159, 1987

84. Ho DD, Hartshorn KL, Rota TR et al: Recombinant human interferon alpha-A suppresses HTLV-III replication in vitro. Lancet 1:602, 1985

85. Yamamoto JK, Barré-Sinoussi F, Bolton V et al: Human alpha- and beta-interferon but not gamma- suppress the in vitro replication of LAV, HTLV-III, and ARV-2. J Interferon Res 6:143, 1986

86. Krown SE, Real FX, Cunningham–Rundles S et al: Preliminary observations on the effect of recombinant leukocyte A interferon in homosexual men with Kaposi's sarcoma. N Engl J Med 308:1071, 1983

87. Groopman JE, Gottlieb MS, Goodman J et al: Recombinant alpha-2 interferon therapy for Kaposi's sarcoma associated with the acquired immunodeficiency syndrome. Ann Intern Med 100:671, 1984

88. Gelmann EP, Preble OT, Steis R et al: Human lymphoblastoid interferon treatment of Kaposi's sarcoma in the acquired immunodeficiency syndrome. Am J Med 78:737, 1985

89. McCormick JB, Getchell JP, Mitchell SW et al: Ribavirin suppresses replication of lymphadenopathy-associated virus in cultures of human adult T lymphocytes. Lancet 2:1367, 1984

90. Ito M, Baba M, Sato A et al: Inhibitory effect of dextran sulfate and heparin on the replication of human immunodeficiency virus (HIV) in vitro. Antiviral Res 7:361, 1987

91. Hammer SM, Gillis JM, Groopman JE et al: In vitro modification of human immunodeficiency virus infection by granulocyte-macrophage colony-stimulating factor and gamma interferon. Proc Natl Acad Sci USA 83:8734, 1986

92. Hammer SM, Gillis JM: Synergistic activity of granulocyte-macrophage colony-stimulating factor and 3'-azido-3'-deoxythymidine against human immunodeficiency virus in vitro. Antimicrob Ag Chemother 31:1046, 1987

93. Dolin R: Antiviral chemotherapy and chemoprophylaxis. Science 227:1296, 1985

94. Vernon A, Schulof RS, the Ribavirin ARC Study Group: Serum HIV core antigen in symptomatic ARC patients taking oral ribavirin or placebo. Proceedings of the III International Conference on AIDS, June 1987, Washington, DC, p 58

95. DeVita VT, Schein PS: The use of drugs in combination for the treatment of cancer: Rationale and results. N Engl J Med 288:998, 1973

96. Hartshorn KL, Vogt MW, Chou T–C et al: Synergistic inhibition of human immunodeficiency virus in vitro by azidothymidine and recombinant interferon alpha-A. Antimicrob Ag Chemother 31:168, 1987

97. Mitchell WM, Montefiori DC, Robinson WE et al: Mismatched ds RNA (Ampligen) reduces the concentration of 3'-azido-3'-deoxythymidine (AZT) required for the in vitro inhibition of human immunodeficiency virus. Lancet 1:890, 1987

98. Ueno R, Kuno S: Dextran sulfate, a potent anti-HIV agent in vitro having synergism with zidovudine. Lancet 1:1379, 1987

99. Vogt MW, Hartshorn KL, Furman PA et al: Ribavirin antagonizes the effect of azidothymidine on HIV replication. Science 235:1376, 1987

100. Carter WA, Strayer DR, Brodsky I et al: Clinical, immunological, and virological effects of Ampligen, a mismatched double stranded RNA, in patients with AIDS or AIDS-related complex. Lancet 1:1286, 1987

101. Danner SA, Schuurman H–J, Lange JMA et al: Implantation of cultured thymic fragments in patients with acquired immunodeficiency syndrome. Arch Intern Med 146:1133, 1986

102. Hong R: Reconstitution of T-cell deficiency by thymic hormone or thymus transplantation therapy. Clin Immunol Immunopathol 40:136, 1986

103. Ernst M, Kern P, Flad H–D et al: Effects of systemic in vivo interleukin-2 (IL-2) reconstitution in patients with acquired immune deficiency syndrome (AIDS) and AIDS-related complex (ARC) on phenotypes and functions of peripheral blood mononuclear cells. J Clin Immunol 6: 170, 1986

104. Dahlberg JE, Mitsuya H, Blam SB et al: Broad spectrum antiretroviral activity of 2',3'-dideoxynucleosides. Proc Natl Acad Sci USA 84:2469, 1987

105. Yarchoan R, Mitsuya H, Matsushita S et al: Implications of the discovery of HTLV-III for the treatment of AIDS. Cancer Res 45:4685S, 1985

106. Matsushita S, Mitsuya H, Reitz M et al: Pharmacological inhibition of the in vitro infectivity of human T lymphotropic virus type I. J Clin Invest 80:394, 1987

107. Bunn PA, Schechter GP, Jaffe E et al: Clinical course of retrovirus-associated adult T-cell lymphoma in the United States. N Engl J Med 309:257, 1983

108. Popovic M, Flomenberg N, Volkman DJ et al: Alteration of T-cell functions by infection with HTLV-I or HTLV-II. Science 226:459, 1984

109. Yarchoan R, Guo H–G, Reitz M et al: Alterations in cytotoxic and helper T cell function after infection of T cell clones with human T cell leukemia virus, type I. J Clin Invest 77:1466, 1986

110. Gessain A, Barin F, Vernant JC et al: Antibodies to human T-lymphotropic virus type-I in patients with tropical spastic paraparesis. Lancet 2:407, 1985

111. Osame M, Usuku K, Izumo S et al: HTLV-I-associated myelopathy: A new clinical entity. Lancet 1:1031, 1986

112. Kanki PJ, Barin F, M'Boup S et al: New human T-lymphotropic retrovirus related to simian T-lymphotropic virus type III (STLV-III$_{AGM}$). Science 232:238, 1986

113. Clavel F, Guétard F, Brun-Vézinet F et al: Isolation of a new human retrovirus from West African patients with AIDS. Science 23:343, 1986

114. Koprowski H, DeFreitas EC, Harper ME et al: Multiple sclerosis and human T-cell lymphotropic viruses. Nature 318:154, 1985

Other Agents in the Treatment of AIDS

Bruce Polsky
Donald Armstrong

17

As discussed in the previous chapter, the only proven effective treatment for human immunodeficiency virus (HIV) infection is zidovudine, a nucleoside analog. However, before HIV was identified as the etiologic agent of AIDS, α-interferon produced clinical responses in some patients with Kaposi's sarcoma;[1] the mechanism underlying this response remains unclear. Zidovudine has been shown to prolong life and decrease the severity and number of opportunistic infections in a subset of patients with AIDS.[2] Indeed, the most promising compounds in preclinical evaluation to date have belonged to the nucleoside analog class.[3] However, compounds other than nucleoside analogs have shown activity against HIV infection *in vitro* and have at least entered the early stages of clinical evaluation. For some of these agents, reproducible assessment of *in vitro* activity has been difficult to obtain, slowing their clinical development. Others, when combined with nucleoside analogs, have resulted in a synergistic anti-HIV effect *in vitro*. For each compound under consideration we will review the *in vitro* evidence for anti-HIV activity and proposed mode of action; for each we will also discuss the status of clinical development.

We have divided the various agents according to the proposed site of action for each in the HIV replicative cycle (Table 17-1) and will use this format in the following discussion.

ATTACHMENT AND PENETRATION

The initial step in the HIV replicative cycle is attachment of the HIV envelope glycoprotein (gp120) to the CD4 molecule on cells bearing this receptor. Following attachment, penetration into the cell occurs, most likely by way of endocytosis. There are several compounds believed to exert an anti-HIV effect at this step.

AL-721

AL-721 (active lipid) is a lipid mixture composed of neutral glycerides, phosphatidylcholine, and phosphatidylethanolamine in a 7:2:1 ratio. This particular combination of lipids is considered responsible for the drug's ability to modify cell membrane lipid composition and act as a "membrane fluidizer."[4] There is a single published report demonstrating an *in vitro* anti-HIV effect in a tissue culture system;[5] others have not succeeded in reproducing the results of these experiments.* Because the HIV envelope is rich in lipid, it is postulated that AL-721 may alter the structure of the viral envelope or the host cell membrane and thus interfere with attachment and penetration.[6] In a preliminary study in eight patients at one center, the drug appeared to be well tolerated.[7] Further phase I studies are planned in the National Institutes of Health AIDS Treatment Evaluation Units (ATEUs).

Peptide T

Peptide T is a synthetic octapeptide sequence (Ala-Ser-Thr-Thr-Thr-Asn-Tyr-Thr) that is believed to be homologous with a region of the HIV envelope (gp120). Since HIV infection appears to require a specific interaction between gp120 and the CD4 molecule,[8] blocking of CD4 by peptide T might inhibit infection of the target cell. In one laboratory, peptide T potently inhibited HIV infection in an *in vitro* tissue culture system.[9] We and others have been unable to duplicate these results.[10] A report of a pilot clinical study from the Karolinska Institute in Sweden found the drug safe in the four subjects studied.[11] The question of *in vitro* anti-HIV activity must

* Polsky B et al: Unpublished data

295

Table 17-1
Proposed Sites of Action of Antiretroviral Agents in the HIV Replicative Cycle

	In Vitro	In Vivo
Attachment and Penetration		
AL721	Limited evidence of activity	Phase I trials
Peptide T	Conflicting evidence for activity	Phase I trials
Castanospermine	Inhibits syncytium formation in CD4-positive cells	Preclinical
? Others (e.g., amphotericin B methyl ester, gossypol)		
Reverse Transcription		
Suramin	Inhibits reverse transcriptase	Phase I/II trials no clinical benefit; marked toxicity
Antimoniotungstate (HPA-23)	Inhibits reverse transcriptase	Phase I/II trials +/− inhibition of viral replication; hematologic toxicity
Phosphonoformate (Foscarnet)	Inhibits reverse transcriptase; synergy with zidovudine	Phase I trials; nephrotoxicity
Rifabutin (ansamycin)	Inhibits reverse transcriptase	Phase I trials; well tolerated; crosses blood–brain barrier
2′,3′-dideoxynucleoside analogs	Inhibits reverse transcriptase	Phase III trials
Transactivation and Transcription		
? "Anti-sense" RNA oligonucleotides	May be targeted to compete with specific genes (e.g., *tat, trs/art*)	Preclinical
Postranscriptional Processing and Translation		
Ribavirin	? Inhibits 5′-capping of messenger RNA	Phase I/II trials
Ampligen	? Cleaves viral RNA or interrupts viral protein synthesis ? Interferon induction	Phase I trials—inhibits virus replication in some cases
? Interferons		
? "Anti-sense" RNA oligonucleotides	Competitive inhibitors of hybridization	Preclinical
Fusidic acid	? Inhibits translocation of ribosomes	Phase I in Europe
Assembly and Release		
Interferons	Alpha-interferon synergistic with zidovudine, dideoxycytidine, phosphonoformate	Alpha interferon effective in KS; phase I trials in combination with zidovudine
Granulocyte–macrophage colony-stimulating factor (GM-CSF)	Inhibits HIV infection of monocytoid cell line; synergistic with zidovudine	Increases leukocytes in leukopenic AIDS patients in phase I/II study
Other or Uncertain		
Biologic response modifiers		Trials in combination with antiretroviral agents planned
Bone marrow transplantation		Preliminary evidence for immune reconstitution when combined with antiretroviral agents

be settled before this agent is studied in larger clinical trials.

Castanospermine

Castanospermine (1,6,7,8-tetrahydroxyoctahydroindolizine) is a plant alkaloid that inhibits glucosidase I, an enzyme important for the normal processing of glycoproteins. In a transfected CD4[+] cell line expressing the *env* gene, castanospermine inhibited syncytium formation.[12] In H9 cells, castanospermine protected against acute HIV infection. Current evidence suggests that this agent induces changes in the HIV envelope glycoprotein rather than the CD4 molecule on the cell membrane.[12] Further *in vitro* work to better define the role of this drug in the treatment of HIV infection, as well as animal toxicology studies, will be necessary prior to planning clinical trials.

Other Drugs

In addition to the drugs discussed above, other compounds have exhibited anti-HIV activity *in vitro* and warrant mention.

Amphotericin B methyl ester (AME) is a derivative of the polyene macrolide antifungal agent amphotericin B. Amphotericin B binds with sterols, causing changes in cell permeability. This is the basis for its antifungal activity. AME has been reported to protect cells in culture from HIV infection at concentrations that were not toxic to uninfected cells.[13] In the same study, amphotericin B also protected the cells from HIV infection, although it was considerably more toxic than AME. It has been proposed that AME binds to sterols of the lipid-enveloped HIV, resulting in a loss of infectivity. Reports of irreversible leukoencephalopathy with AME when used as experimental treatment for systemic mycoses[14] mandates caution in the further development of this agent.

Gossypol is a polyphenolic aldehyde isolated from cottonseed. This drug has been widely studied in China for its male antifertility effects. In our laboratory, high concentrations of gossypol inactivate HIV in an *in vitro* system.[15] Because of its chemical structure, gossypol would most likely bind to the virus envelope.

REVERSE TRANSCRIPTION

Inhibition of reverse transcriptase is the most virus-specific target for the anti-HIV agents currently under investigation. Reverse transcription is necessary for viral replication, allowing HIV genomic RNA to serve as a template for DNA synthesis. Such RNA-directed DNA synthesis does not occur in the host cell; therefore, reverse transciptase activity may be considered a unique function of the virus. For this reason and because of the experience with nucleoside analogs as antiviral and antineoplastic agents, it was logical that this class of drugs, aimed at the enzymes directing DNA synthesis, be the first developed for clinical use. Zidovudine is the prototype for drugs acting at the level of reverse transcriptase inhibition. As discussed in the previous chapter, other nucleoside analogs are in various stages of preclinical and clinical development.[3]

Compounds other than nucleoside analogs inhibit reverse transcriptase. Among these are suramin and antimoniotungstate (HPA-23), two of the earliest drugs studied in clinical trials.

Suramin

Suramin sodium, a hexasodium salt derivative of naphthalenetrisulfonic acid, is a drug that has been used for over 50 years in the treatment of African trypanosomiasis and onchocerciasis. Suramin has been known since 1979 as a strong competitive inhibitor of reverse transcriptase activity in several animal retroviruses.[16] However, suramin may also inhibit certain cellular DNA polymerases and is therefore not a specific reverse transcriptase inhibitor.

Suramin was the first compound identified with anti-HIV activity *in vitro*. In 1984, Mitsuya and co-workers, using an immortalized OKT4[+] T-cell clone (ATH8) highly sensitive to the cytopathic effect of HIV, reported partial protection against this cytopathic effect at 10 and 25 μg/ml and complete protection at 50 μg/ml.[17] No inhibition of ATH8 cell growth or lymphocyte proliferative response to antigens or mitogens was noted until concentrations of 100 μg/ml and greater were studied. Armed with these *in vitro* observations, and the knowledge that *in vivo* suramin concentrations in excess of 100 μg/ml had been achieved during the treatment of parasitic diseases, clinical studies of suramin in patients with AIDS-related Kaposi's sarcoma and AIDS-related complex (ARC) were undertaken.

There have been several clinical studies of suramin in patients with Kaposi's sarcoma and ARC.[18-21] These studies suggest that suramin, in the short term, may decrease detectable HIV viremia in some patients; however, this was not substantiated over the course of these studies. There was no improvement in studies of immune function and 52 of the 98 patients developed progressive disease as evidenced by new opportunistic infections, new or accelerated progression of Kaposi's sarcoma or lymphoma, and encephalopathy while under study. The suramin clinical trials were most remarkable for the toxicity seen in the participants.[21] The most common toxicities observed consisted of fever (78%), rash (48%), malaise (43%), anorexia (35%), nausea (34%), neutropenia (26%), vomiting (20%), elevation of serum creatinine (12%), thrombocytopenia (12%), and stomatitis (5%). Liver dysfunction occurred in 14% of patients with fatal hepatic failure in three patients. Clinical and/or laboratory evidence of adrenal insufficiency as a late complication of suramin treatment developed in 23%. This finding correlates with the observation of adrenal cortical injury seen in guinea pigs treated with suramin.[22] Rat adrenals, however, appear to be resistant to this effect of suramin.[23] The drug was discontinued in 30% of patients because of either toxicity (20%) or noncompliance (10%).

These studies demonstrate that suramin is highly toxic and is without apparent clinical, virologic, or immunologic benefit to individuals with HIV disease. At this point, suramin has no role in the treatment of HIV infection.

Antimoniotungstate (Heteropolyanion-23, HPA-23)

HPA-23 is a mineral-condensed polyanion of ammonium 5-tungsto-2-antimoniate that acts as a competitive inhibitor of the reverse transcriptases of murine oncornaviruses as well as HIV.[24] The drug was developed in the early 1970s as a possible treatment for Creutzfeld–Jacob disease. In phase I studies in patients with AIDS or ARC, HPA-23 was associated with a transient reduction in reverse transcriptase activity in supernatants from peripheral blood mononuclear cell cultures.[25] In these same studies, thrombocytopenia developed consistently and was related to the duration of therapy. Other adverse reactions included leukopenia, elevation of serum transaminases and creatinine, and a metallic taste. In most cases the toxicity was reversed when HPA-23 was discontinued. Clinical trials designed to evaluate efficacy will be required in order to determine the value of HPA-23 in the treatment of HIV infection.

Phosphonoformate (Foscarnet)

Trisodium phosphonoformate, a pyrophosphate analog, is an inhibitor of herpesvirus DNA polymerases and has been studied in Europe for the treatment of herpes simplex and cytomegalovirus (CMV) infections. Oberg has shown that phosphonoformate acts as a noncompetitive inhibitor for templates and substrates of reverse transcriptases from a wide range of animal retroviruses[26] and, more recently, from HIV reverse transcriptase.[27] *In vitro,* dose-dependent inhibition of HIV infection is seen at concentrations easily achieved *in vivo;*[28] and synergistic inhibition is observed *in vitro* when phosphonoformate is combined with α-interferon.[29] In addition, phosphonoformate is known to cross the blood–brain barrier,[30] an important property for candidate anti-HIV drugs. In short-term pilot studies in patients with AIDS and ARC, phosphonoformate was well tolerated and there was a suggestion of anti-HIV activity as measured by virus isolation and circulating HIV antigen.[31,32] Because of the experience with phosphonoformate in bone marrow and renal transplant patients with CMV infections,[30,33] nephrotoxicity was anticipated and was the leading adverse reaction seen in patients with HIV infection.[31,32] Phosphonoformate is of particular interest because of its activity against CMV, one of the major opportunistic infections seen in patients with AIDS.[34] Studies to assess the safety and efficacy of phosphonoformate in CMV retinitis and HIV infection are currently underway in the ATEUs.

Rifabutin

Rifabutin (ansamycin, LM427) is a semisynthetic derivative of rifamycin S and has considerable *in vitro* activity against mycobacteria, including *Mycobacterium avium-intracellulare* (MAI). There has been considerable clinical experience with this drug in the treatment of disseminated MAI infection in patients with AIDS. Although the drug appears to be relatively safe, evidence of efficacy in the treatment of MAI infection in the setting of AIDS is lacking.[35] In one laboratory, rifabutin inhibited HIV infection of peripheral blood mononuclear cells *in vitro.*[36] In animal retrovirus models, rifamycins bind to reverse transcriptase, perhaps inhibiting virus replication.[37] Rifabutin is assumed to inhibit HIV replication by means of a similar mechanism. A phase I study of this drug has revealed that daily doses of 600 mg are not associated with toxicity; however, there does not appear to be any clinical benefit or antiviral effect *in vivo* at this dose.[38] The same investigators have reported that rifabutin crosses the blood–brain barrier.[39] They are currently investigating higher doses of rifabutin.

TRANSACTIVATION AND TRANSCRIPTION

The HIV genome includes two genes, *tat* and *trs/art,* coding for factors that regulate the post-transcriptional or transcriptional expression of the HIV structural genes, *gag, pol,* and *env.*[40–43] The *tat* and *trs/art* genes are required for HIV synthesis; when either gene is inactivated, virus replication is halted.[44] In the future, drugs may be developed that specifically bind to and block the function of these regulatory genes and their products, resulting in decreased HIV replication.

A possible approach to inhibiting specific functions of genes or their products may be the use of oligonucleotides synthesized as complementary sequences targeted at specific regions of HIV genomic RNA or messenger RNA (mRNA). These so-called anti-sense oligonucleotides may serve as competitive inhibitors of hybridization at the level of transcription or translation. One could therefore imagine an "anti-sense RNA" designed to compete with *tat* or *trs/art* function. Although certain anti-sense synthetic oligonucleotides inhibit the replication of HIV *in vitro,*[45] the applicability of such an approach *in vivo* remains uncertain.

POST-TRANSCRIPTIONAL PROCESSING AND TRANSLATION

Following reverse transcription and integration of proviral DNA into host chromosomal DNA, the integrated sequences are transcribed into viral mRNA, which is subsequently translated into viral proteins. During post-transcriptional processing, the viral mRNA is modified. The 5' end is "capped" by methylated guanosine residues and the 3' end is polyadenylated. The 5' triphosphate of ribavirin is known to inhibit guanyl transferase, responsible for the capping of the 5' end of mRNA; this is the proposed site of action for HIV inhibition by ribavirin.[46] Clinical experience with ribavirin, a nucleoside analog, has been covered in detail in the chapter on this class of compounds.

Ampligen

Double-stranded RNAs (dsRNAs) are believed to promote the production of various lymphokines, including tumor necrosis factor, and interferons.[47] Certain cellular enzymes dependent on dsRNAs, such as 2'-5'-oligoadenylate synthetase and a protein kinase, are thought to inhibit the replication of some viruses through the cleavage of viral RNA or by blocking viral protein synthesis.[48] Ampligen, a mismatched double-stranded RNA poly(I):poly(C_{12},U), has been reported to inhibit the replication of HIV *in vitro*.[49] When ampligen was combined with zidovudine, at least additive and perhaps synergistic inhibition of HIV infection was observed.[50] Though its precise mechanism of action is unclear, ampligen is believed to exert its anti-HIV effect through a combination of lymphokine induction and as a co-factor for the synthetase and kinase functions discussed above. In an 18-week pilot study of 10 patients with AIDS, ARC, or persistent generalized lymphadenopathy,[51] treatment with ampligen was associated with a reduction in HIV replication *in vivo* as measured by molecular hybridization, culture of peripheral blood mononuclear cells, or circulating HIV antigens; augmentation of delayed hypersensitivity skin reactions; and a suggestion of clinical improvement in the patients with ARC or lymphadenopathy, but not in the patients with AIDS. No toxicity attributable to ampligen was seen in any of the 10 patients. These preliminary results are promising; however, larger numbers of individuals treated over a longer period of time will be required in order to properly assess the value of ampligen in the treatment of HIV infection. A multicenter phase II study of ampligen in patients with ARC is currently in progress.

Other Drugs

As discussed in the section on transactivation and transcription, the anti-sense RNA approach may have applicability at the level of translation as targeted competitive inhibitors of hybridization at specific regions of mRNA.

Fusidic acid, a steroidal antibiotic product of the fungus *Fusicidium coccineum*[52] with activity against *Mycobacterium tuberculosis,* has recently been reported to inhibit HIV replication *in vitro*.[53] Because fusidic acid inhibits the translocation of ribosomes,[54] it is speculated that it may be acting at the level of HIV protein synthesis. Confirmation of these *in vitro* results will be required before clinical studies of fusidic acid in HIV infection are planned.

ASSEMBLY AND RELEASE

The final steps of the HIV replicative cycle include the processing of viral proteins in the rough endoplasmic reticulum by proteases and enzymes involved in glycosylation and myristylation.[55,56] The processed viral proteins are then transported through the Golgi apparatus to the plasma membrane where they, along with the HIV genomic RNA, are assembled. Ultimately, the virus particles are released by budding from the plasma membrane of the infected host cell. Although the molecular mechanisms are unclear, certain members of the group of naturally occurring substances known generically as "cytokines" are believed to inhibit HIV assembly and release. Inhibitors of glycosylation, such as castanospermine, may have a role at this stage of the HIV life cycle.

Interferons

Interferons are naturally occurring proteins with activity against many DNA and RNA viruses. They are produced endogenously during viral infection and appear to act indirectly through the induction of certain cellular enzymes with antiviral activity. *In vitro* and *in vivo* studies of animal retroviruses have demonstrated that interferons are active as antiviral agents and appear to act at the level of assembly and release of new virus particles.[57] In 1985, Ho and colleagues demonstrated that recombinant interferon α-A (rIFN-α-A), *in vitro*, inhibited HIV replication in peripheral blood mononuclear cells at concentrations that were not toxic to the cells in culture.[58] Since this initial observation, the combination *in vitro* of rIFN-α-A with the antiviral agents phosphonoformate,[29] zidovudine,[59] and 2',3'-dideoxycytidine[60] has resulted in synergistic inhibition of HIV infection.

However, preparations of α-interferon have been studied for the treatment of AIDS-related Kaposi's sarcoma as early as 1981, 2 to 3 years before a retrovirus was identified as the etiologic agent of AIDS. In 1983, Krown and her co-workers at Memorial Sloan–Kettering Cancer Center reported that rIFN-α-A induced various degrees of tumor regression, including complete remission, in several patients with Kaposi's sarcoma.[1] Since this initial study, several investigators have reported similar results with various α-interferon preparations.[61] The precise mechanism(s)—antiviral, immunomodulatory, antiproliferative, or a combination of these—underlying the response of Kaposi's sarcoma to treatment with α-interferon remains unclear. Phase I studies of α-interferon in combination with zidovudine in patients with Kaposi's sarcoma are currently in progress in the ATEUs.

Gamma interferon, a product of sensitized T lymphocytes and a pure immunomodulator, is thought to be an important component of the immune response to microorganisms controlled by the monocyte–macrophage arm of the immune system. It is this group of microorganisms that most commonly causes the infectious complications seen in patients with AIDS.[34] *In vitro,* peripheral blood lymphocytes from certain patients with AIDS failed to proliferate or to produce γ-interferon upon appropriate antigenic stimulation.[62] Results of clinical trials of γ-interferon have been disappointing. When administered to patients at doses at which immunologic enhancement was anticipated, γ-interferon caused unacceptable toxicity.[63]

Infection of the monocyte–macrophage has recently been appreciated as an important component of HIV pathogenesis.[64] Monocytes and macrophages appear to be relatively resistant to the cytopathic effect of HIV and may therefore serve as a reservoir for persistence of the virus in the host or as a vehicle for the transport of HIV to the central nervous system, where it appears to contribute to the wide array of previously unexplained neurologic syndromes associated with AIDS.[64] Recently, in an *in vitro* monocyte model of HIV infection, recombinant interferon γ (rIFN-γ) modified the course of infection in this system,[65] suggesting a possible role for this substance.

Granulocyte–Macrophage Colony-Stimulating Factor (GM-CSF)

Colony-stimulating factors are glycoprotein hormones required for *in vitro* proliferation and differentiation of hematopoietic precursor cells.[66,67] Recombinant human GM-CSF has been studied *in vitro* and *in vivo* in the setting of HIV infection. *In vitro,* inhibition of HIV replication has been reported in the monocytoid cell line, U-937.[65] In the same system, combination of GM-CSF with zidovudine resulted in a synergistic anti-HIV effect.[68] *In vivo,* administration of GM-CSF to leukopenic patients with AIDS resulted in dose-dependent increases in circulating leukocytes with minimal toxicity.[69] Although there is *in vitro* evidence of anti-HIV activity, there is concern that, *in vivo,* GM-CSF may stimulate macrophages persistently infected with HIV to produce large amounts of virus. It is important, therefore, that studies of GM-CSF in the setting of HIV infection be pursued cautiously.

OTHER OR UNCERTAIN SITE OF ACTION

There are several agents or treatment modalities that do not fit conveniently into any of the steps of the HIV replicative cycle. We will consider these in the following discussion.

Biologic Response Modifiers (Immunomodulators)

Several immunomodulators have been studied by various investigators, both *in vitro* and *in vivo.* We will discuss those most widely used in clinical trials.

Interleukin-2 (IL-2)

In vitro, the defective natural killer cell responses of patients with AIDS may be reconstituted to varying degrees by IL-2.[70] Based on their *in vitro* observations, Fauci and his co-workers at the National Institute of Allergy and Infectious Diseases (NIAID) began a phase I study of recombinant IL-2 in patients with AIDS. Over the 8-week study period they observed an initial increase in total T4 lymphocyte counts, followed by a decrease to baseline levels; a decrease in the isolation of HIV; increased spontaneous proliferation of lymphocytes; and minor regressions in Kaposi's sarcoma.[71]

Isoprinosine

Isoprinosine (inosine pranobex) has been reported to have anti-HIV activity *in vitro.*[72] It is an immunomodulator capable of enhancing a variety of cell-mediated immune functions.[73] Unfortunately, these changes have not correlated with consistent improvement of clinical status. Isoprinosine is available without prescription in many countries, including Mexico, and has been a popular agent for self-treatment among patients with HIV infection.

Imuthiol

Imuthiol (sodium diethyldithiocarbamate), a sulfur containing organic compound, is an inducer of T-lymphocytes[73] and has been reported to have anti-HIV activity *in vitro.*[72] Multicenter studies of this agent in patients with AIDS and ARC are underway in the United States.

Imreg

Imreg (leukocyte dialysate) is a natural, leukocyte-derived polypeptide immunomodulator with an ability to enhance the production of various lymphokines *in vitro.*[74] A multicenter trial of this substance is underway.

Studies of the various immunomodulators in combination with an antiviral agent such as zidovudine are planned. As with GM-CSF, there is concern that the immunostimulatory effect of a biologic response modifier may trigger the activation of a latent HIV infection.

D-Penicillamine

D-penicillamine, a chelating agent commercially available for the treatment of various inflammatory and metabolic disorders including Wilson's disease, primary biliary cirrhosis, cysteinuria, and rheumatoid arthritis, has been reported to inhibit the replication of HIV *in vitro*.[75] The mechanism of this inhibition has not been defined; however, chemical inactivation of HIV proteins through cross-linking of disulfide groups has been proposed. In a phase I study in patients with ARC or persistent generalized lymphadenopathy, D-penicillamine suppression of HIV replication was seen at dosage levels associated with a reversible depression of T4 lymphocyte counts.[76] Studies aimed at defining a regimen that preserves the apparent antiviral effect without the toxicity to T-lymphocytes are in progress.

Bone Marrow Transplantation

An ideal approach to the treatment of HIV infection would be complete replacement of the damaged immune system. This has been attempted by Fauci and his colleagues at NIAID, both by the adoptive transfer of syngeneic lymphocytes and by bone marrow transplantation.[71] In 1984, prior to the availability of antiretroviral therapy, these investigators transplanted bone marrow into a patient with AIDS from his healthy identical twin brother.[77] Although a partial, transient reconstitution of the immune response was observed, this patient died several months later of opportunistic infection. Subsequent studies among identical twin pairs have combined pretreatment with an antiretroviral agent (suramin or zidovudine) and syngeneic lymphocyte transfusions, followed by bone marrow transplantation with maintenance antiretroviral therapy and lymphocyte transfusion.[78] Preliminary results of these studies have shown at least partial reconstitution of the immune response in some patients; however, long-term follow-up will be required in order to assess the value of this approach.

CONCLUSIONS

Agents other than nucleoside analogs with activity against HIV have been identified; however, the role for most of these in the treatment of HIV infection and AIDS has yet to be defined. There are, however, a few statements that may be made with relative certainty. Alpha-interferon has clearly found its niche in the treatment of Kaposi's sarcoma and may be of value when used in combination with an antiretroviral agent. Treatment with suramin, the first anti-HIV agent studied, has not been associated with clinical, virologic, or immunologic improvement and is highly toxic; no further studies of suramin in HIV-infected individuals are planned.

For some of the agents discussed, such as AL-721 and peptide T, reproducible evidence of anti-HIV activity *in vitro* is lacking and should be obtained prior to the initiation of clinical studies. And as underscored by the experience with suramin, activity *in vitro* does not necessarily translate into clinical efficacy.

The evidence for synergistic inhibition of HIV *in vitro* is encouraging and paves the way for clinical study of combination chemotherapy for HIV infection. This approach has been used successfully for the treatment of neoplastic disease and some infectious diseases. Such studies are currently in progress.

As with many viral infections, the natural history of HIV infection is variable. Consequently, anecdotal reports of efficacy are difficult to evaluate. For this reason, carefully controlled trials of new agents, first evaluating safety and pharmacokinetics (phase I), and then efficacy (phase II), will be required. Studies of efficacy should be multicenter collaborative trials, usually randomized and double-blind, and new agents should ultimately be tested against the established therapy of the day. In the United States, the NIH-sponsored National Cooperative Drug Discovery Groups for the Treatment of AIDS (NCDDG-AIDS) and the ATEUs provide a mechanism for the development and testing of new treatments for HIV infection and AIDS. We are optimistic that these and other collaborative research efforts will contribute to the successful control of this epidemic.

REFERENCES

1. Krown SE, Real FX, Cunningham–Rundles S et al: Preliminary observations on the effect of recombinant leukocyte A interferon in homosexual men with Kaposi's sarcoma. N Engl J Med 308:1071, 1983
2. Fischl MA, Richman DD, Grieco MH et al: The efficacy of azidothymidine (AZT) in the treatment of patients with AIDS and AIDS-related complex. N Engl J Med 317:185, 1987
3. Yarchoan R, Broder S: Development of antiretroviral therapy for the acquired immunodeficiency syndrome and related disorders: A progress report. N Engl J Med 316:557, 1987
4. Lyte M, Shinitsky M: A special lipid mixture for membrane fluidization. Biochim Biophys Acta 812:133, 1985
5. Sarin PS, Gallo RC, Scheer DI et al: Effects of a novel compound (AL 721) on HTLV-III infectivity in vitro. N Engl J Med 313:1289, 1985
6. Crews FT, Laurence, J, McElhaney R et al: Modification of human immunodeficiency virus envelope lipids, protein structure, and infectivity by AL 721, a unique lipid mixture. Twenty-seventh Interscience Conference on Antimicrobial Agents and Chemotherapy, New York, October 5, 1987 (abstr 371)

7. Grieco MH, Lange M, Klein EB et al: Open study of AL-721 in HIV-infected subjects with generalized lymphade-nopathy syndrome (LAS). III International Conference on AIDS, Washington, DC, June 2, 1987 (abstr TP 223)

8. McDougal JS, Kennedy MS, Sligh JM et al: Binding of HTLV-III/LAV to T4⁺ T cells by a complex of the 110K viral protein and the T4 molecule. Science 231:382, 1986

9. Pert CB, Hill JM, Ruff MR et al: Octapeptides deduced from the neuropeptide receptor-like pattern of antigen T4 in brain potently inhibit human immunodeficiency virus receptor binding and T-cell infectivity. Proc Natl Acad Sci USA 83:9254, 1986

10. Sodroski J, Kowalski M, Dorfman T et al: HIV envelope-CD4 interaction not inhibited by synthetic octapeptides. Lancet 1:1428, 1987

11. Wetterberg L, Alexius B, Saaf J et al: Peptide T in treatment of AIDS. Lancet 1:159, 1987

12. Walker BD, Kowalski M, Goh WC et al: Inhibition of human immunodeficiency virus syncytium formation and repli-cation by castanospermine. Twenty-seventh Interscience Conference on Antimicrobial Agents and Chemotherapy, New York, October 5, 1987 (abstr 373)

13. Schaffner CP, Plescia OJ, Pontani D et al: Anti-viral activity of amphotericin B methyl ester: Inhibition of HTLV-III replication in cell culture. Biochem Pharmacol 35:4110, 1986

14. Ellis WG, Sobel RA, Nielsen SL: Leukoencephalopathy in patients treated with amphotericin B methyl ester. J Infect Dis 146:125, 1982

15. Polsky B, Gold JWM, Baron PA et al: Inactivation of human immunodeficiency virus by gossypol. Clin Res 35:487A, 1987

16. DeClercq E: Suramin: A potent inhibitor of the reverse transcriptase of RNA tumor viruses. Cancer Lett 8:9, 1979

17. Mitsuya H, Popovic M, Yarchoan R et al: Suramin protection of T cells in vitro against infectivity and cytopathic effect of HTLV-III. Science 226:172, 1984

18. Broder S, Yarchoan R, Collins JM et al: Effects of suramin on HTLV-III/LAV infection presenting as Kaposi's sarcoma or AIDS-related complex: Clinical pharmacology and suppression of virus replication in vivo. Lancet 2:627, 1985

19. Levine AM, Gill PS, Cohen J et al: Suramin antiviral therapy in the acquired immunodeficiency syndrome. Ann Intern Med 105:32, 1986

20. Kaplan LD, Wolfe PR, Volberding PA et al: Lack of response to suramin by patients with AIDS and AIDS-related com-plex. Am J Med 82:615, 1987

21. Cheson BD, Levine AM, Mildvan D et al: Suramin therapy in AIDS and related disorders: Report of the US suramin working group. JAMA 258:1347, 1987

22. Humphries EM, Donaldson L: Degeneration of the adrenal cortex produced by germanin. Am J Pathol 17:767, 1941

23. Frisch E, Gardner LI: Failure of suramin (Bayer 205; Ger-manin) to cause changes in the adrenal cortex of the rat. Endocrinology 63:500, 1958

24. Dormont D, Spire B, Barré–Sinoussi FC et al: Inhibition of RNA dependent DNA polymerases of two primate ret-roviruses (LAV and AIDS virus) by ammonium-21-tungsto-9-antimoniate (HPA 23). Ann Virol (Inst Pasteur) 136E:75, 1985

25. McKinley GF, Englard A, Ong K et al: Use of HPA-23 in patients with AIDS: Observed toxicity during an eight week trial. III International Conference on AIDS, Washington, DC, June 3, 1987 (abstr WP 218)

26. Sundquist B, Oberg B: Phosphonoformate inhibits reverse transcriptase. J Gen Virol 45:273, 1979

27. Vrang L, Oberg B: PP$_i$ analogs as inhibitors of human T-lymphotropic virus type III reverse transcriptase. Antim-icrob Agents Chemother 29:867, 1986

28. Sandstrom EG, Kaplan JC, Byington RE et al: Inhibition of human T-cell lymphotropic virus type III in vitro by phosphonoformate. Lancet 1:1480, 1985

29. Hartshorn KL, Sandstrom EG, Neumeyer D et al: Synergistic inhibition of human T-cell lymphotropic virus type III replication in vitro by phosphonoformate and recombinant alpha-A interferon. Antimicrob Agents Chemother 30:189, 1986

30. Ringden O, Lonnqvist B, Paulin T et al: Pharmacokinetics, safety and preliminary experiences using foscarnet in the treatment of cytomegalovirus infections in bone marrow and renal transplant recipients. J Antimicrob Chemother 17:373, 1986

31. Farthing CF, Dalgleish AG, Clark A, McClure M, Chanas A, Gazzard BG: Phosphonoformate (foscarnet): A pilot study in AIDS and AIDS related complex. AIDS 1:21, 1987

32. Gaub J, Pedersen C, Poulsen AG et al: The effect of fos-carnet (phosphonoformate) on human immunodeficiency virus isolation, T-cell subsets and lymphocyte function in AIDS patients. AIDS 1:27, 1987

33. Klintmalm G, Lonnqvist B, Oberg B et al: Intravenous fos-carnet for the treatment of severe cytomegalovirus infec-tion in allograft recipients. Scand J Infect Dis 17:157, 1985

34. Armstrong D, Gold JWM, Dryjanski J et al: Treatment of infections in patients with the acquired immunodeficiency syndrome. Ann Intern Med 103:738, 1985

35. Hawkins CC, Gold JWM, Whimbey E et al: *Mycobacterium avium* complex infections in patients with the acquired immunodeficiency syndrome. Ann Intern Med 105:184, 1986

36. Anand R, Moore J, Feorino P et al: Rifabutine inhibits HTLV-III. Lancet 1:97, 1986

37. Wu AM, Gallo RC: Interaction between murine type-C virus RNA-directed DNA polymerase and rifamycin derivatives. Biochim Biophys Acta 240:419, 1974

38. Burger H, Weiser B, Neff S et al: An antiviral trial of rifabutin in patients with ARC. III International Conference on AIDS, Washington, DC, June 4, 1987 (abstr THP 233)

39. Davidson BP, Siegal FP, Reife RA et al: Ansamycin (rifa-butin), an inhibitor of HIV in vitro, crosses the blood–brain barrier. III International Conference on AIDS, Washington, DC, June 4, 1987 (abstr THP 228)

40. Arya SK, Guo C, Josephs SF et al: *trans*-activator gene of human T-lymphotropic virus type III (HTLV-III). Science 229:69, 1985

41. Sodroski J, Patarca R, Rosen C et al: Location of the *trans*-activating region on the genome of human T-lymphotropic virus type III. Science 229:74, 1985

42. Rosen CA, Sodroski JG, Goh WC et al: Post-transcriptional regulation accounts for the *trans*-activation of the human T-lymphotropic virus type III. Nature 319:555, 1986

43. Sodroski J, Goh WC, Rosen C et al: A second post-tran-scriptional *trans*-activator gene required for HTLV-III replication. Nature 321:412, 1986

44. Fisher AG, Feinberg MB, Josephs SF et al: The *trans*-ac-tivator gene of HTLV-III is essential for virus replication. Nature 320:367, 1986

45. Zamecnik PC, Goodchild J, Taguchi Y et al: Inhibition of replication and expression of human T-cell lymphotropic

virus type III in cultured cells by exogenous synthetic oligonucleotides complementary to viral RNA. Proc Natl Acad Sci USA 83:4143, 1986

46. Shannon WM: Mechanisms of action and pharmacology: Chemical agents. In Galasso GJ, Merigan TC, Buchanan RA (eds): Antiviral Agents and Viral Diseases of Man, 2nd ed, p 55. New York, Raven Press, 1984

47. Marcus PI, Sekellick MJ: Defective interfering particles with covalently linked [±] RNA induce interferon. Nature 266: 815, 1977

48. DeBendetti A, Pytel BA, Baglioni C: Loss of (2′–5′) oligoadenylate synthetase activity by production of antisense RNA results in lack of protection by interferon from viral infections. Proc Natl Acad Sci USA 84:658, 1987

49. Montefiori DC, Mitchell WM: Antiviral activity of mismatched double-stranded RNA against human immunodeficiency virus in vitro. Proc Natl Acad Sci USA 84:2985, 1987

50. Mitchell WM, Montefiori DC, Robinson WE et al: Mismatched double-stranded RNA (ampligen) reduces concentration of zidovudine (azidothymidine) required for in vitro inhibition of human immunodeficiency virus. Lancet 1:890, 1987

51. Carter WA, Strayer DR, Brodsky I et al: Clinical, immunological, and virological effects of ampligen, a mismatched double-stranded RNA, in patients with AIDS or AIDS-related complex. Lancet 1:1286, 1987

52. Godtfredsen W, Roholt K, Tybring L: Fusidin: A new orally active antibiotic. Lancet 1:928, 1962

53. Faber V, Dalgleish AG, Newell A et al: Inhibition of HIV replication in vitro by fusidic acid. Lancet 2:827, 1987

54. Tanaka N: Fusidic acid. Antibiotics 3:436, 1975

55. Schultz AM, Oroszlan, S: In vivo modification of retroviral *gag* gene-encoded polyproteins by myristic acid. J Virol 46:355, 1983

56. Henderson LE, Krutzsch HC, Oroszlan S: Myristyl amino-terminal acylation of murine retrovirus proteins: An unusual post-translational protein modification. Proc Natl Acad Sci USA 80:339, 1983

57. Pitha P, Bilello JA, Riggin CH: Effect of interferon on retrovirus replication. Tex Rep Biol Med 41:603, 1981–2

58. Ho DD, Hartshorn KL, Rota TR et al: Recombinant human interferon alfa-A suppresses HTLV-III replication in vitro. Lancet 1:602, 1985

59. Hartshorn, KL, Vogt MW, Chou TC et al: Synergistic inhibition of human immunodeficiency virus in vitro by azidothymidine and recombinant alpha A interferon. Antimicrob Agents Chemother 31:168, 1987

60. Durno AG, Vogt MW, Chou TC et al: Strong synergistic interactions between 2′,3′-dideoxycytidine and recombinant interferon alpha A. Twenty-seventh Interscience Conference on Antimicrobial Agents and Chemotherapy, New York, October 5, 1987 (abstr 370)

61. Krown SE: AIDS and Kaposi's sarcoma: Interferons in pathogenesis and treatment. In Gressor I (ed): Interferon 7, p 185. London, Academic Press, 1986

62. Murray HW, Rubin BY, Masur H et al: Impaired production of lymphokines and immune (gamma) interferon in the acquired immunodeficiency syndrome. N Engl J Med 310: 883, 1984

63. Lane HC, Sherwin S, Masur H et al: A phase I trial of recombinant immune (gamma) interferon in patients with the acquired immunodeficiency syndrome. Clin Res 33: 408A, 1985

64. Ho DD, Pomerantz RJ, Kaplan JC: Pathogenesis of infection with human immunodeficiency virus. N Engl J Med 317: 278, 1987

65. Hammer SM, Gillis JM, Groopman JE et al: In vitro modification of human immunodeficiency virus infection by granulocyte-macrophage colony-stimulating factor and gamma interferon. Proc Natl Acad Sci USA 83:8734, 1986

66. Metcalf D: The granulocyte-macrophage colony-stimulating factors. Science 229:16, 1985

67. Clark SC, Kamen R: The human hematopoietic colony-stimulating factors. Science 236:1229, 1987

68. Hammer SM, Gillis JM: Synergistic activity of granulocyte-macrophage colony-stimulating factor and 3′-azido-3′-deoxythimidine against human immunodeficiency virus in vitro. Antimicrob Agents Chemother 31:1046, 1987

69. Groopman JE, Mitsuyasu RT, DeLeo MJ et al: Effect of recombinant human granulocyte-macrophage colony-stimulating factor on myelopoiesis in the acquired immunodeficiency syndrome. N Engl J Med 317:593, 1987

70. Rook AH, Masur H, Lane HC et al: Interleukin-2 enhances the depressed natural killer and cytomegalovirus-specific cytotoxic activities of lymphocytes from patients with the acquired immune deficiency syndrome. J Clin Invest 72: 398, 1983

71. Fauci AS: Immunomodulators, p 574. In DeVita VT Jr (moderator): Developmental therapeutics and the acquired immunodeficiency syndrome. Ann Intern Med 106: 568, 1987

72. Pompidou A, Zagury D, Gallo RC et al: In-vitro inhibition of LAV/HTLV-III infected lymphocytes by dithiocarb and inosine pranobex. Lancet 2:1423, 1985

73. Pompidou A, Delsaux MC, Telvi L et al: Isoprinosine and imuthiol, two potentially active compounds in patients with AIDS-related complex symptoms. Cancer Res 45: 4671s, 1985

74. Gottlieb AA, Farmer JL, Matzura CT et al: Modulation of human T cell production of migration inhibitory lymphokines by cytokines derived from human leukocyte dialysates. J Immunol 132:256, 1984

75. Chandra P, Sarin PS: Selective inhibition of replication of the AIDS-associated virus HTLV-III/LAV by synthetic *D*-penicillamine. Arzneim Forsch Drug Res 36:184, 1986

76. Parenti DM, Scheib R, Simon G et al: *D*-Penicillamine (DPA) treatment for lymphadenopathy syndrome (LAS) and AIDS-related complex (ARC). III International Conference on AIDS, Washington, DC, June 2, 1987 (abstr TP 220)

77. Lane HC, Masur H, Longo DL et al: Partial immune reconstitution in a patient with the acquired immunodeficiency syndrome. N Engl J Med 311:1099, 1984

78. Fauci AS, Lane HC: Antiretroviral therapy and immunologic reconstitution in AIDS. In Gluckman JC, Vilmer E (eds): Acquired Immunodeficiency Syndrome: International Conference on AIDS, Paris 1986, p 229. Paris, Elsevier, 1986.

Strategies for the Identification of New Agents for the Treatment of AIDS: A National Program to Facilitate the Discovery and Preclinical Development of New Drug Candidates for Clinical Evaluation

Michael R. Boyd

18

The National Institutes of Health (NIH), the major biomedical research component of the United States Public Health Service (USPHS), has launched a comprehensive set of new programs to confront the burgeoning worldwide epidemic of acquired immune deficiency syndrome (AIDS). Strategies encompassed in these efforts not only include an increased emphasis upon specialized intramural AIDS-related basic and clinical research projects at the NIH, but also include AIDS-targeted efforts of an extensive cross-section of the extramural scientific community.

The extramural programs are supported through NIH grants, cooperative agreements, and contracts. Grant-supported activities focus predominantly upon the development of a critical foundation of scientific knowledge through basic research. AIDS-related activities supported under cooperative agreements give additional emphasis to applied research and development, specifically toward the expeditious application of new scientific discoveries to new treatment strategies. The AIDS National Cooperative Drug Discovery Group (NCDDG) Program, developed jointly by the National Institute of Allergy and Infectious Diseases (NIAID) and the National Cancer Institute (NCI), provides an excellent example of how the cooperative agreement mechanism provides support for extramural investigator-initiated, basic and applied, interdisciplinary, multicenter programs aimed specifically at development of new treatments for AIDS.

Major contract-supported programs encompassed within the NIH strategies for AIDS are intended to provide comprehensive centralized resources for AIDS treatment research. These resources give focus to synergistic, cooperative efforts in AIDS treatment research among the NIH, other government agencies, academia, industry, and other potential collaborators worldwide. Key NIH extramural initiatives in this regard include the implementation of complementary national programs to facilitate the discovery and prompt *preclinical* development of promising new candidate agents for treatment of AIDS and to facilitate the *clinical* evaluation and development of new potential agents and applications. The NIAID is focusing predominantly upon the clinical program, as exemplified by the implementation of the national AIDS treatment/evaluation units (ATEUs), a clinical evaluations network involving major medical centers throughout the United States. The NCI is primarily responsible for the preclinical program and, as described herein, has implemented a contract-based drug development program of a national/international scope, for the support of the worldwide effort to expeditiously discover and develop the most promising candidate agents for clinical evaluation against AIDS.

For the past several years the NCI has played an

active role in supporting certain specialized aspects of AIDS drug development. However, the implementation by the NCI of a more comprehensive program for support of a full preclinical drug development program for AIDS, including a national AIDS drug screening resource, was initiated after the recommendation of the Board of Scientific Counselors of the NCI Division of Cancer Treatment (DCT). The Board formally approved the NCI AIDS drug development program concept in February 1987.[1] The NCI's charge to implement a national AIDS preclinical drug development program was based on the urgent need for such a resource and the Institute's extensive experience and pre-existing program for preclinical development of anticancer agents.

A NATIONAL PROGRAM TO FACILITATE THE DISCOVERY AND PRECLINICAL DEVELOPMENT OF NEW DRUG CANDIDATES FOR CLINICAL EVALUATION AGAINST AIDS

Background: The Drug Development Program of the National Cancer Institute

The NCI's drug development program is a unique entity within the federal government. In both organization and function, it is similar to a large multinational drug corporation, although it is not profit-driven and lacks a marketing component. The rationale for the creation of such a federal program over 30 years ago was a national commitment to enhance the discovery and rapid development of new agents for the treatment of cancer, a disease area where private-sector pharmaceutical industries were, and continue to be, relatively reluctant to engage their greatest efforts. Anticancer drug discovery and development has been generally perceived by industry as a high-risk, exceedingly expensive venture, with relatively limited profit potential compared to other, more accessible pharmaceutical areas. Clearly, therefore, an important function of the NCI program in achieving its goal of expediting the entry of effective new anticancer agents into the population at large has been its role in assuming a major portion of the costs and "risks" involved in the early phases of anticancer drug discovery and development. Ultimately, for any effective new drug or treatment developed either partly or completely by the NCI, the pharmaceutical industry always assumes a critical role in commercialization, marketing, and distribution of the new products to the target populations.

The federal program is in an ideal position to serve as a bridge between academia and industry to bring the best ideas from all sectors to fruition as quickly as possible. The NCI's drug development program has indeed evolved with a rich tradition of highly productive, cooperative efforts among government, academia, and industry on both a national and an international scale. A review of the NCI preclinical drug development program status up to 1982 revealed that half of the current

commercially available anticancer agents discovered since 1955 were initially discovered by the NCI screens and that the NCI has played an important role in the preclinical and/or clinical development of essentially all of the drugs receiving New Drug Application (NDA) approval from the U.S. Food and Drug Administration (FDA) for entry into the marketplace.[2]

It is important to note that a very high percentage of substances acquired by the NCI program for initial testing and/or consideration for potential development come from non-NCI sources. Such materials are obtained under the protection of formal confidentiality documentation to ensure the original suppliers' patent positions. On the other hand, in those less common instances where the drug originates from within the NCI itself (e.g., from an intramural laboratory) or from an outside investigator independent of industry, the NCI seeks to facilitate the negotiation and execution of licensure arrangements with industry, again to ensure the ultimate delivery of a useful new drug product to the population if and when appropriate.

Potential Role and Contribution of a National AIDS Drug Development Program

It is important to consider these precedents in the face of the current AIDS crisis. Regardless of whether the future responsibility for operation of a federal program to facilitate AIDS drug development continues to reside with the NCI, there is clearly ample experience from the NCI anticancer drug development program to illustrate vividly the *potential* impact of such a program on a major public health problem. A federal program providing centralized support for new drug development can indeed provide a critical interface among the best of academia, private industry, and government to enhance the attack on a problem of the potential magnitude of AIDS.

Current industry perspectives regarding AIDS drug development appear to be substantially different than those for anticancer drug development. One of the greatest differences appears to be the perception of a high profit potential for AIDS drugs, making the financial "riskiness" of AIDS drug discovery and development less an obstacle. Clearly there is considerable interest within industry to engage very substantially in AIDS-related drug research and development. To that extent, therefore, the federal program does not appear to be essential to help provide incentive for involvement. For confronting the AIDS epidemic, the federal program should nevertheless make a major contribution by enhancing the pace and efficiency of progress. An effective government program can expedite the process of drug discovery and development from the earliest stages of screening through the point of delivery of the finished pharmaceutical products to the clinical trials specialists. The recent development of dideoxycytidine (DDC), the antiviral activity of which was discovered in an NCI intramural laboratory,[3] exemplifies how the NCI preclinical drug development program can accelerate the progress of a new drug candidate. From the point of entry of DDC into the drug development program described herein, the total time for completion of all the steps of preclinical development (see below) to the point of readiness and FDA approval for clinical testing was an unprecedented 12 months. The NCI program also played a substantial supportive role with industry in expediting the development of azidothymidine (AZT), which was the first drug approved and marketed for the treatment of AIDS.

Organization of Contract-Supported AIDS Preclinical Drug Research and Development Responsibilities Within the National Cancer Institute

To facilitate the most rapid deployment, AIDS program requirements were integrated with the existing NCI extramural contract-based anticancer drug development program, the general organization of which is depicted in Figure 18-1. The NCI preclinical drug development program is a part of the Developmental Therapeutics Program (DTP), located within the Division of Cancer Treatment (DCT). Although it will not be discussed further herein, the DTP organization also encompasses an extramural research component supported by grants and cooperative agreements, as well as an intramural research component with laboratories located in Bethesda, Maryland, and at the Frederick Cancer Research Facility in Frederick, Maryland.

Key extramural program managers within DTP presently have responsibility for organizing and operating both the anticancer and the AIDS-antiviral drug development areas; additional specialized staff are assigned as necessary to meet the more detailed requirements of each area. AIDS program operations described herein are accomplished primarily through a portfolio of specific AIDS-designated contracts. Decision making and/or prioritization responsibilities are performed jointly for AIDS and anticancer drug development by committees strategically placed within the operational/management framework shown schematically in Figure 18-2.

The remainder of this chapter details further the organization, functions, contact points, committee functions, and other specific issues of relevance to the contract-based AIDS preclinical drug discovery and development components of the DTP. The discussion does not encompass non-NCI drug development programs; nor does it cover other areas of related NCI research, such as the intramural AIDS research components described elsewhere (see Chapters 2 and 5). Other NCI AIDS-related contract-based programs, such as vaccine development, also are reviewed in Chapter 6. The purpose of the present discussion is to describe, and to

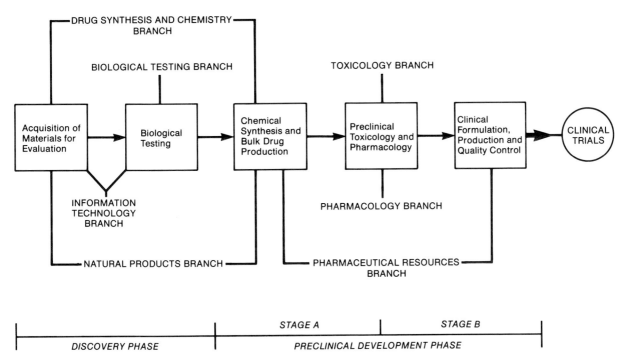

FIG. 18-1.   Organization and functions of the NCI Developmental Therapeutics Program components supporting AIDS drug development.

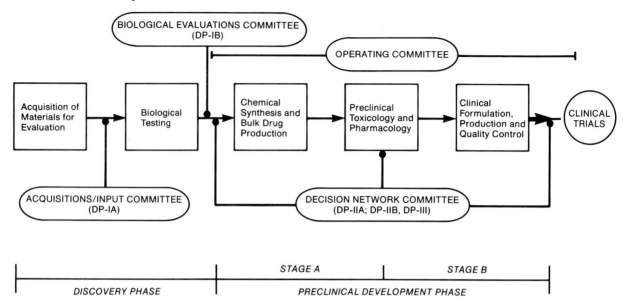

FIG. 18-2. Key committees and decision points for anticancer and AIDS drug development by the NCI Developmental Therapeutics Program.

indicate both the availability and the current status of, NCI resources potentially applicable to AIDS drug research and development, and to invite the input and utilization of this program by responsible members of the academic, private industry, and government sectors.

NATIONAL CANCER INSTITUTE AIDS PRECLINICAL DRUG RESEARCH AND DEVELOPMENT PROGRAM: DRUG DISCOVERY PHASE

Acquisition of Materials for Evaluation

The NCI for many years has operated a worldwide acquisitions program for identifying and obtaining promising substances (more than 10,000 new materials per year), including both synthetic and natural products, for evaluation for potential anticancer activity (Fig. 19-3). Both the Chemical Repository and the Natural Products Repository of the NCI, which contain a broad sampling of previous years' acquisitions, and the nonproprietary portions of their structure/activity databases, are available to support the search for new leads with promising anti-HIV activity. On-going NCI natural products collection projects, currently focusing upon new or relatively unexplored areas (e.g., marine biology, novel plant sources, microbial fermentations including bacteria, cyanobacteria, and fungi) for discovery of active constituents with antitumor/antiviral and other biologic activities, will provide further materials for anti-HIV testing.

To complement the existing NCI repositories and acquisitions programs, an additional AIDS-designated acquisitions program has been implemented to enhance the input of substances specifically for anti-HIV testing. This initiative also includes the development of a separate AIDS-designated chemical/biologic database.

Analogous to the acquisitions component of the anticancer drug program, materials for testing are acquired both through active solicitations and through voluntary submissions from a wide variety of sources including the NIH intramural programs, NIH extramural programs (grantees, contractors, NCDDGs), other government agencies, private research institutes/foundations, individual investigators, universities, pharmaceutical/chemical industries, and international collaborations (see Fig. 19-3). Initial reports of the evaluation of discreet compounds thus acquired are sent to suppliers as soon as the screening data are available.

Suppliers' commercial or other proprietary (e.g., patent) interests are protected, whenever necessary, through written confidentiality agreements, which are preferably formalized prior to acquisition and testing. Testing data and other information produced by the NCI program may be used by the original suppliers or their assignees in support of their publications or patent applications. A copy of the confidentiality agreement used currently for suppliers of compounds to be evaluated is provided in Appendix A. Potential suppliers are encouraged to contact the NCI Developmental Therapeutics Program for further details concerning submission of compounds and the securing of confidentiality documentation.

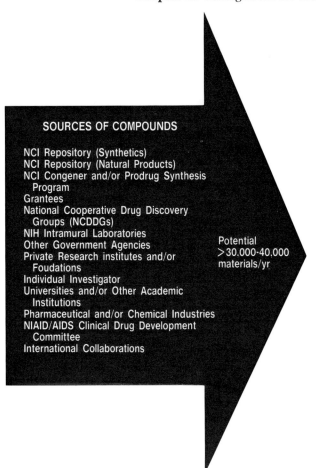

FIG. 18-3. Sources of compounds submitted to the National Cancer Institute for biologic testing.

Biologic Testing

Need for a Centralized Resource

One of the most critical factors determining the potential value of a national program as described in this chapter is the ability to provide investigators throughout the country—indeed, worldwide—with an adequate central standardized resource for rapid initial screening of substances for anti-HIV activities and/or other relevant biologic properties. Based upon the experience of the cancer drug program, it was projected that an initial testing capacity of at least 10,000 substances per year is required to examine an adequate fraction of the total potential new submissions for antiviral activity. Moreover, substantial testing capacity is also required to systematically re-examine for anti-HIV activity the existing NCI synthetic and natural products repositories containing over 200,000 materials, many of which were initially acquired on the basis of known or suspected

"biologic activities," including antiviral, of potential interest.

In vitro anti-HIV tests recently used with success for initial identification of promising new agents such as AZT and DDC[3,4] are conceptually analogous to other commonly used antiviral assays.[5,6] Such tests are based upon the ability of an "active" substance to prevent virus-induced cytopathic effects in appropriate target cells in culture. A test for anti-HIV activity therefore typically utilizes HIV-infected human host cells; an active test shows an enhancement of survival of the virus-infected host cells at drug concentrations that are relatively nontoxic to the uninfected host cells.[3,4]

Unfortunately, the availability of anti-HIV test systems to the research community at large has been exceedingly limited, owing to the low capacities of the few laboratories performing such tests, the difficulties of scale-up, and the reluctance of many investigators to become directly involved with the active AIDS virus. Moreover, there has been considerable variation in the specific test protocols used by various laboratories, substantially compromising meaningful detailed comparisons of compounds among laboratories. For these reasons, a high-capacity national AIDS-antiviral screening resource is essential to serve a variety of drug discovery research needs. The need is further exemplified in the following.

Rational versus Empirical Approaches to Drug Discovery

All so-called rational approaches (e.g., molecular design) for new drug discovery ultimately require the availability of appropriate biologic screening models against which to test the chemical products of the medicinal chemists ideas. Moreover, in the empirical approach to new drug discovery, the biologic screening models *per se* are the primary tools for new drug discovery.

The process of empirical screening of large, chemically diverse sets of organic compounds, recently criticized by some as inefficient[7] yet also encouraged by others[8] as essential for AIDS drug research, is nonetheless *the* most successful drug discovery approach used for many areas of pharmaceuticals. This is nowhere better exemplified than in the area of anticancer drugs where a majority of the clinically useful agents have been initially discovered by the process of empirical screening.[2]

For the natural products area, empirical screening is the primary avenue to the discovery of new leads. Furthermore, the critical process of bioassay directed isolation and structure identification of the active pure constituents from a crude natural product extract frequently requires extensive screening of the partially purified fractions. Many of the most important clinically used drugs, across all pharmaceutical classes, have their origins as natural products discovered predominantly through the empirical process.

Once an initial new lead is identified empirically, regardless of whether it is of synthetic or natural origin, the rational approach may then be applied by the medicinal chemist to modify the structure to improve the lead compound's characteristics (e.g., stability, solubility, biologic potency or selectivity) as a potential pharmaceutical agent. This process of "lead optimization" obviously also depends upon the use of biologic screens to monitor the progress of optimization. Thus, not infrequently the rational drug design approach occurs much later, only after an initial new active lead structure is discovered by empirical screening and the molecular/biochemical basis for its activity in the screen is elucidated. The designer chemist then conceives of ways to improve the lead structure or to develop entirely new molecules to address the new molecular/biochemical targets thus discovered.

The explosion in the knowledge of the molecular biology of the AIDS virus and its effects upon its cellular targets certainly make the prospects for success of rational drug design all the more appealing. However, the record of success for purely *ab initio* rational design of effective antivirals is, as yet, no greater than the slim record for anticancer agents. For the present, the rational and the empirical approaches to drug discovery in both the anticancer and the antiviral areas are most prudently viewed and utilized as complementary and potentially synergistic.

Testing Strategy

Presently, the emphasis for biologic testing is primarily toward the identification of anti-HIV active leads.

Other types of screens to detect other kinds of agents potentially useful against AIDS (e.g., immunomodulatory agents; anti-infectives) may later be incorporated into the program as the available technology and resources allow.

Figure 18-4 illustrates the antiviral screening strategy currently being implemented by the DTP. Although not yet in place, anti-HIV related screening at the biochemical/molecular level will be a part of the integrated AIDS drug discovery resource. Like other retroviral infections, HIV infection of cells involves a series of critical steps including the binding of virus to cellular receptors, internalization of the virus, transcription of the viral RNA into DNA by means of viral enzyme reverse transcriptase, integration of the viral DNA transcript into host chromosomal DNA, and subsequent transcription of viral DNA resulting in synthesis and release of new infective virus particles. Efforts at rational drug design focusing upon these targets are underway in many laboratories; however, a generally available biochemical screening resource specifically addressing such targets has not been available.

The biochemical/molecular screens should be potentially useful not only to support specific target-directed, rational drug design projects, but also to enrich the input of bioactive materials to the other screens. For example, it is anticipated that the biochemical/molecular screening resource will be utilized for empirical screening of widely diverse synthetic molecular structures (e.g., from the existing repositories). Such a resource may not only help preselect for novel drug candidates, but also may yield useful new probes for basic research on HIV and potential molecular targets therein. Moreover, the complementary use of the biochemical prescreens resource, with the cell-culture–based screens

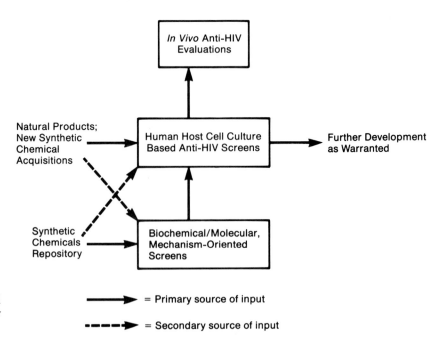

FIG. 18-4. Integrated AIDS-antiviral screening strategy being implemented by the DTP.

⟶ = Primary source of input

┅┅▶ = Secondary source of input

used to identify active leads from crude natural products, also may facilitate the identification and isolation of the most biologically diverse new natural product drug candidates.

In order to address a diversity of molecular targets with the biochemical/molecular screen, a battery of screens will be operated simultaneously and new screens will be added as technology and resources permit and/or as other screens are deleted. On an annual basis it is anticipated that multiple screening models, each addressing unique molecular targets, will be utilized and that each will have a testing capacity of approximately 10,000 compounds. It is anticipated that critical input for the selection and review of potential targets for screening will come from the extramural scientific community by way of NCI advisory groups, such as the DCT Board of Scientific Counselors and Ad Hoc Expert committees, and through national workshops or other suitable forums. Implementation of the biochemical screens project is expected to begin during 1988.

Currently, there do not appear to be any appropriate *in vivo* animal model systems that could have practical application as a primary drug screen. However, as depicted in Figure 18-4, any currently available *in vivo* models will be considered for follow-up testing and secondary evaluations of new leads whenever possible. The development of new *in vivo* models, particularly short-term models employing HIV-infected human host cells, is a current research priority within DTP. Suitable short-term animal models, if adequately validated, would be particularly useful for preclinical experimental therapeutics (e.g., dose route/schedule dependency studies) and further prioritization of promising agents identified by the primary *in vitro* screens.

Presently, the NCI program for initial selection of drug candidates for consideration for preclinical development and possible clinical testing relies principally upon a cell-culture–based assay system (see Fig. 18-4). As described further below, the highly automated, high-capacity assay system currently being deployed for the national AIDS-antiviral drug screening program has evolved directly from technology developed initially by DTP staff and contractor staff (Program Resources, Inc.) for NCI's new cell-culture–based anticancer drug screens at the Frederick Cancer Research Facility.

Development and Implementation of a High-Capacity, Cell-Culture–Based Antiviral Screen

For the past 2 years, DTP has been intensively involved in the development of an entirely new anticancer drug screening program based upon the use of human tumor cell line panels in complementary *in vitro* and *in vivo* testing models.[9-13] The technical goal has been the implementation of a program for the annual *in vitro* evaluation of at least 10,000 substances, each tested over a multi-log range of concentrations against each of 100 or more different kinds of human tumor cell lines.

Therefore, to accomplish this goal it has been necessary to develop new technology amenable to an anticipated operational level of over 10 million cultures per year. The successful implementation of this program is based upon the development of high-flux microculture tetrazolium assay (MTA) technology for the precise, highly reproducible quantitative measurement of cell growth in culture.[14-18]

The MTA technology, although originally developed for the NCI antitumor screen, appears to have many other potential applications in other kinds of assays or drug screens in which the end point involves either an inhibition or an enhancement of cell growth in culture. In addition to the adaptation to use as an antiviral screen as described below, other applications of the MTA technology currently being explored by DTP scientists include new screens for radiomodulators, differentiating agents, and modifiers of drug resistance.

The conceptual basis for the antiviral application of the MTA assay technology is straightforward. Appropriate host cells susceptible to the cytopathic effects of HIV *in vitro* are grown in microtiter plate wells in the presence or absence of virus and in the presence or absence of the test substance of interest (Fig. 18-5). Antiviral activity is indicated by an enhanced growth/survival of the virus-infected cells, measured quantitatively by a colorimetric procedure as described below, in the presence of the drug. The virus-free cells used as controls in the assays provide a measure of the direct growth inhibitory effect of the drug on the host cells.

A new MTA reagent (XTT), currently being used to determine the cell growth end-point in this assay[15,16,18] was developed by DTP staff and contractor colleagues. The basis for its use in the antiviral assay as well as its potentially broader usage in a variety of other cell culture assay systems is depicted in Figure 18-6. The colorless XTT tetrazolium salt is metabolically reduced in the presence of viable cells and an electron coupling reagent (e.g., phenazinemethosulfate [PMS]) to a highly colored formazan. The special feature of the XTT formazan, which makes it attractive for application to the antiviral assay, is its solubility in the culture medium, which allows direct spectrophotometric assay of optical density in the culture wells. Indeed, the entire assay procedure after addition of the XTT reagent is carried out in sealed culture wells, thereby potentially enhancing the safety of the assay as well as simplifying the problems of disposal of the assay plates and contents. All steps of the antiviral assay are carried out under BL3 containment facilities.

This is the general framework from which the particular assay protocol currently in use has been developed. The specific parameters, such as choice of host cell line, viral strain(s) to be used, viral multiplicity, drug exposure times, and numerous other variables, have been the subject of considerable discussion, debate, and experimentation. Indeed, shortly after the DCT Board of Scientific Counselors approval of the DTP plan to proceed with the implementation of an antiviral

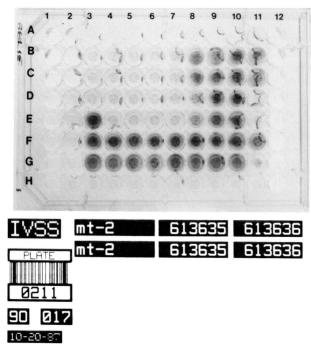

FIG. 18-5. Photograph showing microtiter plate with bar code label used in automated AIDS-antiviral assay. In this example, rows F and G contain virus-free host (MT-2) cells and rows B, C, D, and E contain virus-infected host cells. Columns 4–11 contain increasing concentrations (Log_{10} intervals) of the test drug and a positive control drug. In this example, rows B, C, and F contain AZT and rows D, E, and G contain an unknown. Color density in the wells (see Fig. 18-6 and text discussion of XTT reagent) is proportional to the number of viable host cells remaining at the end of the incubation period. Here, it is readily apparent that both AZT and the unknown drug enhance the survival of the virus-infected host cells at drug concentrations well below those directly toxic to the host cells.

screen, a workshop was organized and held in Bethesda, Maryland on April 8–9, 1987, entitled "Issues for Implementation of a National Anti-HIV Preclinical Drug Evaluation Program; Critical Parameters for an *in Vitro* Human Host–Cell Based Primary Screen." Participants in the workshop included a broad representation of experts from groups actively involved in virology and antiviral research throughout the country. Both the feasibility and the specific assay protocol issues were discussed in great detail. A verbatim transcript of the workshop proceedings is available.[19] Participants at the workshop were in general agreement that the screen proposed by DTP was feasible.

Based upon recommendations from this workshop, a variety of potential host cell lines for the assay, as well as assay protocols, have been under consideration and evaluation. The cell lines include human lymphoblastoid lines such as MT-2, ATH8, CEM, C3-44, LDV-7 and Sup-T1, as well as others such as U937 and HeLa/T4.[19]

The ATH8 line, used by NCI intramural scientists for preclinical studies of agents such as suramin, AZT, and DDC,[3,7] was viewed by workshop participants as useful for follow-up or secondary testing of materials emanating from the primary screen.[22]

Among the individual cell lines evaluated for the primary screen, the MT-2 line originally developed in Japan[20] initially appeared to best meet many of the optimal criteria. However, the simultaneous use of several different host cell lines is feasible with the automated microculture assay technology. A detailed description of the assay protocols evaluated to date, and the basis for the particular selection of "standardized" protocols, and the validation thereof for current use in the primary screen, will be provided in a separate publication. A detailed, periodic review of the primary assay, its further development, and the development of related secondary assays will be the task of an extramural ad hoc review committee for the AIDS screen project.

Currently, screening with the new assay is on-going at both the FCRF and at a contractor laboratory (Southern Research Institute, Birmingham, Alabama). Screening capacity as of fall 1987 is approximately 120 samples per week, which will be further expanded to approximately 250 samples per week in the near future. During 1988 the goal is full implementation of the primary screen to a total capacity of approximately 500 samples per week (24,000/yr).

Appendix B shows a DTP supplier report exemplifying the current format of the screening data provided to the original supplier of the test compound. Presently, each material is evaluated over a wide range of concentrations (8 log_{10} dilutions), in duplicate, for both the control and the virus-infected cells. Sample curves of typical assay responses, including an example of an inactive substance, and two examples of substances with differing patterns of anti-HIV activity, are routinely provided as a part of the report (see Appendix B).

Potential AIDS Antiviral Applications of New in Vivo Models Under Development by NCI

It is of interest to consider other potential applications of new NCI antitumor screening models to antiviral assays. For example, agents identified in the new NCI *in vitro* cancer screen as having antitumor activity in particular cell lines of interest are further evaluated against these same cell lines using novel *in vivo* models specifically developed for this program. One such model is the microencapsulated tumor assay (META).[21] In this model the desired cell line (e.g., any line of interest from the *in vitro* screen) is encapsulated within small (≤1 mm) nutrient- and drug-permeable spheres implanted within the peritoneal cavities of athymic mice. The mice are treated (IV, SC, PO, or as desired) with the test substances, and after the appropriate interval, the microcapsules are recovered, lysed, and cell viability determined (e.g., by cell count and/or by metabolic assay such as XTT).

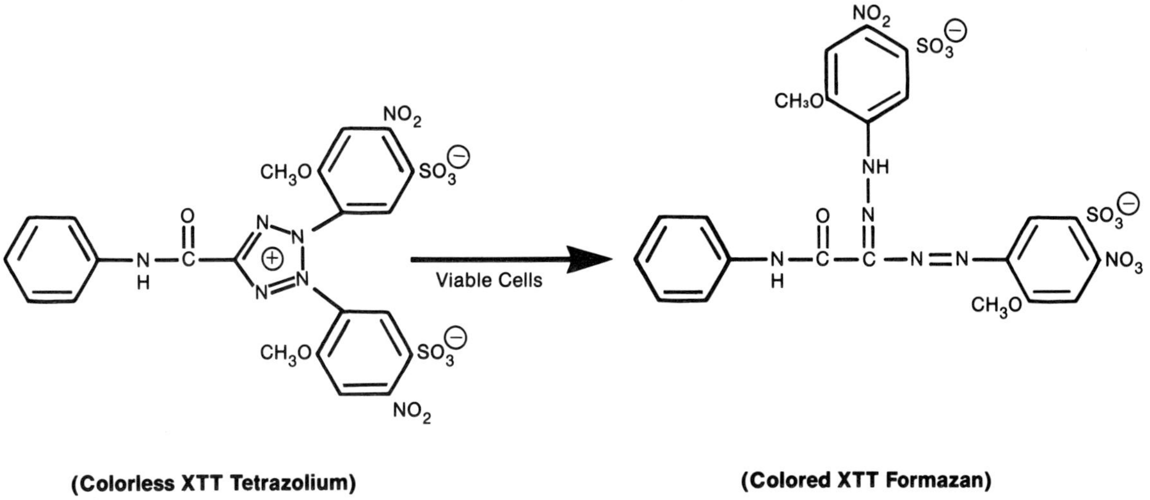

(Colorless XTT Tetrazolium)   **(Colored XTT Formazan)**

FIG. 18-6. New reagent used for the high-flux, automated cell culture assay technology used by DTP for antitumor and AIDS-antiviral screens; the colorless XTT tetrazolium is metabolically reduced, in proportion to the number of viable cells in the culture wells, to a colored formazan derivative that is measured spectrophotometrically. For antitumor or other cell growth inhibition end points, active compounds are detected by a diminished production of XTT formazan. For antiviral or other cell growth enhancement end points, active compounds are detected by an enhanced production of XTT formazan.

An *in vivo* antiviral application of the META appears obvious: to grow the microencapsulated host cells of interest in athymic mice and evaluate the drug effects on host cell survival. As in the *in vitro* antiviral assay, a positive antiviral effect of the test drug is indicated by an enhancement of the growth/survival of the virus-infected human host cells contained in the microcapsules. At its February 1987 meeting, the DCT Board of Scientific Counselors approved a DTP plan to explore application of the META to antiviral testing.[1] Feasibility evaluations of this approach to *in vivo* anti-HIV screening have been encouraging.[22]

NATIONAL CANCER INSTITUTE AIDS PRECLINICAL DRUG RESEARCH AND DEVELOPMENT PROGRAM: DRUG DEVELOPMENT PHASE

Overview

Of the major functions depicted in Figure 18-1, those subsequent to acquisition and biologic testing comprise the preclinical development phase. Most of the activities encompassed therein are generally required for most classes of drugs whether for treatment of AIDS, cancer, or other diseases. These activities include bulk chemical synthesis and drug production, toxicology and pharmacology, clinical formulation production, and quality control. It should be emphasized that, when appropriate and if the necessary resources are available, the pre-

clinical drug development program can be utilized not only for primary anti-HIV agents, but also for rapid development of other high-priority candidate agents (e.g., agents for treatment of opportunistic infections; agents for stimulation of the immune system) of potential value in therapy of AIDS.

The preclinical development phase is subdivided into two stages, A and B.

Stage A Preclinical Development

Stage A (Table 18-1) focuses upon feasibility evaluations relevant to consideration for further development and the elucidation of additional biologic information to further assess merit and relative priority as a drug candidate. Abbreviated toxicologic and pharmacokinetic evaluations are intended to guide the follow-up evaluations of the drug candidates in any relevant *in vivo* disease models available, as well as, where necessary, to provide a basis for selection/prioritization of potential candidates for further development based on *in vitro* preclinical screening data alone.

Stage B Preclinical Development

Stage B (Table 18-2) represents the final phase of preclinical development and is generally undertaken only for agents for which there is a clear commitment to clinical testing. The major tasks include the production of

Table 18-1

Activities Encompassed in Stage A Preclinical Development

1. Develop and optimize method for isolation and/or synthesis; evaluate scale-up feasibility and costs
2. Optimize leads through congener/prodrug synthesis when appropriate
3. Develop method for production of acceptable pharmaceutical formulation
4. Develop qualitative and quantitative analytical methods
5. Prepare radiolabeled drug if feasible
6. Determine maximally tolerated dose (MTD) in one or more animal species; measure relevant body compartmental concentrations of drug at MTD
7. Measure oral bioavailability
8. Test for *in vivo* activity in appropriate model(s) if available

Table 18-2

Activities Encompassed in Stage B Preclinical Development

1. Produce and/or purchase necessary amounts of bulk chemical
2. Prepare suitably formulated drug
3. Monitor purity of bulk chemical and formulated drug
4. Perform route- and schedule-dependency studies in *in vivo* model if feasible
5. Perform detailed pharmacokinetic analyses in at least one species
6. Perform full toxicologic evaluation in rodents and dogs
7. Develop sufficient quantity of formulated drug for clinical distribution; monitor quality control

bulk drug properly formulated for clinical usage, the detailed evaluation of toxicology and pharmacokinetics, and the performance of additional preclinical studies as needed to guide the optimal design of clinical trials protocols.

Stage B also encompasses many activities addressing the complex regulatory requirements that are encountered increasingly as a drug progresses through the late steps of preclinical development and into the clinical arena. Bulk production of synthetic or natural products must be accomplished in facilities meeting rigidly defined regulatory requirements. Likewise, drug formulations and purities must meet established standards and be monitored extensively. Highly defined quality control requirements must be addressed, and detailed drug inventory and distribution protocols, and records thereof, must be managed. Particularly in the area of toxicologic evaluation, the last major preclinical development step, the regulatory requirements are complex. Indeed, DTP staff often work very closely with the FDA to finalize the toxicology database providing the critical support for

filing of the investigational new drug application (INDA) for a new agent.

Approval of the INDA by the FDA marks the beginning of the clinical development phase. Although the primary role of the preclinical program is thus completed, certain difficulties encountered in the early clinical trials may require re-involvement of the preclinical program in additional stage B activities. This most commonly results from unexpected problems with formulations, or stabilities thereof, and unpredicted toxicities. Often, then, the preclinical program and clinical program staff can work effectively together to address and successfully resolve such problems when they arise with an otherwise promising new drug.

KEY DTP/DCT COMMITTEE FUNCTIONS FOR NCI PRECLINICAL DRUG RESEARCH AND DEVELOPMENT PROGRAM

Discovery Phase

Acquisitions/Input Committee

The Acquisitions/Input Committee (AIC) is composed predominantly of senior DTP staff from the acquisitions and biologic testing areas. The focus of the AIC is Decision Point (DP) I-A as depicted in Figure 18-2. This committee regularly reviews the current acquisitions inventory and selects and prioritizes the available agents for initial screening. Relative priorities are determined principally upon criteria of chemical or biologic uniqueness or novelty of the agent, or any other relevant known property (Table 18-3). However, if sufficient screening capacity is available, the policy of the program is to screen essentially all new acquisitions.

The AIC also is responsible for identifying potential "bypass" agents for which there is some reasonable rationale or prior information to recommend immediate entry to a more advanced stage of development. Such "bypass" recommendations go initially to the DTP Operating Committee, then to the DCT Decision Network Committee for further consideration (see below). The AIC chairpersons or their designates serve as the initial contact point for potential entry of new agents to the NCI preclinical drug development program.

Biologic Evaluation Committee

The Biologic Evaluation Committee (BEC), composed predominantly of senior DTP staff, addresses decision point I-A (see Figure 18-2). In so doing, the Committee regularly reviews all screening data emanating from the *in vitro* screens, and selects and prioritizes "active" agents for presentation to the DCT Decision Network Committee (see below). Recommended priorities are likewise based predominantly upon biologic and structural novelty, as well as other potentially

Table 18-3

Responsibilities of DTP Acquisitions/Input Committee: Decision Point (I-A)

1. Recommend and prioritize materials for biologic testing.
2. Recommend potential "bypass" candidates.

Criteria for Recommendations

1. Available testing capacity
2. Uniqueness of structure or source
3. Known or predicted biologic activity of interest
4. Previous performance in screens (e.g., as crude or partially purified product)
5. Relevant other properties (e.g., opportunistic anti-infective; immunostimulatory
6. Rationale for identification as "bypass" candidate

Table 18-4

Responsibilities of DTP Biologic Evaluation Committee: Decision Point (I-B)

1. Recommend and prioritize active drug candidates for presentation to Decision Network Committee (DNC)
2. Recommend additional testing as appropriate

Criteria for Recommendations

1. Appropriate *in vitro* antitumor and/or antiviral activity and/or other relevant bioactivity
2. Relative potency or other potentially favorable characteristics
3. Uniqueness of structure and/or biologic properties

Table 18-5

Responsibilities of DCT Decision Network Committee: Decision Point (II-A)

1. Recommend and prioritize new candidates for stage A development
2. Recommend other supplementary studies as appropriate

Criteria for Recommendations:

1. Appropriate antitumor and/or antiviral activity and/or other relevant bioactivity
2. Uniqueness of structure and/or biologic properties
3. Availability of resources for further preclinical development
4. Consideration of potential options for current and/or future industrial participation in development

favorable pharmacologic characteristics (Table 18-4). At DP II-A, *in vivo* preclinical studies may or may not have yet been undertaken and are not considered obligatory at this point. On an annual basis it is anticipated that the BEC will bring to the Decision Network Committee a maximum of 100 to 200 of the highest priority new leads for further consideration and selection and for prioritization of its subsets for stage A development.

Development Phase

Decision Network Committee

The Decision Network Committee (DNC) functions at three critical decision points, DP II-A, II-B, and III, within the preclinical development phase (see Fig. 19-2). The regular DNC membership includes the DCT director, the DCT associate directors, the chairpersons of the AIC, BEC, DCT operating committee, and selected other senior DCT, NCI, and NIAID staff. Additional ad hoc members with specialized expertise may be appointed by the DNC chairman whenever appropriate for specific DNC meetings.

At DP II-A, the DNC is responsible for selecting and prioritizing new drug candidates for stage A development (see Fig. 18-2). Generally, in accord with current available resources, a maximum of only 10 to 20 agents will be selected annually for stage A. As indicated in Table 18-5, the major criteria considered are similar to those for earlier stages. However, at this point there are additional considerations of potential options for current and/or future industrial participation in development.

It is the policy of the program to encourage maximum industrial participation as soon as possible in the development of a promising new agent. This maintains maximum flexibility and responsiveness of the program to facilitate the development of the most promising agents at any stage, as well as to accommodate the development of other potential agents that may be relative "orphans" (i.e., have no patent positions) with respect to industrial or other interests in development. The resources of the program are finite and the expenses for development escalate rapidly as an agent proceeds to the later stages. Direct contract costs for preclinical development of an agent through stages A and B may be generally expected to average a million or more dollars.

At decision point II-B (Table 18-6; see Fig. 18-2), a positive recommendation by the DNC for stage B development generally is based upon the view that the available biologic information on the agent is of sufficient interest and merit to justify eventual clinical testing. The decision and the priority assigned therewith must also take into account the limits of the available resources for stage B development; currently the program can accommodate four to six new drugs per year through stage B. Decision point III is confronted by the DNC at the completion of stage B development and prior to filing of an INDA. Chief concerns of the DNC at this point are to ensure that the appropriate regulatory, safety, and other issues relevant to the prudent design and execution of the clinical trials have been adequately addressed. Approval of a drug by the DNC at decision point III is followed by a period of intensive interaction between NIH preclinical and clinical program staff for preparation of the INDA. Subsequent approval of the drug by the FDA for clinical testing provides the final impetus for entry into the NIH extramural clinical trials network and/or the NIH intramural clinical programs.

Operating Committee

The Operating Committee (OC) does not have primary responsibilities at any of the specific decision points discussed above. Nonetheless it plays a very important role (Table 18-7) in expediting and monitoring the flow of compounds through the various stages of development encompassed within the DTP. The OC is comprised of senior DTP staff predominantly representing the development area. The committee is responsible for organizing the DNC meeting agenda, as well as for ensuring implementation of its recommendations. DNC agenda candidates are provided to the chairperson of the OC from the AIC (re: "bypass" candidates) and the BEC (re: actives identified from the screens). The OC chairperson also serves as the contact

point for inquiries for consideration of assistance in specific, limited aspects of development.

SUMMARY AND PERSPECTIVE

There has been an urgent need for an adequate national program to which scientists from the broadest possible spectrum of the entire research community can submit materials for rapid evaluation for anti-HIV activity. The need has been similarly urgent for a national program to support the expeditious preclinical development of the most promising new drug candidates through any or all the stages of preclinical development as required. The resource described herein is intended to help provide a focus for the best talents and resources from government, academia, and industry to work effectively in concert toward the rapid discovery and development of new anti-HIV drug candidates. This resource will complement and substantially enrich the expanded AIDS NCDDGs (multi-disciplinary, multi-institutional) and other drug discovery efforts based on rational design and/or screening, located throughout the country—indeed, worldwide. These synergistic approaches to new anti-AIDS drug discovery might also prove to have important ramifications for additional disease areas such as cancer, arthritis, multiple sclerosis, and others for which slow-growing viruses with long incubation times are implicated.

Table 18-6
Responsibilities of DCT Decision Network Committee: Decision Point (II-B)

1. Recommend and prioritize new candidates for stage B development
2. Recommend other supplementary studies as appropriate

Criteria for Recommendations

1. Major technical, time, and cost considerations resolved
2. Peak *in vivo* drug concentrations in plasma and/or other appropriate fluids or tissues (e.g., in cerebrospinal fluid for AIDS-antiviral agents) at MTD in at least one animal species are equal to or greater than those known to give positive *in vitro* antitumor and/or antiviral activity
3. Other potentially favorable characteristics (e.g., activity in *in vivo* model; oral bioavailability)
4. Consideration of potential options for current and/or future industrial participation in development

---

Table 18-7
Responsibilities of DCT Decision Network Committee: Decision Point (III)

1. Recommend and prioritize drug candidates for INDA filing and clinical evaluation
2. Recommend other supplementary studies as appropriate

Criteria for Recommendations

1. Safe starting dose for humans predicted from animal toxicology studies
2. Normal tissue toxicity for humans estimated from animal toxicology studies
3. Drug pharmacokinetic studies in animals allow optimal design of clinical studies in humans

REFERENCES

1. AIDS Update: Division of Cancer Treatment approves 17 AIDS concepts. Cancer Lett 6[Suppl]:5, 1987
2. Driscoll JS: The preclinical new drug research program of the National Cancer Institute. Cancer Treat 68:63, 1984
3. Mitsuya H, Broder S: Inhibition of the *in vitro* infectivity and cytopathic effect of human T-lymphotrophic virus type III/lymphadenopathy-associated virus (HTLV-III/LAV) by 2',3'-dideoxynucleosides. Proc Natl Acad Sci 83:1911, 1986
4. Mitsuya H, Weinhold K, Furman P et al: 3'-Azido-3'-deoxythymidine (BW A509U): An antiviral agent that inhibits the infectivity and cytopathic effect of human T-lymphotropic virus type III/lymphadenopathy-associated virus *in vitro*. Proc Natl Acad Sci 82:7096, 1985
5. Herrmann EC Jr: The detection, assay and evaluation of antiviral drugs. Prog Med Virol 3:158, 1961
6. Ehrlich J, Sloan BJ, Miller FA et al: Detection and evaluation of potential antiviral drugs. Ann NY Acad Sci 130:5, 1965
7. Burns JJ, Groopman JE: AIDS: Strategic considerations for developing antiviral drugs. In Issues in Science and Technology. Natl Acad Sci 3:102, 1987
8. Institute of Medicine, National Academy of Sciences Committee on a National Strategy for AIDS of the Institute of Medicine. Confronting AIDS: Directions for public health, health care, and research. Washington, DC, National Academy Press, 1986
9. Boyd MR: National Cancer Institute Drug Discovery and Development. In Frei EJ, Freireich EJ (eds): Accomplishments in Oncology, vol 1, No 1, Cancer Therapy: Where Do We Go From Here?, p 8. Philadelphia, JB Lippincott, 1986

10. Boyd MR, Shoemaker RH, McLemore TL et al: New drug development. In Roth JA, Ruckdeschel JC, Weisenburger TH (eds): Thoracic Oncology. New York, WB Saunders, in press.

11. DCT Board approves new screening program, natural product concepts. Cancer Lett 1:4, 1985

12. Developmental Therapeutics Program, Division of Cancer Treatment, National Cancer Institute, Bethesda, Maryland: Proceedings of Ad Hoc Review committee for NCI *in vitro/ in vivo* disease-oriented screening project, December 8–9, 1986

13. DCT gets okay to proceed with human cell line drug screening, more drug discovery groups. Cancer Lett 19:1, 1987

14. Alley MC, Scudiero DA, Monks A et al: Feasibility of drug screening with panels of human tumor cell lines using a microculture tetrazolium assay. Cancer Res 48:589, 1988

15. Scudiero DA, Shoemaker RH, Paull KD et al: A new simplified tetrazolium assay for cell growth and drug sensitivity in culture. Cancer Res (In preparation)

16. Paull KD, Shoemaker RH, Boyd M et al: The synthesis of XTT: A new tetrazolium reagent bioreducible to a water-soluble formazan. J Hetero Chem (In press)

17. Monks A, Scudiero D, Shoemaker R et al: Implementation of a pilot-scale anticancer drug screening program utilizing disease-oriented panels of human tumor cell lines. Proc Am Assoc Cancer Res (In press)

18. Weislow OS, Shoemaker RH, Kiser R et al: Application of an automated microculture tetrazolium assay to large-scale AIDS antiviral drug screening. Fed Proc (In preparation)

19. Developmental Therapeutics Program, Division of Cancer Treatment, National Cancer Institute, Bethesda, Maryland: Proceedings of NCI/NIAID workshop on issues for implementation of a national anti-HIV preclinical drug evaluation program; critical parameters for an *in vitro,* human host-cell based, primary screen, April 8–9, 1987

20. Koyanagi Y, Harada S, Takahashi M et al: Selective cytotoxicity of AIDS virus infection towards HTLV-I transformed cell lines. Int J Cancer 36:445, 1985

21. Gorelik E, Ovejera A, Shoemaker R et al: Microencapsulated tumor assay: New short-term assay for *in vivo* evaluation of the effects of anticancer drugs on human tumor cell lines. Cancer Res 47:5739, 1987

22. McMahon J, Camalier R, Shoemaker R et al: Feasibility of microencapsulation technology for the evaluation of anti-HIV drugs *in vivo.* Fed Proc (In press)

APPENDIX A
Document of Confidentiality

Director
Division of Cancer Treatment
National Cancer Institute
National Institutes of Health
Bethesda, Maryland 20892

Dear Sir:

RE: Agreement for Submitting Products
to the Division of Cancer Treatment,
National Cancer Institute.

We submit herewith to you for your approval our understanding of the arrangements to be used as a guide in the confidential screening of our products by the Division of Cancer Treatment. This agreement will serve as a basis for this Company's voluntary cooperation with you in the treatment of AIDS and opportunistic infections associated with AIDS.

1. From time to time we may supply products, patented or unpatented, so that you may proceed to screen and test such products for possible treatment for AIDS and AIDS-related infections. These products are to be used for screening and testing as anti-viral, anti-bacterial, anti-fungal, anti-parasitic, immunomodulating, and biological modifying agents with potential for the treatment of AIDS and associated infections, and for no other purpose.

    The products will be screened by one or more of the National Cancer Institute's contract testing laboratories, or in any other testing laboratory which may from time to time be added to the Program but in any event will not be placed in the laboratories of any company in the pharmaceutical or chemical industries without our permission.

2. In order to facilitate the records keeping and handling of confidential materials, we propose the following procedure:

    a. We shall forward to the Division of Cancer Treatment the products to be tested together with a data sheet for each product, giving pertinent available data as to chemical constitution, solubility, toxicity, and any precautions which need to be followed in handling, storing and shipping.

    b. The Division of Cancer Treatment will inform us which products are new to their program and will provide us with a record of the accession numbers of the products, retaining the data sheets for your files. Duplicate products will be returned to us upon our specific request.

    c. It is clearly understood that no data about the products and the results of the testing will be kept in files open to the public either by the Division of Cancer Treatment, the testing laboratories, or the data processing activities. Only those employees directly engaged in the operation of the Division of Cancer Treatment will have access to the files of information regarding source and nature of confidential materials and results of testing.

    d. Whenever possible we will be given our choice of the National Cancer Institute's contract testing laboratories, although at present we have no preference; and it is understood that the Division of Cancer Treatment reserves the right to send our products to another screening contractor if the need arises. It is furthermore understood that the contracts of the Division of Cancer Treatment with the testing laboratories will contain provisions to safeguard the rights of our Company under this Agreement.

    e. In order that we may submit to you products in which we have a proprietary interest and on which we do not as yet have adequate patent protection we may, if we so desire, submit up to five percent of our products under our code number only. We agree, in this event, to reveal to you the structures or identities of those coded products which subsequently turn out to be positive in any one of your test systems, as judged by whatever standards you have in existence at that time.

    f. You shall return to us any of our products which we may designate at any time before you have started actual screening and testing or within six months if the screening and testing have already started.

3. Though we recognize that the interchange of information is generally desirable in the field of treatment for AIDS, it is our mutual understanding that our Company, in voluntarily supplying a product hereunder, is entitled to protection for the research and development work it has done and for any technical information it may furnish.

    a. You, accordingly, agree that all rights in those compounds or products in which we have a proprietary interest shall remain in our Company. Subject, notwithstanding, to the proviso that, with respect only to those drugs which have been determined by means of the various screening and testing processes to possess such significant AIDS treatment potential to be scheduled for clinical trial by the Division of Cancer Treatment, the Government shall have a royalty-free, irrevocable, nonexclusive license under any patent which the Company may have or obtain on such compound or product or on a process for use of such compound or product, to manufacture and/or use by or for the Government the invention(s) claimed by the patent(s) only for medical research purposes related to or connected with the therapy of AIDS and AIDS-related infections.

    b. We agree that the publication of biological data on products supplied by us is worthwhile and shall be encouraged. Specifically:

        (1) With regard to screening results on compounds in which our Company has a proprietary interest, that you deem significant for the furtherance of treatment of AIDS research, we agree that you may publish such results after a period of twelve months from the date of final reporting of screening and testing results to us. Publication of data within the twelve-month period requires our prior consent. For the purposes of this Agreement, compounds falling in this category are limited to those which the Division of Cancer Treatment has selected to pursue toward clinical trial; and the date of reporting is defined as the date on which you report to us the selection of the compound as a clinical candidate.

        (2) For all other compounds, you may ask our consent periodically to publish screening data along with the available biological and physical data; and such consent shall not be unreasonably withheld.

        (3) In no case will you publish information identifying us as the source of the compound without our written approval.

    c. As soon as tests are completed and reported to the Division of Cancer Treatment, we will receive from you a full report including all screening data. The drugs scheduled for clinical trial, referred to hereinbefore, shall be designated by the Division of Cancer Treatment, and the beforementioned report will specify the compounds so selected. The Division of Cancer Treatment shall be consulted whenever our Company desires to include your screening data in a publication, and appropriate credit shall be given to the U.S. Public Health Service.

4. You agree to screen our products against the appropriate screens for therapy in the treatment of AIDS and associated diseases. It is understood that the Company has no control over the Division of Cancer Treatment's use of the products submitted hereunder and shall not be liable for any damages which the NCI or the U.S. Government may incur as a result of the Division of Cancer Treatment's use or testing of such products.

We are confident that this agreement will lay the basis for mutually satisfactory cooperation in the field of therapy in the treatment of AIDS and associated diseases research. If you agree to the above, we would appreciate your countersigning the attached duplicate of this agreement and returning it to us for our files.

Yours very truly,

_____
Name (Signature)

_____
Name (Print)

_____
Title

_____
Company

_____
Address

_____
Date

_____
Director
Division of Cancer Treatment, NCI

DEPARTMENT OF HEALTH & HUMAN SERVICES　　Public Health Service

National Institutes of Health
National Cancer Institute
Bethesda, Maryland 20892
TLX:908111

Dear Dr.

The compound, with the NSC number cited in the attachment, which you submitted for testing by the National Cancer Institute has been evaluated for *in-vitro* anti-HIV activity.

The protocol used in NCI's Developmental Therapeutics Program AIDS antiviral drug screening program involves plating of susceptible human "host" cells with and without virus in microculture plates, adding various concentrations of test material, incubating the plates for seven days (during which time infected, non-drug treated control cells are largely or totally destroyed by the virus), and then determining the number of remaining viable cells using a colorimetric endpoint. To help put the results for your compound in perspective, we cite the results obtained for AZT (Figure 1), castanospermine, a glycosylation inhibitor currently being followed as a lead by this Program (Figure 2), and a compound which shows no antiviral activity (Figure 3). In Figure 1, dose related antiviral activity which is limited by growth inhibitory activity at high drug concentrations is observed. Two parameters can be extracted from the curves: the EC50, representing the concentration of drug that results in a 50% reduction of the viral cytopathic effect; and the IC50, representing the concentration of drug resulting in 50% growth inhibition (derived from the normal, uninfected cultures). An *in-vitro* therapeutic index (TI) can be calculated as the ratio (IC50/EC50).

At present, we have no strict criteria regarding "activity" in the anti-HIV drug screen. Compounds showing any *in-vitro* anti-HIV activity are considered carefully and may or may not be followed up, depending upon the structural type they represent and also their activity relative to other leads in the program.

Questions regarding these data should be addressed to me at the address below.

Biologist
Biological Testing Branch,
NCI-FCRF,
Building 428, Room 63,
Frederick, MD, 21701-1240
Telephone (301) 698-5605

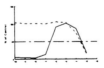

Figure 1

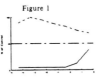

Figure 2

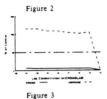

Figure 3

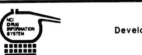

National Cancer Institute

Developmental Therapeutics Program

In-Vitro Testing Results

NSC: 376451-T	COMI: DMK-I-287A	SSPL: 216B	November 9, 1987

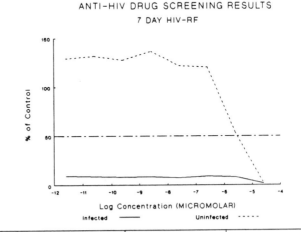

ANTI-HIV DRUG SCREENING RESULTS
7 DAY HIV-RF

% of Control

Log Concentration (MICROMOLAR)

Infected ——　　Uninfected - - - -

Cell Line: MT-2		Plate Number: 0028 Lab: 90	Test Date: 24-Jun-87		
		Uninfected		Infected	
IC50 = 2.97×10⁻⁸		Dose	Response	Dose	Response
EC50 =		Micromolar	% of Control	Micromolar	% of Control
TI50 =					
		2.50E-12	129.10	2.50E-12	9.20
IC90 = 1.73×10⁻⁸		2.50E-11	131.60	2.50E-11	8.70
EC90 =		2.50E-10	127.50	2.50E-10	8.10
TI90 =		2.50E-09	136.50	2.50E-09	8.60
		2.50E-08	121.80	2.50E-08	7.50
IC100 = 2.50×10⁻⁸		2.50E-07	120.30	2.50E-07	9.10
EC100 =		2.50E-06	53.90	2.50E-06	8.10
TI100 =		2.50E-05	1.70	2.50E-05	1.40

Psychosocial Issues: Prevention and Treatment

Grace H. Christ
Karolynn Siegel
Rosemary T. Moynihan

19

The psychosocial effects of AIDS vary at different points along a health–illness continuum ranging from asymptomatic to HIV-positive to symptomatic. Understanding the different psychosocial issues that confront individuals at different points along that continuum can lead to more effective treatments and better ways of helping patients cope with the illness.

First, the psychosocial issues confronting people who have no symptoms of AIDS are reviewed. This group includes individuals who are seronegative, those who have not been tested and who are therefore uncertain about their antibody status, and those who have tested seropositive for the HIV virus but remain asymptomatic. Second, the social and psychological issues that confront AIDS patients, their sexual partners, and their family and friends are discussed. The chapter ends with a description of one intervention program developed to deal with these issues.

ISSUES CONFRONTING ASYMPTOMATIC INDIVIDUALS

Asymptomatic individuals who have not been tested for HIV antibodies represent circumstances ranging from those who run a minimal risk of exposure to AIDS to those who, because of their past sexual or drug-taking behavior, run a strong risk of infection. Regardless of where a person falls on this continuum, three important psychosocial issues are relevant: (1) prevention or reduction of risk, (2) HIV antibody counseling, and (3) coping with uncertainty and the anxiety that uncertainty evokes.

Preventive behaviors that can reduce the risk of infection or transmission of HIV should be addressed with all sexually active people who are not in long-standing, mutually monogamous relationships. The counselor should review the risk-reduction guidelines below in a

nonjudgmental manner. The important task is to help clients understand the following facts:

- Their behavior, not their membership in a particular group, is what places them at risk for infection.
- The virus can be transmitted during vaginal intercourse, anal intercourse, and oral-genital contact as well as through the sharing of contaminated needles.
- Condoms must be used properly and consistently during all sexual encounters where the virus conceivably could be transmitted—for instance, during any casual sexual encounter. Even with condoms there are no guarantees—a small risk of infection is always present.

BARRIERS TO BEHAVIORAL CHANGE

Heterosexuals

Although female-to-male transmission of the HIV virus is not well documented and may be less efficient than male-to-female transmission,[1-8] many heterosexuals are probably infected but are unaware of it and therefore are not protecting their partners. In a random sample of high-risk heterosexuals from the San Francisco area who had two or more sexual partners within the previous 12 months or knowingly had sexual relations with a gay or bisexual male, intravenous (IV) drug user, or prostitute, a study commissioned by the San Francisco AIDS Foundation found that high-risk sexual practices persisted despite the high incidence of AIDS in the area.[9] In other words, a variety of barriers to the widespread adoption of behavioral modification operate among heterosexuals. Among the most prevalent barriers are weak perception of one's vulnerability, a dislike of condoms, ignorance about the magnitude of the threat, the interpersonal nature of sexual activity, the stigma of AIDS.

Misperceptions About the Magnitude of the Threat

Most models of preventive health behavior regard a feeling of susceptibility to an illness as a necessary (although not necessarily sufficient) condition for adopting a preventive health action.[10] Several authors have documented the human tendency to believe that one will not be a victim of negative life events.[11–13] People tend to distort reality in a positive direction to avoid the anxiety that would result from a realistic assessment of their vulnerability. Thus, individuals may falsely appraise their risk for infection. In addition, public health education also must deal with unfounded optimism about one's invulnerability to AIDS and other health threats.

Because of some unfortunate ways we have communicated with the public about AIDS in both the media and public health messages, many heterosexuals believe that they have little cause for concern. For example, the widespread emphasis on anal intercourse as a principal mode of sexual transmission may lead many heterosexuals to believe they are at low risk. Similarly, the early emphasis on a large number of partners as the major factor may lead many who have had few partners to believe they are not threatened. In reality, of course, the possibility of being infected exists even with a single partner if the two practice unsafe sex.[14] The focus on "risk groups" rather than "risk behaviors" is still a feature of health communications, and this focus has contributed to a false sense of security among many who engage in practices associated with transmission of the AIDS virus.

Furthermore, people also evaluate their risk of experiencing a negative life event by using stereotypes, or what Tversky and Kahneman[15] called the "representativeness" heuristic—people tend to have preconceived notions about the kind of person who is prone to a particular kind of negative event such as a sexually transmitted disease. In the case of a venereal disease, the stereotype is usually of a lower-class member of a minority group who has many sexual contacts. To the extent that people perceive themselves as different from such stereotypes, they will regard their risk as low. The same stereotypes are used to evaluate a prospective partner's risk of being infected.

Although the creeping spread of AIDS in the heterosexual community has been discussed intermittently in the media, one also hears periodic reassurances that the proportion of AIDS cases in low-risk groups has remained relatively stable over time. These apparently conflicting messages have confused many heterosexuals about their chances of becoming infected.

Finally, although bidirectional transmission of the virus is accepted as possible, the relatively small number of documented cases of female-to-male transmission has contributed to the perception that heterosexual males probably are at low risk for infection during unprotected intercourse. Because males are still expected to introduce condoms, this poor appreciation of their own vulnerability may be a barrier to using them in a heterosexual relationship.

Antipathy Toward Condoms

Condoms are an important method of controlling the spread of HIV infection as well as other sexually transmitted diseases.[16,17] Preliminary data, although inconclusive, also seem to support the efficacy of condoms in preventing transmission of the HIV virus.[18] Whether heterosexuals will be more motivated to use condoms to prevent AIDS than they have been to prevent other venereal diseases remains to be seen. According to Hart,[16] the proportion of male clinic patients who have sexually transmitted diseases ranges from 3% to 20%, whereas the use of condoms in the general male population does not exceed 25%.

Well-documented barriers to the use of condoms include the following:

- The belief that the device compromises the pleasure of intercourse[19–21]
- The tendency to view the condom as a contraceptive rather than a prophylactic device[22,23]
- The belief that condoms are unnatural[19,20]
- The tendency to underestimate the personal risk of infection and the failure to anticipate or prepare for sexual activity[16,24,25]
- The belief that one's partner will be offended by the introduction of a condom[23–25]
- The use of alcohol or drugs before or during sexual intercourse, which leads to neglecting to use condoms or using them improperly[24,25]
- The association of condoms with promiscuity, prostitution, and extramarital sex[27–29]
- The belief that condoms are ineffective or unreliable[16,27]
- The embarrassment experienced when purchasing condoms,[30,31] and
- The common belief that condoms make sex seem premeditated rather than spontaneous.

The Interpersonal Nature of Sex

Because of the interpersonal nature of sexual intercourse, decisions to engage in or refrain from risky sex must be "negotiated." To practice safe sex effectively, the partners must agree on limits and on the use of condoms whenever the opportunity to exchange body fluids exists. With most preventive health behaviors (such as being vaccinated or practicing breast self-examination), only one person has to be persuaded to change his or her behavior to bring about the desired outcome; when two individuals are involved, both must be persuaded to modify their actions. When one partner is not motivated to practice safe sex, he or she either may not cooperate with the partner or may undermine the partner's resolve by denying that unprotected intercourse is risky or by failing to use condoms properly.

The Stigma Associated With AIDS

Sexually transmitted diseases have always been stigmatized in American society because they are widely regarded as being the result of sexual excess, low moral character, dirt, and uncleanliness.[32] So strongly are these diseases connected with sin and moral depravity in the public mind that victims feel compelled to deny their condition or assert their innocence with statements such as "I got it from a toilet seat."[33]

AIDS, of course, is no exception. The fact that it is associated with two of society's most stigmatized groups—homosexuals and drug users—has only accentuated the stigma attached to the disease. Thus, the need to dissociate oneself from even the implication that one is infected is extremely great. If using a condom could be construed to mean that one might be at risk or is impugning the partner's character, a person may be unwilling to do so. Finally, the fear of stigma may make a person unwilling to seek information about AIDS.

Gay and Bisexual Men

Studies conducted in a number of American cities have found that homosexual men have significantly modified their sexual behavior in response to the threat of AIDS.[9,34-46] For example, the men reported increased use of condoms during anal intercourse and reduced frequency of oral contact and swallowing of semen, fewer sexual partners, and lower attendance at gay baths and backroom bars. Although these findings are based on self-reports and thus may be subject to errors in recall or deliberate misrepresentation, indirect evidence also indicates that significant changes in behavior have occurred in the gay community because of AIDS. The incidence of gonorrhea and syphilis among gay men in New York City and Denver showed a significant decline as early as 1983.[43,44]

Although these changes in sexual behavior are encouraging, the fact that a substantial number of gay men continue to participate in risky sexual behavior is disturbing from a public health viewpoint. As Handsfield[45] pointed out, the prevalence of HIV infections is cumulative. In San Francisco, for example, where two-thirds of gay men may be infected, an 80% reduction in high-risk contacts still means an 89% chance of exposure.

Fortunately, an accumulating body of research and clinical experience permits us to identify a variety of barriers to desirable behavioral adaptations among homosexual men: misperceptions of risk and vulnerability, confusion about the value of modifying sexual behavior, the relationship between high-risk behavior and gay identity, and the existence of health schema.

Misperceptions of Risk

Research indicates that a substantial number of gay men may underestimate the risk of infection that their behavior entails. In their sample of asymptomatic gay men in New York City, Bauman and Siegel[47] found that about 83% of the men who engaged in risky sexual behavior exhibited a variety of misconceptions and cognitive distortions concerning their own chances of contracting AIDS despite their awareness of the guidelines for safer sex. For example, those who engaged in risky practices only with partners they knew were more likely to underestimate the risk associated with their behavior than were those who engaged in the same practices, but with anonymous partners. They genuinely believed that simply knowing their partners reduced their risk of contracting the disease, whereas in reality, knowing one's partners, in and of itself, is no guarantee of protection; one must be certain that the partner is negative for HIV antibodies at the time of the sexual encounter. Because most data for this study were gathered before antibody testing was accessible, few men in the study knew their own or their partners' HIV status. Given the long incubation period of AIDS, one would have to take an extensive sexual history of any untested prospective partner to even begin to assess the risk of engaging in unsafe sexual practices with him. Even that would not be sufficient because few prospective partners could provide the necessary information about the sexual histories of their previous partners.

These findings are important because a perception of personal vulnerability to the disease is a necessary prerequisite to modifying one's behavior. Men who persist in consistently underestimating the danger inherent in risky behavior are unlikely to be motivated to change that behavior.

Confusion About the Value of Modifying Sexual Behavior

At about the same time it became clear that high-risk sexual behavior was related to the transmission of AIDS, the fact that the disease often had a long incubation period also was becoming evident.[48,49] Consequently, some gay men with a history of high-risk behavior with many partners believed that the sudden initiation of safer sex practices was futile because they either were probably infected already or, if they remained asymptomatic, must have some genetic immunity to the disease.

Now that a blood test for antibodies to the HIV virus is available, gay men can determine whether they actually have been exposed. However, widespread opposition to testing has developed within the gay community, primarily because of concerns about confidentiality and the ambiguous meaning of a positive result.

In addition, because the disease cannot be cured, the usefulness of the test seems questionable. Furthermore, a positive result causes severe emotional distress. Thus, many gay men choose not to be tested. Because the factors that distinguish infected individuals who eventually will develop AIDS from those who will not are unknown, it is unclear whether altering one's sexual behavior after infection can influence the outcome of the disease.

Many gay men feel that the epidemiologic evidence about several possible modes of transmission (e.g., kissing or swallowing semen), apart from unprotected anal intercourse, remains inconclusive. In a random study of gay men in San Francisco,[35] only 11% of the men agreed with the following statement: "Medical researchers now know which practices transmit the AIDS virus." As long as scientific evidence is inconclusive, its power to influence behavior is limited.

Conflicting Values

Some men equate refraining from risky sexual practices with an abnegation of their homosexuality. Furthermore, such activities serve the important function of integrating them into the homosexual community. As McKusick and co-workers pointed out, recommending that a gay man modify his sexual behavior may conflict with values acquired during years of struggling for the right to choose among sexual options with externally imposed constraints.[50]

Thus, although gay men presumably value good health as highly as most people do, they may place equal value on risky sexual behavior. Evidence of such competing values was reported in the survey of gay men in San Francisco.[34] Although virtually all the men gave a high rating to the importance of reducing their chances of getting AIDS, half said they would engage in anal sex involving the exchange of semen as often or more often than they had before.

During the early stage of the AIDS epidemic, some segments of the gay community charged that labeling certain homosexual practices such as anal intercourse as high-risk behaviors represented an organized effort to suppress homosexual behavior and to discredit homosexuality as an acceptable lifestyle. Although this attitude currently is not widely held within the gay community as a whole, it is still expressed in some quarters.

Health Schema

People develop various explanations for why some people are susceptible to a disease and why others are not. Kortaba and Lang discovered two such explanations among gay men who engaged in risky sex practices despite the AIDS epidemic.[51] One group of men they studied had a holistic view of the human system—that is, they followed the sensible recommendation to have regular physical examinations, eat well, get adequate exercise and sleep, and minimize stress—believing that

these practices would protect them against AIDS whether they engaged in risky sexual behavior or not. Another group had a fatalistic attitude about AIDS, believing that people who contracted the disease were genetically predisposed or that the gay lifestyle made the risk of AIDS or other sexually transmitted diseases unavoidable.

Intravenous Drug Users

Interest in the relationship between the sexual behavior of IV drug users and the spread of AIDS has focused primarily on the role of drug users in transmitting AIDS to the heterosexual population. So far, most cases of heterosexual transmission involve IV drug users, usually males, who infect their female partners, many of whom do not use drugs.[52] These women are the primary source of infection among newborn babies. In approximately 79% of all pediatric cases of AIDS, at least one parent has the disease and is an IV drug user.[53]

As Friedman, Des Jarlais, and Sotheran pointed out, drug users, like gay men, belong to a subculture associated with specific rituals and ways of interacting.[54] Risky behaviors such as sharing needles must be placed in this context before they can be understood, not to mention modified. Despite the stereotype that drug users are incapable of changing, research indicates that many have modified their behavior because of the AIDS epidemic. In one survey, 60% of the respondents said they had stopped or reduced the sharing of needles, were attempting to sterilize their needles, or had stopped taking drugs.[55] In their study, Friedman, Des Jarlais, and Sotheran noted an increased demand for sterile needles.[54]

Although some IV drug users have modified their sexual behavior, a significant proportion continue to engage in behaviors associated with transmission of the HIV virus. Selwyn and associates[56] surveyed 261 IV drug users from a methadone maintenance program or a detention facility in New York City and found that almost half (48%) had not changed their sexual behavior in response to the threat of AIDS. Among those who had modified their behavior, 5% were monogamous or celibate and 14% used condoms or adopted other hygienic measures such as washing before or after intercourse. (Although some "safer sex" guidelines recommend showering before or after sex, risky sexual practices undoubtedly negate the dubious protective value of this recommendation).

The paucity of research on the sexual behavior of IV drug users makes it difficult to identify the barriers to change. However, several likely ones come to mind. First, because IV drug users, unlike gay men, are members of a group lacking formal structure, educating them about the need to practice safer sex is difficult. Many users can be reached through substance abuse programs or the criminal justice system. However, others are difficult to reach because they use drugs irregularly or are treated for drug-related problems in the general health care system and thus are not labeled as IV drug users.[54,57] Second, even if users as a group could be educated, the fact that many support their habit through prostitution would be a major obstacle to behavioral change—for example, calling attention to AIDS by insisting on the use of a condom would be bad for business. Third, although evidence indicates that IV drug users have assimilated some basic information about AIDS (e.g., the disease can be transmitted through shared needles), misconceptions and gaps in information still exist among a significant proportion.[56,58]

Finally, needle sharing has several important objectives—it is a way of initiating an individual into the subculture of IV drug users; it symbolizes a close, caring, family-like relationship; and in many cases it is an economic necessity.[59] Thus, eradicating the practice will be difficult unless alternative ways of accomplishing these objectives develop.

ISSUES INVOLVING HIV ANTIBODY TESTING AND COUNSELING

Since March 1985, when the Food and Drug Administration licensed the test for detecting antibodies to the HIV virus, some have called for widespread testing as a method of controlling the disease. Others warn that misuse of test results could lead to discrimination in employment and housing, loss of insurance benefits, and social ostracism. The availability of anonymous testing, however, has reduced fears about potential breaches of confidentiality and their consequences. Thus, more and more people are likely to consider the question of whether to learn their antibody status. All these people will need counseling before as well as after testing.

Pretest Counseling

Before people are tested, the counselor should help them to analyze their reasons for wanting the test and to undergo a realistic appraisal of the likelihood that they are infected. In addition, the counselor should inform them about the limitations of the test and what a positive result does—and does not—mean. They also need to understand the relative protections afforded by anonymous, confidential testing; how the disease is transmitted; and the methods required to prevent transmission. Individuals should understand that the test can only detect HIV antibodies; it cannot predict who will ultimately develop AIDS. They should understand the possibility of false positive or false negative results. Finally, people who are considering the test should be informed about the potential benefits and risks of testing.

According to Goldblum and Seymour, the potential benefits of testing for HIV antibodies are as follows:[60]

- It may motivate people who engage in high-risk sexual behavior to reduce or stop such behavior.
- It may reduce the anxiety of those who are unlikely to be infected.
- It can help women who are at high risk to decide whether they should become pregnant, continue a pregnancy, breast feed their infant, or have the infant inoculated with vaccine produced from live virus.
- It can be used to help support a medical diagnosis in those who exhibit unexplained symptoms that their physician believes may be related to an HIV infection.

Among the risks of testing Goldblum and Seymour identify are the following

- Severe anxiety, depression, suicidal ideation, intrusive thoughts, nightmares, and sleep disturbances.
- Interpersonal problems ranging from blaming the partner and sexual dysfunction to homicidal rage.
- Social ostracism.
- Self-imposed withdrawal of tested individuals.
- Discrimination in employment and housing.
- Insurance problems.
- Preoccupation with physical symptoms.

For people who test negative for HIV antibodies, the risk is that they will have a false sense of security and thus continue engaging in high-risk behavior.

Individuals who have a history of high-risk behaviors—especially if they belong to high-risk groups—but who are unwilling to undergo HIV antibody testing may find it extremely difficult to cope with uncertainty about their status. They may alternate between hopelessness and despair, convinced that they are infected, and defensive denial, asserting that they are certain they are seronegative. These individuals need help to adapt to the uncertainty so that they can maintain an acceptable quality of life, continue to function, yet protect their health and avoid spreading the infection. Health educators often advise such people to assume they are negative but to act as if they were positive. In other words, the goal is to maintain a sense of hope and plan for the future while consistently taking precautions to protect oneself and others. Denial can be adaptive in the sense that it permits a person to avoid despair and hopelessness. However, it is maladaptive if it permits rationalizations about the lack of need to take precautions against becoming infected or transmitting the infection to others.

As Forstein pointed out, people who are trying to cope with an ambiguous status need to have a sense of control over their lives.[61] It is sometimes helpful to remind them that even healthy people must deal with uncertainty about the future, yet continue to plan constructively. In addition, it helps to point out that it is useless to dwell on what the person could have done or should not have done in the past. Behavioral techniques such as relaxation exercises and cognitive therapies may help the person manage anxiety. In some cases, however, pharmacologic intervention may be necessary.[62]

Ideally, individuals who are considering testing should go home and think carefully about all the risks and benefits outlined during the pretesting session. In practice, however, counselors often find that clients have already made the decision to be tested or not to be tested before the counseling session or by the end of the counseling session. Because of the possible far-reaching social and psychological consequences of testing, precipitous decisions should be discouraged unless the client has an urgent need to know his or her status.

For individuals who ultimately decide to be tested, the counselor should develop an action plan to prepare them for a positive test result,[60] and should always tell clients the results of their test face to face. Potential sources of social support from family, friends, and the community should be discussed.

Post-Test Counseling

Seronegative Individuals

Because clients who test negative obviously will feel tremendously relieved, the counselor must remind them that if they have engaged in high-risk behaviors within the previous 8 to 10 weeks, they may have been exposed to the virus but have not developed antibodies that can be detected yet. They should be told that because months can elapse between the time of infection and the development of antibodies,[57] they may want to repeat the test after at least 3 months of only safe-sex practices.

If the seronegative client continues to engage in high-risk behavior, he or she may benefit from additional counseling. Coates, Morin, and McKusick suggest that some high-risk individuals who test negative conclude that they must be immune to HIV infection and therefore believe they can engage in high-risk behavior with impunity.[63]

Seropositive Individuals

Clients who test positive need counseling to come to terms with the infection, integrate the implications, and cope with an uncertain future. The counselor should repeatedly emphasize the fact that a positive test result does not mean that the client will develop AIDS-related complex (ARC) or AIDS. However, most clients will experience an initial sense of dread and doom. Learning that one is seropositive for HIV antibodies is profoundly distressing, even among people who anticipated the outcome of the test in advance. In the first few weeks after hearing the test results, most feel hopeless and helpless. They may have suicidal thoughts; thus the risk of suicide should be evaluated if the individual has a history of mental illness, poor coping strategies, or little social support.

Several misunderstandings are common among individuals who test seropositive. One misunderstanding is that they currently have AIDS, are going to die, and therefore are in a medical crisis. The counselor must repeatedly emphasize to such individuals that they are in a psychological and social crisis, not a medical one; therefore, they need time to react and think about how they can handle the information and thus avoid destructive behavior.

The counselor should be aware of the community resources available to people who have disorders associated with HIV infection. Even if the client's family is likely to provide adequate support, the client should be made aware that resources such as self-help groups are available in the community.

Seropositive individuals must acknowledge that they can infect others. Thus, they must practice safer sex and, if they are IV drug users, stop sharing needles as well. The most common reactions to this information are the following. Many people immediately stop all physically intimate behavior, including hugging. Several counseling sessions may be needed to inform them about the options available, help them tell others who need to know about their medical status, learn about alternative sexual practices, and monitor their physical condition appropriately. Unfortunately, people who impulsively reveal their antibody status lose their jobs and insurance coverage and experience other kinds of social discrimination. Whether notifying past and future sexual partners is appropriate or useful also should be discussed. Some individuals need ongoing help to learn safer sex practices and to solve the problems created in their relationships by this change in behavior. Some have difficulty modifying their behavior because of specific cultural or personal reactions to practices such as using condoms. Those who are extremely anxious, depressed, or suicidal need a referral for more intensive therapy.

Unfortunately, most infected individuals are of childbearing age. Thus, infected women must understand the possibility that they can transmit the infection to their baby before birth or during breast feeding.[64] Although the incidence of maternal transmission is unknown, evidence suggests that the risk is substantial[65] and that pregnancy itself may accelerate the development of AIDS.[57] Women who may have been infected at the time of their pregnancy or while breast feeding may want to have the infant tested. If an infected woman is in the first trimester of pregnancy, the risks and benefits of terminating the pregnancy should be discussed. Limitations on childbearing cause extreme distress in both men and women. Some women who view children as their only opportunity to be fulfilled and to contribute to society may feel that a 50% chance of having a normal child is an acceptable risk even if pregnancy will jeopardize their own health.

Counselors must understand that a person may need weeks or months to come to terms with his or her seropositive status. Because denial is often the initial response, one counseling session after the test is rarely adequate. Provisions must be made for the person to have access to some ongoing form of individual or group support.

The fear experienced by seropositive individuals about whether they will develop the symptoms of AIDS is much the same as that experienced by the cancer patient who fears that the disease will recur or metastasize. Initially, the rate of conversion from seropositive status to AIDS was believed to be about 10%. However, recent data indicate that approximately 50% of seropositive individuals will convert, and this information has vastly increased anxiety.[66] Thus, they need help to become hopeful about their health and about scientific progress that will prevent progression of the disease. They can be encouraged to maintain their health by avoiding practices that may activate the disease—for example, pregnancy, reinfection by continuing to engage in high-risk behaviors, and use of "recreational drugs" that may suppress the immune system. Such clients often need continuous reassurance, support, and access to consistent health care to maintain an optimal degree of concern about their condition—to ensure regular monitoring and preventive health behaviors—yet avoid excessive anxiety that could lead to destructive behavior such as acting without regard for their own safety or that of others or attempting suicide.

Because of their potential ability to infect others, seropositive individuals have major problems in their sexual relationships. For example, a young nurse was unaware that she was seropositive until she gave birth to a baby that had AIDS. She had stopped taking drugs five years before, had obtained her nursing degree, and had married a devoted family man. After the baby's diagnosis, she was afraid of hurting anyone and behaved in ways that alienated her husband because she was afraid of hurting anyone. Because of his strong commitment to the marriage and his child, he was distraught and confused, had difficulty concentrating at work, and eventually lost his job. A long period of family counseling was needed to limit the destructiveness of the situation.

Finally, people who know they are seropositive struggle with lowered self-esteem and social isolation that are often self-inflicted. They feel like social pariahs and may withdraw from people who are important to them for fear of infecting them even through casual contact. Although there are no easy solutions to these problems, clients should be encouraged to meet with groups or individuals who are in the same situation to share their concerns and learn better ways of coping with the limitations imposed on them.

ISSUES CONFRONTING AIDS PATIENTS

When people who are seropositive for HIV antibodies begin showing symptoms of active disease, they experience all the social and psychological stresses associated with AIDS. Two important sources of stress are the high mortality rate associated with the disease and the youth of the population it affects. Other sources of stress are the contagious nature of AIDS, its debilitating and disfiguring effects, and its symptoms. The psychosocial ramifications of these stresses are different at each stage of the disease.

The social conditions of the people who usually contract the disease add to the complexity of disease-related stress. The groups that are currently affected most often are homosexual and bisexual men, IV drug users, women who contract the disease from heterosexual contacts, and hemophiliacs and others who contract the disease from blood transfusions.

Gay and Bisexual Men

The largest group of AIDS patients, homosexual and bisexual men, now accounts for 71% of the total population of AIDS patients.[66] The gay community has developed a culture, network, and language that protects its members from the hostility of the general population. The gay patient with AIDS must share intimate personal information with health care professionals who usually are heterosexual and whose unconscious prejudices may make them emotionally distant at a time when the patient is already struggling with guilt, shame, and fear. Bisexual men, especially, tend to be secretive about their homosexual activities. Thus, revealing those activities to spouses or heterosexual partners can cause enormous conflict.

Because the disease has become epidemic, most gay men know at least one person who has died of AIDS and are in contact with many AIDS patients. The cumulative impact of watching numerous friends and acquaintances deteriorate and die can be as great as the impact of a family member's death. The newly diagnosed patient's anxiety is based on observations of how the disease progresses in other patients and on the fear that his own disease will progress in the same way. Thus, he should be encouraged to focus on how the course of his disease differs from that of others to diminish his negative identification, reduce his anxiety, and increase his sense of control.

Intravenous Drug Users

IV drug users, the second largest group at risk for AIDS, makes 29% of the total population of AIDS patients.[48] Unlike gay men, addicts have no organized community that can rally to their support. Many are only marginally functional, have poor support resources, and have limited ability to cope with the stresses of the disease and its treatment. However, professionals must avoid acting on stereotypic views and approach these patients as individuals who have different backgrounds, vocations, and life situations and have chosen to use drugs as a way of solving life's problems.[54]

Like gay men, IV drug users are concerned about sexual relations, but they also are concerned about endangering their future children, despite the stereotype that they are personally and socially irresponsible. Furthermore, the drugs to which they are addicted affect the efficacy of drugs prescribed for pain, depression, anxiety, and nausea, and it is difficult to maintain addicts on methadone while giving them drugs used to treat AIDS.

Effective treatment for AIDS requires a high degree of compliance in return for a limited benefit, and people who are impulsive and have little tolerance for emotional and physical frustration have problems complying with treatment. Therefore, they are likely to have difficulty staying off drugs while coping with physical deterioration, energy loss, neurologic impairment, and inactivity.

In most cases, a long, debilitating illness depletes the drug user's personal and financial resources. For example, Luis stopped taking drugs while serving a prison term, then returned to his wife, Maria, and their two teenage sons. When Luis was diagnosed as having AIDS, Maria quit her job and applied for public assistance so that she could take care of him. A year later, she had to return to work, and Luis watched his sons' behavior deteriorate, in part because of stress related to his history of drug abuse and in part because of his debilitating illness.

Working with patients who are or were addicts presents special problems. Therefore, close liaison with drug rehabilitation programs and self-help groups of former addicts is required for ongoing consultation about drug-related difficulties and referrals for additional counseling.

Hemophiliacs and Other Patients

Hemophiliacs and other patients who have contracted the virus from blood transfusions can be expected to exhibit anger and mistrust of physicians and other health care personnel that may seem unjustified. Understanding the source of their anger and fear can help staff respond effectively.

PATIENTS' REACTIONS AT DIFFERENT STAGES OF THE DISEASE

Diagnosis

The diagnosis of AIDS has been identified as a critical, but often neglected, time for psychosocial intervention.[67–69] Because of the high mortality rate associated with the disease, the patient is immediately confronted with the inevitability of dying. As mentioned earlier, denial can be a useful defense for patients confronted with a potentially fatal condition because it gives them some control over when and how they will confront their own mortality. For patients diagnosed with AIDS, however, denial is less likely to be effective for two reasons: the publicity the disease has received, and the demoralizing experience of knowing other AIDS patients who have died.

The age at which AIDS strikes is another traumatic factor. Most AIDS patients are between 25 and 49 years old—an age group that does not expect to develop a potentially fatal illness. As Rossi pointed out, stress is often "a manifestation of asynchrony in the timing of life events. It is the unanticipated event, not the anticipated, which is likely to represent the traumatic event."[70]

The ability to fulfill the developmental tasks of young adulthood—choosing an occupation, establishing a career, forming long-term relationships, solidifying one's sense of identity, and establishing and refining a pattern of adult life—is profoundly affected by the demands of AIDS and its treatment. Yet, young adults often make a supreme effort to continue their development in these areas until their physical condition deteriorates to the point where they cannot do so. For example, patients often say that their work not only protects their medical insurance but also makes them feel normal. Therefore, they desperately try to conceal the signs of their disease so that they can work as long as possible.

Patients who were unaware of their seropositive status until the diagnosis are suddenly confronted with the following issues: transmitting the disease to others; protecting themselves from opportunistic infections; revealing their homosexuality or drug use to family, friends, and colleagues; and dealing with the fears of lovers, friends, family, and the public. One of their greatest fears is being "found out" and consequently being labeled and discriminated against. In fact, they must now tell people about the disease to obtain financial benefits and explain their absences from work because of the illness and its treatment and the physical changes associated with the disease. They worry about whom to tell, who suspects, and who will reject them. In addition, when talking with health professionals, they must discuss sexual and drug behaviors that they have kept hidden—discussions that are particularly difficult for bisexual men. For example, when a successful 40-year-old businessman who had kept his bisexuality a secret from his wife, child, parents, and business associates became ill and needed people to help him, he worried about whom to tell and what they would think of him.

Some patients will not talk openly with a health professional until they are certain that confidentiality will be maintained and that they are respected and accepted. The professional can help patients identify people in their social network who are most likely to be trustworthy and to develop ways of communicating with them that will result in support but maximize confidentiality. The professional also can encourage patients to ventilate their fears and anger about discrimination and can intercede on their behalf with employers and financial entitlement agencies.

Maylon and Pinka noted that, at diagnosis, health care professionals often fail to appreciate the AIDS patient's immediate and long-term need for psychological support.[67] Although referrals to community support services may be appropriate during the course of the illness, psychosocial intervention by mental health professionals, in collaboration with physicians, should begin immediately to resolve practical problems such as how patients will support themselves if they cannot work, how their medical treatment will be paid for, and what they should say to family and friends about their condition. For example, all patients must apply soon after their diagnosis for financial entitlements such as Social Security Disability Insurance, Supplemental Security Income, and Medicaid. Because the onset of opportunistic infections or dementia is often sudden,[71] they also need to consider establishing durable power of attorney for health care. Since discussing these possibilities is frightening, applications for financial and legal assistance at this early stage should be presented as an insurance to fall back on in case it is needed.

Development of Clinical Syndromes

The debilitating and often disfiguring effects of AIDS are another cause of stress among patients. For example, a patient may literally waste away, be profoundly fatigued and lethargic, suffer from opportunistic infections, exhibit the symptoms of central nervous system (CNS) disease, or develop lymphomas or other cancers such as Kaposi's sarcoma, the reddish-purple macules of which are readily identifiable. Each clinical syndrome creates a different kind of stress.

Opportunistic Infections

Until new chemotherapeutic agents such as AZT were developed, AIDS patients with opportunistic infections such as *P. carinii* pneumonia had no structured treatment regimen to follow that would help them cope with the progressive effects of the disease. Opportunistic infections were treated as they occurred. Now, reinfections can be treated more effectively, but uncertainty about the course of the disease remains. Patients say they feel like a "walking time bomb"—that they are waiting for the next explosion. Because of this uncertainty, they have difficulty making decisions about whether to continue working or to apply for disability benefits even if they feel well. If they are experiencing mild physical effects of the disease, they often keep on working because it gives them a sense of purpose.

As multiple reinfections become more relentless, however, patients are chronically fatigued and uncomfortable and rarely experience signs of improvement or plateaus. They can cope better with uncertainty by concentrating on the aspects of their condition that are within their control; for example, by closely monitoring the course of the disease and by tracking the results of their blood tests, the number of bouts of pneumonia, fluctuations in weight, and so forth. Such monitoring not only gives them a sense of control but also helps them anticipate changes in their health. Relaxation exercises also can be helpful in controlling their anxiety.

Central Nervous System Disease

More and more AIDS patients are exhibiting symptoms of CNS disease characterized by progressive, incapacitating dementia. Early symptoms may include loss of memory for names, historical details, and appointments; difficulty concentrating; mental slowing; confusion of time and person; and apathy, withdrawal, and depression.[72] Some patients become agitated and hyperactive and behave inappropriately. Others develop an unsteady gait, weakness of the legs, lack of coordination, impaired handwriting, and tremors. As the disease progresses, the patient may need extensive help with daily activities such as traveling to and from the hospital, preparing meals, and caring for his personal needs.

Patients usually fear CNS disease more than any other manifestation of AIDS, and the loss of memory and mood changes associated with the disease elicit deep sadness and intense anger. As a result, they may try to conceal the symptoms from their physician and avoid situations where the condition might be exposed. However, they may allude to their symptoms when talking with another member of the health care team or their caretaker. For example, a 35-year-old patient yelled at his friends, then refused to talk to them on the phone and discouraged them from visiting. When the social worker asked him about this behavior, he said: "I just don't have the patience to figure out their questions, and I don't remember what the doctor says to me."

Useful methods of managing CNS-related symptoms include (1) discussing the possibility of CNS symptoms realistically with patients, (2) emphasizing the symptoms that respond to treatment, and (3) avoiding frightening terms such as "dementia." In addition, close communication between the patient's caretaker and members of the health-care team may enable early identification of such symptoms. Thus, the physician should determine as soon as possible after the diagnosis who will be responsible for health decisions if the patient becomes mentally incapacitated. Obviously, this sensitive issue must be approached in a manner that acknowledges the patient's adaptive denial. Once the symptoms emerge, the adequacy of the patient's care at home must be monitored constantly.

The cognitive changes associated with CNS disease also have a tremendous impact on health care staff and patients' friends, caretakers, and others. Thus, early identification is important so that patients will be cared for adequately at home, can be given psychotropic drugs to control psychiatric symptoms, and will receive timely supportive treatment. In the terminal stages of AIDS, patients with CNS disease can be so difficult to care for that they must be institutionalized. They can be virtually mute,[72] partially paralyzed, incontinent, stare vacantly, and be capable of only rudimentary social or intellectual interaction.

Kaposi's Sarcoma, Lymphomas, and Other Cancers

Patients with Kaposi's sarcoma live with a constant visual reminder of their disease—a circumstance that interferes with their use of adaptive denial. The lesions also heighten the feeling of stigma and evoke rejection by others. The loss of work and social isolation caused by such visible and aversive signs of disease is profoundly disturbing to patients. Thus, they may try to cover the lesions with makeup, which can be effective but sometimes makes the lesions look even more conspicuous. They mourn the loss of their physical and social desirability. For example, a 28-year-old architect said, "I can't look at myself in the mirror. I don't know whose face that is, I look ugly and dead already." Encouraging such patients to mourn openly about their grief can provide some relief.

When anticancer drugs are withdrawn because the patient's immune system is compromised, lesions suddenly appear all over the body—a terrifying reminder that the immune system is failing and the disease is progressing. At this point, some patients demand further chemotherapy even though their bodies are exhausted from it, or they may demand radiation of the lesions before starting chemotherapy.

The lymphomas and other cancers diagnosed in patients who are HIV-positive is a relatively new phenomenon.[73] Although these patients must acknowledge their HIV status and their potential for infecting others, they often deny that the cancer is related to AIDS, preferring instead to view themselves as cancer patients. For example, a 40-year-old postal clerk was so convinced he had cancer rather than AIDS that he confused physicians who met him for the first time. His lover had died of AIDS, which was so horrifying that he could not accept his own diagnosis. Patients who exhibit strong denial in the early stages of AIDS often become increasingly distressed as the symptoms become more apparent. However, some manage to deny the disease until it reaches the terminal stage.

Health professionals must respect this type of defensive denial until the patient's coping patterns and strengths have been assessed—a difficult situation because the patient must simultaneously accept his or her potential for spreading AIDS. Patients who deny their AIDS-related condition also have difficulty because of their need to apply for benefits specifically designed for AIDS patients. Again, the professional is in a difficult situation because intervention strategies with such patients often need to accept the patient's denial to a certain extent and at the same time assist the patient in realistic planning for his present and future care.

Treatment

Many young AIDS patients desperately try to find some active treatment for their disease. Therefore, those who are medically ineligible for research protocols may seek an alternative treatment, no matter how unscientific it may be, and those who are medically eligible may turn to unproved treatments while on research protocols to increase, in their view, their chances of prolonged survival.

Treatments such as interferon and some antibiotics have side-effects such as weakness and depression, which only add to the AIDS patient's misery. In addition, treatment often involves repeated clinic visits, uncomfortable or painful tests and procedures, and prolonged hospitalizations with isolation precautions.

Isolation is stressful because the patient is confronted with sensory deprivation at a time when closeness to others is comforting. As one AIDS patient said: "I haven't been touched without rubber gloves in 6 months. Will I ever be touched again?" However, isolation is especially difficult because of the discrimination and alienation the patient may have experienced earlier. Thus, some patients and their friends may misinterpret the isolation precautions as a punishment. In addition, isolation tends to dissuade visitors, who may be frightened by the precautions and worried about contracting an infection themselves or giving one to the patient. Thus, family members and friends must understand the importance of maintaining maximum contact with the patient within the limits of these precautions.

Termination of Treatment

Termination of treatment is another particularly stressful time for AIDS patients. When a treatment protocol is completed successfully, patients become anxious because they are stopping an activity that controls the disease and will no longer be under intense medical surveillance. Thus, their fears of renewed progression of the disease are greatly increased. If treatment is stopped because it is ineffective or its side effects are life threatening, the patient is confronted with feelings of helplessness about the possibility that few treatment options remain. Finally, at a time of intense anxiety and a need for intimacy, the patient is faced with making major changes in his or her lifestyle without the support provided by regular involvement with health care staff.

EMOTIONAL REACTIONS OF PATIENTS

In the early stages of the disease, patients may concentrate on the problems of living—on keeping their job and maintaining their home and their relationships with friends and family. When treatment proves ineffective and the disease progresses, the patient experiences all the feelings associated with approaching death, including denial, fear, anger, ambivalence, and a search for meaning. When patients are young adults, they are depressed about the loss of potential, of what they could have accomplished, and they mourn the loss of their dreams.

Fear

It is difficult to overestimate the degree of fear experienced by patients who have an intractable disease such as AIDS. Because of the fear, many become excessively dependent on health care staff. For example, physicians report that patients call them repeatedly at all hours regarding control of symptoms. Their dependency and demands can be even more excessive if they mistrust the health care system. The overwhelming nature of the psychological reactions to AIDS and its treatment often impedes compliance with treatment, resolution of practical problems, and social functioning and thus obstructs the provision of care.

Patients also fear being rejected by their colleagues and casual acquaintances and being abandoned by their close friends and lovers. Because of the stigma attached to AIDS, this fear is real. When a Kaposi's sarcoma patient with visible lesions on his arms entered an elevator in a large city hospital, the other 15 passengers stepped out at the next stop. Such experiences are not uncommon among AIDS patients. Patients often say they feel like a leper. Ambivalent responses in the community, especially to the sexual and drug-related aspects of AIDS, often means that patients do not receive some of the usual benefits of the sick role and have great difficulty obtaining employment, insurance coverage, and care.

Denial

Denial can be a useful and necessary defense for patients who have a fatal illness because it gives them some control over when and how they will confront their own mortality. For AIDS patients, however, denial is less likely to be effective because of the publicity the disease has received. Unfortunately, health professionals may limit a patient's ability to use adaptive denial by acting on naive and often romantic views of death. Although society has become more open about discussing emotion-laden issues such as death, most people focus on their own death only for brief periods and with only a few people such as a spouse, clergyman, or lover. Even at the terminal stage of illness, some patients choose not to discuss their thoughts and fears about death with professional staff. In fact, most AIDS patients say they are more afraid of the pain, disfigurement, and CNS symptoms of AIDS than of death, and management of these manifestations may be the focus of their discussions.

Suicidal Thoughts

Suicidal thoughts are common among patients and are usually related to anger, fear of isolation, and concern about the inability to manage the symptoms and progress of the disease. For example, patients often make statements such as the following: "I will kill myself if I get much sicker (am unable to work, am in pain, or if AIDS goes to my brain)." Fears of the symptoms of an incurable illness can provoke intense feelings of helplessness and hopelessness. Although professionals are always apprehensive about the possibility, AIDS patients seldom commit suicide if they can ventilate their feelings, feel certain that the medical staff is concerned about them and will take care of them, and clearly understand that they will have options at all stages of the illness—that drugs for pain will be available, that they can make choices about treatment, and so forth. In addition, it is important to help them maintain social contacts in the community to limit their sense of isolation.

Guilt About High-Risk Behaviors

Guilt about past sexual or drug behaviors that may have led to contracting the disease is another common psychological problem among AIDS patients. IV drug use, specific high-risk sexual practices, and the number of anonymous sexual partners were recognized early as risk factors. Because of the prolonged incubation period, a patient may have been involved in this type of sexual activity months or years before the diagnosis.

Five different patterns of response to such guilt have been identified: celibacy, denial or rejection of one's positive HIV status and thus continuing one's former level of sexual activity, celibacy with close friends while engaging in sex with multiple anonymous partners, increased use of drugs and alcohol, and development of small groups of sexual contacts. Some gay patients internalize society's homophobia and may even believe that homosexuality caused their disease. Others blame their lover or those who "led" them into homosexual behavior.

SPECIAL PROBLEMS OF PATIENTS, FAMILIES, AND PARTNERS

During a pilot study involving 42 of the first 58 AIDS patients treated at Memorial Sloan-Kettering Cancer Center between April 1981 and December 1982, Christ,

Wiener, and Moynihan identified several characteristics that make AIDS patients more vulnerable than other patients to social and psychological dysfunction.[74] These patients were far more likely to have employment and insurance problems, limited support networks, and severe difficulties with their sexual partners and families.

Patients

Employment and Insurance

The 42 patients represented a broad range of occupations and professions such as architecture, education, finance, health care, interior design, and skilled labor. Many were self-employed and thus had less financial and job security than those who worked for an organization. However, early in the epidemic, many patients were fired from long-standing, secure jobs because of pervasive fears about the disease. Although many cases have been challenged successfully in court, employment remains a problem because of the reactions of co-workers and employers.

Insurance also is a major problem for AIDS patients. Over one-third of the patients in the study either had no insurance or their insurance had been terminated when they were fired from their jobs after diagnosis or when they could no longer afford private coverage. Even when there is insurance, limitations or inadequate structures mean that it seldom covers the amount of home care AIDS patients need. As a result, patients often must stay in an acute care facility much longer than is medically required. Applying for Medicaid and Social Security disability is a new experience for most patients, and the requirement that they must divest themselves of most resources to be eligible often means leaving familiar surroundings and drastically changing their lifestyle.

Limited Support Networks

Unlike most other young adults who have a life-threatening illness, most AIDS patients do not become intensely reinvolved with their families of origin or have a family or spouse to rely on for financial and emotional support. (Twenty-six of the 42 patients who participated in the pilot study had minimal or no contact with their families, and a third lived alone and had no one to turn to for help.) Instead, patients tend to be more dependent on lovers or a wider network of friends; some live in "reconstituted" families made up of close friends. For patients who lack a support network, support from gay or drug rehabilitation organizations and hospital staff can be vital to their ability to cope with the stresses of AIDS.

Sexual Partners

The sexual partners of AIDS patients are confronted with losing someone they love and depend on. Yet, they un-

derstandably fear they have been exposed to the virus and, if married, are concerned about the possible risk to their children. For example, a 32-year-old real estate agent, upon learning that her boyfriend had AIDS, began screaming that she wanted to be ill too so they could "die" together. Several weeks later, when she agreed to be tested for exposure to the virus, she said she hoped God had not heard her first request.

Developing safer sex practices is a tremendous challenge to a relationship in the presence of such fear. Initially, these practices seem artificial, lacking in spontaneity, and "too clinical." Couples often need help in discussing ways to remain physically close. Furthermore, as the disease progresses, the patient's sexual needs and abilities diminish and generate fear that the partner will leave. Finally, all sexually transmitted diseases involve guilt and blame. Unless such issues are discussed openly, they can erode the couple's relationship and make both feel isolated, angry, and fearful about the future. The need to change sexual patterns is a special problem for women, especially those from certain ethnic groups. Women from such groups tend to lack a sense of their right to direct the sexual relationship, often seeing no alternative to sexual surrender. Furthermore, refusing sex often means losing income, housing, and child care. For some, it also means losing their only close human contact.

As mentioned earlier, decisions about childbearing are extremely troubling for individuals who are HIV positive. Many women choose to have a child, risking their own and their child's life, for religious or cultural reasons or as a source of fulfillment; others chose to have an abortion or decide to remain childless—a profound psychological challenge for women of childbearing age as well as their partners.

Sexual partners can help contain their worry about contracting AIDS and gain a sense of control by maintaining and monitoring their own health. It is essential that they be able to discuss any symptoms confidentially with a physician as a way of containing anxiety and gaining a sense of control.

Families

In many cases, the families of AIDS patients are in great need of supportive care. They not only have the same fears and anxieties that everyone who has frequent contact with patients does; they also face rejection by society just as patients do. Many families are confronted with the news that a son, brother, or spouse is a homosexual at the same time they learn the person is dying. Major conflicts can arise as a result. For example, the family may be angry because they were not told about the patient's lifestyle and wonder which family member knew about it. Or the family may blame the patient for what he did to himself. Rather than focus on these issues immediately, and thus intensify the conflict, the family needs to look for ways to help the patient cope and assist in his or her care.

If intense conflict existed between patient and family before the diagnosis, the family may feel responsible for the illness. They can be reassured that their negative or conflicted feelings did not cause the patient's illness, but their ability to respond to this crisis can affect the patient's remaining future and the family's future as well. If they tried to be supportive to the patient in the past—especially if the patient was an IV drug user—they may be afraid the patient will manipulate and overwhelm them with ungrateful, demanding behavior. Health professionals need to respect the past experiences of such families rather than criticize them.

Many families are able to get beyond their disagreements about the patient's lifestyle and become involved in caretaking. However, they must learn to communicate meaningfully with the patient again after years of emotional distance. A helpful approach includes the following elements: (1) clear and consistent information about the disease, its treatment, and its potential for contagion, (2) a focus on the family's values and strengths, and (3) early definition of the roles of family members and friends in caring for the patient. Misconceptions about how the disease is transmitted need to be clarified; thus, specific information about food handling, laundry, cleaning of bathrooms, and casual physical contact with the patient is required. Families also need to know how to negotiate the hospital system; for example, which physicians they should contact and how they can get information about the disease and treatment throughout the illness. Families also need advice about whom and how much to tell about the patient's condition and often need assistance in negotiating with community organizations that provide supportive help or financial assistance to AIDS patients.

Families frequently get into conflict with the patient's lover, nontraditional partner, or friends because they perceive these individuals as having more control in vital treatment decisions. The family may have difficulty accepting the lover as a person who is as significant as a spouse. Since the roles and responsibilities of both lover and family are ambiguous, they require clarification. This can be facilitated by bringing the lover and family together as a unit to define and distribute the tasks involved in the patient's care, by minimizing the lack of legally defined roles, and by focusing on the need for making realistic decisions about the patient's care.

A PSYCHOSOCIAL INTERVENTION MODEL

The pilot study described earlier revealed a major lack of home and supportive care for AIDS patients as well as a lack of coordination between acute care facilities and community groups.[74] It was clear that activities designed to reduce emotional, social, and physical stress among AIDS patients and their caregivers and to foster public attitudes that facilitated patient management would result in more effective delivery of treatment and strengthen preventive efforts. Therefore, in 1982 the Social Work Department at Memorial Sloan-Kettering Cancer Center developed a psychosocial intervention program for patients, their friends and relatives, and the center's staff. The program has been modified over time as the needs of patients and staff have changed. The remainder of this section describes the various facets of the program.

Orienting Patients to the Center

An effort is made to do a psychosocial assessment of all patients at the time of their first visit to the hospital, either before or after they are seen by a physician. The purpose of the initial social work contact is to engage them with the hospital in a way that meets their needs for information and personal acceptance and meets the staff's need for information. The social worker prepares the patients for what will happen that day, gives them a booklet that answers many of their questions, and describes the services and resources available to them, their friends, and their family. These services include financial resources, community support services, and counseling. At this time, patients also are introduced to the clinic nurse who facilitates the management of their treatment and the negotiations with the health care system.

The worker also briefly assesses the patient's need for psychosocial intervention in the future. This assessment includes information about demographics; the nature and stability of the patient's living and occupational arrangements; the quality of his or her relationships with family, partners, and significant others; the amount of emotional support these individuals can provide; the patient's behavior patterns, knowledge of reactions to the disease, and beliefs, attitudes, and expectations about treatment and outcome; and preliminary information about the patient's ability to cope. The patient's support systems are assessed specifically concerning his or her ability to manage physical deterioration and neurological impairment. This information is shared with the treating physician.

Depending on information obtained before or during the medical examination, the social worker may begin individual counseling immediately to resolve urgent problems. If a patient has a drug problem, seems to have severe psychopathology, is potentially suicidal, or requests specialized services, the worker makes the appropriate referrals. The worker also makes referrals to appropriate community resources such as drug rehabilitation centers and self-help groups, gay service organizations, Social Security, public assistance, Medicaid, and legal services and invites the patient to join a weekly support group conducted at the center.

Providing Ongoing Intervention and Support

The same social worker provides patients with case management and counseling services throughout their treatment. Knowing that someone will direct their questions and concerns to the appropriate staff and help them obtain financial and other concrete services greatly reduces their anxiety, conserves the physician's time, and results in more continuous care.

In addition to immediate crisis intervention and individual counseling, the program provides the following ongoing psychosocial support activities: (1) support groups for patients, lovers, and families, (2) patient education, (3) instruction in relaxation and other behavioral techniques, and (4) liaison with community resources such as gay- or drug-related service agencies, cancer counseling agencies, and the Social Security Administration.

Support Groups

After patients' basic needs have been met and their individual problems have been addressed, support groups are highly effective. The center currently conducts a number of psychoeducationally oriented support groups for AIDS patients organized around specific phases of the illness, disease symptoms, or treatment regimens: for instance, one for individuals who are HIV positive, one for patients who have Kaposi's sarcoma, a third for those with opportunistic infections, and a fourth for those on the AZT protocol.

New patients have an immense need for reassurance and for a chance to observe and speak with other patients who have the same illness. A support group reduces patients' feelings of isolation and loneliness, enables them to share their experiences, and offers a wide range of people with whom they can interact and solve problems. A professional skilled in group dynamics serves as facilitator. The self-help approach is an acknowledgment that experiential knowledge is different from professional knowledge and offers a unique contribution. Individual group members not only serve as models for others but also reinforce their perceptions as people capable of controlling their own lives and situations.

Although all groups have a flexible membership and attendance, patients are encouraged to attend regularly. A support group is a vitally important, cost-effective intervention, but it should not be viewed as the only ongoing intervention.[75] Some patients are reluctant to participate in a group or do so only when they are not acutely upset; others use the group continuously for encouragement and support. Individual crises and a vast range of practical problems usually cannot be handled adequately in a group.

The death of a group member is a special problem in a group of potentially terminally ill patients. The group facilitator informs the other members about the patient's death during the subsequent group meeting rather than let them hear about it informally. She tells them about the care the patient received, who was present when the patient died, and other pertinent information. She encourages the group to discuss their reactions and to ask questions; then she helps the group

refocus on the present and how members can cope with the disease.

Patient Education

Education is an integral part of the group treatment program. At times, group facilitators adopt an active educative technique or use outside speakers to present information on topics such as the results of medical and psychiatric research on AIDS, legal issues, relaxation techniques, infectious diseases, and community resources. The group process gives members an opportunity to ask questions in an informal and supportive atmosphere, to have contact with physicians, and to gain information that they can relay to friends and family. The emphasis on education gives them a greater sense of control through improved access to information.

Individual Instruction

Individual instruction and printed materials have proved to be of vital importance in helping patients cope. The printed materials provide information about AIDS, its symptoms, and its treatment; self-care and ways of preventing the spread of the disease; and methods of obtaining appropriate medical and nonmedical services. Many drug treatment centers, gay organizations, and government agencies have developed educational materials in all of these areas.

Methods of cognitive control over anxiety, such as relaxation techniques, help patients cope with extreme anxiety related to medical procedures, pain, and chronic stress. These methods can be taught individually or in groups and are especially helpful to patients who have previously relied on drugs or compulsive sexual behavior to reduce tension.

Meeting the Needs of Staff

Physicians, nurses, and others involved in patient care are prone to occupational stress, fear and anxiety, prejudices, and guilt feelings as a result of working with AIDS patients. Thus, education, multidisciplinary patient care rounds, crisis intervention, and ongoing stress-reduction groups have proved to be effective with the center's staff.

Educational materials and programs that present detailed information about the disease are available to physicians and other professionals. For example, information that helps sensitize staff to the gay lifestyle is provided, and complementary measures to improve communication between staff and patients are offered. Poor communication contributes to staff discomfort with AIDS patients—a problem related in part to the extreme anxiety exhibited by many patients and their tremendous need for contact, encouragement, and reassurance. These factors, together with the different lifestyles of the two groups, often lead to mutual suspicion and uneasiness.

Crisis intervention also has become necessary for staff. Crises are usually precipitated by a sudden resurgence of acute fear about contracting AIDS, by pressure from spouses about contagion, by pregnancy, by pressure from social contacts, or by a confrontation with a patient's lifestyle, deteriorating condition, or death. Either time-limited or ongoing staff support groups that focus on emotional abreaction, problem solving, and development of mutually supportive relationships are used to reduce stress and increase productivity. For example, when the media announced that three health care workers had contracted the HIV virus during their work, open meetings for all hospital staff were initiated four times a week for several weeks. These meetings were led by the chief of the infectious disease service and by the assistant director of social work, who heads the AIDS support program. The leaders discussed the specific circumstances of all three infected workers to correct misinformation, reviewed the effective safety precautions available, and encouraged the staff to express their fears about their own vulnerability to the disease. In such meetings, the role of the mental health professional is to draw out and respond to the staff's anxiety, fears, and other emotions; clarify misconceptions, which are often based on stereotypes; and encourage a realistic approach to the management of risk.

CONCLUSION

There is a growing awareness that perceptions of the nature of the AIDS epidemic have reached a watershed. The disease is no longer viewed as one that only affects isolated groups; it is recognized as a potential threat to everyone. In other words, AIDS is, or should be, of major concern to every sexually active person who is not in a long-standing, mutually monogamous relationship; every person who is a parent or is thinking of having a child; every person who is a sexually inexperienced teenager; and every person who has AIDS.

This chapter has examined the psychological and social effects of AIDS at different points along the health-illness continuum from asymptomatic to HIV-positive to symptomatic. Clearly, the social, psychological, ethical, and legal consequences of AIDS are far more complex and challenging than anyone imagined when the first cases were diagnosed. These psychosocial consequences are as complex as the scientific issues that remain unresolved and are perhaps even more challenging to the American national character. Effective collaboration between government groups and traditional and nontraditional service agencies and organizations has created a structure within which many service issues can be productively addressed. Finally, major social and psychological research programs on AIDS have greatly increased the likelihood that the problems concerning the changes in human behavior needed to prevent the further spread of the disease will be solved.

REFERENCES

1. Centers for Disease Control: Heterosexual transmission of human T-lymphotropic virus type III/lymphadenopathy-associated virus. Morbid Mortal Weekly Rep 34:561, 1985
2. Jones P, Hamilton PG, Bird G, et al: AIDS and hemophilia: Morbidity and mortality in a well defined population. Br Med J 291:695, 1985
3. Redfield R, Markham P, Salahuddin SZ, et al: Heterosexual acquired HTLV/III/LAV disease (AIDS-related complex and AIDS): Epidemiologic evidence for female-to-male transmission. JAMA 254:2094, 1985
4. Calabrese LH, Gopalakrishna KV: Transmission of HTLV-III infection from man to woman to man. N Engl J Med 314:1352, 1985
5. Padian N, Pickering J: Female-to-male transmission of AIDS: A reexamination of the African sex-ratio of cases (Letter to the Editor). JAMA 255:590, 1986
6. Schultz S, Milberg JA, Kristal AR, et al: Female-to-male transmission of HTLV-III (Letter to the Editor). JAMA 255:1703, 1986
7. Wykoff RF: Female-to-male transmission of HTLV-III (Letter to the Editor). JAMA 255:1704–1705, 1986
8. Redfield RR, Wright DC, Markham PD, et al: Female-to-male transmission of HTLV-III (Letter to the Editor). JAMA 255:1705, 1986
9. Research and Decisions Corporation: Designing an Effective AIDS Risk Reduction Program for San Francisco: Results from the First Probability Sample of Multiple/High-Risk Partner Heterosexual Adults. San Francisco, 1986
10. Cummings KM, Becker MH, Maile MC: Bringing the models together: An empirical approach to combining variables used to explain health actions. J Behav Med 3:123, 1980
11. Weinstein ND: Unrealistic optimism about future life events. J Pers Soc Psychol 39:806, 1980
12. Weinstein ND: Unrealistic optimism about susceptibility to health problems. J Behav Med 5:441–460, 1982
13. Perloff LS: Social comparison and illusions of invulnerability to negative events. In Snyder CR, Forc C (eds): Clinical Social Psychological Perspectives on Negative Life Events. New York, Plenum Press (in press)
14. Francis DP, Chin J: The prevention of acquired immunodeficiency syndrome in the United States: An objective strategy for medicine, public health, business and the community. JAMA 257:1357, 1987
15. Tversky A, Kahneman D: Judgement under uncertainty: Heuristics and biases. Science 185:1124, 1974
16. Hart G: Role of preventive methods in the control of venereal disease. Clin Obstet Gynecol 18:243, 1983
17. Stone KM, Grimes DA, Madgar LS: Personal protection against sexually transmitted diseases. Am J Obstet Gynecol 155:180, 1986
18. Conant M, Hardy D, Sernatinger J, et al: Condoms prevent transmission of AIDS-associated retrovirus. JAMA 255:1706, 1986
19. Darrow WW: Attitudes toward condom use and the acceptance of venereal disease prophylactics. In Redford MH, Duncan GW, Prager DJ (eds): The Condom: Increasing Utilization in the United States, pp. 173–185. San Francisco, San Francisco Press, 1974

20. Felman Y, Santora FJ: The use of condoms by VD clinic patients: A survey. Cutis 27:330, 1981
21. Condoms. Consumer Reports 44:583, 1979
22. Cutler JC: Prophylaxis in the venereal diseases. Med Clin North Am 56:1211, 1972
23. Arnold CB: The sexual behavior of inner city adolescent condom users. J Sex Res 8:298, 1972
24. Curjel RN: An analysis of the human reasons underlying the failure to use a condom in 723 cases of venereal disease. J Royal Navy Med Serv 50:203, 1964
25. Wittkower ED, Cowan JL: Some psychological aspects of promiscuity. Psychosomat Med 6:287, 1944
26. Yacenda JA: Knowledge and attitudes of college students about venereal disease and its prevention. Health Serv Rep 89:170, 1974
27. Armonker RG: What teens know about the facts of life. J School Health 50:527, 1980
28. Free MJ, Alexander NJ: Male contraception without prescription: A reevaluation of the condom and coitus interruptus. Public Health Rep 91:437, 1976
29. Sherris JD, Lewison D, Fox G: Update on condoms: Products, protection and promotion. Popul Rep September–October:121–156, 1982
30. Yarber YL: Teenage girls and venereal disease prophylaxis. Br J Venereal Dis 53:135, 1977
31. Yarber WL, Williams CE: Venereal disease prevention and a selected group of college students. J Am Venereal Dis Assoc 2:17, 1975
32. Brandt AM: No Magic Bullet: A Social History of Venereal Diseases in the United States Since 1880. New York, Oxford University Press, 1985
33. Darrow WW, Pauli ML: Health behavior and sexually transmitted diseases. In Holmes KK, Mardin PA, Sparling PF, (eds): Sexually Transmitted Diseases, pp. 65–73. New York, McGraw Hill, 1984
34. Research and Decisions Corporation: Designing an Effective AIDS Prevention Campaign Strategy for San Francisco: Results From the First Probability Sample of an Urban Gay Male Community. San Francisco, 1984
35. Research and Decisions Corporation: Designing an Effective AIDS Prevention Campaign Strategy for San Francisco: Results From the Second Probability Sample of an Urban Gay Male Community. San Francisco, San Francisco AIDS Foundation, 1985
36. McKusick L, Horstman W, Coates TJ: AIDS and sexual behavior reported by gay men in San Francisco. Am J Public Health 75:493, 1985
37. McKusick L, Wiley JA, Coates TJ, et al: Reported changes in sexual behavior of men at risk for AIDS, San Francisco, 1982–1984: The AIDS Behavioral Research Project. Public Health Rep 100:622, 1985
38. Ostrow DG, Emmons CA, O'Brien K, et al: Magnitude and predictors of behavioral risk reduction in a cohort of homosexual men. Paper presented at the International Conference on AIDS, Paris, June 1986
39. Feldman DA: AIDS health promotion and clinically applied anthropology. In Feldman DA, Johnson TM (eds): The Social Dimensions of AIDS: Method and Theory, pp. 145–159. New York, Praeger Publishers, 1986
40. Martin JL: The impact of AIDS on gay male sexual behavior patterns in New York City. Am J Public Health 77:578, 1987
41. Siegel K, Christ GH, Moynihan RM, et al: Patterns and correlates of change in sexual behavior among homosexual men at risk for AIDS. Paper presented at the annual meeting of the American Society of Clinical Oncologists, Atlanta GA, May 1987
42. Jones CC, Waskin H, Gerety B, et al: Persistence in high risk sexual activity among homosexual men in an area of low incidence of acquired immunodeficiency syndrome. Sex Transm Dis 14:79, 1987
43. Schultz S, Friedman S, Kristal A, et al: Declining rates of rectal and pharyngeal gonorrhea among men—New York City. JAMA 252:327, 1984
44. Judson FN: Fear of AIDS and gonorrhea rates in homosexual men. Lancet ii:159, 1983
45. Handsfield HH: AIDS and sexual behavior in gay men. Am J Public Health 75:329, 1987
46. Valdiserri RO, Lyter DW, Kingsley LA, et al: The effect of group education on improving attitudes about AIDS risk reduction. NY State J Med 87:272, 1987
47. Bauman LJ, Siegel K: Misperceptions among gay men of the risk for AIDS associated with their sexual behavior. J Applied Soc Psychol 17:329, 1987
48. Curran JW, Morgan WM, Hardy AM, et al: The epidemiology of AIDS: Current status and future prospects. Science 229:1352, 1985
49. Goedert JJ, Blattner WA: The epidemiology of AIDS and related conditions. In DeVita VT, Hellman S, Rosenberg SH (eds): AIDS: Etiology, Diagnosis, Treatment, and Prevention. Philadelphia, JB Lippincott, 1985
50. McKusick L, Conant M, Coates T: The AIDS epidemic: A model for developing intervention strategies for reducing high risk behavior in gay men. Sex Transm Dis 12:229, 1985
51. Kortaba JA, Lang NG: Gay lifestyle change and AIDS: Preventive health care. In Feldman DA, Johnson TM (eds): The Social Dimensions of AIDS: Method and Theory, pp. 127–143. New York, Praeger, 1986
52. Des Jarlais DC, Friedman SR: AIDS among intravenous drug users: Current research in epidemiology, natural history and prevention strategies. Paper prepared for the Committee on a National Strategy for AIDS, Institute of Medicine, National Academy of Sciences, Washington, D.C., 1986
53. Centers for Disease Control: Update. Acquired immunodeficiency syndrome—United States. Morbid Mortal Weekly Rep 35:757, 1986
54. Friedman SR, Des Jarlais D, Sotheran JL: AIDS health education for intravenous drug users. Health Educ Q 13:383–393, 1986
55. Selwyn PA, Cox CP, Feiner C, et al: Knowledge about AIDS and high-risk behavior among intravenous drug abusers in New York City. Paper presented at the annual meeting of the American Public Health Association, Washington, D.C., November 1985
56. Selwyn PA, Cox CP, Feiner C, et al: Knowledge about AIDS and high-risk behavior among intravenous drug abusers in New York City. Paper presented at the International Conference on AIDS, Paris, June 1986
57. Institute of Medicine: Confronting AIDS: Directions for Public Health, Health Care and Research. Washington, D.C., National Academy Press, 1986
58. Ginzburg HM, French J, Jackson J, et al: Health education and knowledge assessment of HTLV-III diseases among intravenous drug users. Health Educ Q 13:373, 1986
59. Des Jarlais DC, Friedman SR, Strug D: AIDS and needle sharing within the IV drug use subculture. In Feldman DA, Johnson TM (eds): The Social Dimensions of AIDS: Method and Theory, pp. 111–125. New York, Praeger, 1986

60. Goldblum P, Seymour N: Whether to take the test: Counseling guidelines. Focus: A Guide to AIDS Research 2:1, 1987

61. Forstein M: AIDS anxiety in the worried well. In Nichols SE, Ostrow DG (eds): Psychiatric Implications of Acquired Immune Deficiency Syndrome, pp. 122. Washington, D.C., American Psychiatry Press, 1985

62. Perry SW, Markowitz J: Psychiatric interventions for AIDS spectrum disorders. Hosp Community Psychiat 37:1001, 1986

63. Coates T, Morin S, McKusick L: The psychological and behavioral consequences of AIDS antibody testing. Paper presented at the NIMH AIDS Methodology Conference, Bethesda, MD, September 1986

64. Ziegler JB, Cooper DA, Johnson RO, et al: Postnatal transmission of AIDS-associated retrovirus from mother to infant. Lancet i:896, 1985

65. Scott GB, Fischl MA, Klimas N, et al: Mothers of infants with acquired immunodeficiency syndrome: Evidence for both symptomatic and asymptomatic carriers. JAMA 253: 363, 1985

66. AIDS Surveillance Unit: AIDS surveillance update: Preliminary data. New York City Department of Health, August 26, 1987

67. Maylan AK, Pinka AT: Acquired immune deficiency syndrome: A challenge to psychology. Professional Psychologist 7(4):1, 1983

68. Nichols SE: Psychiatric aspects of AIDS. Psychosomatics 24:1083, 1983

69. Grossman RJ: Psychosocial support in AIDS: A practitioner's view. In Friedman-Klein A, Lambenstein LJ (eds): AIDS. New York, Masson, 1984

70. Rossi AS: The middle years of parenting. In Baltes P, Brim OG (eds): Lifespan Development and Behavior, vol. 3. New York, Academic Press, 1980

71. Steinbrook R, Lo B, Moulton J, et al: Preferences of homosexual men with AIDS for life-sustaining treatment. N Engl J Med 314:457, 1986

72. Navia PA, Jordan BD, Price RW: The AIDS dementia complex: I. Clinical features. Ann Neurol 19:517, 1986

73. Leventhal DA, Straus DG, Campbell SW, et al: AIDS-related lymphoid neoplasia: The Memorial Hospital experience. (Unpublished) Memorial Sloan-Kettering Cancer Center, New York, June 1987

74. Christ GH, Wiener LS, Moynihan RT: Psychosocial issues in AIDS. Psychiatr Ann 16:173, 1986

75. Weinberg S, William CJ: Male Homosexuals: Their Problems and Adaptations. New York, Oxford University Press, 1974

AIDS in the Pediatric Population

Judith Falloon
Janie Eddy
Maryann Roper
Philip A. Pizzo

20

Soon after the acquired immunodeficiency syndrome (AIDS) was recognized in homosexual males and intravenous drug abusers in 1981, cases of an immunodeficiency with similar features were observed in children.[1-6] The immunologic abnormalities were not typical of known immunodeficiencies, and it was suspected that these children had AIDS.[1] With the recognition that the retrovirus now called the human immunodeficiency virus or HIV-1 is the etiologic agent of AIDS, and with the development of culture and serodiagnostic techniques, it has become evident that children with HIV infection can develop disease manifestations both similar to and different from those seen in adults. With time, increasing numbers of HIV-infected children are being observed, making HIV infection a leading cause of immunodeficiency in the infant and child.[7-12]

ROUTES OF TRANSMISSION

Although some children have acquired HIV infection by routes similar to those well established in adults, such as sexually (including by sexual abuse), by intravenous drug abuse, or through the transfusion of infected blood or the use of contaminated clotting factor replacement in the treatment of hemophilia,[12-17] these routes account for a minority of infected children. Cases related to blood-product transfusion account for only 13% of reported cases of AIDS in childhood.[18,19] Another 5% of children with AIDS have become infected during the treatment of hemophilia or other coagulation disorder.[19] The majority of the children, however, have acquired HIV infection from their mothers, transplacentally or perinatally.[7,19]

Since most children have been infected *in utero* or perinatally, HIV infection is an illness of young children. Of children with AIDS, 50% were diagnosed during the first year of life and 82% by 3 years of age.[20] Symptoms generally become evident between the ages of 4 and 6 months.[5,9,11,13,14] In fact, abnormalities such as lymphadenopathy and hepatomegaly can be seen at birth, and some children have had opportunistic infections in the first month of life.[5,14]

Mother to Child Transmission of HIV

Epidemiologic features support the concept of mother to child transmission. The majority (80%) of HIV-infected children have a parent who is at risk for AIDS or who has ARC or AIDS.[18,19] Frequently, the mother is asymptomatic but has T-cell functional defects *in vitro* and antibodies to HIV.[2,10,21,22] Such mothers usually have a history that suggests the route by which they have become infected. In the United States, a history of intravenous drug abuse or sexual contact with an intravenous drug abuser is the most common. Other histories include sexual contact with a bisexual, hemophiliac, or otherwise infected man, origin from regions such as Haiti or Central Africa where heterosexual transmission appears common, multiple sexual partners or prostitution, or transfusion with contaminated blood.[12,19,20,23] Because such women are disproportionately Black or Hispanic, poor and urban, most infected children belong to such groups.[12,18,23,24] In addition, most infected children (and infected women) are from New York, California, New Jersey, or Florida, but the proportion of children from these areas is decreasing.[12,18]

The timing of infection *in utero* is not known; however, virus and viral antigens have been detected in 14- to 20-week fetuses,[14,25,26] and dysmorphic craniofacial features suggesting early antenatal infection have been described.[27,28] HIV has been grown from cord blood and HIV antigens demonstrated in the thymus of a 20-day-old baby born at 28 weeks of gestation.[13,29] Such data

339

suggest that infection occurs early during gestation in at least some cases.

Transmission during birth is possible since there is exposure of the infant to potentially infected maternal blood or genital tract secretions.[30] Such transmission, however, has been difficult to document. Children born by cesarean section have been infected,[7,29,31,32] and no data suggest a role for cesarean delivery in the prevention of transmission of HIV infection.

Postpartum transmission by infected breast milk may be possible. Virus has been isolated from cell-free breast milk,[33] and transmission through breast-feeding is suggested by the case of a breast-fed infected child who had been born to a woman infected by postpartum transfusion.[34]

The rate of *in utero* or perinatal transmission from an infected mother is not yet defined but appears to be approximately 50%. Reported transmission rates are quite variable, however, and follow-up times are short.[13,14,20–22,35–39] Cases in which only one of a pair of monozygotic twins was infected *in utero* have also been described.[10,13,14,31] Further studies should better delineate the risk to fetus and infant, and perhaps identify features predisposing to fetal infection.[38]

Transmission Within Families

There is no evidence that casual contact or even the more intimate contact common among family members can spread infection.[40,41] Several studies have failed to demonstrate risk to family members or schoolmates, and few cases that suggest infection of family members have been described.[13,14,42–48] In one of these cases, a mother was presumed infected through care of her transfusion-infected infant that involved heavy exposure to blood, secretions, and excreta without gloving or adequate handwashing.[46] In another case, the brother of a boy with transfusion-acquired AIDS was found to be seropositive; exposure to the infected brother, including a bite that did not cause apparent bleeding, was presumed but not proven to be the route of acquisition of infection.[47] Because of the special needs of infants, larger studies of the risks to caretakers and families of small infants are warranted.

DEFINITION OF AIDS IN CHILDREN

The recognition that AIDS exists in children led the Centers for Disease Control (CDC) to develop a definition of pediatric AIDS for its surveillance purposes (Table 20-1).[9,49] This definition, despite its modification in 1985,[50] excluded an estimated 50% to 75% of symptomatic HIV-infected children.[10,13,51] In this original definition, those infections and malignancies used to identify AIDS in an adult were also used to identify AIDS in a child. In addition, children with histologically confirmed lymphocytic interstitial pneumonitis (LIP) met the criteria for AIDS unless tests for HIV were negative.

Table 20-1

Provisional Case Definition for AIDS Surveillance of Children (Used Prior to September 1987)

For the limited purposes of epidemiologic surveillance, CDC defines a case of pediatric acquired immunodeficiency syndrome (AIDS) as a child who has had:

1. A reliably diagnosed disease at least moderately indicative of underlying cellular immunodeficiency, and
2. No known cause of underlying cellular immunodeficiency or any other reduced resistance reported to be associated with that disease.

The diseases accepted as sufficiently indicative of underlying cellular immunodeficiency are the same as those used in defining AIDS in adults. In the absence of these opportunistic diseases, a histologically confirmed diagnosis of chronic lymphoid interstitial pneumonitis will be considered indicative of AIDS unless test(s) for HIV are negative. Congenital infections, e.g. toxoplasmosis or herpes simplex virus infection in the first month after birth or cytomegalovirus infection in the first 6 months after birth must be excluded.

Specific conditions that must be excluded in a child are:
1. Primary immunodeficiency diseases—severe combined immunodeficiency, DiGeorge syndrome, Wiskott-Aldrich syndrome, ataxia-telangiectasia, graft versus host disease, neutropenia, neutrophil function abnormality, agammaglobulinemia, or hypogammaglobulinemia with raised IgM.
2. Secondary immunodeficiency associated with immunosuppressive therapy, lymphoreticular malignancy, or starvation.

(From reference 40.)

Children with identified primary or secondary immunodeficiency diseases or congenital infections were specifically excluded. AIDS was thus separated from the other manifestations of HIV infection in children commonly called AIDS-related complex or ARC.

The most recent CDC definition of AIDS (Table 20-2) has broadened the criteria so that a larger range of manifestations are included, and there are fewer exclusions for underlying immunodeficiency.[52] In this definition, employed as of September 1987, the manifestations required for the diagnosis of AIDS vary according to the patient's anti-HIV antibody status. When laboratory evidence for HIV infection is present, encephalopathy, wasting syndrome, a broader range of specific AIDS-indicative diseases (including recurrent serious bacterial infections in children), and AIDS-indicative diseases that were presumptively but not definitively diagnosed are included. Patients with other causes of immunodeficiency are no longer excluded.

Patients whose laboratory tests for HIV are negative or inconclusive may still be categorized as having AIDS. If laboratory tests for HIV are negative, patients without other reasons for immunodeficiency who have had one of the listed AIDS indicator diseases and have a depressed helper T-lymphocyte count or who have had *Pneumocystis carinii* pneumonia (PCP) definitively di-

Table 20-2

Summary of the 1987 Revision of the CDC Surveillance Case Definition for AIDS

I. Without laboratory evidence of HIV infection (tests not done or inconclusive*), a case of AIDS
   - does not have another cause of underlying immunodeficiency, *and*
   - has had one of a list of AIDS "indicator diseases"† definitively diagnosed.

II. With laboratory evidence of HIV infection, a case of AIDS
   - has had one of a list of AIDS "indicator diseases"† definitively diagnosed, *or*
   - has had one of a list of AIDS "indicator diseases"† diagnosed presumptively.

III. With laboratory evidence against HIV infection (tests negative), a case of AIDS
   - does not have another cause of underlying immunodeficiency, *and*
   - had had PCP definitively diagnosed, *or* one of a list of AIDS "indicator diseases"† definitively diagnosed *and* a helper T-lymphocyte count of $<400/mm^3$.

---

* Includes seropositive children <15 months of age with an HIV-infected mother who do not have other evidence for immunodeficiency or for HIV infection.
†The list of AIDS indicator diseases differs for each category of laboratory evidence and for definitively versus presumptively diagnosed diseases.
(Modified from reference 52; see this reference for specifics.)

Table 20-3

CDC Definition of HIV Infection in Children

Children <15 months of age with perinatal infection have
   - HIV in blood or tissues*, *or*
   - symptoms meeting CDC case definition for AIDS, *or*
   - antibody to HIV† *and* evidence of both cellular and humoral immunodeficiency‡ *and* symptoms§

Older perinatally infected children or children who acquired infection through another mode of transmission have
   - HIV in blood or tissues,* *or*
   - antibody to HIV,† *or*
   - symptoms meeting CDC case definition for AIDS

---

*Confirmed by culture or other laboratory detection method.
†Repeatedly reactive screening test plus confirmatory test.
‡↑ Immunoglobulin levels, ↓ helper T-lymphocyte count, ↓ helper/suppressor T-lymphocyte ratio, absolute lymphopenia.
§Class P-2, Table 5.
(Modified from reference 51.)

---

agnosed are now considered to have AIDS.[52] If tests for IIIV arc inconclusive or not done, and if other causes of immunodeficiency are excluded, one of a list of definitively diagnosed indicator diseases provides a diagnosis of AIDS.

Although this latest revision in the definition of AIDS is complex and will probably result in the inclusion of some patients who have not been infected with HIV, it will also result in more complete reporting and better representation of the spectrum of HIV-related diseases. Nonetheless, clinicians must recognize that patients with serious HIV-related illness may still be excluded from the CDC's revised definition of AIDS.

According to CDC statistics, 558 cases of AIDS had been reported in children under 13 years of age as of August 12, 1987. New cases of AIDS in children continue to be reported, and the Public Health Service estimates that the number of pediatric AIDS cases, even according to the earlier definition, will exceed 3000 by 1991.[53] The number of symptomatic HIV-infected children will be even greater. Since seroprevalence studies have not yet been performed in children in the United States, the number of asymptomatic infected children is unknown.

DIAGNOSIS OF HIV INFECTION IN CHILDREN

The CDC has also addressed the issue of defining HIV infection in children (Table 20-3).[51] Although serologic testing has been very helpful in defining the spectrum of disease in adults, the situation is more complicated in infants because of the transplacental transfer of maternal antibodies.[13,51,54] In young children, culturing HIV from blood or body fluid can confirm infection.[13,51] Antigen testing on blood, body fluid, or tissue is not yet fully evaluated or generally available but may provide a simpler and less expensive method to detect virus and to establish a diagnosis of infection.[55] Other methods that may prove useful include the use of HIV cDNA probes for *in situ* hybridization on the mononuclear cells of neonates, the detection of HIV antigen on neonatal lymphocytes, the use of serial western blot analyses showing acquisition of new bands of antibody to viral proteins, and the use of sequential changes in the quantity of antibody of specific IgG subclass.[54,56-58] Although IgM antibodies have been used as evidence of antibody production by the infant in other congenital infections, no consistently useful IgM anti-HIV testing exists at present.[54,59-61]

Passively acquired antibody may persist for long periods in HIV-infected children, so that the CDC considers possibly perinatally infected children under 15 months to be definitely infected only if their symptoms meet CDC criteria for AIDS, they have HIV in blood or tissues, or if they have antibody to HIV, immunodeficiency, and symptoms.[51] In older children or in children infected by other routes, evidence of a repeatedly positive ELISA anti-HIV test with a positive confirmatory test such as western blot is enough to define HIV infection.[51]

Differential Diagnosis

Since it can present so early in infancy, HIV infection must be differentiated from other known immunodeficiencies, both congenital and acquired.[14,49] Suspicion of HIV infection is raised when typical clinical manifestations are seen, especially in a child thought to be at epidemiologic risk. The discovery of elevated serum immunoglobulins paired with T-cell immunodeficiency in such a child can usually lead to a diagnosis.[59,62] For example, in one study of 68 immunodeficient children, all except seven fit established criteria for known immunodeficiencies.[62] These seven children had elevated serum immunoglobulins and abnormal cell-mediated immunity. Six were seropositive for HIV. Only one of these children, a girl first seen in 1973, was seronegative for HIV.

Serodiagnosis

Excessive reliance on serodiagnosis may be misleading. While ELISA serology has proved very useful in children, false negatives and false positives occur, and the experience in children is not extensive. Samples that are ELISA-positive must, after repeat ELISA testing, be confirmed by a more specific test such as western blot. Children who are seronegative but in whom suspicion is high should also be evaluated further, since some testing negative on ELISA have had positive western blot tests or virologic evidence of HIV infection.[10,44,63–65] In one series of 85 children with documented HIV infection, 9 were seronegative by ELISA.[63] In some children, especially those with hypogammaglobulinemia or those who are critically ill, the diagnosis of HIV infection must be made in the absence of antibody to HIV.[10,14,16,17,66,67] Children reverting from seropositive to seronegative despite HIV infection have also been described, so that not all such children have simply cleared maternal antibody.[38,56] False seronegatives could also be seen in children who have recently received large volumes of seronegative transfused blood, and false seropositives seen in children who have received therapeutic immunoglobulin preparations containing anti-HIV antibodies.[68,69] The timing of testing may be critical as well, since it is clear that seroconversion after infection can be delayed in adults; the time to seroconversion in children is unknown. When available, culture or antigen tests are useful in confirming the diagnosis in children with confusing results on antibody testing.[10,51,63]

CLINICAL MANIFESTATIONS

As in adults, there is a spectrum of clinical manifestations of HIV infection in children. Infected children range from asymptomatic to critically ill.[10] An understanding of the natural history of HIV-related disease is still evolving.

The interval from HIV infection to the onset of symptoms or overt AIDS is shorter in children than in adults, and shorter in children infected perinatally than in those infected through transfusion.[5,9,12] Although the age at diagnosis of AIDS has increased over time, perinatally infected children have a median age at diagnosis

of 9 months, whereas in children acquiring AIDS through transfusion the interval between transfusion and diagnosis is a median of 17 months.[12] The onset of AIDS has been quite delayed (up to 7½ years) in some transfusion-infected children.[70]

Nonspecific Manifestations

Most children with HIV infection have nonspecific findings, including lymphadenopathy, hepatosplenomegaly, oral candidiasis, low birth weight or failure to thrive and weight loss, diarrhea, chronic eczematoid dermatitis, or fevers (Table 20-4).[2–5,10,11,13] The pathophysiology underlying these manifestations is not clearly understood.

Bacterial Infections

One common presenting manifestation of HIV infection in children is bacterial infection.[2,14] Serious bacterial infections such as sepsis, pneumonia, meningitis, abscess, and cellulitis are often seen in children before other manifestations of AIDS.[4,10,13,14,17,71,72] In one study of 46 HIV-infected children who were evaluated for bacterial infections, there were 27 episodes of sepsis, 5 of meningitis, and 6 of pneumonia.[71] Common infecting organisms are *Streptococcus pneumoniae, Hemophilus influenzae,* and salmonella.[11,71] Gram-negative organisms including enterobacteriaceae and pseudomonas, generally seen in hospitalized children or those on antibiotics, are the cause of death in a number of cases.[4,17,71] A wide range of pathogens has been isolated from blood,

Table 20-4
Clinical Manifestations in 29 Children with HIV Infection

Feature	Incidence (%)
Lymphadenopathy	90
Hepatomegaly	86
Splenomegaly	69
Failure to thrive	62
Serious bacterial infections	55
Thrush/monilial diaper rash	48
Recurrent otitis media	45
Neurologic abnormalities	34
Opportunistic infections	31
Lymphocytic interstitial pneumonitis	28
Diarrhea	17
Microcephaly	17
Clubbing of nails	10
Salivary gland enlargement	10
Lymphoma	7

(Modified from reference 10.)

including lactobacillus, Group D streptococci, *Staphylococcus aureus,* and *Staphylococcus epidermidis.*[71] Less severe bacterial infections are also quite common, especially chronic otitis media, skin and soft-tissue infections, and urinary tract infections.[2,11,71] Since fever is common, hospitalization for antibiotic therapy can be a repeated event in children with ARC or AIDS. The role, if any, of prophylactic antibiotics is not known.

Encephalopathy

One of the more tragic manifestations of HIV infection in children is a characteristic encephalopathy resulting in developmental delay or in a deterioration of motor skills and intellectual functioning.[10,14,73–76] The incidence is uncertain, but the majority of HIV-infected children may be affected to varying degrees. Encephalopathy can be the primary manifestation of a child's HIV infection. The encephalopathy is often accompanied by neurologic abnormalities such as paresis, pyramidal tract signs, ataxia, abnormal tone, or pseudobulbar palsy.[14,73–75] Among younger children, acquired microcephaly is common.[27,73,74,77] Seizures can occur but are not typical.[73,75] Cerebrospinal fluid (CSF) can be normal or demonstrate a mild pleocytosis or protein elevation.[73–75] Computed tomographic scans generally show atrophy of the brain with ventricular enlargement and often calcification in the basal ganglia and frontal white matter or attenuation of the white matter.[73–75] Contrast enhancement of the basal ganglia has been noted in association with these calcifications. Electroencephalograms show diffuse background slowing.[74,75] At autopsy, cerebral atrophy with decreased brain weight, inflammatory cell infiltrates, microglial nodules, multinucleated cells, inflammation and calcification of vessels, especially those of the basal ganglia and frontal lobes, and changes in white matter are seen.[73–75,77,78] HIV viral particles, DNA, and RNA can be demonstrated in central nervous system tissues or in CSF.[75,78–80] Virus has been isolated from both CSF and brain tissues, and HIV antigen demonstrated in CSF.[55,65,81] Specific antibody to HIV is synthesized within the blood-brain barrier of the central nervous system.[73,81] These data suggest that this encephalopathy is the result of HIV infection of the brain.

Lymphocytic Interstitial Pneumonitis (LIP)

One of the most characteristic features of pediatric HIV infection is LIP, an entity occurring in 51% of children with AIDS but rare in adults.[12] A more nodular variant has been called pulmonary lymphoid hyperplasia.[13,14,82–84] In this chronic, progressive, interstitial pulmonary disease, children develop bilateral diffuse reticulonodular infiltrates, sometimes with hilar and mediastinal adenopathy.[14,84] The definitive diagnosis of LIP is made by biopsy, in which nodular peribronchiolar lymphoid aggregates, some with germinal centers, or a diffuse infiltration of the alveolar septae and peribronchiolar areas by lymphocytes and plasma cells are demonstrated.[83] The clinical and radiographic findings appear to be so typical, however, that a presumptive diagnosis can sometimes be made without histologic confirmation.[84]

Children with LIP represent a subset of children with AIDS. They often have generalized lymphadenopathy, salivary gland enlargement, and digital clubbing.[84] They may have higher elevations of serum immunoglobulins and lesser elevations of serum lactate dehydrogenase (LDH) than are seen in HIV-infected children with PCP.[84] The prognosis for children with LIP, who have a median survival of 91 months, is better than for those with opportunistic infection.[85]

The etiology of LIP is not clear. Both Epstein-Barr virus (EBV) DNA and HIV RNA have been demonstrated in lung tissues from affected children.[14,84,86–88] Such children often have high titers and atypical antibody responses to EBV, but the roles of these viruses in the pathogenesis of LIP are not clearly delineated.[83,84,86–88]

There is no established therapy for LIP, although the use of corticosteroids for progressive LIP has been advocated.[14] Anecdotal reports of improvements after such therapy exist, but the toxicities and benefits of corticosteroid therapy for LIP are unknown.

Opportunistic Infections

Like adults, HIV-infected children develop opportunistic infections with those pathogens associated with defects in cell-mediated immunity.[14,89] In children, PCP is the most common infection; it has occurred in 52% of the childhood AIDS cases reported to the CDC.[18] Other important opportunistic infections in children are disseminated cytomegalovirus, candida esophagitis, disseminated *Mycobacterium avium-intracellulare,* cryptosporidiosis, and chronic herpes simplex infection.[12] There are no specific studies of the therapies of opportunistic infections in children, but in practice such therapies have been similar to those used in adults.[90] Trimethoprim-sulfamethoxazole prophylaxis against PCP has been suggested,[11] but no studies documenting benefit or assessing toxicity in this population exist.

Malignancies

Kaposi's sarcoma, a common manifestation of AIDS in adults, has been seen in only 4% of children with AIDS and has occurred mostly in children with Haitian parents.[12] Children with the lymphadenopathic form of Kaposi's sarcoma, discovered at autopsy, have been described.[4,91] HIV-associated lymphomas are also uncommon in childhood.[44,86,92] Long-range epidemiologic studies to define the type and incidence of malignancies in pediatric AIDS patients are in progress.

Other Manifestations

Less well defined HIV-related syndromes include hepatitis with elevated transaminases, renal disease, and a carditis or cardiomyopathy that may be a cause of death.[4,51,93–95] An HIV-associated embryopathy has been described, but its specificity has not been confirmed.[27,28] The craniofacial features noted include microcephaly, prominent boxlike forehead, ocular hypertelorism, flat nasal bridge, obliquity of the eyes, long palpebral fissures with blue sclerae, short nose with flattened columella, well-formed triangular philtrum, and patulous lips with a prominent upper vermilion border. Older children may manifest the acute HIV infection syndromes seen in adults. Persistent salivary gland enlargement or parotitis is another feature seen in children but not adults with HIV infection.[2,14,84] On biopsy, affected glands have a lymphocytic infiltrate. Ophthalmologic disease including perivasculitis of the retinal vessels has also been described in HIV-infected children.[96] As in adults, thrombocytopenia is a feature of HIV infection in children[4,10,11,14,17,97]; this is usually an immune thrombocytopenia although one case of amegakaryocytic thrombocytopenia in an HIV-infected child has been described.[98] Anemia, including Coombs-positive anemia, and immune leukopenias and neutropenias have also been reported.[3,99]

Table 20-5
Classification System for HIV Infection in Children Under 13 Years of Age.

P-0*   Indeterminate infection in perinatally exposed children <15 months of age with antibody to HIV (Table 20-3).
P-1   Asymptomatic infection
    †A   Normal immune function
    B   Abnormal immune function
    C   Immune function not tested
P-2   Symptomatic infection
    A   Nonspecific findings
    B   Progressive neurologic disease
    C   Lymphoid interstitial pneumonitis
    D   Secondary infectious diseases
       ‡D-1   Those listed in CDC definition of AIDS
       D-2   Recurrent serious bacterial infections
       D-3   Others (persistent oral candidiasis, recurrent herpes stomatitis, multidermatomal or disseminated herpes zoster)
    E   Secondary cancers
       E-1   Those listed in CDC definition of AIDS
       E-2   Others
    F   Other diseases possibly due to HIV infection (hepatitis, cardiopathy, nephropathy, anemia, thrombocytopenia, dermatologic disease)

---
* Pediatric class.
† Subclass.
‡ Category.
(From reference 51 with modifications.)

Viral infections other than those listed as opportunistic infections are important causes of morbidity in HIV-infected children. Primary varicella can be unusually severe, and atypical recurrent ulcerative herpes zoster can occur so that acyclovir therapy is important in at least some HIV-infected children with varicella zoster virus infection.[14,90] Evidence for EBV infection is commonly found in HIV-infected children, often with atypical antibody responses such as high titer antibody to viral capsid antigens and early antigens and abnormal nuclear antigen responses.[86,87,92] The EBV genome has been found in a number of tissues in these children, including lymph node, lung, and salivary gland.[14,86] An evaluation of the role of EBV in the lymphocytic infiltrates and lymphocytic tumors in these children requires further study.[86,87]

CLASSIFICATION SCHEME

The CDC has devised a classification scheme for HIV infection in children (Table 20-5).[51] Symptomatic children fall into class P-2 and are further separated into subclasses and categories by clinical manifestations. This classification system should facilitate the collection of much-needed data on the incidence of such features in infected children.

BIOPSY AND AUTOPSY DATA

From limited autopsy and biopsy data, characteristic features of some involved organs in HIV-infected children have been described.[82,83,100–102] The thymus can be normal but is often small, with lymphocyte depletion, obscured corticomedullary differentiation, and fewer Hassall's corpuscles or calcification or microcystic changes of Hassall's corpuscles.[102–104] In some glands, lymphoid follicles with germinal centers and multinucleated giant cells are seen in the medulla, or a mononuclear or plasmacytic cell infiltrate obscuring corticomedullary differentiation is seen.[104] The thymic epithelium can demonstrate abnormal morphology, necrosis, decrease in thymulin and differentiation antigens, and the presence of immunoglobulin and complement.[105] HIV antigen has been demonstrated in the thymus, and virus has been isolated from the thymus of both fetuses and infants.[25,104]

In lymph nodes, follicular hyperplasia with or without lymphocyte depletion of the paracortical zone and atrophy of follicles with lymphocyte depletion have been described.[100] Progression from an initial follicular hyperplasia to an atrophic pattern has been seen.[14] Lymphocytic infiltrates or follicular hyperplasia have also been seen in spleen, kidneys, stomach, intestine, liver, adrenals, skeletal muscle, epicardium, bone marrow, and salivary glands of HIV-infected children.[100,101] In some HIV-infected children, lymphoid tissues such as Peyer's patches, lymph nodes, spleen, and appendix

Table 20-6

Immunologic Abnormalities in Symptomatic HIV-Infected Children

Abnormality	Number Abnormal/ Number Tested
↓Thymulin	14/14 (100%)
Hypergammaglobulinemia	27/29 (93%)
↓Lymphoproliferative responses	12/15 (80%)
T4/T8 ratio <1.0	21/27 (78%)
T4 lymphopenia (<400/mm³)	12/29 (41%)
Lymphopenia (<1500/mm³)	1/29 (3%)
Hypogammaglobulinemia	1/29 (3%)

(Modified from reference 10.)

have shown lymphocyte depletion.[100] Abnormalities described in the livers of infected children include nodular lymphoid aggregates in the portal triads, hepatocellular and bile duct damage, sinusoidal cell hyperplasia, endothelialitis, lobular and portal triad lymphocytic infiltrates, and changes suggestive of chronic active hepatitis.[83,95,100] In some HIV-infected children, a polyclonal polymorphic B-cell lymphoproliferative disorder with nodular lymphoid lesions in the lung and other organs and lymphoid infiltrates in nodal and extranodal sites, sometimes with blood vessel invasion, has been seen.[83,101] An arteriopathy with abnormalities of the intima and media including fibrosis and calcification as well as vasculitis and perivasculitis has been described in children with AIDS.[106]

LABORATORY FINDINGS

The unique feature of the immunologic evaluation in HIV-infected children is the frequency of normal values in the face of severe illness (See Table 20-6).[10,13] Children are often not lymphopenic, for example, and may not have abnormal helper to suppressor T-cell ratios or diminished numbers of helper T-lymphocytes.[2-4,10,14,59] Depending on which mitogen or antigen is used, lymphocyte proliferation testing can be normal.[14] Pokeweed mitogen (PWM) appears to be the most sensitive in detecting abnormalities.[11,14,59] Laboratory testing does not distinguish AIDS from ARC nor are immune abnormalities alone diagnostic of HIV infection.[10,71,103] In children with hemophilia or a history of chronic transfusion, in particular, immune abnormalities may be present in the absence of HIV infection.[70]

B-Cell Immunity

Abnormalities in humoral immunity are typical of HIV infection in children. In fact, it has been proposed that serum immunoglobulin levels be used as a screening test, since of 8000 samples from one immunodeficiency clinic, only children with HIV infection had an IgG over 1800 mg/dl at the age of one year or over 2300 mg/dl at age two.[14] Of the HIV-infected children seen in this clinic, only 14% had serum immunoglobulin levels that were not above these levels.[14] In addition to elevated IgG, other immunoglobulins (IgD, IgA, or IgM) can be increased.[4,5,71,107] In some infected children, IgG subclass deficiency or hypogammaglobulinemia has been noted or has developed.[10,17,66,71,108,109]

Further investigations into the humoral immunity of infected children have revealed that they respond abnormally to new and to recall antigens with diminished primary and secondary responses. These have been demonstrated after immunization with diphtheria or tetanus toxoid or pneumococcal polysaccharide vaccine.[20,107,110,111] Blunted responses with absence of IgM-to-IgG class switch were seen in HIV-infected children who had been immunized with bacteriophage phiX174.[107] B-cell numbers can be elevated and spontaneous secretion of immunoglobulin increased, but secretion after stimulation is diminished.[3,5,112] In vitro responses to PWM and *Staphyloccus aureus* Cowan A are often abnormal.[13] Deficiencies in isoagglutinins have been described, as have antinuclear antibodies and circulating immune complexes.[2,4,71,107,110]

T-Cell Immunity

Impairment of T-cell immunity is a hallmark of HIV infection, although it may be manifested later than B-cell deficiency in infected children. Lymphocyte subsets can be abnormal with a reversal of the ratio of helper to suppressor lymphocytes in the blood; this reflects both a decrease in helper cells and an increase in suppressor cells.[2,3,5,10,59] Lymphocyte proliferative responses to phytohemagglutinin, concanavalin A (Con A) or specific antigens can be abnormal.[2,103,111] Cutaneous anergy is common.[3,59] Suppressor T-cell functions are defective *in vitro,* as demonstrated by abnormal suppression of PWM-driven immunoglobulin secretion and Con A generation of cells that suppress T-cell mitogenic functions.[113] As in adults, an increase in circulating thymosin-α_1 is seen, probably caused by the recognition of an HIV protein by a cross-reacting antithymosin antibody.[103] Circulating thymulin activity is very low or absent in HIV-infected children; this abnormality may be present when other *in vitro* evaluations of cell-mediated immunity are normal.[10,103,114] Interferon production and natural killer cell activity can also be abnormal.[59]

PROGNOSIS

Over 60% of the children with AIDS have died.[12,18] HIV-infected children not meeting the original CDC criteria for AIDS have also had a high mortality. No clearcut predictors of poor prognosis have been developed, although symptomatic children are more likely to have immunologic abnormalities.[10,110] Which children or what proportion of infected children will progress to symptoms, opportunistic infections, malignancy, or death cannot now be predicted. It appears that children who develop PCP present with symptoms at a younger age than those with other opportunistic infections and have a shorter median survival.[115] Children diagnosed before 1 year of age and children with encephalopathy also appear to have a shorter survival.[12,73]

Children with abnormal antigen-induced lymphocyte proliferative responses or anergy may also have a poorer prognosis.[110] The numbers of circulating T4 lymphocytes, the pattern of antibody responses on western blot, the presence of HIV antigen in serum or cerebrospinal fluid, and the presence of neutralizing antibodies in serum are being evaluated as predictors of prognosis.[16,55,73,81,110,116]

MANAGEMENT AND THERAPY

The current mainstay of therapy of HIV-infected children remains close observation and good general medical and supportive care with prompt therapy for bacterial infections and treatable opportunistic infections. As in adults, adverse reactions to drugs are common. Nutrition can be a serious problem, and some children require intravenous hyperalimentation.

Immunization

The issues related to the immunization of HIV-infected children are complex, and the risks of acquiring childhood diseases must be weighed against the potential risks of live vaccines or of antigenic stimulation. In addition, serologic responses and vaccine efficacy may be poor in some HIV infected children, including those receiving intravenous immunoglobulin.[20,111] The Immunization Practices Advisory Committee (ACIP) has published guidelines for the immunization of children with HIV infection. These suggest that asymptomatic children receive diphtheria and tetanus toxoids and pertussis vaccine (DTP); live measles, mumps, and rubella viruses in a combined vaccine (MMR); *Haemophilus influenzae* type b conjugate vaccine (HbCV); and inactivated poliovirus vaccine (IPV) but not oral attenuated poliovirus vaccine (OPV).[20,117] Vaccination of symptomatic children should be considered, and vaccines should include DTP, IPV, MMR, HbCV, and pneumococcal and influenza vaccines. In addition, the use of OPV should be avoided in healthy children with HIV-infected siblings or other family members; such children can receive IPV.[20]

Although the original ACIP recommendations[20] suggested omitting the MMR in symptomatic HIV-infected children to avoid the use of live viral vaccines in immunosuppressed patients, current recommendations are to administer MMR. There have not been reports of serious adverse effects caused by the administration of the MMR vaccine, and serious and fatal measles infections have occurred in HIV-infected children.[118] Of note, some of these children did not manifest the typical rash of measles. Even though vaccinated, however, these children should receive immune globulin after known measles exposure because vaccine efficacy in this setting is suspect. In addition, varicella-zoster immune globulin should be administered for exposures to this virus.[20]

Intravenous Immunoglobulin

Thus far, the most extensively administered therapy in the symptomatic HIV-infected child has been intravenous immunoglobulin (IVIG), which was initially used in an attempt to decrease the incidence of bacterial infections with such organisms as *Hemophilus influenzae* and *Streptococcus pneumoniae*.[11,113,119–121] No randomized controlled trials have yet been performed, so firm support for the use of IVIG does not now exist. It has been reported that children treated with IVIG had fewer febrile episodes and fewer episodes of sepsis, and that they have stabilized or improved clinically.[72,119,120] In one study, one of 14 IVIG-treated children developed sepsis during a period of observation that averaged 20 months, as compared with 18 of 27 untreated patients from a non-randomly selected control population.[120] Some laboratory improvements have been noted in IVIG-treated children, including increases in helper T-lymphocytes and lymphocyte proliferative responses, decreases in circulating immune complexes and LDH, and a normalization of the suppression of PWM-driven immunoglobulin secretion.[113,119,120] Because of the lack of controlled data and long-term follow-up, however, the safety and efficacy of the routine use of IVIG in HIV-infected patients are unknown. However, a multicenter trial comparing intravenous gamma globulins to a placebo is currently in progress under the auspices of the National Institute of Child Health and Human Development.

Antiretroviral Therapy

The use of antiretroviral agents in infants and children has lagged significantly behind their use in adults. In spite of this, a concerted effort is now being made to develop a comprehensive strategy for the evaluation and treatment of children with HIV disease. Thus far, children were treated with ribavirin in a small trial performed in France; although the details of the trial have not been reported, no benefit was seen.[122] Other trials of ribavirin in HIV-infected children are in progress. We and others are currently completing Phase I studies of azidothymidine (AZT) in children. In these studies, AZT is administered either by intermittent or continuous intravenous infusion or orally in some older children. Two objectives guide our NCI study of AZT administered by continuous intravenous infusion. First, by providing steady state levels of AZT in both plasma and the CSF, it may be possible to inhibit HIV replication constantly. This is based on the short-half life of AZT in the plasma (one hour in adults) indicating that, even if administered on an every four-hour basis the level of AZT would be below the theoretical virostatic level of 1 μM. Second, although the oral route is more convenient, compliance may become a problem, especially in younger children. Thus, a continuous intravenous administration provides an optimized pharmocologic way to assess AZT efficacy and toxicity in children.

In this study, AZT is delivered through a Hickman-Broviac catheter using a programmable portable infusion pump. Four dosages are being studied: 0.5 mg/kg/hr (level 1); 0.9 mg/kg/hr (level 2); 1.4 mg/kg/hr (level 3) and 1.8 mg/kg/hr (level 4). The starting dosage (0.5 mg/kg/hr) is approximately 25% of the maximally tolerated dose that was used in adults. Between December 16, 1986, and November 16, 1987, 22 children ranging in age from 14 months to 12 years have been entered into this trial. Steady-state levels have been determined at the four dosages indicating plasma concentration of 1.9 μM at level 1, 3.0 μM at level 2, 3.3 μM at level 3, and 5 μM at level 4. The steady-state CSF-to-plasma ratio is 28% ±7%. Although results are preliminary, the patients enrolled in this Phase I study have had demonstrable clinical improvement, including weight gain, improved appetite, increased sense of well-being, increased helper T-lymphocyte counts, decreased immunoglobulin levels, and decreased adenopathy and organomegaly. Most notable has been the improvement in children who had evidence of encephalopathy at the time of entry to the study; all have shown improvements in neurological function or interactiveness or have regained lost developmental milestones. These results, albeit preliminary, are encouraging and suggest that agents such as AZT will play a role in the management of children with HIV-related infections.

A second Phase I study of AZT administered on an intermittent basis (every 6 hours) has also been completed. When given orally, AZT's pharmacokinetic profile in children is similar to that in adults. As with the continuous infusion regimen, improvements in immune function and recovery from neurodevelopmental deficits have been observed.[124–126] It is not established whether the maintenance of HIV levels at constantly inhibitory concentrations (as achieved in the continuous infusion regimen) will offer a benefit beyond that achieved with the intermittent dosing schedule. A comparative evaluation to assess this will soon be underway. In addition, Phase II evaluation of AZT in symptomatic HIV children is also underway.

There is an urgent need for trials of promising agents in symptomatic HIV-infected children, in asymptomatic children, and in neonates in whom infection can be documented by culture or other method.

Currently, Phase I testing of AZT in seropositive neonates is underway to determine whether its pharmacokinetics will differ from those observed in infants older than 3 months of age. Pending these results, studies will be initiated by the Pediatric AIDS Clinical Trials Group to evaluate whether AZT begun at birth in infants born to seropositive mothers can alter the course of infection. Furthermore, trials in which an anti-retroviral agent like AZT might be given to a seropositive mother just prior to delivery, or even during pregnancy, are also likely to be initiated.

For older HIV-infected children who are already symptomatic, a study evaluating AZT with or without intravenous gammaglobulin infusions will follow the Phase II evaluation of AZT. This study will delineate whether gammaglobulin can add to the benefits accrued with AZT alone. For less symptomatic children, including patients with LIP alone, and patients with hemophilia, the potenial benefit of anti-retroviral therapy prior to the onset of more full-blown HIV-related disease manifestations will also be studied.

Because of the hematologic toxicity associated with AZT, as well as the need to improve its efficacy, combination regimens will need to be developed. The success of combination chemotherapy in treating both peripheral and central nervous system leukemia in children serves as a good model on which to base developmental strategies for HIV infection in children. Accordingly, new agents must be evaluated and regimens combining them with existing therapies developed. At present, the anti-retroviral agent dideoxycytidine (DDC) is undergoing Phase I testing at the NCI and will also be evaluated in combination with AZT. Studies to evaluate other promising anti-retroviral agents (e.g., DDA/DDI or CD4 blockers) will also soon be initiated in children. Similarly, methods to improve host defenses or to stimulate bone marrow production to overcome the myelosuppression associated with agents like AZT also need to be evaluated. A trial combining AZT with the cytokine GM-CSF (granulocyte-macrophage colony stimulating factor) is currently in progress at the NCI. Future studies are also likely to evaluate other cytokines (e.g., IL3 and other interleukins) together with anti-retroviral agents.

Immune Reconstitution

There are few data on immune reconstitution in the pediatric age group. A limited number of agents have been tried, such as thymic factors, without success.[103]

Education

The issue of the schooling of HIV-infected children is one surrounded by strong emotions and fears. The guidelines established by the CDC, which take into consideration what is known about the routes of transmission of the virus, appear to be prudent.[40] In each case the risks and benefits of school attendance should be assessed. It is suggested that infected children attend school unless they lack control of body secretions, have uncoverable oozing lesions, have unacceptable behaviors such as biting, or unless their risks of contracting infectious disease at school is felt to be unacceptable.[40,127] Very young infants and children present a special problem because of their lack of control of body secretions and their oral behavior; current recommendations are that such children not be placed into day care.[40,128,129] Those likely to be exposed to an infected child's body fluids or secretions as in feeding or diaper changing should be aware of the child's HIV infection and should be educated as to proper precautions.[40]

PREVENTION

The key to the control of future HIV infections now lies in prevention. Although blood-product–related HIV infection will continue to be seen because of the long interval between transfusion and illness, new blood-related infections will be few now that donor-deferred antibody-negative blood is used for transfusion and for the production of heat-treated clotting factor concentrates. Since most affected children are transplacentally or perinatally infected, the control of infection in the adult population, especially in women of childbearing age, is crucial.[35] In order to interrupt transmission, testing and counseling must be easily and confidentially available, especially to those in high-risk groups, and effective education programs aimed at altering behaviors that promote transmission must be instituted.[35] The identification of infected women through antibody screening programs is essential to the interruption of perinatal transmission, especially since infected women are often asymptomatic and a child may be the index case in a family. Infected women need to be effectively counseled to avoid pregnancy. If pregnant, they must understand the risks to their infants, including the potential risk of breastfeeding. Uninfected women must avoid behaviors that could facilitate their acquisition of infection.

FUTURE ISSUES

There are now several major ongoing studies that will define more precisely the spectrum of pediatric AIDS. These studies will examine the epidemiologic characteristics of children with the infection, transmission patterns, the natural history of the disease in maternally acquired infection, seroprevalence in newborns, rates of perinatal transmission, and the developmental outcome of perinatally infected children. With a better understanding of the disease and with the development of effective anti-retroviral therapies, we will be better prepared to care for the large numbers of HIV-infected children who will be born in the coming years.

REFERENCES

1. Unexplained immunodeficiency and opportunistic infections in infants—New York, New Jersey, California. MMWR 31:665, 1982
2. Rubinstein A, Sicklick M, Gupta A, et al: Acquired immunodeficiency with reversed T4/T8 ratios in infants born to promiscuous and drug-addicted mothers. JAMA 249:2350, 1983
3. Oleske J, Minnefor A, Cooper R, et al: Immune deficiency syndrome in children. JAMA 249:2345, 1983
4. Scott GB, Buck BE, Leterman JG, et al. Acquired immunodeficiency syndrome in infants. N Engl J Med 310:76, 1984
5. Thomas PA, Jaffe HW, Spira TJ, et al: Unexplained immunodeficiency in children. A surveillance report. JAMA 252:639, 1984
6. Ammann AJ, Cowan MJ, Wara DW, et al. Acquired immunodeficiency in an infant: Possible transmission by means of blood products. Lancet i:956, 1983
7. Cowan MJ, Hellman D, Chudwin D, et al: Maternal transmission of acquired immune deficiency syndrome. Pediatrics 73:382, 1984
8. Church JA, Isaacs H: Transfusion-associated acquired immune deficiency syndrome in infants. J Pediatr 105:731, 1984
9. Rogers MF: AIDS in children: a review of the clinical, epidemiologic and public health aspects. Pediatr Infect Dis 4:230, 1985
10. Pahwa S, Kaplan M, Fikrig S, et al: Spectrum of human T-cell lymphotropic virus type III infection in children. Recognition of symptomatic, asymptomatic, and seronegative patients. JAMA 255:2299, 1986
11. Shannon KM, Ammann AJ: Acquired immune deficiency syndrome in childhood. J Pediatr 106:332, 1985
12. Rogers MF, Thomas PA, Starcher ET, et al: Acquired immunodeficiency syndrome in children: Report of the Centers for Disease Control national surveillance, 1982 to 1985. Pediatrics 79:1008, 1987
13. Rubinstein A, Bernstein L: The epidemiology of pediatric acquired immunodeficiency syndrome. Clin Immunol Immunopathol 40:115, 1986
14. Rubinstein A: Pediatric AIDS. Curr Probl Pediatr 16:361, 1986
15. Wykoff RF, Pearl ER, Saulsbury FT: Immunologic dysfunction in infants infected through transfusion with HTLV-III. N Engl J Med 312:294, 1985
16. Lange JMA, van den Berg H, Dooren LJ, et al: HTLV-III/LAV infection in nine children infected by a single plasma donor: clinical outcome and recognition patterns of viral proteins. J Infect Dis 154:171, 1986
17. Saulsbury FT, Wykoff RF, Boyle RJ: Transfusion-acquired human immunodeficiency virus infection in twelve neonates: Epidemiologic, clinical and immunologic features. Pediatr Infect Dis J 6:544, 1987
18. Update: Acquired immunodeficiency syndrome—United States. MMWR 35:757, 1986
19. Lifson AR, Rogers MF, White C, et al: Unrecognized modes of transmission of HIV: Acquired immunodeficiency syndrome in children reported without risk factors. Pediatr Infect Dis 6:292, 1987
20. Immunization of children infected with human T-lymphotropic virus type III/lymphadenopathy-associated virus. MMWR 35:595, 1986

21. Scott GB, Fischl MA, Klimas N, et al: Mothers of infants with the acquired immunodeficiency syndrome. Evidence for both symptomatic and asymptomatic carriers. JAMA 253:363, 1985

22. Minkoff H, Nanda D, Menez R, et al: Pregnancies resulting in infants with acquired immunodeficiency syndrome or AIDS-related complex: Follow-up of mothers, children and subsequently born siblings. Obstet Gynecol 69:288, 1987

23. Guinan ME, Hardy A: Epidemiology of AIDS in women in the United States, 1981 through 1986. JAMA 257:2039, 1987

24. Acquired immunodeficiency syndrome (AIDS) among Blacks and Hispanics—United States. MMWR 35:655, 1986

25. Jovaisas E, Koch MA, Schafer A, et al: LAV/HTLV-III in 20-week fetus. Lancet ii:1129, 1985

26. Sprecher S, Soumenkoff G, Puissant F, et al: Vertical transmission of HIV in 15-week fetus. Lancet ii:288, 1986

27. Marion RW, Wiznia AA, Hutcheon RG, et al: Human T-cell lymphotropic virus type III (HTLV-III) embryopathy. A new dysmorphic syndrome associated with intrauterine HTLV-III infection. Am J Dis Child 140:638, 1986

28. Marion RW, Wiznia AA, Hutcheon RG, et al: Fetal AIDS syndrome score: Correlation between severity of dysmorphism and age at diagnosis of immunodeficiency. Am J Dis Child 141:429, 1987

29. Lapointe N, Michaud J, Pekovic D, et al: Transplacental transmission of HTLV-III virus. N Engl J Med 312:1325, 1985

30. Vogt MW, Witt DJ, Craven DE, et al: Isolation patterns of the human immunodeficiency virus from cervical secretions during the menstrual cycle of women at risk for the acquired immunodeficiency syndrome. Ann Intern Med 106:380, 1987

31. Menez-Bautista R, Fikrig SM, Pahwa S, et al: Monozygotic twins discordant for the acquired immunodeficiency syndrome. Am J Dis Child 140:678, 1986

32. Minkoff H, Nanda D, Menez R, et al: Pregnancies resulting in infants with acquired immunodeficiency syndrome or AIDS-related complex. Obstet Gynecol 691:285, 1987

33. Thiry L, Sprecher-Goldberger S, Jonckheer T, et al: Isolation of AIDS virus from cell-free breast milk of three healthy virus carriers. Lancet ii:891, 1985

34. Ziegler JB, Cooper DA, Johnson RO, et al: Postnatal transmission of AIDS-associated retrovirus from mother to infant. Lancet i:896, 1985

35. Recommendations for assisting in the prevention of perinatal transmission of human T-lymphotropic virus type III/lymphadenopathy-associated virus and acquired immunodeficiency syndrome. MMWR 34:721, 1985

36. Chiodo F, Ricchi E, Costigliola P, et al: Vertical transmission of HTLV-III. Lancet i:739, 1986

37. Luzi G, Ensoli B, Turbessi G, et al: Transmission of HTLV-III infection by heterosexual contact. Lancet ii:1018, 1985

38. Mok JQ, Giaquinto C, De Rossi A, et al: Infants born to mothers seropositive for human immunodeficiency virus: Preliminary findings from a multicentre European study. Lancet i:1164, 1987

39. Semprini AE, Vucetich A, Pardi G, et al: HIV infection and AIDS in newborn babies of mothers positive for HIV antibody. Br Med J 294:610, 1987

40. Education and foster care of children infected with human T-lymphotrophic virus type III/lymphadenopathy-associated virus. MMWR 34:517, 1985

41. MacDonald KL, Danila RN, Osterholm MT: Infection with human T-lymphotropic virus type III/lymphadenopathy-associated virus: Considerations for transmission in the child day care setting. Rev Infect Dis 8:606, 1986

42. Kaplan JE, Oleske JM, Getchell JP, et al: Evidence against transmission of human T-lymphotropic virus/lymphadenopathy-associated virus (HTLV-III/LAV) in families of children with the acquired immunodeficiency syndrome. Pediatr Infect Dis 4:468, 1985

43. Friedland GH, Saltzman BR, Rogers MF, et al: Lack of transmission of HTLV-III/LAV infection to household contacts of patients with AIDS or AIDS-related complex with oral candidiasis. N Engl J Med 314:344, 1986

44. Martin K, Katz BZ, Miller G: AIDS and antibodies to human immunodeficiency virus (HIV) in children and their families. J Infect Dis 155:54, 1987

45. Fischl MA, Dickinson GM, Scott GB, et al: Evaluation of heterosexual partners, children and household contacts of adults with AIDS. JAMA 257:640, 1987

46. Apparent transmission of human T-lymphotropic virus type III/lymphadenopathy-associated virus from child to mother providing health care. MMWR 35:75, 1986

47. Wahn V, Kramer HH, Voit T, et al: Horizontal transmission of HIV infection between two siblings. Lancet ii:694, 1986

48. Berthier A, Chamaret S, Fauchet R, et al: Transmissibility of human immunodeficiency virus in hemophiliac and non-hemophiliac children living in a private school in France. Lancet ii:598, 1987

49. Update: Acquired immunodeficiency syndrome (AIDS)—United States. MMWR 32:688, 1984

50. Revision of the case definition of acquired immunodeficiency syndrome for national reporting—United States. MMWR 34:373, 1985

51. Classification system for human immunodeficiency virus (HIV) infection in children under 13 years of age. MMWR 36:225, 1987

52. Revision of the CDC surveillance case definition for acquired immunodeficiency syndrome. MMWR 36:1S, 1987

53. Coolfont report: a PHS plan for prevention and control of AIDS and the AIDS virus. Public Health Rep 101:341, 1986

54. Pyun KH, Ochs HD, Dufford MTW, et al: Perinatal infection with human immunodeficiency virus: Specific antibody responses by the neonate. N Engl J Med 317:611, 1987

55. Goudsmit J, de Wolf F, Paul DA, et al: Expression of human immunodeficiency virus antigen (HIV-Ag) in serum and cerebrospinal fluid during acute and chronic infection. Lancet ii:177, 1986

56. Tovo P-A, Gabiano C, Riva C, et al: Specific antibody and virus antigen expression in congenital HIV infection. Lancet i:1201, 1987

57. Johnson JP, Nair P, Alexander S: Early diagnosis of HIV infection in the neonate. N Engl J Med 316:273, 1987

58. Harnish DG, Hammerberg O, Walker IR, et al: Early detection of HIV infection in a newborn. N Engl J Med 316: 272, 1987

59. Ammann AJ, Levy J: Laboratory investigation of pediatric acquired immunodeficiency syndrome. Clin Immunol Immunopathol 40:122, 1986

60. Di Maria H, Courpotin C, Rouzioux C, et al: Transplacental transmission of human immunodeficiency virus. Lancet ii:215, 1986

61. Gaetano C, Scano G, Carbonari M, et al: Delayed and

defective anti-HIV IgM response in infants. Lancet i:631, 1987

62. Ammann AJ, Kaminsky L, Cowan M, et al: Antibodies to AIDS-associated retrovirus distinguish between pediatric primary and acquired immunodeficiency diseases. JAMA 253:3116, 1985

63. Borkowsky W, Krasinski K, Paul D, et al: Human-immunodeficiency-virus infections in infants negative for anti-HIV by enzyme-linked immunoassay. Lancet i:1168, 1987

64. Shanks GD, Redfield RR, Fischer GW: *Toxoplasma* encephalitis in an infant with acquired immunodeficiency syndrome. Pediatr Infect Dis 6:70, 1987

65. Ragni MV, Urbach AH, Taylor S, et al: Isolation of human immunodeficiency virus and detection of HIV DNA sequences in the brain of an ELISA antibody-negative child with acquired immune deficiency syndrome and progressive encephalopathy. J Pediatr 110:892, 1987

66. Maloney MJ, Guill MF, Wray BB, et al: Pediatric acquired immune deficiency syndrome with panhypogammaglobulinemia. J Pediatr 110:266, 1987

67. Pyu KH, Ochs HD, Wedgwood RJ, et al: Seronegativity and paediatric AIDS. Lancet i:1152, 1987

68. Human immunodeficiency virus infection transmitted from an organ donor screened for HIV antibody—North Carolina. MMWR 36:306, 1987

69. Safety of therapeutic immune globulin preparations with respect to transmission of human T-lymphotropic virus type III/lymphadenopathy-associated virus infection. MMWR 35:231, 1986

70. Hilgartner MW: AIDS in the transfused patient. Am J Dis Child 141:194, 1987

71. Bernstein LJ, Krieger BZ, Novick B, et al: Bacterial infection in the acquired immunodeficiency syndrome of children. Pediatr Infect Dis 4:472, 1985

72. Wood CC, McNamara JG, Schwarz DF, et al: Prevention of pneumococcal bacteremia in a child with acquired immunodeficiency syndrome-related complex. Pediatr Infect Dis J 6:564, 1987

73. Epstein LG, Sharer LR, Oleske JM, et al: Neurologic manifestations of human immunodeficiency virus infection in children. Pediatrics 78:678, 1986

74. Belman AL, Ultmann MH, Horoupian D, et al: Neurological complications in infants and children with acquired immune deficiency syndrome. Ann Neurol 18:560, 1985

75. Epstein LG, Sharer LR, Joshi VV, et al: Progressive encephalopathy in children with acquired immune deficiency syndrome. Ann Neurol 17:488, 1985

76. Ultmann MH, Belman AL, Ruff HA, et al: Developmental abnormalities in infants and children with acquired immune deficiency syndrome (AIDS) and AIDS-related complex. Devel Med Child Neurol 27:563, 1985

77. Belman AL, Lantos G, Horoupian D, et al: AIDS: Calcification of the basal ganglia in infants and children. Neurology 36:1192, 1986

78. Sharer LR, Epstein LG, Cho E-S, et al: Pathologic features of AIDS encephalopathy in children: evidence for LAV/HTLV-III infection of brain. Human Pathol 17:271, 1986

79. Epstein LG, Sharer LR, Cho E-S, et al: HTLV-III/LAV-like retrovirus particles in the brains of patients with AIDS encephalopathy. AIDS Research 1:447, 1984

80. Shaw GM, Harper ME, Hahn BH, et al: HTLV-III infection in brains of children and adults with AIDS encephalopathy. Science 227:177, 1985

81. Epstein LG, Goudsmit J, Paul DA, et al: Expression of human immunodeficiency virus in cerebrospinal fluid of children with progressive encephalopathy. Ann Neurol 21:397, 1987

82. Joshi VV, Oleske JM, Minnefor AB, et al: Pathologic pulmonary findings in children with the acquired immunodeficiency syndrome: A study of ten cases. Human Pathol 16:241, 1985

83. Joshi VV, Oleske JM: Pulmonary lesions in children with acquired immunodeficiency syndrome: A reappraisal based on data in additional cases and follow-up study of previously reported cases. Human Pathol 17:641, 1986

84. Rubinstein A, Morecki R, Silverman B, et al: Pulmonary disease in children with acquired immune deficiency syndrome and AIDS-related complex. J Pediatr 108:498, 1986

85. Thomas PA, O'Donnell RE, Lessner L: Survival analysis of children reported with AIDS in New York City, 1982–1986. Abstract TP.76. In Third International Conference on Acquired Immunodeficiency Syndrome (AIDS), Washington, DC, June 1–5, 1987

86. Andiman WA, Eastman R, Martin K, et al: Opportunistic lymphoproliferations associated with Epstein-Barr viral DNA in infants and children with AIDS. Lancet ii:1390, 1985

87. Fackler JC, Nagel JE, Adler WH, et al: Epstein-Barr virus infection in a child with the acquired immune deficiency syndrome. Am J Dis Child 139:1000, 1985

88. Chayt KJ, Harper ME, Marselle LM, et al: Detection of HTLV-III RNA in lungs of patients with AIDS and pulmonary involvement. JAMA 256:2356, 1986

89. Joshi VV, Oleske JM, Saad S, et al: Pathology of opportunistic infections in children with acquired immune deficiency syndrome. Pediatr Pathol 6:145, 1986

90. United States Department of Health and Human Services: Report of the Surgeon General's workshop on children with HIV infection and their families, April 6–9, 1987. DHHS Publication No. HRS-D-MC 87-1, pp 53–55

91. Buck BE, Scott GB, Valdes-Dapena M, et al: Kaposi sarcoma in two infants with acquired immune deficiency syndrome. J Pediatr 103:911, 1983

92. Katz BZ, Andiman WA, Eastman R, et al: Infection with two genotypes of Epstein-Barr virus in an infant with AIDS and lymphoma of the central nervous system. J Infect Dis 153:601, 1986

93. Steinherz LJ, Brochstein JA, Robins J: Cardiac involvement in congenital acquired immunodeficiency syndrome. Am J Dis Child 140:1241, 1986

94. Joshi V, Gadol C, Connor E, et al: Congestive cardiomyopathy in association with acquired immune deficiency syndrome in children. Abstract TP.170. In Third International Conference on Acquired Immunodeficiency Syndrome (AIDS), Washington, DC, June 1–5, 1987

95. Duffy LF, Daum F, Kahn E, et al: Hepatitis in children with acquired immune deficiency syndrome. Histopathologic and immunocytologic features. Gastroenterology 90:173, 1986

96. Kestelyn P, Lepage P, Van de Perre P: Perivasculitis of the retinal vessels as an important sign in children with AIDS-related complex. Am J Ophthalmol 100:614, 1985

97. Saulsbury FT, Boyle RJ, Wykoff RF, et al: Thrombocytopenia as the presenting manifestation of human T-lymphotropic virus type III infection in infants. J Pediatr 109:30, 1986

98. Weinblatt ME, Scimeca PG, James-Herry AG, et al: Thrombocytopenia in an infant with AIDS. Am J Dis Child 141:15, 1987

99. McCance-Katz EF, Hoeker JL, Vitale NB: Severe neutropenia associated with anti-neutrophil antibody in a patient with acquired immunodeficiency syndrome-related complex. Pediatr Infect Dis 6:417, 1987

100. Joshi VV, Oleske JM, Minnefor AB, et al: Pathology of suspected acquired immune deficiency syndrome in children: A study of eight cases. Pediatr Pathol 2:71, 1984

101. Joshi VV, Kauffman S, Oleske JM, et al: Polyclonal polymorphic B-cell lymphoproliferative disorder with prominent pulmonary involvement in children with acquired immune deficiency syndrome. Cancer 59:1455, 1987

102. Joshi VV, Oleske JM: Pathologic appraisal of the thymus gland in acquired immunodeficiency syndrome in children: A study of four cases and a review of the literature. Arch Pathol Lab Med 109:142, 1985

103. Rubinstein A, Novick BE, Sicklick MJ, et al: Circulating thymulin and thymosin-alpha-1 activity in pediatric acquired immune deficiency syndrome: In vivo and in vitro studies. J Pediatr 109:422, 1986

104. Joshi VV, Oleske JM, Saad S, et al: Thymus biopsy in children with acquired immunodeficiency syndrome. Arch Pathol Lab Med 110:837, 1986

105. Savino W, Dardenne M, Marche C, et al: Thymic epithelium in AIDS: An immunohistologic study. Am J Pathol 122:302, 1986

106. Joshi V, Pawel B, Connor E, et al: Arteriopathy in children with AIDS. Abstract MP.170. In Third International Conference on Acquired Immunodeficiency Syndrome (AIDS), Washington, DC, June 1–5, 1987

107. Bernstein LJ, Ochs HD, Wedgwood RJ, et al: Defective humoral immunity in pediatric acquired immunodeficiency syndrome. J Pediatr 107:352, 1985

108. Honda NS, Sun NCJ, Heiner DC: Isolated IgG$_4$ subclass deficiency and malignant lymphoma in a child with acquired immunodeficiency syndrome. Am J Dis Child 141:378, 1987

109. Church JA, Lewis J, Spotkov JM: IgG subclass deficiencies in children with suspected AIDS. Lancet i:279, 1984

110. Blanche S, Le Deist F, Fischer A, et al: Longitudinal study of 18 children with perinatal LAV/HTLV III infection: Attempt at prognostic evaluation. J Pediatr 109:965, 1986

111. Borkowsky W, Steele CJ, Grubman S, et al: Antibody responses to bacterial toxoids in children infected with human immunodeficiency virus. J Pediatr 110:563, 1987

112. Pahwa S, Fikrig S, Menez R, et al: Pediatric acquired immunodeficiency syndrome: Demonstration of B-lymphocyte defects in vitro. Diag Immunol 4:24, 1986

113. Gupta A, Novick BE, Rubinstein A: Restoration of suppressor T-cell functions in children with AIDS following intravenous gammaglobulin treatment. Am J Dis Child 140:143, 1986

114. Incefy GS, Pahwa S, Pahwa R, et al: Low circulating thymulin-like activity in children with AIDS and AIDS-related complex. AIDS Research 2:109, 1986

115. Lampert R, Milberg J, O'Donnell R, et al: Life table analysis of children with acquired immunodeficiency syndrome. Pediatr Infect Dis 5:374, 1986

116. Lange JMA, Paul DA, Huisman HG, et al: Persistent HIV antigenaemia and decline of HIV core antibodies associated with transition to AIDS. Br Med J 293:1459, 1986

117. Immunization of children infected with human immunodeficiency virus—supplementary ACIP statement. MMWR 37:181, 1988

118. Measles in HIV-infected children, United States. MMWR 37:183, 1988

119. Silverman BA, Rubinstein A: Serum lactate dehydrogenase levels in adults and children with acquired immune deficiency syndrome (AIDS) and AIDS-related complex: Possible indicator of B-cell lymphoproliferation and disease activity. Am J Med 78:728, 1985

120. Calvelli TA, Rubinstein A: Intravenous gammaglobulin in infant acquired immunodeficiency syndrome. Pediatr Infect Dis 5:S207, 1986

121. Ochs HD: Intravenous immunoglobulin in the treatment and prevention of acute infections in pediatric acquired immunodeficiency syndrome patients. Pediatr Infect Dis J 6:509, 1987

122. Blanche S, Fischer A, Le Deist F, et al: Ribavirin in HTLV-III/LAV infection of infants. Lancet i:863, 1986

123. Pizzo PA, Eddy J, Falloon J, et al: Administration of Azidothymidine by continuous inravenous infusion in children with symptomatic HIV infection. Improvement in neurodevelopmental deficits. (Submitted)

124. Pediatric Zidovudine Study Group: Pharmacokinetics of zidovudine in children 14 years or less. Pediatr Res 23:378A, 1988

125. Pediatric Zidovudine Study Group: Safety and tolerance of zidovudine during a Phase I study in children. Pediatr Res 23:379A, 1988

126. Pediatric Zidovudine Study Group: Indices of neurological status during a pediatric Phase I trial of zidovudine. Pediatr Res 23:379A, 1988

127. American Academy of Pediatrics, Committee on School Health, Committee on Infectious Diseases: School attendance of children and adolescents with human T lymphotropic virus III/lymphadenopathy-associated virus infection. Pediatrics 77:430, 1986

128. American Academy of Pediatrics, Committee on Infectious Diseases. Health guidelines for the attendance in day-care and foster care settings of children infected with human immunodeficiency virus. Pediatrics 79:466, 1987

129. Additional recommendations to reduce sexual and drug abuse-related transmission of human T-lymphotropic virus type III/lymphadenopathy-associated virus. MMWR 35:152, 1986

PART III

Public Health Issues

High-Risk Sexual Practices in the Transmission of AIDS

Marianne Glasel

21

Since the first cases of acquired immune deficiency syndrome (AIDS) were identified in 1981,[1] there has been a growing body of evidence indicating that this is in large part a sexually transmitted disease. More than with other venereal diseases, such as syphilis or gonorrhea, a variety of what may be considered nonstandard sexual practices have been implicated in the transmission of AIDS. Although some of these practices have been traditionally associated primarily with male homosexual behavior, it has become apparent that heterosexuals may also engage in them. Furthermore, conventional heterosexual practices have also been identified as placing people at risk for becoming infected with the human immunodeficiency virus (HIV). It is the purpose of this chapter to outline the high-risk sexual practices that have been implicated in the transmission of AIDS and to discuss the physician's role in assessment, education, and counseling for the identification and reduction of patients' risks of becoming infected with HIV.

With little hope, at the present time, for a cure or vaccine for AIDS, risk reduction becomes a public health problem that must be addressed by primary prevention.[2] In the case of AIDS, primary prevention—the prevention of infection or disease in an apparently healthy population—is directed toward preventing the disease in the sexual partners of those who are infected with the virus. Public education must be a major focus in these preventive efforts. Since the exact mode of transmission of HIV has not been conclusively determined, recommendations must be based on the practical interpretation of current information. Moreover, these recommendations need to be made to all people, including those who are at high risk, those who engage in high-risk sexual practices (especially in epidemic areas), and those who are at apparently low risk, sexually and demographically. The general public needs and wants this information. In a survey by the National AIDS Hotline, 89% of their callers requested information about AIDS, with the highest demand (33%) being for information on transmission.[3]

Before health professionals can educate their clients, they need to receive the information necessary to carry out this education. This is apparent when we look at the results of a recent survey of medical students.[4] Twenty-six percent of those questioned believed that mosquitoes could transmit AIDS, and 18% thought AIDS could be transmitted by sweat. Physicians will be on the front line of caring for people who are worried whether they may have been infected with HIV or might have already contracted AIDS. One of their responsibilities will be to counsel these people about lowering their risk of transmitting or becoming reinfected with the AIDS virus. Education and counseling on transmission and risk reduction can be effective in changing behavior.[5-8] However, sex educators and counselors have long known that advising people to refrain from having sex simply does not work as a preventive measure for sexually transmitted diseases (or unwanted pregnancy). Furthermore, it is unrealistic to expect that moral injunctions will persuade people to cease to engage in any behavior, especially one as pleasurable and central to human beings as sexual activities. However, in the face of an epidemic of a potentially fatal disease that is in part sexually transmitted, it is important for individuals to remain sexually active only in responsible ways. To do this, people need to be provided with the information that can best enable them to take appropriate precautionary measures to avoid infection. The positive relationship that most people have with their physicians is conducive to the acquisition of this information.

HUMAN SEXUAL BEHAVIOR

Sexual practices have been recorded in art and literature throughout history. In pre-seventeenth century China, fellatio and anal intercourse were permitted as long as there was no ejaculation of semen, since the loss of this precious body fluid was considered detrimental to health. Cunnilingus was a widely accepted practice, as well. Homosexuality and bisexuality among both males and females was also common among the ancient Chinese during certain periods in their history. These sexual orientations or practices were known to have been condoned.[9]

One only has to examine a copy of the *Kamasutra* to see a chronicle of the varied sexual practices in India during that period in its history. For instance, eight stages of oral intercourse are represented in this, the first sex manual. In medieval and post-medieval France and Greece, anal intercourse was commonly used as a method of birth control. In the Western hemisphere, pre-Columbian people of the Andes apparently also practiced heterosexual and homosexual anal intercourse, and oral-genital sex, too, as evidenced by the depictions of these acts in the pottery art of that period.[9]

Human sexual behavior in the United States was first studied by Alfred Kinsey and his colleagues,[10,11] beginning in 1938 and continuing until 1949. These sex researchers interviewed 11,200 men and women for the landmark books that would come to be known as "The Kinsey Report." Oral sex, they found, was commonly practiced by heterosexual Americans; over 50% of men and women had experienced fellatio or cunnilingus. Of the males who identified themselves as homosexual, 13% engaged in oral sex as the active participant, and 35% in the passive role. Data on the occurrence of anal intercourse in the sample were not pursued or examined in depth. Only 8% admitted to ever having engaged in this sexual practice. However, when questioned about anal stimulation, some men and women stated that they were as aroused by anal as by genital stimulation, if not more so.

It was not until 1972 that more data were gathered on sexual behavior in the United States. Morton Hunt published his findings as *Sexual Behavior in the 1970s,* where he reported on a nearly equal sample of 2026 American males and females.[12] The reported prevalence of oral sex increased in the approximately three decades since Kinsey and his associates conducted their research; nearly 70% of the subjects reported engaging in oral sex. Twenty-five percent of males and females between the ages of 25 and 34 years admitted to having experienced anal intercourse, and 50% of homosexual males reported engaging in anal intercourse.

The sexual revolution of the 1970s brought with it the beginning of a flurry of sex surveys which continued into the 1980s. Popular magazines such as *Redbook, Cosmopolitan,* and *Playboy* hired researchers to survey readers about their sexual behavior and practices.[13-15] Bell and Weinberg examined only male and female homosexuals.[16] Blumstein and Schwartz published their research in *American Couples: Money, Work, and Sex.*[17] The effect of the sexual revolution, and perhaps the women's liberation movement, is evident in the findings from these surveys (see Table 21-1). Oral sex continued

to increase in popularity; anal intercourse was reported by a moderate to sizable number of American males and females, heterosexual as well as homosexual; and for the first time, in the *Playboy* survey, anal-oral contact and the use of sexual devices were found to be not uncommon practices.[18]

It is clear from the findings of these studies that men and women in the United States have become increasingly more experimental and non-traditional in their approach to the achievement of sexual stimulation and gratification. Sexual practices that were, and still are by some, looked upon as being "perverted" or "deviant" are more widely practiced. Now that the sexual revolution is over and some of these revolutionary behaviors have been incorporated into sexual scripts, it is evident that many of these practices may put people at risk for becoming infected with the new and devastating sexually transmitted disease known as AIDS.

HIGH-RISK SEXUAL PRACTICES

Numerous case-control and cohort studies have examined risk factors in the development of AIDS. Central to many of these studies has been the identification of certain sexual practices that appear to increase the risk of infection with HIV. These high-risk sexual practices and behaviors include receptive anal intercourse, insertive anal intercourse, brachioproctic eroticism ("fisting"), rectal douching/enemas, use of anal sexual devices, analingus, genital sexual intercourse, oral-genital contact, and ancillary sexual practices (i.e., mutual masturbation, kissing). Other sexual practices which may also present a risk are brachiovaginal eroticism, use of vaginal sexual devices, and contact with urine. Sexual contact where there is exposure to semen or blood, appears to carry the highest risk. Contact with vaginal/cervical secretions or menstrual blood may be associated with infection. The risk of contact with saliva is lower; exposure to urine and feces has not been investigated, but is presumed to be a risk.

Anal Sexual Practices

Studies of human sexual behavior have presented evidence that anal sexual stimulation is perceived as erotic by members of both sexes. As Kinsey and associates reported in 1953, the perineum and anus are sexually sensitive areas.[11] The perineum shares several important nerves and muscles with the anus and genitals and manipulation of one can cause a reaction in the other. Pressure on the perineum can cause an erection in the male, and may also be sexually stimulating for the female. Anal stimulation, either by touching, manipulation, use of the tongue, enemas, insertion of devices, or insertion of a penis can be interpreted as erotic and produce orgasm in some men and women. Variations in anatomy, as well as psychological differences, will influence the

Table 21-1

Percentage of Heterosexual and Homosexual Males and Females Who Have Experienced, or Sometimes to Regularly Engage In, Sexual Practices Other Than Genital Sexual Intercourse.

	Kinsey et al (1948, 1953)	Hunt (1974)	Redbook (1974)*	Bell, Weinberg (1978)†	Cosmo (1981)*	Playboy (1983)	Blumstein, Schwartz (1983)‡
Fellatio							72
Females	52	72	85		84	95	
Males	59	61				95	
Gay males	13 active 35 passive	66		87		75	84
Cunnilingus							74
Males	51	66				95	
Females	58	72	87		84	95	
Gay females	no data	no data	no data	64	no data	70	77
Anal Intercourse	8% of all				13	61	no data
Females		25 (age	21			47	no data
Males		25–34)		71 (active)		75	27 (reciprocal)
Gay males		50		54 (passive)			43 (non-reciprocal)
Anal-Oral Contact	no data	no data			no data		no data
Males				no data		36	
Females			no data			39	
Use of Sexual Devices	no data	no data	no data	no data	no data	66	no data

* Females only.
† Homosexual males and females.
‡ Heterosexual and homosexual couples.

ability of a person to enjoy anal stimulation. Masters and Johnson observed that the anus was an erogenous zone for some heterosexual people in their study.[19] This capacity for anal eroticism may be explained by the fact that the external anal sphincter contains many nerves that make it a very sensitive area. Also, insertion of a device or penis in the anus may cause pain, which for some individuals increases sexual pleasure.[20] The sensitivity of the rectum in anal sexual practices is not so clearly defined, since this area, or at least about the distal three centimeters, is essentially devoid of nerves. However, dilation and deep penetration of the rectum may stimulate the perineal nerves and produce erotic sensations.

Trauma may result from anal sexual practices. This can range from rectal irritation to abrasions, ulcerations, fissures, lacerations, and perforations of the bowel. The lining of the rectum is thin (unlike that of the vagina) and does not offer protection against injury and penetration by microorganisms into other tissues and the bloodstream. Semen, which has been found to contain HIV,[21] may enter the blood and lymphatic system during anal intercourse. It has also been hypothesized that genital or anorectal ulcers, as from herpes simplex virus infection or syphilis, may facilitate infection with HIV. Handsfield and associates showed an association of anogenital ulcer disease with HIV infection in homosexual

men.[22] The trauma of rectal douching or use of enemas before receptive anal intercourse or brachioproctic eroticism and the use of anal sexual devices as an accompanying sexual practice may also compromise the anal mucosa and contribute to the transmission of HIV by facilitating contact with blood and semen.

Receptive Anal Intercourse

Receptive/passive anal intercourse between males is hypothesized to be the major sexual risk factor for becoming infected with HIV and probably for developing AIDS in the United States. An early investigation of homosexual men examined passive anal intercourse as a risk factor for AIDS.[23] This and other subsequent studies[24–33] have identified receptive anal intercourse (alone or with ejaculation) with large numbers of homosexual partners or with increasing frequency as the highest-risk sexual practice. The risk may be increased if the sexual partner subsequently develops AIDS[34] or resides in a city where AIDS is common.[35] Evidence that refraining from this behavior may reduce one's risk for HIV seroconversion has recently been demonstrated.[36] It should be noted, however, that not all partners of persons with HIV/AIDS have become infected. Discordant pairs of HIV seronegative and seropositive homosexual male partners have been observed.[37] Among the sample subjects, 40% were concordant seronegative, 27% were concordant seropositive, but 33% were discordant. None of the discordant pairs who returned for follow-up became infected, although some of them reportedly had engaged in unprotected receptive anal and oral intercourse with their infected partners in the preceding period.

Heterosexual anal intercourse, active or passive, has only begun to be investigated as a risk factor for HIV seroconversion, but should be considered as potentially a high-risk sexual practice until such time as further research clarifies the risk.[38] One study found that the rate of infection for women who engaged in anal intercourse was nearly 1.8 times higher than that for women who practiced vaginal or oral sex.[39] Another group conducted a prospective investigation of women without other risk factors who were steady partners of patients with AIDS or AIDS-related complex (ARC).[40] They report that "only anal intercourse was found to be a significant independent predictor of HIV seropositivity" among these women. Conversely, in a study of risk factors for HIV seropositivity in southern Florida prostitutes, there was no correlation with anal intercourse, oral sexual practices, or the use of sexual devices.[41] The most recent investigation of sexual practices among heterosexuals found an association between anal intercourse and HIV infection in the female partners.[42] The likelihood of infection among women who practiced anal intercourse was twice as high as among uninfected women who did not.

Insertive Anal Intercourse

Insertive anal intercourse carries with it a certain degree of risk but apparently represents a less efficient, and as yet unknown, mode of transmission of HIV. An inflamed urethra because of sexually transmitted disease or a lesion on the penis may be the route of infectivity in the male. In studies examining the sexual practices of homosexual males seropositivity has been associated primarily with receptive anal intercourse, but insertive anal intercourse is also a significant risk factor according to some studies.[25,31,36,43] One seropositive male in a study reported usually practicing only insertive anal intercourse and rarely engaging in orogenital or oral-anal sex.[44] Some studies have suggested a lower level of transmission efficiency for insertive anal intercourse[25,36,43]; in another study, no associated risk was found among homosexual and bisexual men.[29] Since the evidence is conflicting, the risk of transmitting HIV to the active partner in insertive anal intercourse cannot be eliminated.

Brachioproctic Eroticism (BPE)

The anus may be used for other heterosexual or homosexual erotic activities. Anal manipulation or foreplay may consist of brachioproctic eroticism (insertion of the fist or forearm into a partner's rectum), commonly called "fisting." Although this practice is generally associated with male homosexual or bisexual behavior, it may also be practiced by female homosexuals, who may use vaginal as well as anal penetration.[45] Reports from sex educators and therapists indicate that some heterosexual couples also engage in brachioproctic and brachiovaginal sexual practices.

Because of the pain or discomfort involved in brachioproctic eroticism, many individuals report the use of drugs to facilitate relaxation and analgesia before insertion of the hand. One survey found the most common drugs used to be marijuana, amyl nitrite, methylene dioxyamphetamine (MDA), alcohol, and cocaine.[45]

"Fisting" carries with it the risk of anal tears and fissures, muscle tears, and bowel perforations, which offer a suitable portal of entry for HIV. Marmor and associates found that "fisting" was a significant risk factor for the development of Kaposi's sarcoma in homosexual men, along with receptive anal intercourse and cytomegalovirus antibody titers.[25] They postulate that this practice might represent exposure through feces to the putative agent causing AIDS or "might be an indicator of involvement in activities leading to abrasions of the anal mucosa and enhanced uptake by that route."

In a previous study, more AIDS patients than matched controls reported having participated in insertive "fisting," as well as active analingus.[46] One investigation found that receptive "fisting" correlated with seropositivity, but that the greatest risk factor was the combination of large numbers of homosexual partners and the practice of receptive anal intercourse.[24] The Vancouver Lymphadenopathy-AIDS Study group found that insertive and receptive "fisting" and receptive anal intercourse were the greatest risk factors for HIV seropositivity.[44] In another study, insertive and receptive "fisting" was associated with HIV seropositivity in homosexual men.[28]

A group in Sydney, Australia, recently reported a case of AIDS apparently transmitted through insertive brachioproctic eroticism.[47] The patient had breaks in the skin of his hands and face (solar keratoses with ulceration for many years and a syphilis chancre on his hand 3 years ago). The evidence for this transmission by insertive "fisting" is confounded by other sexual practices of the patient and his partner who was HIV-antibody–positive and showed symptoms of AIDS-related complex (ARC). These practices included "dry" kissing and mutual masturbation with ejaculation. However, because the patient reported being exposed to his partner's rectal blood during brachioproctic eroticism, the authors believe that the patient probably acquired HIV infection through this activity over a long period of exposure. HIV has been isolated from blood,[49,50] and contact with blood may place one at risk for becoming infected with the AIDS virus.

Although insertive and receptive brachioproctic eroticism has been identified as a high-risk sexual practice for males, it is difficult to single out this behavior as an independent risk factor because most homosexual or bisexual men who practice brachioproctic eroticism also engage in anal intercourse or oral-genital contact.

Enemas/Rectal Douches

Rectal douches or enemas can be sexually arousing for some persons. Agnew reports:

> For males, dilation of the rectum while receiving enemas causes increasing pressure on the prostate gland and seminal vesicles, thus producing sensations that may be interpreted as sexual by some individuals. For females, dilation of the rectum during an enema procedure may produce the same pressure on internal organs reported by Kinsey et al. (1953) to produce erotic sensations upon deep penetration of the vagina or rectum during sexual intercourse.[20]

Enemas may be used as a masturbatory technique by males and females. The dilation of the rectum may be pleasurable, and peristalsis during expulsion of the enema may stimulate the genitals and even produce an orgasm.[20] More commonly, an enema is used to cleanse the rectum prior to anal intercourse or brachioproctic eroticism. Often, mineral oil enemas are used because they have the added benefit of facilitating penetration of the rectum.

Rectal douches/enemas have been associated with HIV infection in a cohort of homosexual males, along with the number of episodes of receptive anal intercourse and sexual contact with males with AIDS or ARC.[32] A statistically significant elevation in risk with rectal douching among homosexual men was also found in the San Francisco Men's Health Study.[33] This risk probably arises because the anal mucosa is compromised by the enema, thus increasing the likelihood of infection with HIV during the high-risk sexual practices that follow. There may also be a risk involved in sharing enema equipment.

Use of Anal Sexual Devices

Sexual devices or fingers may be used for anal masturbation, a practice which some individuals find erotically stimulating. Dildoes (phallic-shaped devices) are used for anal (or vaginal) sexual arousal, usually with genital stimulation. Depending on the nature of the device, the depth of penetration, and the method and force used, sexual devices can cause anal and rectal trauma that may permit passage of the human immunodeficiency virus

(and other organisms) into the bloodstream. (Educators instructing people in safer sexual practices suggest that if these devices are used they should be disinfected before being shared or that a fresh condom be placed on the device before insertion.) In one study, history of use of a dildo was a statistically significant risk factor for HIV seroconversion in a group of homosexual and bisexual men.[33]

Analingus (Analinctus)

Use of the tongue to stimulate the anus is commonly referred to as "rimming." This behavior is usually not practiced to the exclusion of other erotic activities. The risk of acquiring the human immunodeficiency virus through analingus may result because of contact with infectious feces, with or without blood. Two of the studies that evaluated this risk found that analingus was correlated with low helper T-cell counts in homosexual males.[27,50] An investigation of sexual practices among another group of homosexual males found a statistically significant increase in risk of HIV infection with receptive analingus but not with insertive analingus.[29] No explanation was offered for this finding.

GENITAL SEXUAL TRANSMISSION AMONG MALES AND FEMALES

Sexual encounters between men and women can involve a variety of activities, including penis-vagina intercourse, oral-genital contact, anal sexual practices, and kissing. Because sexual activities often represent a group of behaviors, it is difficult to separate out those that place the female or male at high risk for becoming infected with HIV. This effort may be impeded, in certain instances, by the reluctance of individuals to give an accurate and forthright account of their sexual practices because of the perceived taboos surrounding some of these behaviors.

Only a small proportion of HIV seroconversions or cases of AIDS have been generally attributed to heterosexual contact in the United States and Europe. In August 1987, the Centers for Disease Control classified only 4% of all AIDS cases as transmitted by heterosexual contact.[51] In Africa, however, AIDS appears to be primarily a heterosexually transmitted disease.[52-55] These geographical differences are not fully understood.

The first report of male-to-female transmission of HIV in the United States occurred in 1983 when two women with AIDS were identified as steady sexual partners of men who had been diagnosed with AIDS.[56] Since then, an increasing number of women have become infected through sexual contact.[57] Heterosexual transmission from female-to-male has been rarely reported in the United States. However, it is a common mode of infection in Africa, where the ratio of male cases to female cases is nearly 1:1.[53,54]

The most recent studies involving both male-to-female and female-to-male transmission of HIV have conflicting findings. A continuing study is examining a group of men and women in New York City who have no identified risk factors in themselves or their partners, other than heterosexual contact.[58] Of the 76 males and 53 females, HIV seropositivity has been detected in two of each gender group. In another investigation, among a sample of 64 males and 25 females attending a sexually transmitted disease clinic in New York City, none of 65 heterosexuals who were not intravenous drug abusers was positive for HIV antibody. This study included five men and five women who reported sexual contact with an intravenous drug abuser (IVDA). The other 55 individuals had multiple sex partners, many had a history of sexually transmitted disease (STD), some had practiced anal intercourse, most rarely or never used condoms, and some men had sex with prostitutes. These investigators conclude that the findings "suggest low prevalence of HIV infection among sexually active heterosexual adults who are not IVDA." Partners of patients with AIDS or ARC appear to be at higher risk for becoming infected through heterosexual contact. Investigators studied 100 healthy heterosexual contacts (male and female), with no risk factors, who were steady sexual partners of 97 patients with AIDS or ARC.[40] Since 1982, 48% of the subjects (almost equal numbers of males and females) have seroconverted; two of these have developed AIDS. The sexual practices significantly associated with seropositivity in this study were anal intercourse, recipience of analingus (among females), and oral contact with semen (among females); none of these activities, however, was a prerequisite for seropositivity. The researchers conclude that "both male and female steady heterosexual partners of patients with AIDS or ARC are at substantial risk for HIV infection and related disease."

Sexual Transmission From Male to Female

Women who have become infected with HIV through sexual contact are primarily those who are heterosexual partners of intravenous drug abusers,[60-62] men with AIDS or ARC,[40,61] bisexual men,[39,42,63] hemophiliacs,[64-68] and men from areas of the world where heterosexual transmission is common.[69] In one report, infection was acquired through artificial insemination with infected donor semen.[70] The CDC reported on a female sexual partner of a transfusion recipient who developed AIDS.[71] Although the largest numbers of infected females have been partners of IVDA, Goedert believes that female partners of hemophiliacs are at extremely high risk and will represent a significant number of infected women in the future.[72] Some female partners of hemophiliacs who receive therapy with blood products have become infected with HIV and a number of these women have developed AIDS, apparently through sexual activities.[65,67,68]

The proportion of heterosexual AIDS patients who are female has risen from 12% to 26% since 1982.[57] According to Guinan and Hardy:

> Heterosexual contact is the only transmission category where women with AIDS outnumber men with AIDS. . . . In the United States, at the present time, a heterosexual woman is at greater risk for acquiring AIDS through sexual intercourse than is a heterosexual man.[57]

It has been demonstrated that HIV can be found in lymphocytes in the seminal fluid of infected men.[73] Women may acquire HIV during penis-vagina, and possibly anal, intercourse (which may be used as a method of birth control by some people) through contact with infected semen. Anal intercourse as a mode of transmission for females has only begun to be assessed and may be an under-reported practice in some investigations. Because receptive anal intercourse in males has been identified as the greatest risk factor for the transmission of AIDS, the role of this practice in male-to-female transmission should not be overlooked or underestimated. In a recent study by Padian and colleagues, a significant association between anal intercourse and HIV infection was found for women who engaged in this sexual practice.[42] However, some women who engaged only in vaginal intercourse were also seropositive. Until heterosexual anal intercourse has been clearly established as a risk, penis-vagina intercourse with exposure to infected semen is considered to be the greatest risk factor for females.

Sexual Transmission from Female to Male

Evidence for the efficient transmission of HIV from females to males is not strong, except in Africa[53,54,74,75] and possibly Haiti.[76] Those who propose female-to-male transmission argue that since other sexually transmitted diseases are bidirectional in nature, we should presume that AIDS can be spread in this manner.[77,78] One study cites evidence that 10 males became seropositive as a result of heterosexual contact with either prostitutes, multiple sexual partners, or a Haitian immigrant.[78] In another study, the same investigators reported that two of three women with transfusion-acquired AIDS infected their husbands through sexual contact.[61] Other reports of seropositivity among American males attributed to heterosexual contact have appeared recently.[40,58] Epidemiologic studies from Africa would appear to support female-to-male transmission to a greater degree than studies conducted in the United States and Europe.[53,55,75,79,80] African men who have multiple female sex partners or sexual contact with prostitutes have been found to be at higher risk for becoming infected with HIV.[74,80,81] Cofactors, as yet unidentified, have been suggested as an explanation for the higher heterosexual transmission rates in Africa.[82]

Possible sources of HIV in the female are vaginal and cervical secretions and menstrual blood. Glands in the cervix normally secrete varying amounts of mucus, and acidic secretions are found in the vagina. During sexual arousal a different type of vaginal secretion is present. Masters and Johnson first identified this "sweating" phenomenon of the vaginal walls.[19] They observed that the blood vessels in the walls become engorged during arousal, causing tiny droplets of fluid to be squeezed through the vessels and producing copious amounts of an alkaline lubricant that coats the inside of the vagina. Small amounts of HIV have been isolated from the cervical and vaginal secretions of some high-risk or HIV-seropositive women.[83,85] One researcher postulates that because there are increased vaginal secretions during sexual arousal, there may be more retrovirus present at that time.[84] Vogt and co-workers recently reported recovering HIV from the cervical secretions of some menstruating seropositive women.[86] Therefore, contact with menstrual blood could represent a possible source of infection. Sexual intercourse during menses is not an uncommon practice, and may be used as a method of birth control. Furthermore, many women report an increase in sexual desire just prior to and during menstruation.[87]

The Role of Prostitutes in Transmission

In Africa, HIV has been detected in a high number of prostitutes who are not intravenous drug abusers: 88% in Rwanda,[88] and up to 66% in Nairobi.[74] HIV-antibody–positive heterosexual males in Rwanda more often report sexual contact with prostitutes than do controls.[79] Prostitutes in Rwanda reported many sexual contacts and practiced primarily penis-vagina intercourse; anal intercourse was rare.[88] In January 1985, 65% of prostitutes tested in Nairobi were HIV seropositive; 2 years later, 56% of the sample who had been seronegative had converted to positive.[89] Generally, seroprevalence rates among prostitutes in Central Africa are lower for women who use condoms.[90]

Some prostitutes in Europe, usually intravenous drug abusers (IVDA), have been found to be HIV positive.[91] However, none of the non-IVDA prostitutes studied in London, Paris, and Poland have been seropositive.[91] In a sample of male and female prostitutes in Italy, none of the female non-IVDAs were HIV positive, whereas one of the homosexual male prostitutes tested positive.[92] Sexual contact with prostitutes in Germany has been implicated in the transmission of HIV in one study of American men.[78]

In the United States, a large multicenter study is underway to determine the prevalence of HIV seropositivity in prostitutes.[93] The seven research sites are Las Vegas, Colorado Springs, Atlanta, Los Angeles, San Francisco, Miami, and the Newark–Jersey City–Paterson area. To date, the highest proportion of seropositive prostitutes has been found in the northern New Jersey area (69.2%). The seroprevalence rates in the other locations are: Miami, 19.1%; San Francisco, 5.6%; Los Angeles, 5.2%; Colorado Springs, 1.5%; Atlanta, 1.1%; and Las Vegas, 0%. The greatest risk factor for seropositivity in this study is intravenous drug abuse. Unprotected sexual intercourse with many partners is also significantly associated with a positive HIV antibody test. Among the prostitutes who always use condoms, HIV positivity rates are lower.

Fischl and colleagues evaluated the seroprevalence of HIV infection in a group of prostitutes in the south Florida/Miami area.[41] Of the 90 prostitutes studied, 41% were HIV antibody positive—46% of IVDAs, and 30% of those who were not IVDAs. They found no correlation with oral-genital contact, anal intercourse, use of sexual devices, or condom use. There was a correlation with a history of hepatitis B infection, syphilis, and gynecologic surgery. The women in the study were also more sexually active and more likely to have participated in vaginal intercourse in areas where there was a high incidence of AIDS.

The implications of these studies are that female prostitutes in any area of the world are at high risk for acquiring HIV and may represent a potential and important source of infection for heterosexual males.

ORAL-GENITAL SEXUAL PRACTICES

Oral-genital sexual contact is commonly practiced among peoples of South Pacific islands, industrialized Asian nations, the northern regions of Africa, and the Western hemisphere.[94]

Both the mouth and the genitals are erogenous zones, and, therefore, it may be pleasurable to give as well as to receive oral-genital stimulation. Cunnilingus or fellatio may precede sexual intercourse or other sexual activities, or may be practiced to the exclusion of other acts. Furthermore, oral-genital sex may be performed by only one partner or simultaneously by both individuals.

Fellatio

Fellatio is the oral stimulation of the penis (and scrotum); it is sometimes accompanied by anal stimulation. The penis and scrotum are very sensitive to sexual stimulation and many males find this practice erotically pleasurable. Often, this activity is carried to orgasm, at which time the ejaculate may be ingested. Even if ejaculation does not occur, some pre-ejaculate fluid, which may contain sperm, can enter the mouth of the active partner. During fellatio, vigorous thrusting of the penis in the partner's mouth may result in lacerations of the partner's lips as he or she tries to protect the penis from the teeth. Transmission of the human immunodeficiency virus may occur with ingestion of semen or contact of semen with compromised mucous membranes of the mouth. The degree of risk for this sexual practice is not clear; epidemiologic evidence is conflicting regarding the risk of transmission by this route. One group of investigators found an association with HIV seropositivity and receptive oral-genital contact with ejaculation in homosexual men.[30] In a study of heterosexual couples, female spouses of patients with AIDS who were seropositive for HIV "were more likely to have participated in receptive oral sex and not to use barrier contraceptives [during vaginal intercourse]."[95] Other studies have observed no evidence of risk, or minimal risk, for HIV infection associated with oral-genital sexual contact, with and without ejaculation.[27,96] Furthermore, one study reported that of 21 homosexual men who refrained from receptive anal intercourse but continued to practice active anal intercourse and oral-genital, oral-anal, or oral-oral sexual activities, only one person became seropositive.[43] This man reported practicing active anal intercourse.

Cunnilingus

Cunnilingus is oral stimulation of the clitoris, labia minora, vestibule, and vaginal opening. This sexual practice is often combined with manual stimulation of the vaginal opening. Cunnilingus can produce sexual arousal in the female, at which time copious amounts of vaginal secretions may be present. Also, the Bartholin's glands secrete a few drops of fluid near the vaginal opening during the excitement phase of the sexual response cycle.[19] As has been noted previously, HIV has been isolated from cervical/vaginal secretions, including during menses, of some seropositive or high-risk women.[83–86] Transmission of HIV could theoretically occur during contact with these secretions or menstrual blood. To date, there have been no studies implicating cunnilingus alone as a high-risk sexual practice. However, there is one case report of HIV infection in a lesbian who gave a history of oral-genital contact with many women in Europe.[97] In another case report a "non-IVDA, non-Haitian" woman with Kaposi's sarcoma was described as being exclusively homosexual, but no sexual practices were described.[98] An additional case may or may not implicate oral-genital contact in transmission. A woman became infected with HIV, possibly as a result of a lesbian relationship with a IVDA partner who had Kaposi's sarcoma.[99] She reported digital and oral contact with her partner's vagina and oral-anal contact during her partner's menses, and both women experienced vaginal bleeding as a result of trauma during their sexual activities. The subject also had vaginal intercourse with a bisexual male without using a condom, but after developing lymphadenopathy. Lesbians may practice cunnilingus but as often engage in mutual masturbation, sometimes with shared sexual devices which can cause bleeding and transmission of HIV.

ANCILLARY SEXUAL PRACTICES

Ancillary sexual practices may include the use of vaginal (as well as anal) sexual devices, mutual masturbation, kissing, and contact with urine on the skin or in the mouth. The risk associated with some of these behaviors is not clear, either because they have not been studied or, more often, because it is difficult to isolate these (and other) sexual practices for evaluation of risk. Vaginal sexual devices may cause trauma and bleeding of the genitals and vagina and increase the risk of transmission of HIV from an infected partner. Mutual masturbation with ejaculation may present a risk because of exposure through openings in the skin to infected semen. "Deep" kissing with the exchange of significant amounts of saliva may allow passage of the virus through intact or compromised tissues of the mouth. Infected urine may transmit HIV through broken skin or the oral cavity.

Kissing

Kissing is usually the first phase of sexual contact among Americans. In other cultures, sensuous ("deep") kissing is rarely practiced in sexual interactions.[94] Blumstein and Schwartz found that the majority of American couples engage in kissing, usually, or every time, they have sexual contact: 99% of lesbians, 96% of heterosexuals, and 87% of gay males.[17] HIV has been isolated from the saliva of some homosexual men.[100,101] However, in one study, only one of 83 saliva samples was seropositive for HIV, whereas 56% of the males had HIV-positive blood samples.[101] Furthermore, the HIV titer of the saliva from that subject was much lower than that of his blood, and only small amounts of the virus were found in his saliva sample. One report cites the case of an elderly woman who became infected with HIV apparently solely through contact by kissing her HIV-positive husband (a transfusion recipient).[102] The evidence for a causal relationship in this case has been challenged, though, because of incomplete information on other risk factors.[103] At this time, it appears that the risk of transmission of HIV by saliva is low, but not zero.

Contact with Urine

Some individuals include contact with urine (on the skin or in the mouth) in their sexual behaviors. Certain persons find this practice psychologically erotic or merely use it as an adjunct to other sexual activities. This practice is commonly referred to as "water sports."

In 1986, The Centers for Disease Control recommended that HIV-negative persons who are at high risk take "appropriate precautions to prevent contact with . . . blood, semen, urine, feces, saliva, cervical secretions, or vaginal secretions."[104] HIV has been isolated from the urine of some persons with AIDS or at high risk for AIDS.[105] Investigators found that one of five urine samples was positive for HIV, but in low titers. Therefore, it would appear that there is a risk, although perhaps small, of contact with infected urine on non-intact skin or mucous membranes.

ASSESSMENT AND COUNSELING FOR SEXUAL RISKS

Every physician has an ethical and social responsibility to help prevent the spread of AIDS by educating and counseling patients about their sexual risks of becoming infected with HIV. However, physicians often receive little or no education or training in sexuality and may be ill-equipped to obtain sexual histories and counsel patients about such matters.[106] Three prerequisites are necessary for sexual assessment and counseling: comfort in discussing sexuality, knowledge of human sexuality, and skill in interviewing and counseling about sexual issues.[107]

Before physicians can carry out sexual assessment and counseling for the prevention of AIDS, they need to examine their own attitudes, values, and beliefs about various sexual behaviors and orientations, as well as their level of comfort, knowledge, and skill in counseling others about high-risk sexual practices. Those physicians who wish to discuss the sexual transmission of AIDS and counsel for risk reduction will also need to have accurate, current knowledge about high-risk sexual practices and skill in obtaining a sexual history.

Increased comfort in discussing sexuality will come with practice. If a physician feels that he or she will not be able to achieve the necessary comfort level and may have difficulty accepting the sexual orientation and practices of patients, he or she should recognize this fact and refer to resources where the appropriate education and counseling can be implemented.

Acquisition of knowledge about high-risk sexual practices will be an ongoing process. Recommendations, based on epidemiologic investigations, have changed and may be revised in the future. At present, there are no clear guidelines for advising about some of these practices. This complicates the education and counseling tasks of practitioners and presents a challenge for physicians whose patients expect precise information about what to do or what to avoid.

The following list[108] includes some of the sexual information that physicians need to know:

- Kinsey and associates found that 25% of American females and 46% of American males had extramarital sexual contact by the time they were 40 years old.[10,11]
- According to Kinsey, 37% of men who identified themselves as heterosexuals had sexual contact with another male by age 45.[10]
- Married or supposedly monogamous or heterosexual

patients may be at risk. Monogamy does not necessarily protect one from becoming infected.
- Because heterosexual transmission of HIV infection is increasing, the danger of even one high-risk contact cannot be minimized.

Only by taking a detailed sexual history of past and present practices can physicians determine if their patients are at risk for acquiring AIDS. However, patients may be reluctant to reveal the sexual behaviors or lifestyle that places them at high risk. They may fear rejection or discrimination by their physician.[108] It is clear that time, sensitivity, and skill are necessary in interviewing and counseling these individuals—more so than when questioning persons at low or no risk who are merely seeking advice. Counseling should be individualized to meet patients' needs: consideration should be given to people's values, beliefs, culture, ethnicity, religion, sexual orientation, and level of risk.[108] A common vocabulary of sexual terms needs to be established between patients and practitioners. Medical terms for sexual practices may not be understood by some patients, and many physicians may not be familiar with "street" names for behaviors or body parts. If these terms are not clarified, the counseling session can be ineffective.[109] Patients who sense a level of trust and respect and a nonjudgmental attitude on the part of physicians will be more likely to give an open and candid sexual history. In addition, if physicians assure confidentiality regarding these discussions, patients are more apt to answer questions about sexual practices and drug use honestly. It has been suggested that a questionnaire that does not become part of the patient's record can be an aid in determining an individual's level of risk.[108] Pamphlets and informational posters on AIDS and its transmission can also be used in the office or clinic setting to facilitate discussions. It is extremely important, however, that even if patients do not admit to any risk behaviors, they should receive education about sexual practices that may place them at risk for becoming infected with HIV.

It may be unrealistic (although idealistic) to expect that all physicians will have the time or inclination to acquire the necessary comfort, knowledge, and skills needed to counsel patients about high-risk sexual practices. Whether or not physicians choose to involve themselves in sexual counseling for AIDS prevention, they should know how to use referral resources for patients. These resources include community groups, public health agencies, HIV counseling and testing sites, and advocacy organizations such as those that have been established by the gay community in many areas of the United States. Other health care professionals who have an interest in education and counseling for risk reduction should be identified. These may be other physicians, nurses, social workers, or public health workers. This type of networking is essential for the preventive effort against the transmission of AIDS.

SUMMARY

A number of high-risk sexual practices in the transmission of AIDS have been identified. Those that place a person at highest risk are practices that involve contact with infected blood or semen: receptive anal intercourse, especially with ejaculation; receptive vaginal intercourse with ejaculation; and fellatio involving contact with semen.[110] Other sexual practices that have been associated with HIV infection are insertive anal or vaginal intercourse, brachioproctic (or brachiovaginal) eroticism, use of enemas/rectal douches (preceding anal sexual practices), use of sexual devices, oral-anal contact, and fellatio without contact with semen. Contact with urine, mutual masturbation with ejaculation on partner, "deep" kissing, and cunnilingus may also entail some, albeit lower, risk (see Table 21-2.).[108,110] Until the exact mode of transmission of HIV has been clearly defined, proscriptions regarding high-risk sexual practices should be based on the practical interpretation of available evidence.

In order to implement preventive measures against the sexual transmission of AIDS, physicians need to be comfortable, knowledgeable, and skilled in counseling for risk identification and risk reduction in their patients. This crucial public health effort requires a commitment on the part of practitioners to involve themselves. A physician may be the first one that an individual will turn to for information and advice on AIDS transmission. This physician should ideally be equipped to carry out the necessary sex education and counseling but may wish to refer the client to other health professionals with a special interest or training in sexual counseling for AIDS prevention. The health care team involved with AIDS education is an ever-expanding group that will play a vital part in the prevention of the spread of this disease.

The author would like to acknowledge Michael Shernoff, MSW, ACSW, adjunct faculty member, Department of Education, Gay Men's Health Crisis, for his critical review, sensitive suggestions, and valuable contribution to this chapter.

REFERENCES

1. Gottlieb MS, Schroff R, Schanker HM, et al: *Pneumocytis carinii* pneumonia and mucosal candidiasis in previously healthy homosexual men: Evidence of a new acquired cellular immunodeficiency. N Engl J Med 305:1425, 1981
2. Shernoff M, Palacios-Jimenez L: AIDS: Prevention is the only vaccine available. J Soc Work Hum Sex 6(2): 1988
3. Rosenberg MJ, Kohmescher R, Bonhomme M, et al: What the public wants to know: The national AIDS hotline (abst). III International Conference on Acquired Immunodeficiency Syndrome (AIDS), Washington D.C., June 1–5, 1987
4. Barthof H, Mandel J, Grade M, et al: AIDS education in medical and nursing students: knowledge and attitude correlates (abst). III International Conference on Acquired Immunodeficiency Syndrome (AIDS), Washington D.C., June 1–5, 1987
5. Emmons C, Joseph JG, Kessler RC, et al: Psychosocial predictors of reported behavior change in homosexual men at risk for AIDS. Health Educ Q 13:331, 1986
6. Martin JL: AIDS risk reduction recommendations and sexual behavior patterns among gay men: A multi-factorial categorical approach to assessing change. Health Educ Q 13:347, 1986
7. Martin JL: Prevention of HIV infection through sexual behavior change (abst). III International Conference on Acquired Immunodeficiency Syndrome (AIDS), Washington D.C., June 1–5, 1987
8. Nyanjom D, Greaves W, Delapenha R, et al: Sexual behavior change among HIV seropositive individuals (abst). III International Conference on Acquired Immunodeficiency Syndrome (AIDS), Washington D.C., June 1–5, 1987
9. Tannahill R: Sex in History. New York, Stein and Day, 1980
10. Kinsey AC, Pomeroy WB, Martin C: Sexual Behavior in the Human Male. Philadelphia, WB Saunders, 1948
11. Kinsey AC, Pomeroy WB, Martin CE, et al: Sexual Behavior in the Human Female. Philadelphia, WB Saunders, 1953
12. Hunt M: Sexual Behavior in the 1970s. Chicago, Playboy Press, 1974
13. Tavris C, Sadd S: The Redbook Report on Female Sexuality. New York, Delacorte, 1975
14. Wolfe L: The Cosmo Report. New York, Arbor House, 1981
15. Petersen JR: The Playboy readers' sex survey (Parts 1–4). Playboy, Jan, Mar, May, July, 1983
16. Bell AP, Weinberg MS: Homosexualities: A study of Diversity Among Men and Women. New York, Simon and Schuster, 1978
17. Blumstein P, Schwartz P: American Couples: Money, Work and Sex. New York, Morrow, 1983

Table 21-2
Sexual Practices Associated With Increased Risk of Infection With HIV

Highest Risk Factors*
Contact with infected semen or blood
- Receptive anal intercourse (especially with ejaculation)
- Receptive vaginal intercourse (especially with ejaculation)
- Fellatio involving contact with semen

Moderate/Significant Risk Factors*
- Insertive anal intercourse
- Insertive vaginal intercourse
- Brachioproctic eroticism
- Use of enemas/rectal douches
- Use of sexual devices
- Oral-anal contact
- Fellatio without contact with semen

***Lesser Risk Factors*†**
- Contact with urine
- Mutual masturbation with ejaculation on partner
- "Deep" kissing
- Cunnilingus

---

* Based on current epidemiologic evidence.
† Based on weaker evidence and/or presumed risk.

18. Petersen JR: The Playboy readers' sex survey (parts three-four). Playboy, May, July, 1983

19. Masters WH, Johnson VE: Human Sexual Response. Boston, Little, Brown and Company, 1966

20. Agnew J: Some anatomical and physiological aspects of anal sexual practices. J Homosex 12:75, 1985

21. Ho DD, Schooberg RT, Rota JR, et al: HTLV-III in the semen and blood of a healthy homosexual man. Science 226:451, 1984

22. Handsfield HH, Ashley RL, Rompalo AM, et al: Association of anogenital ulcer disease with human immunodeficiency virus infection in homosexual men (abst). III International Conference on Acquired Immunodeficiency Syndrome (AIDS), Washington D.C., June 1–5, 1987

23. Darrow WW, Jaffe HW, Curran JW: Passive anal intercourse as a risk factor for AIDS in homosexual men. Lancet ii: 160, 1983

24. Goedert JJ, Sarngadharan MG, Biggar RJ, et al: Determinants of retrovirus (HTLV-III) antibody and immunodeficiency conditions in homosexual men. Lancet ii: 711, 1984

25. Marmor M, Friedman-Kien AE, Zolla-Pazner, et al: Kaposi's sarcoma in homosexual men. Ann Intern Med 100: 809, 1984

26. Melbye M, Biggar RJ, Ebbesen P, et al: Sero-epidemiology of HTLV-III antibody in Danish homosexual men: Prevalence, transmission, and disease outcome. Br Med J 289: 573, 1984

27. Goedert JJ, Biggar RJ, Winn DM, et al: Decreased helper T lymphocytes in homosexual men. II. Sexual Practices. Am J Epidemiol 121:637, 1985

28. Nicholson JKA, McDougal JS, Jaffe HW, et al: Exposure to human T-lymphotropic virus type III/lymphadenopathy-associated virus and immunologic abnormalities in asymptomatic homosexual men. Ann Intern Med 103:37, 1985

29. Evans BA, Dawson SG, McLean KA, et al: Sexual lifestyle and clinical findings related to HTLV-III/LAV status in homosexual men. Genitourin Med 62:384, 1986

30. Mayer KH, Ayotte D, Groopman JE, et al: Association of human T lymphotropic virus antibodies with sexual and other behaviors in a cohort of homosexual men from Boston with and without generalized lymphadenopathy. Am J Med 80:357, 1986

31. Coates RA, Calzavara SE, Read MM, et al: Risk of seropositivity in relation to specific sexual activities of sexual contacts of men with AIDS or ARC (abst). III International Conference on Acquired Immunodeficiency Syndrome (AIDS), Washington D.C., June 1–5, 1987

32. Cornelis AM, Rietmeyer KA, Penley DL, et al: Factors influencing the risk of infection with human immunodeficiency virus in a cohort of homosexual men—Denver 1983–1985 (abst). III International Conference on AIDS, Washington D.C., June 1–5, 1987

33. Winkelstein W Jr, Lyman DL, Padian N, et al: Sexual practices and risk of infection by the human immunodeficiency virus: The San Francisco Men's Health Study. JAMA 257:321, 1987

34. Polk BF, Fox R, Brookmeyer R, et al: Predictors of the acquired immunodeficiency syndrome developing in a cohort of seropositive homosexual men. N Engl J Med 316:61, 1987

35. Goedert JJ, Biggar RJ, Winn DM, et al: Decreased helper T lymphocytes in homosexual men. I. Sexual contact in high incidence areas for the acquired immunodeficiency syndrome. Am J Epidemiol 121:629, 1985

36. Detels R, Visscher B, Kingsley L, et al: No HIV seroconversion among men refraining from anal-genital intercourse (abst). III International Conference on Acquired Immunodeficiency Syndrome (AIDS), Washington D.C., June 1–5, 1987

37. Seage GR III, Hardy A, Mayer K, et al: HIV transmission among homosexual male partners: evidence of the inefficiency of transmission (abst). III International Conference on Acquired Immunodeficiency Syndrome (AIDS), Washington D.C., June 1–5, 1987

38. Melbye M, Ingerslev J, Biggar RJ, et al: Anal intercourse as a possible factor in heterosexual transmission of HTLV-III to spouses of hemophiliacs (letter). N Engl J Med 312:857, 1985

39. Padian N, Wiley J, Winkelstein W Jr: Male to female transmission of human immunodeficiency virus (HIV): Current results, infectivity rates, and San Francisco seroprevalence estimates (abst). III International Conference on Acquired Immunodeficiency Syndrome (AIDS), Washington D.C., June 1–5, 1987

40. Steigbigel NH: Heterosexual transmission of infection and disease by human immunodeficiency virus (abst). III International Conference on Acquired Immunodeficiency Syndrome (AIDS), Washington D.C., June 3, 1987

41. Fischl MA: Human immunodeficiency virus among prostitutes in South Florida (abst). III International Conference on Acquired Immunodeficiency Syndrome (AIDS), Washington D.C., June 3, 1987

42. Padian N, Marquis L, Francis DP, et al: Male-to-female transmission of human immunodeficiency virus. JAMA 258:788, 1987

43. Schechter MT, Boyko WJ, Douglas WJ: Can HTLV-III be transmitted orally? (letter) Lancet i:379, 1986

44. Jeffries E, Willoughby B, Boyko WJ, et al: The Vancouver lymphadenopathy-AIDS study. 2. Seroepidemiology of HTLV-III antibody. Can Med Assoc J 132:1373, 1985

45. Lowry JP, Williams GR: Brachioproctic eroticism. J Sex Educ Ther 9:50, 1983

46. Jaffe HW, Choi K, Thomas PA, et al: National case-control study of Kaposi's sarcoma and *Pneumocystis carinii* pneumonia in homosexual men. I: Epidemiologic results. Ann Intern Med 99:145, 1983

47. Donovan B, Tindall B, Cooper D: Brachioproctic eroticism and transmission of retrovirus associated with acquired immune deficiency syndrome (AIDS). Genitourin Med 62:390, 1986

48. Barré-Sinoussi F, Chermann JC, Rey F, et al: Isolation of a T-lymphotropic retrovirus from a patient at risk for acquired immune deficiency syndrome (AIDS). Science 220:868, 1983

49. Gallo RC, Salahuddin SZ, Popovic M, et al: Frequent detection and isolation of cytopathic retroviruses (HTLV-III) from patients with AIDS and at risk for AIDS. Science 224:500, 1984

50. Rogers MF, Morens DM, Stewart JA, et al: National case-control study of Kaposi's sarcoma and *Pneumocystis carinii* pneumonia in homosexual men. 2: Laboratory results. Ann Intern Med 99:151, 1983

51. Centers for Disease Control: AIDS Weekly Surveillance Report-United States. August 10, 1987

52. Clumeck N, Sonnet J, Taelman H, et al: Acquired immunodeficiency syndrome in African patients. N Engl J Med 310:492, 1984

53. Piot P, Quinn TC, Taelman H, et al: Acquired immunodeficiency syndrome in a heterosexual population in Zaire. Lancet ii:65–69, 1984

54. Biggar RJ: The AIDS problem in Africa. Lancet i:79–83, 1986

55. Taelman H, Bonneux L, Cornet P, et al: Transmission of HIV to partners of seropositive heterosexuals from Africa (abst). III International Conference on Acquired Immunodeficiency Syndrome (AIDS), Washington D.C., June 1–5, 1987

56. Centers for Disease Control: Immunodeficiency among female sexual partners of males with acquired immune deficiency syndrome—New York. MMWR 31:697, 1983

57. Guinan ME, Hardy A: Epidemiology of AIDS in women in the United States. JAMA 257:2039, 1987

58. Marmor M, Sanchez M, Krasinski K, et al: Risk factors for human immunodeficiency virus (HIV) infection among heterosexuals in New York City (abst). III International Conference on Acquired Immunodeficiency Syndrome (AIDS), Washington D.C., June 1–5, 1987

59. Lifson AR, Stoneburner RJ, Chiasson MA, et al: HIV infection in sexually active heterosexual adults (abst). III International Conference on Acquired Immunodeficiency Virus (AIDS), Washington D.C., June 1–5, 1987

60. Harris C, Small CB, Klein RS, et al: Immunodeficiency in female sexual partners of men with the acquired immunodeficiency syndrome. N Engl J Med 308:1181, 1983

61. Redfield RR, Markham PD, Salahuddin SZ, et al: Frequent transmission of HTLV-III among spouses of patients with AIDS-related complex and AIDS. JAMA 253:1571, 1985

62. Chiasson MA, Fleisher E, Petrus D, Miller B: Epidemiologic characteristics of women with AIDS in New York City (abst). III International Conference on Acquired Immunodeficiency Syndrome (AIDS), Washington D.C., June 1–5, 1987

63. Miller SN, DeLuca PS, Ringler RP: AIDS in the wife of a bisexual man (letter), NY State J Med 86:158, 1986

64. Pitchenik AE, Fischl MA, Spira TJ: Acquired immune deficiency syndrome in low-risk patients: Evidence for possible transmission by an asymptomatic carrier. JAMA 250:1310, 1983

65. Pitchenik AE, Shafron RD, Glasser RM, Spira TJ: The acquired immunodeficiency syndrome in the wife of a hemophiliac. Ann Intern Med 100:62, 1984

66. Ratnoff DD, Lederman MM, Jenkins J: Lymphadenopathy in a hemophiliac patient and his sexual partner (letter). Ann Intern Med 100:915, 1984

67. Kreiss JK, Kitchen LW, Prince HE, et al: Antibody to human T-lymphotropic virus type III in wives of hemophiliacs: Evidence for heterosexual transmission. Ann Intern Med 102:623, 1985

68. Jason JM, McDougal S, Dixon G: HTLV-III/LAV antibody and immune status of household contacts and sexual partners of persons with hemophilia. JAMA 255:212, 1986

69. Chamberland M, White C, Lifson A, et al: AIDS in heterosexual contacts: A small but increasing group of cases (abst). III International Conference on Acquired Immunodeficiency Syndrome (AIDS), Washington D.C., June 1–5, 1987

70. Stewart GJ, Tyler JPP, Cunningham AL, et al: Transmission of human T-cell lymphotropic virus type III (HTLV-III) by artificial insemination by donor. Lancet ii:581, 1985

71. Centers for Disease Control: Human immunodeficiency virus infections in transfusion recipients and their family members. MMWR 36:137, 1987

72. Goedert JJ: Transmission of human immunodeficiency virus associated with severe T-cell depletion in male hemophiliacs (abst). Presented at the III International Conference on Acquired Immunodeficiency Syndrome (AIDS). Washington D.C., June 3, 1987

73. Zagury D, Bernard J, Leibowitch J, Safai B, et al: HTLV-III in cells cultured from semen of two patients with AIDS. Science 226:449, 1984

74. Kreiss JK, Koech D, Plummer FA, et al: AIDS virus infection in Nairobi prostitutes: Spread of the epidemic in East Africa. N Engl J Med 314:414, 1986

75. Katzenstein DA, Latif A, Bassett MT, et al: Risks for heterosexual transmission of HIV in Zimbabwe (abst). III International Conference on Acquired Immunodeficiency Syndrome (AIDS), Washington D.C., June 1–5, 1987

76. Pape JW, Liautaud B, Thomas F, et al: The acquired immunodeficiency syndrome in Haiti. Ann Intern Med 103:674, 1985

77. Centers for Disease Control: Heterosexual transmission of human T lymphotropic virus type III/lymphadenopathy-associated virus. MMWR 34:561, 1985

78. Redfield RR, Markham PD, Salahuddin SZ, et al: Heterosexually acquired HTLV-III/LAV disease (AIDS-related complex and AIDS): Epidemiologic evidence for female-to-male transmission. JAMA 254:2094, 1985

79. Van de Perre P, Rouvroy D, Lepage P, et al: Acquired immunodeficiency syndrome in Rwanda. Lancet ii:62–5, 1984

80. Cameron DW, Plummer FA, Simonsen JN, et al: Female to male heterosexual transmission of HIV infection in Nairobi (abst). III International Conference on Acquired Immunodeficiency Syndrome (AIDS), Washington D.C., June 1–5, 1987

81. Clumeck N, Robert-Guroff M, Van de Perre P, et al: Seroepidemiological studies of HTLV-III antibody prevalence among selected groups of heterosexual Africans. JAMA 254:2599, 1985

82. Clumeck N, Van de Perre P, Carael M, et al: Heterosexual promiscuity among African patients with AIDS (letter). N Engl J Med 313:182, 1985

83. Vogt NW, Witt DJ, Craven DE, Byington R, et al: Isolation of HTLV-III/LAV from cervical secretions of women at risk for AIDS. Lancet i:525, 1986

84. Wofsy CB, Cohen JB, Hauer LB, et al: Isolation of AIDS-associated retrovirus from genital secretions of women with antibodies to the virus. Lancet i:527, 1986

85. Archibald DW, Essex M, Sauk J, et al: Antibodies to HIV in cervical and oral secretions of female prostitutes in Zaire (abst). III International Conference on Acquired Immunodeficiency Syndrome (AIDS), Washington D.C., June 1–5, 1987

86. Vogt MW, Witt DJ, Craven DE, et al: Isolation patterns of the human immunodeficiency virus from cervical secretions during the menstrual cycle of women at risk for the acquired immune deficiency syndrome. Ann Intern Med 106:380, 1987

87. Friedman R, Hurt S, Arnoff M, et al: Behavior and the menstrual cycle. Signs 5:719, 1980

88. Van de Perre P, Clumeck N, Carael M, et al: Female prostitutes: A risk group for infection with human T-cell lymphotropic virus type III. Lancet ii:524, 1985

89. Plummer FA, Simonsen JN, Ngugi EN, et al: Incidence of human immunodeficiency virus (HIV) infection and related disease in a cohort of Nairobi prostitutes (abst). III International Conference on Acquired Immunodeficiency Syndrome (AIDS), Washington D.C., June 1–5, 1987

90. Mann J, Quinn TC, Piot P, et al: Condom use and HIV

infection among prostitutes in Zaire (letter). N Engl J Med 316:345, 1987

91. Centers for Disease Control: Antibody to human immunodeficiency virus in female prostitutes. MMWR 36:157, 1987
92. Tirelli U, Vaccher E, Diodato S, et al: HIV infection among female and male prostitutes (abst). III International Conference on Acquired Immunodeficiency Syndrome (AIDS), Washington D.C., June 1–5, 1987
93. Darrow WW: Multicenter study of HIV antibody in U.S. prostitutes (abst). Presented at the III International Conference on Acquired Immunodeficiency Syndrome (AIDS), Washington D.C., June 3, 1987
94. Allgeier ER, Allgeier AR: Sexual Interactions. Lexington, MA, D.C. Health and Co, 1986
95. Fischl MA, Dickinson GM, Scott GB, et al: Evaluation of heterosexual partners, children, and household contacts of adults with AIDS. JAMA 257:640, 1987
96. Lyman D, Winkelstein W Jr, Ascher M, Levy JA: Minimal risk of AIDS-associated retrovirus infection by oral genital-contact (letter). JAMA 255:1703, 1986
97. Monzon OT, Capellan JMB: Female-to-female transmission of HIV (letter). Lancet ii:40–1, 1987
98. Sabatini MT, Patel K, Hirschman R: Kaposi's sarcoma and T-cell lymphoma in an immunodeficient woman: A case report. AIDS Res 1:135, 1984
99. Marmor MM, Weiss LR, Lyden M, et al: Possible female-to-female transmission of human immunodeficiency virus. Ann Intern Med 105:969, 1986
100. Groopman JE, Salahuddin SZ, Sarngadharan MG, et al: HTLV-III in saliva of people with AIDS-related complex and healthy homosexual men at risk for AIDS. Science 226:447, 1984
101. Ho DD, Byington RE, Schooley RT, et al: Infrequency of isolation of HTLV-III virus from saliva in AIDS (letter). N Engl J Med 313:1606, 1985
102. Salahuddin SZ, Groopman JE, Markham PD, et al: HTLV-III symptom-free seronegative persons. Lancet ii:1418, 1984
103. Smith JWG: HIV transmitted by sexual intercourse but not by kissing (letter). Br Med J 294:446, 1987
104. Centers for Disease Control: Additional recommendations to reduce sexual and drug abuse-related transmission of human T-lymphotropic virus type III/lymphadenopathy-associated virus. MMWR 35:152, 1986
105. Levy JA, Kaminsky LS, Morrow WJW, et al: Infection by the retroviruses associated with the acquired immunodeficiency syndrome. Ann Intern Med 103:694, 1985
106. Committee on Medical Education: Assessment of Sexual Function: A Guide to Interviewing. New York, Group for the Advancement of Psychiatry, 1977
107. World Health Organization: Education and treatment in human sexuality: The training of health professionals. (Report of WHO meeting, Technical Report series No. 572). Geneva, WHO, 1975
108. Roundtable Discussion: Encouraging physician counseling for AIDS prevention. III International Conference on Acquired Immunodeficiency Syndrome (AIDS). Washington D.C., June 1–5, 1987
109. Marcotte DB: Sexual history taking. In Nadelson CC, Marcotte DB (eds): Treatment Interventions in Human Sexuality. New York, Plenum, 1977
110. New York Physicians for Human Rights: Policy Statement on HIV transmissability. October 12, 1986, p. 88

Prevention of Transmission of AIDS During Sexual Intercourse

Margaret A. Fischl

22

SEXUAL TRANSMISSION OF HIV

When the acquired immunodeficiency syndrome (AIDS) was first described among homosexual or bisexual men and intravenous drug users in 1981, sexual and parenteral transmission of an infectious agent was postulated. Since that time, human immunodeficiency virus (HIV) has been shown to be effectively transmitted through sexual contact between men and between men and women. Sexual contacts continue to account for more than 75% of all the reported cases of AIDS in the United States.[1] Epidemiologic studies have shown that the sexual acquisition of HIV among homosexual or bisexual men is related predominantly to the number of sexual partners and the practice of receptive anal-genital intercourse.[2,3] In evaluating varying types of rectal trauma, only douching or an enema before sexual contact contributed to the risk of HIV infection through receptive anal-genital intercourse. Data related to brachio-anal contact are less conclusive,[4-6] and the significance of insertive anal-genital contact or oral-genital contact has not been resolved.[7] Although these practices may not transmit HIV as readily as insertive anal-genital contact, nonetheless, they have been associated with transmission of the virus.

The heterosexual transmission of HIV was first recognized among women whose sexual partners were at risk for HIV infection.[8] Subsequently, the transmission of HIV to female spouses of male partners with AIDS or AIDS-related complex has been well established, demonstrating that repeated, long-term heterosexual contact is associated with substantial male-to-female transmission of HIV.[9-11] Several reports have also demonstrated HIV infection and seroconversion among male spouses of female partners with AIDS and AIDS-related complex, documenting male-to-female transmission of HIV.[12-14] Although less than 4% of all the cases of AIDS reported in the United States is attributed to the het-

erosexual transmission of the virus, studies have shown that spouses of partners with AIDS or AIDS-related illnesses are at a considerable risk for acquiring infection (Table 22-1).

In addition, women with multiple sexual partners— prostitutes—have been noted to have an increased rate of infection with HIV.[15-18] Female prostitutes in Nairobi, for example, have a seroprevalence rate of antibody to HIV as high as 65%, demonstrating that HIV infection is already spread extensively among urban prostitutes in Kenya. Further, the seroconversion rate for HIV among seronegative prostitutes over a 2-year period was also high: 56%. Similarly in Rwanda, 88% of female prostitutes screened for antibody to HIV were seropositive. In the United States, seroprevalence rates of antibody to HIV have varied from 0% in Las Vegas to 69% in Newark. In south Florida, 41% of female prostitutes tested had antibody to HIV. In countries reporting a low incidence of AIDS, 20% of unlicensed prostitutes in West Germany and 6% of prostitutes in Greece were found to have antibody to HIV. Moreover, several studies done in Africa, the United States, and Haiti have demonstrated that frequent heterosexual contact with prostitutes is associated with an increasing rate of infection with HIV among sexually active heterosexual men.[18-20]

The prevalence and incidence of HIV infection in the sexually active heterosexual community have not been well studied. The most current information on seroprevalence rates comes indirectly from HIV screening programs of all recruit applicants or active duty personnel in the United States Armed Forces.[21] The mean prevalence of antibody to HIV was 1.5 per 1000 recruit applicants during the first 18 months of the testing program. Seroprevalence was highest among recruits from metropolitan areas reporting a high incidence of AIDS and among blacks. The rate increased with age. The ratio of seropositive men to women was approximately 3 to 1. This is not strikingly different from the nationally

Table 22-1
Seroprevalence of Antibody to HIV Among Spouses
and Heterosexual Partners of Persons
with HIV Infection

	Total Number Studied	Number Seropositive	Percentage Seropositive
Pape et al.	174	95	55
Steibigel et al.	100	48	48
Padron et al.	97	22	23
Fischl et al.	88	47	53
Redfield et al.	41	15	38
Biberfeld et al.	40	4	10*
Goedert et al.	24	4	17*
Kreiss et al.	21	2	10*

* Spouses of patients with hemophilia.

reported ratio of 4:1 among cases of AIDS related to heterosexual contact with a person at risk for HIV infection.

The risk factors or mechanisms associated with the heterosexual transmission of HIV are not completely understood. It is apparent that vaginal intercourse alone is sufficient for the sexual transmission of HIV, and that the rates of male-to-female and female-to-male transmission may well be similar.[14] Preliminary data also suggest that couples who participate in anal-genital intercourse in addition to vaginal intercourse or oral-genital intercourse may be at a greater risk for HIV infection.[22,23] Similar trends have also been noted for women in relation to receptive oral-genital contact.

The exact risk of HIV infection for a person having a single sexual contact with an infected partner is not known. However, there are individuals who remain seronegative for the virus despite repeated long-term sexual contact with an infected partner or partners. Likewise, there are individuals who have AIDS or HIV infection and report only a single sexual contact with an infected partner. A report that 4 of 8 women developed antibody to HIV after being artificially inseminated with semen from an infected donor suggests that a single "sexual" exposure to the virus can result in infection.[24]

It has been suggested that other sexually transmitted diseases may be associated with an increased risk for the sexual acquisition of HIV, whether this be related to an increased exposure rate to HIV, increase in HIV viral replication or expression, activation of T cells, or breaks in epithelial barriers. Several studies among homosexual and bisexual men have shown a significant correlation between syphilis, gonorrhea, hepatitis, and infection with HIV. Similarly, studies evaluating risk factors for the heterosexual transmission of HIV have also demonstrated a significant association between other sexually transmitted diseases, including syphilis, gonnorhea, or genital ulcers and HIV infection.

PREVENTION MEASURES

On the basis of the current information about the sexual transmission of HIV, it appears that couples without any other independent risk factor for HIV infection, who have been mutually monogomous since the introduction of the virus in the United States in 1979, are not at risk for infection.[25] Further, individuals who are at risk for HIV infection through sexual contacts and who have not yet been infected can completely avoid future infection by practicing sexual abstinence. Individuals who are at risk for HIV infection and continue to have sexual contacts place themselves and their partners at an increased risk for infection with HIV.

The risk of HIV infection among sexually active men and women may be decreased by limiting the number of sexual partners and selecting partners who do not have multiple partners. However, in major urban areas reporting AIDS, the prevalence of HIV among homosexual men is high. Even with decreases in the number of sexual partners, the risk of HIV infection in this group still remains substantial because of a greater chance that a single sexual partner will be infected with the virus. Therefore, men and women who are at risk for HIV and who remain sexually active should avoid all contact with semen, genital secretions, and blood. Such contact may occur not only during genital intercourse, anal-genital contacts, brachio-anal contacts, or oral-genital contacts but through extensive foreplay when lesions are present or contact with secretions occurs.

Homosexual Activity

For sexually active homosexual men, the greatest risk for HIV infection is receptive anal-genital contact with an infected partner. Therefore, this practice should be avoided. Those individuals who continue to practice anal-genital intercourse, however, should use latex condoms and avoid douching or enemas before receptive anal-genital contact. Since more than one study has shown a significant correlation between brachio-anal contact and an increased risk of HIV infection, this practice should be avoided. Although the risk of oral-genital contact may be low, semen does harbor HIV and oral-genital contact may therefore carry a risk for infection with HIV. For those individuals who continue to practice oral-genital intercourse, correct and regular use of condoms may decrease contact with semen, pre-ejaculated fluids, and oral or genital lesions and thereby potentially decrease the risk of HIV infection. Since the skin and the oral mucosa appear to be more resistent to the passage of HIV than other body surfaces, hugging, caressing, and genital manipulation have been recommended to reduce the risk of HIV if no lesions are present. Similarly, kissing has also been suggested if no lesions are present. Since saliva has been reported to harbor HIV, deep kissing has been discouraged, although no data exist that HIV has been transmitted by this route.

Heterosexual Activity

With reference to heterosexual transmission of HIV, the number of sexual partners, sexual contact with female prostitutes, and the presence of other sexually transmitted diseases have been associated with an increased risk for HIV infection. Therefore, the total number of sexual partners should be decreased, as every sexual partner or sexual contact increases the risk of infection with HIV. Sexual contact with partners who have multiple partners and sexual contacts with prostitutes or individuals at risk for HIV infection should be avoided. Further, it appears that vaginal intercourse alone is sufficient for the transmission of HIV. However, anal-genital intercourse may well represent an increased risk for the acquisition of HIV, and this practice should be avoided. Again, although the risk for HIV infection from oral-genital intercourse may be low, transmission of virus may occur. Heterosexual men and women who are at an increased risk for HIV infection can avoid transmission and acquisition of HIV by practicing sexual abstinence. Individuals who remain sexually active are at an increased risk for HIV infection and in addition to limiting their sexual partners should use latex condoms during all sexual contacts, including vaginal intercourse, anal-genital intercourse, and oral-genital contact. Caution should also be used during foreplay if lesions or a vaginal or urethral discharge are present.

BARRIER CONTRACEPTIVES

Barrier contraceptives—in particular, condoms—have been shown to provide some protection against the transmission and acquisition of several sexually transmitted diseases. Condom use has been shown, for example, to decrease the risk of transmission of organisms that may be present in semen, including *Chlamydia trachomatis,* hepatitis B virus, *Mycoplasma hominis, Neisseria gonorrhea, Trichomonas vaginalis,* and *Ureaplasma urealyticum.*[26] In vitro studies have demonstrated that herpes simplex virus 1, herpes simplex virus 2, cytomegalovirus, and hepatitis B virus will not pass through stretched latex condoms.[27-31] Herpes simplex virus, human papillomavirus, *Treponema pallidum,* and *Haemophilus ducreyi* are transmitted by direct contact with the skin or mucous membranes and are not typically found in semen. However, condoms may be helpful in the prevention of these sexually transmitted diseases if lesions are on the penis or female genitalia or if an infectious discharge is present. In addition, a condom may also protect the sexual partner from an infectious urethral discharge or an infectious lesion on the genitalia of the user, as well as from an unrecognized infection or from asymptomatic viral shedding. Clinical trials have shown that men who use condoms have a significantly lower risk of acquiring urethral gonorrhea, *U. urealyticum,* and self-reported venereal diseases than those who do not use condoms.[32-36] Use of condoms, however, has not been shown to confer a similar protection against nongonococcal urethritis. Decreases in the incidence of pelvic inflammatory disease and cervical gonorrhea have also been reported among women whose partners use condoms.[37,38]

Condoms and HIV Infection

Since condoms have been shown to be effective in the prevention of several sexually transmitted diseases due to bacteria and viruses similar in size to HIV (such as the herpes simplex virus and cytomegalovirus), condoms have been recommended to members of groups at risk for HIV infection as a potential barrier against the sexual transmission and acquisition of HIV. However, data about the effectiveness of condoms in the prevention of HIV infection are limited.

Several in vitro studies in mechanical models simulating sexual intercourse have shown that latex condoms do not allow the leakage of HIV.[39,40] However, several natural membrane condoms have been shown to allow a significant passage of retroviral antigen. Further, preliminary data suggest that HIV may be inactivated at various degrees inside the condom. The reason for this is not clear and may be related to chemical disinfectants, particularly nonoxynal-9. Thus, there is sufficient *in vitro* data to suggest the latex condoms are not permeable to HIV. (This is not true for natural membrane condoms.) However, even a minute break, as small as a needle puncture, in a latex condom is sufficient to allow a significant passage of HIV across the membrane. Since breakage of condoms is reported during sexual activity, the risk of HIV infection under these circumstances is not known, and use of condoms, therefore, does not "guarantee" prevention of infection with HIV.

HIV has been isolated from cervical secretions, vaginal secretions, and semen. It appears that women can harbor HIV in genital secretions at varying times during the menstrual cycle.[41-43] Further, isolation of virus from genital secretions may not necessarily reflect viremia. The source of HIV in genital secretions is not entirely known. It appears that virus may be derived from blood lymphocytes during menstruation or sequestered in inflammatory lesions. HIV can also be found in monocyte macrophages and Langerhans' cells, which can be found in genital tract epithelium. Similarly, HIV can be readily isolated from semen of men with HIV infection[44-45] and may be harbored in cells in pre-ejaculated fluids or sequestered in inflammatory lesions. Therefore, if condoms are to be the least bit effective in decreasing the transmission of HIV, they must be used to avoid all contact with semen, pre-ejaculated fluids, vaginal and cervical secretions, any genital or oral lesions, and the genital tract in general.

Only preliminary data about condoms in the actual prevention of the sexual transmission or acquisition of HIV are available. Several studies to date have not demonstrated a significant correlation between condom use and the heterosexual transmission of HIV. However, in many instances, couples were not aware of the HIV status of their partner, and prior regular use of condoms was uncommon. Typically, condom use was erratic or occurred after recognition of HIV infection in a partner and, in several instances, after transmission to the partner had already occurred. Therefore, the effectiveness of condoms cannot be determined from many of these studies.

Licensed prostitutes in West Germany have been reported to have a seroprevalence rate of antibody to HIV of approximately 1%, compared to a 20% rate among unlicensed prostitutes.[46] Higher socioeconomic class, the absence of intravenous drug use, and the frequent use of condoms were felt to contribute to the major difference between the two groups. Further, condom use among licensed prostitutes was common not only during vaginal intercourse but also during anal-genital and oral-genital contacts. Among female prostitutes in Kinshasa, Zaire, there was a significant difference in the rate of acquisition of HIV among female prostitutes reporting condom use by 50% or more of their partners as compared with women reporting less frequent use of condoms among their partners.[47]

In a study of monogomous heterosexual couples in which one spouse was infected with HIV, continued sexual contacts and lack of condom use correlated with the acquisition of HIV, as shown in Table 22-2. These data strongly suggest that spouses who have been exposed heterosexually to HIV and have not acquired the virus remain at no risk if they abstain from any further form of sexual contact, whereas spouses who continue to have sexual contacts with an infected partner remain at a considerable risk for HIV infection. Among couples who used condoms appropriately, there was a decrease in the incidence of HIV infection. However, three initially seronegative spouses did subsequently develop infection with HIV despite the regular use of condoms, suggesting a 13% failure rate of condoms in the prevention of HIV. This figure does not differ greatly from the

condom failure rate for pregnancy. The reasons for the failure of condoms to protect against HIV infection were unclear, but may have been related to inadvertent slippage or breakage of condoms and in one couple may have been related to exposure to infected semen through oral-genital intercourse.

Since acquisition of HIV infection through a single sexual encounter has been reported, breakage rates of condoms and factors associated with breakage became important. According to preliminary data from an on-going study in Miami evaluating condom usage in the prevention of HIV infection,[48] approximately 46% of couples evaluated reported slippage or breakage of condoms during a 6-month interval. Based on the mean number of sexual encounters, a breakage ratio of 1:300 to 1:500 contacts occurred. Breakage was more commonly associated with anal-genital intercourse and with use of natural membrane condoms. Breakage was also associated with lack of adequate lubrication and with reuse of condoms.

Another issue related to condom use is compliance with both regular and correct usage. Surveys done in sexually active heterosexual couples and sexually active men at risk for HIV infection still show a relatively high rate of non-usage of condoms. Major reasons for non-use include decreased sensation, unacceptability to the partner, unavailability, embarrassment associated with purchasing condoms, or lack of knowledge or interest in condom use. However, there are studies among sexually active homosexual men and prostitutes in areas reporting a high incidence of AIDS in which use of condoms during sexual contacts is increasing as a result of intensive educational programs.

To be effective, condoms must be used routinely and correctly and must remain intact. The following guidelines have been adapted for use in decreasing the risk of HIV infection among sexually active men and women.[49]

- Condoms *must* be used each and every time one has genital, anal, or oral sexual contact.
- Condoms *must* be put on as soon as an erection occurs and before the penis is inserted into the partner. Any contact with the vagina, penis, mouth, or rectum before a condom is put on is considered *unsafe*.
- The rim of the condom should be rolled carefully to the base of the penis before insertion into the partner. If a condom lacks a reservoir tip, a half-inch of empty space should be left at the tip to catch semen.
- Petroleum jelly (Vaseline), vegetable shortening (Crisco), or oils may cause deterioration of latex and should *not* be used as lubricants. Sufficient lubrication is needed so condoms will not tear or cause trauma to the partner. Water-base jellies (K-Y), spermicide jellies, or spermicide foams can be used as lubricants. Saliva is *not* recommended.
- The condom should be used only *once*. Under no circumstances should condoms be reused. Condoms should be disposed of safely.

Table 22-2

Relationship of Sexual Activity to Development of HIV Antibody Among 58 Seronegative Spouses at Study Entry

Sexual Activity	Total Number	HIV Positive	HIG Negative	Percent Converted
Abstinence	13	0	13	0
Sexual contact with condoms	23	3	20	13
Sexual contact without condoms	22	14	8	64

- The penis should be withdrawn soon after ejaculation. If loss of erection occurs, the condom may slip off. After sexual contact, the penis should be withdrawn carefully, holding the rim of the condom to protect against slippage and contact with semen or the partner's genitalia or secretions.
- Condoms should be checked to see if they are still intact. If condoms tear or come off in the vagina, use of spermicide foams or jellies may be helpful.*
- Condoms should be stored in a cool, dry place. If condoms are kept in a relatively dry environment which is not excessively hot, condom life probably exceeds 5 years.

SPERMICIDES

Spermicides have been shown to potentially provide a chemical barrier for the prevention of sexually transmitted diseases. In vitro studies have demonstrated that spermicides can inactivate several sexually transmitted pathogens, including herpes simplex virus, *N. gonorrhea, T. pallidum, T. vaginalis,* and *U. urealyticum.*[50-53] Further, epidemiologic studies suggest that the use of vaginal spermicides may decrease the risk of acquiring cervical gonorrhea. Contraceptive sponges impregnated with nonoxynol-9 have also been shown to decrease the incidence of infection with *C. trachomatis* and gonorrhea but increase the risk of infection with *Candida.*[54] Although spermicides are generally not irritating to the urethral mucosa or vagina, allergic reactions and irritation have been described.

The effectiveness of spermicide use with condoms in the prevention of HIV infection is not known. Preliminary data suggest that nonoxynol-9 can inhibit HIV replication and kill lymphocytes.[55] Whether its use with condoms will further decrease the risk of HIV infection is unknown. Questions have been raised as to whether spermicides can cause deterioration of latex and therefore potentially increase the risk of breakage of latex condoms.

REFERENCES

1. Centers for Disease Control: Update: Acquired Immunodeficiency Syndrome (AIDS). MMWR 35:17, 1986
2. Curran JW, Morgan WM, Hardy AM, et al: The epidemiology of AIDS: Current status and future prospects. Science 229:1352, 1985
3. Winkelstein W, Jr., Lyman DM, Padian N, et al: Sexual practices and risk of infection by the human immunodeficiency virus: The San Francisco Men's Health Study. JAMA 257(3):321, 1987

* Douching has not been shown to be effective in decreasing the incidence of sexually transmitted disease, and douching or enemas before receptive anal-genital intercourse among men has been shown to increase the risk of HIV infection.

4. Jaffe HW, Keewhan C, Thomas PA, et al: National case-control study of Kaposi's sarcoma and *Pneumocystis carinii* pneumonia in homosexual men: Part 1, epidemiologic results. Ann Intern Med 99:145, 1983
5. Marmor M, Freidman-Kein AE, Zolla-Pazner Z, et al: Kaposi's sarcoma in homosexual men. Ann Intern Med 100:809, 1984
6. Jeffries E, Willoughby B, Boyko WJ, et al: The Vancouver lymphadenopathy-AIDS study. II. Seroepidemiology of HTLV-III antibody. Can Med Assoc J 132:1373, 1985
7. Lyman D, Winkelstein W, Jr., Ascher M, et al: Minimal risk of AIDS-associated retrovirus infection by oral-genital contact. JAMA 255:1703, 1986
8. Harris C, Small CB, Klein RS, et al: Immunodeficiency in female sexual partners of men with the acquired immune deficiency syndrome. N Engl J Med 308:1181, 1983
9. Redfield RR, Markham PD, Salahuddin SZ, et al: Frequent transmission of HTLV-III among spouses of patients with AIDS-related complex (ARC) and the acquired immune deficiency syndrome (AIDS): a family study. JAMA 253:1571, 1985
10. Hadsfeld H, Kobayashi J, Fischl MA, et al: Heterosexual transmission of human lymphotropic virus type III/lymphadenopathy-associated virus. MMWR 34:561, 1985
11. Kreiss JK, Kitchen LW, Prince HE, et al: Antibody to human T-lymphotropic virus type III in wives of hemophiliacs: evidence of heterosexual transmission. Ann Intern Med 102:623, 1985
12. Redfield RR, Markham PD, Salahuddin SZ, et al: Heterosexually acquired HTLV-III/LAV disease (AIDS-related complex and AIDS): epidemiologic evidence for female-to-male transmission. JAMA 254:2094, 1985
13. Calabrese LH, Gopalakrishna KV: Transmission of HTLV-III infection from man to woman to man. N Engl J Med 314:987, 1986
14. Fischl MA, Dickinson GM, Scott GB, et al: Evaluation of heterosexual, partners, children, and household contacts of adults with AIDS. JAMA 257:640, 1987
15. Kreiss JK, Koech D, Plummer FA, et al: AIDS virus infection in Nairobi prostitutes: spread of the epidemic to east Africa. N Engl J Med 314:414, 1986
16. Fischl MA, Dickinson GM, Flanagan S, et al: Human immunodeficiency virus (HIV) among female prostitutes in south Florida. III International Conference on AIDS, Washington, D.C. 105, 1987
17. Darrow WW, Cohen JB, Gill FP, et al: Multicenter study of HIV antibody in U.S. prostitutes. III International Conference on AIDS, Washington, D.C., 105, 1987
18. Van de Perre P, Clumeck N, Carael M, et al: Female prostitutes: A risk group for infection with human T-cell lymphotropic virus type III. Lancet ii:254, 1985
19. Pape JW, Liautaud B, Thomas F, et al: The acquired immunodeficiency syndrome in Haiti. Ann Intern Med 103:674, 1985
20. Collaborative Study Group of AIDS in Haitian-Americans: Risk factors for AIDS among Haitians residing in the United States: Evidence of heterosexual transmission. JAMA 257:635, 1987
21. Burke DSR, Brundage JF, Herbold JR, et al: Human immunodeficiency virus infections among civilian applicants for United States Military service, October 1985 to March 1986: Demographic factors associated with seropositivity. N Engl J Med 317:131, 1987
22. Steigbigel NH, Maude DW, Feiner CJ, et al: Heterosexual transmission of infection and disease by the human im-

munodeficiency virus (HIV). III International Conference on AIDS, Washington, D.C., 106, 1987

23. Padron N, Berkeley M, Francis DP, et al: Male-to-female transmission of human immunodeficiency virus. JAMA 258: 788, 1987

24. Stewart GJ, Tyler JPP, Cunningham AL, et al: Transmission of human T-cell lymphotropic virus type III (HTLV-III) by artificial insemination by donor. Lancet i:581, 1985

25. Francis DP, Chin J: The prevention of acquired immunodeficiency syndrome in the United States: An objective strategy for medicine, public health, business, and the community. JAMA 1357, 1987

26. Stone KM, Grimes DA, Magder LS: Primary prevention of sexually transmitted diseases: a primer for clinicians. JAMA 255:1763, 1986

27. Smith L Jr, Oleske J, Cooper R, et al: Efficacy of condoms as barriers to HSV-2 and gonorrhea: An *in vitro* model. First Sexually Transmitted Diseases World Congress, San Juan, Puerto Rico, 77, 1981

28. Judson FN, Bodin GF, Levin MJ, et al: *In vitro* tests demonstrate condoms provide an effective barrier against *Chlamydia trachomatis* and herpes simplex virus. Fifth International Meeting of the International Society for Sexually Transmitted Diseases, Seattle, Washington; 176, 1983

29. Conant MA, Spicer DW, Smith CD: Herpes simplex virus transmission: Condom studies. Sex Transm Dis 11:94, 1984

30. Katznelson S, Drew WL, Mintz L: Efficacy of the condom as a barrier to the transmission of cytomegalovirus. J Infect Dis 150:155, 1984

31. Minuk GY, Bohme CE, Bowen TJ: Condoms and hepatitis B virus infection. Ann Intern Med 104:584, 1986

32. Pemberton J, McCann JS, Mahony DH, et al: Socio-medical characteristics of patients attending a VD clinic and the circumstances of infection. Br J Vener Dis 48:391, 1972

33. McCormack WM, Lee Y, Zinner SH: Sexual experience and urethral colonization with genital mycoplasmas: A study in normal men. Ann Intern Med 78:696, 1973

34. Hart G: Factors influencing venereal infection in a war environment. Br J Vener Dis 50:68, 1974

35. Barlow D: The condom and gonorrhea. Lancet ii:811, 1977

36. Hooper RR, Reynolds GH, Jones OG, et al: Cohort study of venereal disease: I. The risk of gonorrhea transmission from infected women to men. Am J Epidemiol 108:136, 1978

37. Kelaghan J, Rubin GL, Ory HW, et al: Barrier-method contraceptives and pelvic inflammatory disease. JAMA 248: 184, 1982

38. Austin H, Louv WC, Alexander WJ: A case-control study of spermicides and gonorrhea. JAMA 251:2822, 1984

39. Conant M, Hardy D, Sernatinger J, et al: Condoms prevent transmission of AIDS-associated retrovirus. JAMA 255:1706, 1986

40. Van de Perre P, Jacobs D, Sprecher-Goldberger S: The latex condom, an efficient barrier against sexual transmission of AIDS-related viruses. AIDS 1:49, 1987

41. Vogt MW, Witt DJ, Craven DE, et al: Isolation of HTLV-III/LAV from cervical secretions of women at risk for AIDS. Lancet 1:525, 1986

42. Wofsy CB, Cohen JB, Hauer LB, et al: Isolation of AIDS-associated retrovirus from genital secretions of women with antibodies to the virus. Lancet i:527, 1986

43. Vogt MW, Witt DJ, Craven DE, et al: Isolation patterns of the human immunodeficiency virus from cervical secretions during the menstrual cycle of women at risk for the acquired immunodeficiency syndrome. Ann Intern Med 106:380, 1987

44. Ho DD, Schooley RT, Rota TR, et al: HTLV-III in the semen and blood of a healthy homosexual man. Science 226:451, 1984

45. Zagury D, Bernard J, Leibowitch J, et al: HTLV-III in cells cultured from semen of two patients with AIDS. Science 226:449, 1984

46. Smith GL, Smith KF: Lack of HIV infection and condom use in licensed prostitutes. Lancet 1392, 1986

47. Mann J, Guinn T, Post P, et al: Condom use and HIV infection among prostitutes in Zaire. N Engl J Med 316:345, 1987

48. Fischl MA, Richman GM, Segal et al: Heterosexual transmission of human immunodeficiency virus (HIV): Relationship of sexual practices to seroconversion. III International Conference on AIDS, Washington, D.C., 178, 1987

49. Hatcher R. Contraceptive Technology 1986–1987, 13th ed. New York, Irving Publishers, 1987

50. Bolch OH Jr, Warren JC: *In-vitro* effects of Emko on *Neisseria gonorrhoeae* and *Trichomonas vaginalis*. Am J Obstet Gynecol 115:1145, 1973

51. Singh B, Postic B, Cutler JC: Virucidal effect of certain chemical contraceptives on type 2 herpesvirus. Am J Obstet Gynecol 126:422, 1976

52. Singh B, Cutler JC: Demonstration of a spirocheticidal effect by chemical contraceptives on *Treponema pallidum*. Bull Pan Am Health Organ 16:59, 1982

53. Amortegui AJ, Melder RJ, Meyer MP, et al: The effect of chemical intravaginal contraceptives and Betadine on *Ureaplasma urealyticum*. Contraception 30:135, 1984

54. Rosenberg MJ, Roganapithayakorn W, Feldblum PJ, et al: Effect of the contraceptive sponge on chlamydial infection, gonorrhea and candidiasis: A comparative clinical trial. JAMA 17:2308, 1987

55. Hicks DR, Martin LS, Voeller B, et al: Inactivation of LAV/HTLV-III infected cultures of normal human lymphocytes by nonoxynol-9 *in-vitro*. Lancet ii:1422, 1985

The Safety of Blood and Blood Products

Klaus Mayer
Johanna Pindyck

23

Each year more than three million patients in the United States require therapy with blood or blood products. The discovery that the new disease acquired immunodeficiency syndrome (AIDS) was transmissible by transfusion galvanized the blood service system into action to prevent this from occurring. It also focused the attention of physicians and patients on the safety of blood transfusion, especially with respect to AIDS transmission. This led to increased concern among physicians about the judicious use of blood products, improved awareness of the value of autologous blood transfusion, and demands by some patients to select their own donors for transfusion. The purpose of this chapter is to (1) examine the steps that have been taken to prevent AIDS transmission by transfusion; (2) evaluate the effectiveness of these preventive measures; (3) review the program that has been established to detect persons who may have been exposed to AIDS by prior transfusion; (4) review the transfusion options and recommend procedures that physicians should follow when administering transfusions to their patients.

BACKGROUND

Blood is a complex mixture of cellular elements suspended in liquid plasma, which itself is a solution of salts, hormones, and proteins. There are two major categories of blood products prepared for therapeutic purposes. One group is whole blood or its components—namely, packed red cells, platelets, fresh frozen plasma, cryoprecipitate, and leukocytes. These are collected primarily from volunteer donors to blood centers and hospitals. The elements of the blood are separated into their components by physical means, including centrifugation and freezing. Each unit of whole blood or blood component comes from an individual donor.

The second group of products comprises protein derivatives of plasma, such as albumin, Factor VIII, Factor IX, and immunoglobulin preparations. These are derived by chemical fractionation of plasma pools, sometimes from as many as 20,000 plasma donations. Unlike whole blood and its components, many plasma derivatives can be subjected to procedures, such as heating, that are capable of inactivating viruses and that minimize the risk of virus transmission by these products.

Both blood components and plasma derivatives have the potential to transmit disease to transfusion recipients. The important transfusion-transmissible diseases have two major characteristics in common—a long incubation period and an asymptomatic carrier state. Hepatitis B serves as a paradigm of transfusion-transmissible diseases. Its transmissibility by blood was documented when large outbreaks of hepatitis occurred in the late 1930s and early 1940s among recipients of yellow fever vaccine after human serum was used to stabilize the yellow fever virus in the vaccine.[1] The outbreak of hepatitis in vaccine recipients highlighted the serum transmissibility of this disease. Several studies of transfusion recipients and volunteers resulted in the recognition that serum hepatitis could occur after blood transfusion.[2,3,4,5] It was also noted that paid donors were more likely to transmit serum hepatitis than volunteer donors. A change from paid blood donors to volunteer donors as the source of whole blood and its components is credited with being a major factor in reducing the spread of hepatitis by transfusion.[6] Individual blood donors are also screened for a history of hepatitis as a preventive measure. The discovery of the hepatitis B virus as the causative agent of serum hepatitis and the identification of hepatitis B surface antigen (HBsAg) as a marker for infectivity led to the introduction, in 1972, of the requirement to screen all donated blood for HBsAg as an additional measure to prevent the transmission of hepatitis B virus by this route. Thus selection of donor source, screening of individual donors, and testing of donated units are all used to prevent transmission of hepatitis B by transfusion. At present the risk of contracting hepatitis B by transfusion of whole blood or its components is considered to be very low—probably less than 1:1,000—but its exact incidence is not known.[7] With current methods for inactivation of blood derivatives, the risk from most of these products is even lower.

It is useful to keep in mind the history of the control of hepatitis B transmission by transfusion when evaluating the measures that have been taken to prevent the spread of transfusion-associated AIDS.

RECOGNITION OF THE TRANSMISSIBILITY OF AIDS BY TRANSFUSION

AIDS was first described in 1981. Evidence that it was transmissible by transfusion accumulated in parallel with information suggesting that the disease was, in fact, caused by a transmissible agent. Three lines of evidence converged to pinpoint a transmissible agent as the most likely cause of AIDS: (1) the development of the disease in sexual contacts of gay men with the disease[8]; (2) the recognition of its occurrence in intravenous drug abusers[9]; (3) the report of AIDS in three patients with hemophilia A.[10]

In evaluating the fact that the first indication of transfusion transmissibility was in patients with Factor VIII deficiency, it is important to keep in mind that, as noted above, these patients were treated with products derived from large plasma pools and were therefore exposed to plasma from several thousand donors. Also, at that time, the Factor VIII used to treat hemophilia A patients was not virus-inactivated. Thus, although the number of patients with hemophilia A is relatively small, their individual exposure risk was extremely high compared to recipients of whole blood or components.

By early 1983, it had become clear that AIDS was most likely caused by a transmissible agent and that one route of transmission was transfusion, but the agent had not as yet been identified. Epidemiologic measures to protect the blood supply were applied to donor screening to eliminate blood donation by persons at risk of AIDS. In March of 1983, the Food and Drug Administration (FDA) issued guidelines identifying persons in risk groups for AIDS for donor screening to prevent its transmission by transfusion.

SCREENING BLOOD DONORS TO PROTECT THE BLOOD SUPPLY FROM AIDS

The major risk groups in which AIDS was first recognized were gay men, intravenous drug abusers, and persons from Haiti. These individuals, and their sexual partners, needed to be restricted from blood donation. Intravenous drug users had been interdicted from do-

nation for many years because of their risk of transmitting hepatitis B. The blood service system was now confronted with requiring that gay or bisexual men—a group whose personal sexual behaviors were often unknown to their families, colleagues, and peers—not give blood. As evidence has accumulated indicating the transmissibility of HIV from females to males, contact with prostitutes has been added to the factors warranting inclusion in a risk group category. Table 23-1 lists persons in risk groups currently excluded from blood donation.

Three educational approaches have been employed by blood collection agencies to screen out persons at high risk of exposure to HIV. First, persons in risk groups are requested not to give blood. Two studies have indicated the success of this measure.[11,12] Both studies found a significant decrease in the number of male donors after it was requested that gay men not give blood. Second, all donors are asked if they feel well at the time of the donation. The educational materials provided to prospective donors instruct persons in risk groups to say "no" and indicates that they will be privately excused from donation by the person taking the medical history. Third, donors of whole blood and components are offered an additional compliance mechanism after the medical history. Each blood donor is given a confidential form that asks the donor to decide whether his or her blood donation may be used "for transfusion" or only "for laboratory studies."

Table 23-1

1987 Criteria Defining Persons Who Should Not Give Blood

Any man who has had any sexual contact with another man since 1977

Any woman who has sexual contact with a man who has had sex with another man since 1977

Men and women who have used intravenous drugs—past or present

Men and women who have been sexual partners of male or female intravenous drug users

Homophiliacs

Sexual partners of hemophiliacs

Residents of Haiti, Zaire, Rwanda, Burundi, Kenya, Uganda, Tanzania who have entered the United States since 1977.

Men and women who have been sexual partners of people who were living in any of the above countries at any time since 1977

Men and women who have been sexual partners of persons with AIDS, ARC, or HIV infection—before or after they were diagnosed

Men and women who have engaged in prostitution since 1977

Anyone who has had sex with a prostitute*

Anyone who has had sexual contact with a person who has had sexual contact with a prostitute, an IV drug user, a hemophiliac, or a bisexual man

---

* 6-month deferral after contact

Confidential unit exclusion was pioneered by the New York Blood Center in 1983 at the time of introduction of measures to screen out donors at risk of AIDS exposure. Markers of infection with viruses prevalent in gay men, such as hepatitis B, were found to be significantly higher in persons who advised that their blood should be used only for "laboratory studies."[11] When HIV was identified and antibody tests became available, this testing confirmed that individuals who donated for laboratory studies only had a 24 to 100 times greater prevalence than donors "for transfusion" to the same collection agency,[13,14] indicating that this is a useful additional compliance mechanism. Until the development of anti-HIV testing, donor screening was the only means available to eliminate donors at risk of HIV infection.

SCREENING OF ALL DONATED BLOOD FOR ANTIBODIES TO HIV

In 1983 and 1984 the causative agent of AIDS, now known as the human immunodeficiency virus (HIV), was identified. The concerted action of the federal government and pharmaceutical companies led to the rapid development of enzyme-linked immunoassay (ELISA) methods to screen for antibody to HIV in all donated blood. The available ELISA methods are extremely sensitive and are estimated to detect 96% to 98% of all infected samples. They have, however, two drawbacks. In the first place, there is a significant false-positive rate in normal healthy persons because of antibody reactions to antigens on the cells in which the virus is grown[15] or perhaps to antibody cross reactions with other viruses. In a normal donor population, the false-positive rate may be as high as 78% of all repeatable ELISA reactive tests.[16] A second, more specific test, the Western blot, is used to confirm the presence of anti-HIV antibodies. Even the Western blot test, recently licensed by the FDA, does not completely eliminate the problem of false-positive reactions. Only Western blot tests with no bands present can be interpreted as negative.[17] Those with bands specific for HIV are interpreted as positive. However, a substantial number of Western blots have band patterns that are not clearly specific for HIV infection and that, according to the licensed procedures, must be regarded as "indeterminate." Clinical evaluation and repeat testing of the person's blood after an interval of time, usually 3 to 6 months, is then conducted to determine whether or not the pattern has evolved into one specific for infection with HIV.

Upon the introduction of anti-HIV testing, 0.04% of blood donors in the United States (4 per 10,000) were found to have specific antibodies to HIV.[18] Consent to perform anti-HIV testing is obtained from all donors prior to donation, and they are also advised that they will be informed of positive test results. When notified, donors with positive tests are given public health recommendations as to how to protect their own health and that of their sexual partners, and are advised not to

donate blood. The rate of donations positive for antibodies to HIV has fallen to approximately 0.01% (1 per 10,000 donations) since the introduction of testing and the notification of anti-HIV–positive donors.[7]

As good as the antibody test is as a means for detecting persons with HIV infection, it does have the second drawback that the antibody test does not usually become positive for 6 to 8 weeks after infection, and may not become positive for up to 6 months.[19,20] Therefore, it is still essential to keep donations from persons who are in the early stages of HIV infection out of the blood supply. For this reason, continued rigorous donor screening, in addition to anti-HIV testing, is critical as a means of preventing AIDS transmission by transfusion.

New tests to screen for HIV antigen are being evaluated as a means to at least partially close the gap between infection and antibody development, but none has yet been found efficacious. As with hepatitis B, the prevention of HIV transmission depends on selection of donor source, individual donor screening, and testing of all donated units.

THE RISK OF ACQUIRING HIV INFECTION BY TRANSFUSION OF WHOLE BLOOD OR COMPONENTS

The combination of donor screening and anti-HIV testing of all donated blood has reduced the risk of contracting HIV infection by transfusion with blood or its components to approximately 1:250,000.[7] Maintenance of this low risk level depends on donor cooperation with exclusion guidelines, careful testing, and notification of anti-HIV positive donors not to give blood.

Risk Prior to Anti-HIV Testing

The availability of the anti-HIV test has increased our understanding of the clinical course of HIV infection. It has become clear that persons may have asymptomatic infection for a prolonged period of time. Therefore, when donors of blood or components are seropositive, it has become standard practice for blood centers and hospitals to trace the recipients of past donations to determine whether transmission of HIV had occurred due to transfusion of the earlier donation. This program, known as "Lookback," was of particular importance immediately after the introduction of testing because most donors are repeat donors, no test had been available previously, and it was likely that a significant number of these prior donations were infectious. This has been found to be true, and as many as 70% of prior recipients of components from these donors have themselves been found to be seropositive.[21] It has also been found that the longer the interval between a positive test in the donor and the prior donation, the less likely the chance of infection transmission.[22]

Lookback programs depend on repeat donation by persons in order to detect seropositivity. On the basis of mathematical projections, the Centers for Disease Control (CDC) estimated that as many as 12,000 people living in the United States in early 1987 had acquired HIV infection by transfusion.[23] The risk of infection being transmitted to a recipient is greatest in multiply-transfused recipients, in those transfused closer to the time period when antibody testing for HIV was introduced, and in those transfused with blood drawn from donors in regions with the largest numbers of AIDS cases. For these reasons, the CDC has recommended that physicians "offer HIV antibody testing for some patients who received transfusions between 1978 and late Spring of 1985." The decision about whether to offer testing to a patient should be based on the likelihood of HIV exposure, as noted above, on whether the patient is sexually active, and on the degree of concern expressed by the patient. For patients who are extremely distressed, antibody testing may need to be offered even if the likelihood of exposure was small. If testing is offered to patients who are not in the Lookback program, it is important to recognize that the finding of a positive test may not be at all related to prior transfusion, and a careful risk history is essential to rule out other exposure routes. Any patient for whom testing is performed requires careful pre- and post-test counseling regardless of the test result.

As anti-HIV testing continues, the number of recipients sought through the Lookback program will diminish. It is likely, however, that an occasional patient will have been exposed from a seronegative donation by an infectious donor, as has already been reported.[24] However, it must be remembered that the chances of this occurring at the present time are only 1:250,000 for recipients of blood or its components, as has been noted earlier.

THE RISK OF ACQUIRING HIV INFECTION BY TRANSFUSION WITH PLASMA DERIVATIVES

The plasma derivatives in common therapeutic use include Factor VIII for treatment of patients with hemophilia A; Factor IX for treatment of patients with hemophilia B; various immunoglobulin preparations primarily used to prevent infection before or after exposure to an infectious agent or in patients with immunodeficiency disorders; and albumin or plasma protein fraction, which is used as a plasma volume expander or to replace albumin in certain protein-losing states. Each of these protein concentrates is prepared from a starting pool of several thousand plasma units, obtained largely from paid plasmapheresis donors. These donors are required to undergo essentially the same donor screening procedures which have been described for volunteer donors, and their plasma donations are screened for antibody to HIV prior to pooling. Each of these plasma derivatives will be discussed separately in the following sections.

Albumin and Plasma Protein Factor

The safety of albumin and plasma protein factor has been demonstrated through long use as volume expanders in surgery, for the treatment of burns and septic shock, and for the replacement of protein loss in patients with burns and liver disease. Pasteurization of the products by heating at 60°C for 10 hours essentially renders it sterile. This heat treatment procedure was in effect long before HIV entered the United States, and therefore there is no risk of contracting HIV infection by transfusion of these products.

Despite their safety, there is controversy as to the efficacy of these products, and questions have been raised as to the legitimacy of their widespread use in clinical practice. Experience in Vietnam produced convincing evidence that shock is best treated with massive quantities of crystalloid solutions. Indeed, wounded soldiers were resuscitated more successfully with the crystalloid solution Ringer's lactate, than with colloids such as albumin.[25] These observations have subsequently been extended and confirmed in patients in an older age group, who also did better with infusion of crystalloid solutions.[26] These data have not as yet been widely accepted and a substantial amount of albumin and plasma protein fraction is transfused in the United States annually. Their safety with respect to HIV transmission is not in question.

Immune Globulin Preparations

Unlike albumin and plasma protein fraction preparations, immune globulin cannot be subjected to heat treatment without denaturation of the globulin proteins. Questions have been raised as to the safety of these preparations—which include immune globulin (human), hepatitis B immune globulin; Rh immune globulin; and Varicella zoster immune globulin—with respect to HIV transmission. To determine whether the multiple steps in the Cohn-Oncley process used to prepare immunoglobulins were efficient in partitioning and inactivating HIV, investigators at the FDA have conducted studies examining material "spiked" with HIV at various steps in the fractionation process. These studies demonstrated a potential efficiency of virus removal of 10^{15} infectious units per milliliter in the combined steps of the Cohn-Oncley fractionation process, which was considered to be several orders of magnitude greater than that needed to eliminate the small amount of virus that might be present in a plasma pool used for immune globulin preparation.[27] In addition, prospective studies of immunocompetent recipients of gamma globulin have not been shown to produce antibodies to HIV.[28] These data permit the conclusion that immune globulin therapy is not associated with the risk of developing HIV infection. Rh-negative women at risk for Rh sensitization require therapy, and may require reassurance about the safety of the product. These patients—as well as those in need of passive immunization to prevent hepatitis B, chicken pox, or other infectious agents—can be so reassured, on the basis of current data, that there is no risk of HIV transmission from these products.

Coagulation Factors VIII and IX

The most problematic group of recipients remains that composed of patients with hemophilia A or B. When HIV first entered the United States, coagulation factor concentrates were not subjected to virus inactivation procedures, HIV infection had not as yet been recognized as transfusion transmissible, and neither donor screening nor antibody testing of donated blood were in effect. It is unfortunate that large numbers of hemophilia patients were therefore exposed to the virus by the transfusion route.

It is estimated that there are 20,000 hemophiliacs in the United States. As of the spring of 1987, there were 327 cases reported to the CDC of AIDS in patients with coagulation factor disorders. Of these, 294 were in patients with Factor VIII deficiency (hemophilia A), 20 were in patients with Factor IX deficiency (hemophilia B), 8 were in patients with von Willebrand disease, and 5 in patients with other coagulopathies. Antibody testing of patients with hemophilia has offered further documentation of the risk of exposure of these patients. As many as 90% of hemophilia A patients who required frequent infusion of Factor VIII concentrate have been documented to be seropositive for anti-HIV antibodies.[29] The prevalence of seroconversion in hemophilia B patients (who require Factor IX) has been lower, but in this group as well, 83% of patients with severe disease have been found to be seropositive.[30] It has become clear that there is a close association between the dose of factor concentrate required by the patient during the period before donor screening, testing, and virus inactivation and the patient's chances of having been exposed to HIV.

The situation is now substantially improved. Studies of patients who received only donor-screened, heat-treated coagulation factor products have failed to demonstrate seroconversion in these patients.[31] In addition to heat inactivation, a chemical inactivation method has also been developed that shows great promise in preventing HIV transmission.[32] Unfortunately these methods have not been used for a long enough time to provide absolute answers about the extent to which the risk of HIV infection has been reduced. These products do, however, show indication of providing safe coagulation Factor VIII and IX products for hemophilia A and B patients, and are the recommended therapy at the present time.[31]

THE CONCERNS AND RIGHTS OF TRANSFUSION RECIPIENTS

Despite the current low risk of developing HIV infection or AIDS from the transfusion of whole blood, its components, or plasma derivatives, many persons who require these therapies are gravely concerned about possible exposure to this deadly disease. The extensive public awareness that AIDS could be contracted from transfusion has led to an understandable fear that grips patients who contemplate surgery, require transfusion for other reasons, or require treatment with coagulation products. Hemophiliacs may be among the most fearful recipients and may be inclined to postpone needed therapy during a bleeding episode or to refuse surgery that can only be undertaken with concurrent administration of coagulation factor concentrate. Concerns about transfusion safety have led physicians to be more cautious when ordering transfusion therapy. Although these changes are welcome in that they can improve the utilization of blood products, they may also go too far and compromise patient care. For example, those who truly need transfusion may refuse it, or may refuse or delay needed surgery. Thus, the problems faced by physicians when caring for patients who do or may require transfusion have been enormously increased by the need to more fully explain the reasons for the transfusion, the options available to the patient, and the relative risks and benefits of these options. The risks of homologous transfusion of blood and components from volunteer donors have been detailed above, as have those of blood derivatives. Patients need this information to make a reasonable decision about how to proceed. It is important for the physician to point out that some patients have an alternative to homologous blood transfusion—that is, autologous transfusion—and when that option is available it should be exercised. In addition, physicians may be confronted with patients who require homologous transfusion but cannot be convinced as to the safety of the volunteer donor blood that provides the community blood supply, and instead demand the right to select their own donors—that is, directed donors. Here again the physician is called upon to explain the relative benefits and risks of a patient selected donor source. These alternative donor sources are described in the following sections.

Autologous Transfusion

It has long been recognized by transfusionists that the safest blood for transfusion is the patient's own blood (i.e., autologous blood). Unlike homologous transfusion (i.e., blood from another person), there is no risk of viral or protozoal infection transmission from the donor, since patient and donor are one and the same. The only infection risk is that related to the potential bacterial contamination of the unit, which should be no more than the almost-zero risk of this occurring from homologous transfusion if appropriate precautions are observed. In addition, sensitization to foreign antigens in blood or on the cells of a homologous donor is prevented. There are two categories of autologous transfusion: predeposit donation prior to an elective surgical procedure, and intraoperative autotransfusion of blood collected from the body cavity or wound, processed, and then returned to the patient. When possible autologous donation of whole blood by patients scheduled to undergo elective surgery is recommended, as is intraoperative salvage of blood when appropriate.

Predeposit Autologous Transfusion

The safety and efficacy of predeposit autologous transfusion has been demonstrated by extensive clinical experience,[33,34] although no prospective, controlled, double-blind studies have been done to prove this point. The advantages of autologous transfusion are considered so apparent and so well established that it is unlikely that such a randomized controlled trial will ever be conducted. The major risk of autologous transfusion is administrative error. How often this occurs is not known, but extensive precautions must be taken to prevent it. Blood collected before surgery is primarily for red cell replacement, and only rarely are platelets or plasma prepared for the patient. Many patients who are scheduled for elective surgery are stable enough before surgery to serve as autologous donors. The age limit for donation is established by the collecting facility; usually, many patients, both young and old, can be considered for autologous donation as long as they have sufficiently good veins to collect the blood, have a hematocrit of 34, are not suffering from serious cardiac disease, and are not considered by their physician at risk of being impaired by having undergone phlebotomy in the immediate pre-operative period. Blood can be collected every 72 hours as long as the hematocrit remains acceptable. The last predeposit donation is usually collected 72 hours before the surgery to permit time for volume restoration and stabilization of the patient. For patients requiring more than four units of blood, storage in the frozen state can be arranged. Frozen blood has a storage life of 3 years.

At the Hospital for Special Surgery (HSS) in New York City, three thousand autologous units of blood have been transfused during or after surgery. This hospital specializes in the care of patients with orthopedic and rheumatic diseases, almost all surgery is elective, and most patients are medically stable. Orthopedic patients are prime candidates for this form of transfusion. The autologous transfusion program at HSS has been a striking success, as evidenced by the fact that more than half of all transfusions are now from autologous sources. Both patients and physicians have accepted the program wholeheartedly.

It is important to emphasize that, to be successful, a predeposit autologous transfusion program requires close cooperation between attending physicians, surgeons, and blood bank staff. Patients must be informed of the procedure and its ramifications. They must be made aware that no matter how many units of blood are drawn before surgery, conditions at the time of surgery may require the use of additional blood. In this case the surgeon must have a free hand to transfuse homologous blood. The autologous blood is tested in the same way as all donated blood. Since this includes the test for the antibody to HIV, the patient should be willing to give up confidentiality in that the surgeon and referring physician should be informed of positive test results. The process is somewhat cumbersome and time consuming, but most patients readily accept such inconvenience to be assured of greater blood safety.

"Speculative" Storage of Frozen Autologous Blood

The fear of AIDS from blood transfusion has generated such intense concern in some individuals that a new form of autologous donation has developed in which healthy people store blood in the frozen state in case of future need. It has been termed "speculative" storage of frozen autologous blood. Several commercial enterprises have developed in the United States to cater to these fears by providing long-term frozen storage of autologous blood, and a few non-profit institutions are also offering this form of blood storage for persons who desire it. Most transfusionists do not recommend this form of blood donation and storage because of the small likelihood that the person will need the blood within the storage time limit, and the fact that, if the person does need transfusions, they will most likely be required in an emergency situation. The processes of locating, thawing, transporting, and crossmatching a frozen autologous unit can take many hours. Depending on how close the patient is to the frozen unit, it can take from a minimum of 4–6 hours to more than 24 hours for the unit to reach the patient. In emergency situations this delay is unacceptable, and there is concern that persons may be misled into feeling a false sense of security that they will not receive homologous transfusion because they have stored autologous blood. These services are also very costly to the individual, reaching several hundreds of dollars a year, without providing a real health benefit. A comment about these programs is included here for completeness, not as an endorsement.

Intraoperative Autotransfusion

The process of collecting blood that has been shed from a wound or into a body cavity is termed "intraoperative autotransfusion." After collection, the blood is processed by filtration and reinfused into the patient as whole blood, or is washed prior to reinfusion. Patients eligible for intraoperative autotransfusion include those who have suffered trauma[35,36] and those undergoing a variety of surgical interventions, including cardiovascular surgery,[37,38] vascular procedures, hip replacement, spinal surgery,[39] and several others. Intraoperative autotransfusion is contraindicated in situations in which blood is exposed to bacteria or malignant cells.[40] Increased use of intraoperative autotransfusion in appropriate situations can be expected to occur both because of its ability to reduce the risks of homologous transfusions and its cost effectiveness.[40]

Directed Donations

Fearing transmission of AIDS, patients frequently request, even demand, that they choose their own blood donors. Many patients are persuaded by the seeming logic that a known friend or relative would be a much safer donor than the unknown and anonymous volunteer blood donor. But, in fact, the question arises whether the directed donor, under these circumstances, can be as truthful about his "risk" status as the volunteer donor.

The true volunteer donor has no incentive to donate blood other than to help his fellow man. The community-recruited donor is not paid, receives no material reward, and, not knowing the recipient, does not even receive gratitude directly from a patient. The donor is recruited individually or as a member of a donor group. Community-recruited donors are, as noted earlier, even given the opportunity to donate blood but may prevent its being transfused, by confidentially designating its use for laboratory studies. All these measures are for the purpose of eliminating blood donations from people who are in high-risk groups and may have been exposed to the AIDS virus.[41]

In contrast, the donor selected by a patient, the potential recipient, is chosen for the very reason that the patient and donor know each other. There is at least an implied obligation that the person give blood. If the donor has personal reasons that should cause him to exclude himself, he may not dare to do so for fear of arousing suspicion that he may be in a high-risk group. Since the practices of high-risk groups are socially unacceptable to many people, candor is often sacrificed. There is a real risk that persons in risk groups will feel compelled to donate, hoping that they will test negative. The data available from San Francisco, where almost 12,000 directed donors were compared with a similar number of community recruited donors, suggests that the number of confirmed HIV antibody positives is by no means less in the directed group than in those recruited on a community-wide basis.[42] In fact, the hepatitis markers were found to be higher in the directed-donor group.

Another good reason for patients to avoid transfusions from genetically related donors is that they may cause sensitization to human leukocyte antigens (HLA). For the patient, this may render transplants more difficult if needed in the future. The same warning with respect to exposure to genetically related designated donors applies to patients receiving chemotherapy. They may require HLA-matched platelet transfusions in the future, and sensitization from prior transfusion from these donors will preclude their serving as a matched platelet donor.

Physicians confronted by a patient who does demand directed donations may be unable to dissuade the patient.[42] The provision of directed donors has been viewed by some as a patient's rights issue, and in such cases it may be necessary for the physician to accede to the patient's demand.[43] In this situation, informed consent should be obtained from the patient. Also, donors to the patient should be made aware that they have lost their confidentiality should an infectious post-transfusion illness develop in the recipient. Directed donors are potentially liable to direct litigation by a transfusion recipient, whereas the confidentiality of community volunteer donors is vigorously protected by blood banks throughout the United States.

It is clear that physicians bear a significant responsibility when transfusing blood or blood products, as will be expanded on below; but this responsibility is a shared one.

RESPONSIBILITY OF HOSPITALS

Hospitals have a legal and moral responsibility to ensure that procedures to assure safety of the transfusions are in place in the institution. Some transmission of AIDS by transfusion was unavoidable before the disease was described and before its mode of transmission was clarified; now, however, that risk can be reduced to a minimum. To ensure the safety of the hospital's blood supply; the hospital must monitor the performance of the Transfusion Service and its Director and be certain that blood transfused at the hospital is from the safest available sources. Only true unpaid volunteer donors should be accepted. There should be no material incentive of any kind to the donor. If blood is collected in-hospital, procedures to protect the anonymity of the donor must be in place. Directed donors should be informed of the inability to provide this protection. Most blood is obtained from a blood center, and the hospital should be informed about the procedures in use at the center that serves it. Hospitals, through their lay boards or administration, should not exert pressure on transfusion committees or Transfusion Service Directors to encourage designated or directed donors, since this practice may in fact increase risks to patients. If a directed-donor program is established as hospital policy, it should be available to all patients who request it, either through the hospital blood bank or the regional blood center serving the hospital. If directed donations are accepted, they should be accepted only after appropriate informed consent from the recipient and donor is received. It is strongly recommended that directed donations not be released to other than the designated recipient unless informed consent is also received from any other recipient of the product.

Hospitals should also cooperate in promoting follow-up of transfused patients in the Lookback program, who may have been exposed to HIV. To do this job well means expenditure of time, effort, and money.

PROFESSIONAL ORGANIZATIONS

The American Association of Blood Banks (AABB), American National Red Cross (ANRC), Council of Community Blood Centers (CCBC), American Blood Commission, American Medical Association, and National Hemophilia Foundation have all, from the beginning of the AIDS crisis, worked to contain the spread of AIDS by transfusion. Federal and local standards have been established that require tests for the antibody to HIV on all donors since the spring of 1985, when these tests were first licensed. These standards have been backed up by strict inspection and accreditation programs by licensing agencies and by professional organizations. Recently, surrogate testing to prevent the most common complication of blood transfusion—non-A, non-B hepatitis—has also been widely introduced, using ALT testing and hepatitis B core antibody testing of donated blood. Thus, AABB, ANRC, and CCBC blood banks routinely test for HBsAg, Hepatitis B core antibody, ALT, HIV antibody, and syphilis. Strict rules are in force to maintain donor confidentiality to assure candor with respect to possible exposure to infection. These organizations all have developed extensive educational material directed to the physician to advocate judicious use of transfusions to meet the actual needs of the patient. Through the professional organizations, Blood Bank and Transfusion Service Directors are kept appraised of new developments in donor screening and testing procedures. The organizations also seek to inform donors, patients, physicians, and the public and to present the most current and realistic picture with respect to transfusion-associated AIDS.

The organizations have advisory committees through which they repeatedly make experts available for advice and testimony to governmental bodies such as Congress, the CDC, the FDA, and the National Institutes of Health, as well as Federal and state agencies.

The American Medical Association as well as state and county medical societies also plays an active role in encouraging proper blood utilization, supporting autologous transfusion, and discouraging directed transfusion.

RESPONSIBILITY OF THE PHYSICIAN

In the last analysis, the penultimate consumer of blood and blood products is the patient's physician. It is to his physician that the patient will turn for advice and counsel, and it is to the physician that he will bring his questions and concerns. The last section summarizes the physician's responsibilities.

The physician should be aware of the risks of transfusion versus the benefits. Exaggeration of the incidence of transfusion-related AIDS may unnecessarily deprive a patient of needed blood products. Cancer surgery, chemotherapy, surgery to correct debilitating disease, or correction of coagulation factor deficiencies, may be essential and justify the risks of transfusion. The physician should explain these risks and benefits to the patient, and assure the patient that he or she, too, is conscious of the risks and will carefully consider the need for each unit transfused. By knowing that blood components came from carefully screened donors whose blood has been tested and found negative for antibody to HIV, the physician can give reasonable assurance of the safety of the blood components to be transfused. Similarly, the hemophiliac can be assured that coagulation factor concentrates now come from screened and tested donors and that the product is treated to inactivate viruses, rendering it as safe as possible. Physicians can in good conscience assure patients that transfusions in the late 1980s are given with greater discretion and are far safer than in the beginning of the decade.

To further improve patient safety, predeposit autologous transfusions should be offered whenever appropriate. This entails extra effort on the part of the physician. Surgery must be planned far enough ahead to collect sufficient blood and soon enough for blood not to have become outdated. The physician must also be aware of the autologous donor's medical history and be sure that the patient can tolerate phlebotomy on an ambulatory basis. Although it may be true that if a patient is cleared for surgery he or she should be able to tolerate the loss of a unit of blood, there is a difference in that the patient undergoing surgery is constantly monitored. That is not the case with blood donation in a blood bank. Whenever possible, intraoperative autologous transfusion should be employed by surgeons.

If confronted with a patient demanding directed donors, the physician also has to educate the patient why designation of his or her own donors does not contribute to safety but may in fact lead to other adverse effects discussed above. When necessary, the physician may have to acquiesce to the patient's demands.

Finally, all physicians who transfused patients in the early 1980s are concerned with the problem of recipients whose only apparent exposure to AIDS was through transfusion. Patients who received very few units in the earliest years are at least risk, while those who were massively transfused in 1983–85 are at far greater risk.[23] For those most anxious and at most risk, the test for antibody to HIV should be offered. Patients with negative results can be reassured, as can their sexual partners and families. Patients who test positive need counseling as to their chances for developing AIDS in the future, and they must be advised about safer sexual practices. In particular, women contemplating pregnancy must be informed that if they harbor the virus it may be transmitted to the child.

Patients' physicians have also been called upon to

participate in the Lookback Program. It is they who must decide whether the patient should be told of his potential exposure. Such information may do harm in a moribund individual. No useful purpose will be served if the patient will not live long enough to develop the disease and if he is unable to infect others. In the healthy, sexually active, infected patient, every effort should be made to protect sexual partners. Testing of these partners and counseling should be offered. In these situations, physicians may be able to avail themselves of the services of experienced and knowledgeable social workers, psychiatrists, or psychologists who can continue a program of follow-up and counseling, and should determine the resources that are available. Despite its rarity as a transfusion-transmissible disease, AIDS has significantly altered every aspect of transfusion medicine and promises to continue to do so in the foreseeable future.

REFERENCES

1. Zuckerman AJ: The chronicle of viral hepatitis. Abstr. Hygiene 54:1113, 1979
2. Beeson PB: Jaundice occurring one to four months after transfusion of blood or plasma: Report of seven cases. JAMA 121:1332, 1943
3. Neefe JR, Norris RF, Reinhold JG, et al: Carriers of hepatitis virus in the blood and viral hepatitis in whole blood recipients: Studies of donors suspected as carriers of hepatitis virus and as sources of post-transfusion viral hepatitis. JAMA 154:1066, 1954
4. Murray R, Diefenbach WCL, Ratner F, et al: Carriers of hepatitis virus in the blood and viral hepatitis in whole blood recipients: Confirmation of carrier state by transmission experiments to volunteers. JAMA 154:1072, 1954
5. Allen JG, Saynor WA: Serum hepatitis from transfusions of blood. JAMA 180:1079, 1962
6. Alter HJ, Holland PV, Purcell RH, et al: Post-transfusion hepatitis after exclusion of commercial and hepatitis B–antigen-positive donors. Ann Int Med 77:691, 1972
7. Bove JR: Transfusion-associated hepatitis and AIDS: What is the risk? N Engl J Med 317:242, 1987
8. A cluster of Kaposi's sarcoma and *Pneumocystis carinii* pneumonia among homosexual male residents of Los Angeles and Orange Counties, California. MMWR 31:305, 1982
9. Update on acquired immune deficiency (AIDS)—United States. MMWR 31:507, 1987
10. *Pneumocystis carinii* pneumonia among persons with hemophilia A. MMWR 31:365, 1982
11. Pindyck J, Waldman A, Zang E, et al: Measures to decrease the risk of acquired immunodeficiency syndrome transmission by blood transfusion: Evidence of volunteer blood donor cooperation. Transfusion 25:3, 1985
12. Dahlke MB: Designated blood donations (letter). N Engl J Med 310:1195, 1984
13. Pindyck J, Avorn J, Cleary P, et al: Notification of anti-LAV/HTLV-III positive blood donors: Psychosocial, counseling and care issues. In Petricciani JE, Gust ID, Hoppe PA, et al (eds): AIDS: The Safety of Blood and Blood Products, p 275. New York, World Health Organization, John Wiley & Sons, 1987
14. Nusbacher J, Chiavetta J, Naiman R, et al: Evaluation of a confidential method of excluding blood donors exposed to human immunodeficiency virus. Transfusion 26:539, 1986
15. Kuhne P, Seidl S, Holzberger G: HLA DR4 antibodies cause positive-HTLV-III antibody ELISA results (letter). Lancet i:1222, 1985
16. Fang CT, Darr F, Kleinnan P, et al: Relative specificity of enzyme-linked immunosorbent assays for antibodies to human T-lymphotropic virus, type III, and their relationship to Western blot. Transfusion 26:208, 1986
17. Human Immunodeficiency Virus (HIV). Biotech/Dupont HIV Western blot kit for detection of antibodies to HIV. Manufacturer's instructions.
18. Schorr JB, Berkowitz A, Cumming PD, et al: Prevalence of HTLV-III antibody in American blood donors (letter). N Engl J Med 313:384, 1985
19. Cooper DA, Imrie AA, Penny R: Antibody response to human immunodeficiency virus after primary infection. J Infect Dis 55:1113, 1987
20. Marlink RG, Allen JG, McLane MF, et al: Low sensitivity of ELISA testing in early HIV infection (letter). N Engl J Med 315:1549, 1986
21. Menitove JE: Status of recipients of blood from donors subsequently found to have antibody to HIV. N Engl J Med 315:1095, 1986
22. Pindyck J: Unpublished observations
23. Human immunodeficiency virus infection in transfusion recipients and their family members. MMWR 36:137, 1987
24. Transfusion-associated human T-lymphotropic virus type III/lymphadenopathy-associated virus infection from a seronegative donor—Colorado. MMWR 35:389, 1986
25. Collins JA: Hemorrhage, shock and burns: Pathophysiology and treatment. In Petz LD, Swisher SN (eds): Clinical Practice of Blood Transfusion, p 425. New York, Churchill Livingstone, 1981
26. Virgilio RW, Rice CL, Smith DE, et al: Crystalloid vs colloid resuscitation: Is one better? Surgery 85:129, 1981
27. Wells MA, Wittek AE, Epstein JD, et al: Inactivation and partitioning of human T-cell lymphotropic virus type III during ethanol fractionation of plasma. Transfusion 26:210, 1986
28. Zuck TF, Preston MS, Tankersley DL, et al: More partitioning and inactivation of AIDS virus in immune globulin preparations (letter). N Engl J Med 314:1454, 1986
29. Goldert JJ, Sarngadharan MG, Eyster ME, et al: Antibodies reactive with human T-cell leukemia viruses in the serum of hemophiliacs receiving Factor VIII concentrate. Blood 65:492, 1985
30. Jason J, McDougal JS, Holman RC, et al: Human T-lymphotropic retrovirus type III/lymphadenopathy-associated virus antibody: association with hemophiliacs' immune status and blood component usage. JAMA 253:3409, 1985
31. Survey of non-U.S. hemophilia treatment centers for HIV seroconversions following therapy with heat-treated factor concentrates. MMWR 36:121, 1987
32. Prince AM, Horowitz B, Brothman B: Sterilization of hepatitis and HTLV-III viruses by exposure to tri (n-butyl) phosphate and sodium chlorate. Lancet i:706, 1986
33. Mann M, Sacks HG, Goldfinger D: Safety of autologous blood donation prior to elective surgery for a variety of potentially "high risk" patients. Transfusion 23:229, 1983
34. Milles G, Browne WH, Barrick RG: Autologous transfusions for elective caesarean section. Am J Obstet Gynecol 103:1166, 1969

35. Mattox KL: Autotransfusion in an emergency department. J Am Coll Emerg Phys 4:218, 1975

36. Carter RF, McArdle B, Morrett GM: Autologous transfusion of mediastinal drainage blood. Anesthesia 36:54, 1981

37. Cordell AR, Lavender SW: An appraisal of blood salvage techniques in vascular and cardiac operations. Ann Thorac Surg 31:421, 1981

38. Johnson RG, Rosenkrantz KR, Preston RA, et al: The efficacy of postoperative autotransfusion in patients undergoing cardiac operations. Ann Thorac Surg 36:173, 1983

39. Young JN, Ecker RA, Moretti RL, et al: Autologous blood retrieval in thoracic, cardiovascular, and orthopedic surgery. Am J Surg 144:48, 1982

40. Council on Scientific Affairs, American Medical Association: Autologous blood transfusions. JAMA 256:2378, 1986

41. Mayer K: The community: Still the best source of blood. Hastings Center Report, p 5, April 1987

42. Cordell RR, Yalon VA, Cigahn-Haskell C, et al: Experience with 11,916 designated donors. Transfusion 26:484, 1986

43. Reiss RF, Pindyck J: Reconciling patients' wishes with the public good. Hastings Center Report, p 9, April 1987

Transmission of Human Immunodeficiency Virus among Intravenous Drug Users

Don C. Des Jarlais
Samuel R. Friedman

24

Intravenous drug users are a critical group in the AIDS epidemic in the United States and Europe. They are the second largest group to have developed AIDS. Intravenous (IV) drug use is a risk factor in 10,762/44,795 (24%) of the adult cases in the United States (data through 1 December 1986).[1] Among these patients, 7368 (16%) had IV drug use as their primary risk behavior and another 3394 (8%) also had both male homosexual activity and IV drug use as risk behaviors. In Europe, 1315/6700 (20%) of the adult patients had IV drug use as a risk behavior, 1136 (17%) with IV drug use as their primary risk behavior, and 179 (3%) with both IV drug use and male homosexuality as risk behaviors (data through 30 June 1987).[2] The percentage of American AIDS patients in whom IV drug use was the risk behavior has been quite stable over the last several years. The percentage of European cases attributable to IV drug use has been increasing rapidly—in September 1984, only 2% of adult European cases had IV drug use as the primary risk behavior; in September 1985, 6%; and in September 1986, 13%.

In addition to spreading human immunodeficiency virus (HIV) among themselves, IV drug users are an important source for spread of the virus to their non–drug-injecting heterosexual partners and their newborn children. In New York City, IV drug users are the apparent source of the virus in 93% of the cases in which heterosexual activity is believed to be the mode of transmission and in 80% of the cases of maternally transmitted AIDS.[3] Control of the AIDS epidemic in the United States and Europe will thus require control of HIV infection among intravenous drug users.

The purpose of this chapter is to review the potential for control of the transmission of HIV among IV drug users and their sexual partners. The transmission of HIV among IV drug users and their sexual partners is highly social behavior—it occurs through the sharing of drug injection equipment and through intimate sexual activity. We will first outline some of the major components of the social organization that has contributed to the rapid spread of HIV in some geographic areas and serves as the context within which AIDS prevention efforts will occur. We will then briefly examine the current geographic variation in HIV seroprevalence rates among IV drug users, the potential for rapid spread within a geographic area, and the behavioral factors that have been associated with spread within a local geographic area. The next sections will examine three different AIDS prevention strategies for IV drug users and the current findings regarding the effectiveness of each. Finally, we will discuss certain aspects of the natural history of HIV infection among IV drug users that are relevant to prevention efforts. (The natural history of HIV infection is examined in more detail in other sections of this volume.)

SOCIAL ORGANIZATION OF IV DRUG USE

Because there are very few formal organizations of IV drug users there is a common misperception of IV drug users as not organized. A multi-billion-dollar industry such as the illicit drug trade does not persist over time without social organization.* Sociologists and anthropologists have conceptualized the organization of IV drug use as a "deviant subculture"[4,5,6] with shared values,

---

* Much of the research on the behavior of IV drug users has been conducted in New York City, simply because New York has always had more IV drug users than any other American or European city. Hence, much of this section will be based on studies conducted in New York. There is important variation in different geographic/cultural areas. Full consideration of this variation is beyond the scope of this chapter, but we will note particular sources of variation that are directly relevant to the spread of HIV among IV drug users and their sexual partners.

a common argot, and rules for allocating status. The primary value is "getting high" and the primary basis for having high status within the group is the ability to obtain and use large quantities of high-quality drugs while minimizing adverse social, legal and health consequences of such drug use.

There is strong, often brutal, competition within the IV drug use subculture. There is competition for customers among persons distributing the illicit drugs for injection, and competition between dealers and customers over the price and quality of the drugs being sold. Among IV drug users there is competition for the money needed to purchase drugs, for access to the limited supply of drugs, and sometimes even for the equipment needed to inject the drugs. The illegal status of the drugs keeps prices high, reinforcing economic competition and often leading to a reliance on illegal methods of obtaining money to purchase drugs. The illegal nature of IV drug use also leads to a reliance on threatened or actual violence as the means for resolving disputes.

As will be discussed later, this multi-faceted competition within the IV drug use subculture creates great obstacles to self-organization among IV drug users to take collective action to promote AIDS risk reduction. The intensity of the competition within the group appears related to the extent that IV drug use is criminalized within a society. The greater the law enforcement pressure on IV drug users, the greater the mistrust and competition within the group.

The IV drug use subculture would not be able to persist over time without some positive social relationships to balance the mistrusting, often violent, interactions associated with the illegal nature of IV drug use. There is some degree of common identity as persons allied against "straight" (conventional) society. This encourages the sharing of information about drug availability, about actions of the police, and about new developments that affect the group. This sharing of information is almost totally oral, with very little communication through written or broadcast material. The oral information network often spreads inaccurate news, but is efficient enough to maintain the substantial economic scale of IV drug use in the United States, Europe, and several developing countries.

The primary positive social relationship within the IV drug use subculture is the small friendship group. The high price and limited supply of drugs makes it effective for IV drug users to work together in pairs or small groups to obtain money and drugs. Teamwork provides more opportunities for obtaining money and protection against others who might use force against one. Sharing resources within a friendship group provides a greater likelihood that an individual IV drug user will be able to obtain drugs on any given day.

The social structure of the IV drug subculture promotes the sharing of equipment for injecting drugs in two ways. The ethic of cooperation within small friendship groups is applied to the sharing of the equipment for injecting drugs. To refuse to share drug injection equipment within the small friendship group (without a socially legitimated reason) would call into question the reliability of the person with respect to other cooperative actions.

Limited supplies of drug injection equipment can also lead to sharing among casual acquaintances or complete strangers. Legal restrictions on the sale of needles and syringes, refusal of pharmacists to sell them even when they are permitted to do so, and laws against the possession of narcotics paraphernalia all serve to reduce the availability of sterile equipment for injecting illicit drugs. Even where there are no legal restrictions on drug injection equipment, sterile equipment is often not available at the times and places where IV drug users want to inject.

Persons who have drugs to inject but do not have injection equipment readily available may borrow equipment from acquaintances, sometimes in trade for a small quantity of the drug. Such sharing contains elements of both social solidarity and economic cooperation.

The widest possible sharing occurs through the use of "shooting galleries" or "house works." Shooting galleries are places where one can rent drug injection equipment for a small fee (typically $1 or $2 in New York City). After use, the equipment is returned to the proprietor of the shooting gallery for rental to the next customer. The needle and syringe are used until they become clogged or the needle too dull for further use. Thus the virus can be transmitted among large numbers of IV drug users who do not even know each other. This breaks the limited protection that would occur if sharing occurred only within friendship groups. Shooting galleries are typically located in or near "copping areas" (places where illicit drugs can be easily purchased).

Shooting galleries, as a specialized economic activity, are most often found in areas that have very large numbers of IV drug users. Areas with relatively few IV drug users generally cannot support shooting galleries, but these areas will usually have a functional equivalent to shooting galleries with respect to HIV transmission. "House works" are an extra set of drug injection equipment that a small scale "dealer" (drug distributor) will maintain for lending to customers. These works are then returned to the dealer for lending to the next customer who wants to borrow them.

Both shooting galleries and house works provide the opportunity to inject very soon after the drugs have been obtained. This temporal proximity may be a critical variable in reducing the sharing of drug injection equipment. Currently addicted heroin users often have entered withdrawal by the time they obtain their next dose of the drug (the duration of action of injected heroin in an addicted person is typically 4 to 6 hours). Through classical conditioning, the possession of heroin can in itself trigger withdrawal symptoms in a very experienced heroin user.[7] Withdrawal from heroin is not life-threatening but is extremely unpleasant both physically and psychologically. Relief from this distress is almost instantaneous with the injection of heroin. IV drug users report that almost all of them will use whatever injection equipment is readily available when possessing heroin and experiencing withdrawal.[4]

Two aspects of sexual behavior are of particular importance for the transmission of HIV. The first is the sex ratio among IV drug users in the United States and Western Europe. There are approximately three male IV drug users for every female IV drug user. Thus, most male IV drug users will have to seek their primary sexual relationship with a female who does not inject drugs, leading to a large number of females who do not inject drugs but are at risk for sexually transmitted HIV infection from a male IV drug user. Estimates from New York suggest that the number of females who do not inject drugs themselves but are regular sexual partners of male IV drug users is more than half the total number of IV drug users.[8] Rather than thinking that IV drug users have their primary sexual relationships only with other IV drug users, it would be better to use an analogy with heavy alcohol users. Just as the wives of alcoholics are not likely to be alcoholics themselves, the regular sexual partners of male IV drug users are also not likely to be injecting drugs themselves.

These female sexual partners not only provide a very important psychological relationship for the IV drug user, they often provide needed food, shelter, clothing and money. Thus, the IV drug user usually can ill afford to have the relationship end, and, as will be discussed later, there are special problems in the prevention of heterosexual transmission from IV drug users to regular sexual partners who do not inject drugs.

The second aspect of sexual behavior in the IV drug use subculture that has important implications for the transmission of HIV is prostitution. The selling of sexual services for money to purchase drugs is quite common among female IV drug users. In New York, an estimated one-half of the "street" prostitutes have histories of injecting drugs.[9] Estimates for other cities are not readily available, but there is substantial drug injection among female prostitutes in other American cities[10] and in European cities, such as Amsterdam[11] and Berlin.[12]

Many male IV drug users also sell sexual services, although this is much less well documented. From our observations in New York, much of this occurs without any self-labeling by the IV drug user as a "prostitute" (or as "gay" or "homosexual" even if male-to-male sex is involved).

The potential extent of HIV transmission from prostitutes to their customers in the United States and Europe is currently a matter of intense study, without definitive results. There are clearly many sexual encounters between HIV-infected prostitutes and customers, but there are not yet sufficient data to determine the likelihood of transmission. In New York City, which probably has more HIV-infected prostitutes than any other American or European city, there have been very few cases of AIDS in which contact with a prostitute was the likely source of infection.[9] This may be a result of prostitutes' using specific sexual practices that are unlikely to involve viral transmission. There is probably substantial geographic variation in the frequency of these practices. This is one topic where many local studies will be needed before any conclusions can be safely drawn.

In sum, prior to concern about AIDS, the sharing of drug injection equipment was "normal" behavior among IV drug users. There were many reasons for sharing, from the social norms within the small friendship groups to the greater availability of used equipment when a person had drugs to inject. Although there was some concern about hepatitis, there were no overriding reasons not to share drug injection equipment. The potential for sexual transmission of a virus from IV drug users to persons who did not inject drugs was also a "normal" part of the IV drug use subculture prior to AIDS. These sexual relationships included both relatively long-term interpersonal commitments and transactions for the sole purpose of earning money.

CURRENT EXTENT OF HIV INFECTION AMONG IV DRUG USERS

There are wide variations in seroprevalence rates among IV drug users studied in different locations. In the United States, the New York City–northern New Jersey area clearly has the highest seroprevalence rate. Most studies from this area show seroprevalence rates of 50% or higher.[13,14] Other cities in the Northeast (e.g., Boston,[15] New Haven[16]) tend to have moderate seroprevalence rates—between 20% and 30%. Cities on the West Coast and in the Southeast tend to have lower rates; for example, Los Angeles[17] and New Orleans[18] at less than 5%, San Francisco at 16%.[19,20]

Studies of HIV seroprevalence among IV drug users in Europe also show a wide range. There is a general north-south difference, with higher rates among IV drug users in southern Europe. Italy[21,22] and Spain[23,24] have reported very high rates—approaching 70% in some cities. Rates in Germany,[25] Switzerland,[26] and Holland[11] tend to be in the 25% to 50% range. Low rates, under 10% seropositive, have been reported from London[27] and Glasgow,[28] though Edinburgh has a rate over 50%.[28]

Explaining the great differences in HIV seroprevalence rates within the United States and Europe is a major problem in the epidemiology of HIV among IV drug users. Part of the explanation clearly is the date of first introduction of the virus into the local group of IV drug users. Analysis of historically collected sera from IV drug users show that the first seropositive sample from New York City was collected in 1978,[29] from northern Italy in 1979,[22] from the Federal Republic of Germany in 1982,[30] and from Denmark in 1984.[31]

The studies of historically collected sera also show that, once the virus has been introduced into a local community of IV drug users, very rapid spread is possible. In southern Manhattan, seroprevalence rose to over 40% by 2 years after the first seropositive sample.[29] In Edinburgh, seroprevalence rose to approximately 50% within 2 years of the first seropositive sample,[32] and in Milan to approximately 50% within 4 years after the first seropositive sample.[22] Thus, a currently low seroprevalence rate is no guarantee that the rate will not rise substantially in several years.

Only a few studies have examined the behavioral factors associated with sharing of injection equipment and HIV seropositivity.[11,19,33,34,36] Most of these have been conducted in the New York City area, so that caution is needed in making any generalizations across geographic areas.

The frequency of drug injection was associated with seropositivity in the three studies from the New York area.[33,34,35] Greater levels of drug injection were associated with a greater likelihood of having used contaminated equipment.

The second behavioral factor that has been associated with HIV exposure in different studies has been the use of "shooting galleries" as a place to inject drugs.[33,34,37] As noted above, shooting galleries provide for sharing drug injection equipment with large numbers of other drug users.

Although IV drug users are at risk for infection with HIV from sexual activity, there is little evidence that sexual behavior is an important source of infection in the group. One study did find that homosexual activity was related to HIV seropositivity among male IV drug users,[13] but this may reflect homosexual IV drug users serving as a bridge between HIV infection in gay men and in heterosexual IV drug users in New York City. Two studies[9,37] found prostitutes to have higher seropositivity rates, though in the first of these prostitution was not significant in a multivariate analysis.

Studies in New York,[13,35] Connecticut,[16] and San Francisco[19] found higher rates among blacks and hispanics than whites, but in one of these statistical significance was lost in the multivariate analysis, and a second study from San Francisco[20] did not find ethnic differences.* Europe, with groups of *gastarbeiters* and relatively easy travel across national boundaries, also has the potential for ethnic differences in seroprevalence rates within a single geographic location. One study from Amsterdam[11] did find that German IV drug users in that city had higher seroprevalence rates. The sharing of drug injection equipment, like many other forms of social behavior, may be subject to social segregation by ethnic groups. To date, however, the findings on ethnicity as a predictor of seroprevalence are inconsistent. This may reflect a higher degree of ethnic integration within the IV drug use subculture than in Western societies as a whole. Further research on the relationships between HIV seroprevalence and ethnicity are needed, however, since ethnic and cross-national concerns will be very relevant to mounting effective AIDS prevention programs.

Despite the wide variation in seroprevalence rates in the United States and Western Europe, the risk factor studies conducted to date show a limited number of behavioral factors that are typically associated with HIV exposure. Frequency of drug injection and use of shooting galleries (sharing equipment with large numbers of other IV drug users) appear to be associated with HIV exposure, suggesting that effective prevention programs need to focus on reducing these two factors. Belonging to an ethnic minority group among which the incidence of IV drug use is high and engaging in prostitution may be additional risk factors, indicating the need for prevention programs that include special components for prostitutes and incorporate ethnic differences. Before considering prevention strategies, however, it is necessary to consider the question of whether IV drug users are capable of changing AIDS-related risk behavior.

AIDS PREVENTION FOR IV DRUG USERS

The potential for rapid spread of the virus among IV drug users in a local area suggests urgency is needed in attempts to prevent HIV infection among current IV drug users. In considering AIDS prevention among IV drug users, it is imperative to avoid simplistic solutions. The IV drug use subculture is characterized by a mutual hostility with the dominant society, and a balance of antagonistic competition within the subculture as a whole and intense solidarity among small groups of IV drug users. These factors will affect what types of prevention programs can be established and the effectiveness of those programs. There are also important differences among current and potential IV drug users that will require different strategies for AIDS prevention. We will consider several foci for AIDS prevention efforts among IV drug users: reduction/elimination of drug injection among current IV drug users, promoting "safer injection" among persons who are likely to continue injecting, reducing the number of persons who start injecting drugs, and promoting "safer" sexual practices in communities with high rates of IV drug use. We will relate each of these to the characteristics of the IV drug use subculture, and to the currently known risk factors for HIV infection among IV drug users.

Reducing/Eliminating Drug Injection Among Current IV Drug Users

As noted above, the frequency of injecting drugs has been consistently shown to be related to exposure to HIV. In part this is a simple probability statement (at least prior to any awareness of AIDS): the more one

---

* We will not examine the relationships among ethnic/minority status and IV drug use and HIV infection in detail in this chapter, since they are discussed in depth in the chapter on HIV epidemiology. We do wish to emphasize that the great majority of the IV drug use cases in the United States have occurred among blacks (approximately 50% of the cases) and hispanics (approximately 30% of the cases). Prevention of further HIV infection among IV drug users in the United States will undoubtedly require consideration of a number of issues related to ethnic/racial minority status. Our concerns in this area are discussed in detail in Reference 58.

injects, the more one is likely to use contaminated equipment. A second part of this relationship is that if one is injecting to the point where one is physically addicted to heroin, the distress associated with entering withdrawal will likely lead one to use whatever injection equipment is readily available, even if one is concerned about HIV infection.[4]

Although some IV drug users can be expected to reduce or eliminate drug injection after basic AIDS education, it is likely that drug abuse treatment will be needed for many, especially those who are physically addicted. Provision of additional drug abuse treatment as an explicit means of AIDS prevention has been started in New York and New Jersey, and has been proposed for the United States as a whole,[38] and in several European countries, including the United Kingdom and Sweden. Current data indicate that substantial numbers of IV drug users will enter treatment because of their concerns about AIDS.

In New York, the demand among IV drug users for treatment was greater than the available supply even before the AIDS epidemic. Rather than being taken immediately into treatment after applying, an IV drug user typically had to wait 2 to 3 months for an open treatment position. As of the summer of 1987, approximately three thousand new treatment positions have been opened in response to the AIDS epidemic. All of those have been filled, and there is still more demand for new treatment capability. The waiting time has not been appreciably reduced. An additional five thousand treatment positions are currently planned.

New Jersey has perhaps the best documentation on entering treatment in response to concerns about AIDS. Persons coming into treatment are interviewed as to why they are entering. Approximately half of the recent entrants note fear of AIDS as one of their reasons for entering treatment. New Jersey also operates an "outreach program" that has ex-addicts working as AIDS educators in neighborhoods where drug use is high. Among other AIDS prevention activities, the outreach workers have been distributing coupons that can be redeemed for free detoxification treatment. Approximately 80% of the first 1000 thousand coupons were redeemed.[39]

Drug abuse treatment generally leads to dramatic reductions in the frequency of drug injection,[40] so that the increased willingness of IV drug users to enter treatment because of concern about AIDS indicates that providing additional treatment should be an effective means of reducing HIV infection among IV drug users. Because reducing drug injection would not only serve as a means of preventing AIDS but also would reduce the other individual and social costs associated with IV drug use, it will be a relatively popular method for AIDS prevention among the general public and some segments of the IV drug–using population. There are, however, a number of limitations on the use of drug abuse treatment as an AIDS prevention measure.

First, even though drug abuse treatment will be a relatively popular prevention measure, there are restric-

tions on its potential popularity. Drug abuse treatment tends to have widespread general support in Western societies, but can be very unpopular within a particular neighborhood. It is very susceptible to the "not in my backyard" type of community opposition. Methadone maintenance, which may be the only form of treatment for heroin addiction that can be operated on a public health scale, is particularly unpopular because of philosophical opposition to the use of a psychoactive drug to treat drug abuse. (Note also that we currently do not have any public health scale treatment for cocaine addiction.) Associating the opening of new drug abuse treatment programs with AIDS is not likely to increase the popularity of drug abuse treatment programs.

Drug abuse treatment, while generally leading to dramatic reductions in illicit drug injection, is not a perfected medical/psychological treatment. Our ability to treat heroin and cocaine injection successfully is probably not much better than our ability to treat alcohol and nicotine addiction. A single episode of treatment is not likely to be permanently effective, and even when successful, the treatment process will typically take a year or longer, with intermittent drug injection occurring during that time.

Although many IV drug users have been seeking treatment as a result of their concerns about AIDS, the great majority of current IV drug users probably still hold the value of "getting high" as primary and see entering treatment as a failure to uphold the norms of the IV drug use subculture. AIDS and the other problems associated with frequent IV drug use may eventually lead the great majority of current IV drug users to enter treatment, but there is a very real likelihood that a great number of them will become infected with HIV before they are successfully treated.

"Safer Injection" Among IV Drug Users Who Continue to Inject

Because of the limitations on providing drug abuse treatment as a means of preventing AIDS, some form of "safer injection" practices will be needed for IV drug users who do not eliminate their drug injection. Studies in New York and elsewhere indicate that IV drug users not in treatment and those who have been in treatment but continue to inject at reduced levels have been adopting "safer injection" procedures because of their concerns about AIDS.

In 1984, all of a sample of 59 methadone maintenance patients whom we interviewed had heard of AIDS; 55 (93%) of them knew that IV drug use is a mode of transmission of the disease. Fifty-nine per cent of the subjects reported some form of risk reduction to avoid AIDS; 54% reported changes in injection-related behavior. The most common changes were increased use of clean needles or the cleaning of needles, reported by 31%, and reducing needle sharing, reported by 29%. (These subjects were primarily injecting cocaine, for which methadone has no chemotherapeutic effect.) Fifty-one per cent of the group also reported that friends had changed their behaviors to avoid AIDS.[41]

In the summer of 1985, Selwyn and associates studied IV drug users in jail ($n = 115$) and methadone maintenance clients ($n = 146$) with findings remarkably similar to those from our methadone maintenance subjects.[42] Ninety seven per cent of the two Selwyn samples knew that sharing needles could transmit AIDS. Over 60% of these subjects reported risk reduction. Reducing or eliminating needle sharing was the most common form of risk reduction in both samples.

A 1986 study of IV drug users not in treatment who were interviewed in their natural "street" settings found similar results with respect to AIDS risk reduction.[43] Over 60% reported that they had changed their behavior to reduce the chances of developing AIDS.

Validation of the self-reported "safer injection" practices comes from studies of the marketing of illicit needles and syringes in New York City. These studies show evidence of a large-scale change in the demand for sterile needles and syringes for injecting drugs. In interviews with persons selling needles and syringes in the drug dealing areas of New York City in 1985, almost 90% (18/22) reported that sales had increased over the previous year.[44] The increased demand for sterile needles and syringes was strong enough to support a market in "counterfeit" sterile needles. The persons selling needles and syringes were also asked if they had ever sold used needles as new; 10/21 (48%) reported that they occasionally repackaged used equipment and then sold it as new. This "counterfeit" sterile needle phenomenon had not been observed in the city prior to AIDS, and indicates both the strength of the increased demand for sterile equipment and the hazards of relying on an illicit market for sterile drug injection equipment.

In the fall of 1985, we observed other AIDS-related changes in the marketing of needles and syringes for illicit drug injection. Some needle sellers were including an extra needle with the sale of a "set" of a needle and syringe. If the first needle gets clogged, it can immediately be replaced with the extra needle. This reduces the chances that a clogged needle would lead an IV drug user to rent or borrow a used needle. Finally, some drug dealers have been including a new set of works as a marketing device with $25 and $50 bags of heroin.[45]

The movement in New York City towards "safer injection" preceded any formal prevention efforts aimed at reducing HIV transmission among persons who continue to inject drugs. The information about AIDS was conveyed through the mass media and the oral communication networks of the drug subculture. One means for behavior change—a greater (but not perfect) supply of sterile needles and syringes—was provided by the illicit market. Social support for AIDS risk reduction appeared to be developing, in that the best predictor of AIDS risk reduction by an individual IV drug user was whether or not his or her friends were also practicing AIDS risk reduction.[41]

Officially sponsored AIDS prevention efforts aimed at movement towards "safer injection" should be able to improve on the risk reduction noted above. There is evidence from Amsterdam and San Francisco that AIDS prevention efforts aimed at "safer injection" do lead to large changes in the behavior of IV drug users. In Amsterdam, as in several other Dutch cities, a "needle exchange" has been operating as an AIDS prevention measure. The needle exchanges permit IV drug users to exchange used needles and syringes for new sterile ones at no cost. The exchange system permits safe disposal of potentially contaminated injection equipment as well as providing free injection equipment to the IV drug user. It also permits the possibility of non-threatening therapeutic contact between the IV drug user and health care workers. The needle exchanges were originally established by the Dutch *Junkiebonden* (drug users' associations) as control measures for hepatitis B prior to the AIDS epidemic. (The sale of needles and syringes without prescriptions is legal in Holland, but many pharmacists refused to sell to suspected IV drug users.) The needle exchanges have been greatly expanded by public health authorities in order to reduce the spread of HIV. The Amsterdam exchange has gone from distributing 25,000 sterile needles and syringes per year to 700,000 per year. Between 80% and 90% of the needles and syringes distributed are returned to the exchange. The increase in the needle exchange program is explicitly for AIDS control, and the increased use of the exchanges by IV drug users is attributed to their knowledge of and concern about AIDS.[46]

Needle exchange programs have also been established in the United Kingdom and Australia. It is too early to determine the scale of these programs, but the earliest reports from Liverpool and Sydney[47] indicate that they have met with acceptance from the local IV drug users.

Currently there are no needle exchange programs operating in the United States. Programs have been proposed in New York, New Jersey, California and Massachusetts but have not received enough support to be established. Opposition centers on the belief that public officials should not do anything that could be seen as encouraging IV drug use. (All of these states are among the 12 that currently require prescriptions for the sale of needles and syringes, so the degree of political support needed for a needle exchange program is relatively great.)

There are several programs in the United States that provide IV drug users with information on how to sterilize their injection equipment. Pamphlets containing such information are being distributed as part of "street outreach" programs in New York City, New Jersey, Baltimore, Washington, Chicago, and San Francisco. Most of the street outreach workers are ex-addicts who have been trained as AIDS educators. They emphasize that stopping injection is the safest way of avoiding AIDS, but also provide detailed information on sterilizing equipment prior to injection. In San Francisco and Chicago, the street outreach workers provide small bottles of bleach that can be used for sterilizing needles and syringes. A first evaluation of the San Francisco bleach distribution project showed a great increase in the percentage of IV drug users using bleach, from less than 5% in the pre-distribution survey to over 60% in the post-distribution survey.[48] Only one evaluation of street outreach workers not distributing bleach has been reported. Preliminary findings from a study in Baltimore showed that the street outreach program had led to some increase in knowledge of AIDS, but did not lead to any increase in prevailing levels of risk reduction.[49] While much more study of street outreach programs is needed, it is probable that the major obstacle to increased risk reduction among IV drug users not in treatment is not lack of basic information about AIDS, but either lack of easy methods of risk reduction (readily available treatment, readily available sterile equipment or means of sterilizing equipment) or perceived social support for behavior change.

Clearly, it will not be possible to rely on drug abuse treatment as the only method of reducing the spread of HIV among IV drug users. Some means of "safer injection" also will be needed. Studies of IV drug users who continue to inject show that movement toward safer injection began before any public health programs were begun in this area. Many IV drug users clearly want to adopt safer injection procedures. Some, but not all, prevention programs have shown encouraging preliminary results in terms of increased use of sterile injection equipment in the needle exchanges or in easily applied techniques for sterilizing equipment—the bleach distribution.

One of the major obstacles to any AIDS prevention program that includes safer injection as a legitimate form of AIDS risk reduction is the public resistance to anything that may be seen as "encouraging drug abuse." The question of what does and does not encourage IV drug use will require much more research, since it is an area where there are very strong opinions and very little conclusive data. Additional discussion of this topic will be presented below.

Persons Who Have Not Begun IV Drug Use

The large number of current IV drug users presents an immediate problem for preventing transmission of HIV. Unless a successful vaccine is developed or IV drug users universally adopt safe injection procedures, AIDS prevention efforts will need to include programs to reduce initiation into IV drug use. This type of AIDS prevention would also serve to reduce the individual and social costs associated with illicit drug injection. To date, however, there has been very little effort in this area of prevention programming. There has been general mass media attention to AIDS, some "AIDS education" movies and videotapes, and a few programs developed for use in schools that specifically mention the sharing of drug injection equipment as a means of becoming exposed to the AIDS virus.

While this information clearly needs to be disseminated, there are likely to be great limitations on the effectiveness of these efforts to prevent AIDS through reducing initiation into IV drug use. First, providing information about adverse effects of drug use (using "scare tactics" or "fear arousal") has not been generally effective as a way of reducing drug abuse.[50] While AIDS may invoke greater/different fears leading to different responses, the weight of available evidence suggests that we can expect fear arousal to have only a very limited effect on reducing initiation into IV drug use. Second, many persons who become IV drug users often have left school well before they make decisions about injecting drugs. Thus, the programs are not likely to reach potential new IV drug users at the times when the program would be most relevant to drug injection behavior.

The limited data available on AIDS and initiation into IV drug use is consistent with the idea that information-only or fear arousal efforts will have limited effectiveness, alone or in combination. In studies of persons who were using heroin and cocaine intensively without injecting, the subjects knew about AIDS but only infrequently mentioned concern about AIDS as a reason why they were not injecting.[51] (Fear of the pain associated with injecting and fear of a loss of social respect were the two dominant reasons for not injecting in this group.) A study of IV drug users not in treatment also showed that new IV drug users were much less likely to be practicing "safer injection" procedures than more experienced IV drug users.[43] While 69% of persons who had injected for 10 years or more reported AIDS risk reduction, only 16% of those who had injected for two years or less reported risk reduction.

The experience with information-only/fear arousal tactics in previous drug abuse prevention programs and the limited data on knowledge of AIDS and initiation into drug injection suggest that new and more intensive types of programs will have to be developed. These programs will undoubtedly have to do more than simply provide information about AIDS. They will have to teach skills needed to resist social pressures to begin injecting drugs and skills needed for negotiating safer sex, and they will have to begin to address the psychological and social (and sometimes financial) problems that put adolescents and young adults at increased risk for drug abuse. The programs will also have to operate outside of school settings in order to reach those at highest risk for beginning to inject drugs.

It is important to distinguish this new type of outreach and counseling program from both "AIDS education" and drug abuse treatment programs. The outreach and counseling would involve much more than providing basic information about AIDS. While much of what would be done in this new type of program would be similar to what is done in a drug treatment program, our present drug abuse treatment programs require that the drug abuser recognize that his or her drug use has gotten out of control. This is the first therapeutic task (typically termed "overcoming denial") in drug treatment and forms the basis for all later therapeutic work. An AIDS prevention program focused on preventing initiation into drug injecting will have to work with drug users much earlier in their drug use careers, before their drug use is fully out of control and before they have had the accumulated negative experiences that lead drug users to recognize a need for treatment. Waiting until the drug user is fully ready for a conventional drug abuse treatment regimen may mean waiting until he or she has already begun injecting and possibly is already exposed to HIV. AIDS prevention programs aimed at preventing initiation into drug injection will thus have to develop a new structure appropriate to the earlier stages of drug use.

INTERACTIONS AMONG PREVENTION PROGRAMS

The above discussion of strategies for preventing HIV infection among current and potential IV drug users is based on the belief that IV drug users are not a homogeneous group. Thus, multiple prevention programs are needed; there is no single type of program that will be sufficient by itself, there may not even be a single "most effective" way of preventing HIV infection among IV drug users. The use of multiple prevention strategies raises questions about how they might interact with each other. In particular, will prevention programs that provide for "safer injection" serve to undermine strategies that reduce IV drug use by providing treatment or by discouraging persons from starting to inject drugs? This hypothesis has served as the basis for opposition to a variety of strategies for "safer injection," from the distribution of free needles and syringes to merely informing IV drug users that it is the sharing of injection equipment and not injecting itself that constitutes the risk for AIDS.

At present, there is only limited information on interaction among the strategies discussed above. The available data, however, consistently indicate that the different strategies are complementary rather than conflicting. City-wide information is available for Amsterdam, which has the largest needle exchange program and a treatment system that actively seeks out drug users and offers a wide variety of types of treatment.[52] As noted above, the needle exchange system has been expanded greatly over the last few years. During this time there has been no reduction in the numbers of persons entering treatment; if anything the numbers have been increasing, while the number of IV drug users has remained relatively stable during the time period.[46] Data collected from individual IV drug users show both an increased use of the needle exchange and a decreased frequency of injection as they became more concerned about AIDS.[53]

Data from American programs that include the promotion of "safer injection" practices are less complete, but again suggest that the programs are complementary to efforts to provide treatment to reduce the levels of drug injection. The New Jersey ex-addict street outreach program mentioned above started as an effort to promote safer injection practices. The expanded treatment component of the program evolved in response to IV drug users telling the outreach workers that what they needed was more access to treatment in order to reduce their levels of drug injection.[39] Outreach workers in New York[54] and San Francisco[20] have reported that they need to be able to place IV drug users into treatment programs in order to maintain their AIDS prevention credibility on the streets.

While the available data are clearly preliminary, they also consistently show that programs that promote reduction in drug injection and programs that promote safer injection tend to complement each other. Upon reflection, this should not be considered surprising. Previously, efforts to reduce drug abuse through reducing the supply of illicit drugs (through law enforcement) and through reducing demand for illicit drugs (through treatment) were considered contradictory. These two approaches of supply and demand reduction are currently considered complementary—neither is likely to be successful by itself in reducing drug abuse in society.

HIV ANTIBODY TESTING AND AIDS PREVENTION

HIV antibody testing has been advocated as a potentially powerful technique for reducing the transmission of HIV.[38] There are few data on the effects of HIV testing on AIDS-related behavior in IV drug users. Two papers were presented at the Paris AIDS conference[55,56] and one at the Washington AIDS conference on post-test behavior among IV drug users.[57] All three studies showed reductions in AIDS risk behavior among the subjects who voluntarily underwent counseling and testing. Seropositives showed a period of acute distress/anxiety/depression on learning their serologic status, although this stress generally resolved within several weeks. Over the time lengths measured in these studies—from 2 to 9 months—seronegatives who learned their status showed less risk reduction than seropositives who learned their status. While there was consistency in the findings from these three studies, caution is needed in any generalization. These studies were conducted within treatment settings, the decision to provide counseling was supported by the treatment staff, there was extensive pre-and post-test counseling, the testing was totally voluntary, and extensive precautions were taken to assure confidentiality of the test results. When HIV antibody testing is done without these extensive supports, there appears to be no net positive effect on

AIDS risk behavior, and a potential for harm to the individuals participating.[57] In terms of reducing AIDS risk behavior, it is probably a mistake to think of "antibody testing" as a prevention technique. Instead, one should think of intensive counseling with testing as an adjunct to the counseling as a possible method of facilitating risk reduction among IV drug users.

SUMMARY

There are many obstacles to the prevention of HIV infection among IV drug users. The IV drug use subculture as a whole is in opposition to the majority culture in society. The internal organization of the subculture is characterized by competition both between drug sellers and users and among the users themselves, so that the bases for collective action to support risk reduction are limited. The primary positive social relationships within the subculture—"running buddies" (IV drug users who work together to obtain drugs) and sexual partners—are often undermined by AIDS risk behavior. Withdrawal, which may occur every 4 to 6 hours among heroin addicts and every 20 to 30 minutes among persons who use cocaine intensively, creates a state of sufficient distress that tends to override concerns about AIDS.

Research on the transmission of HIV among IV drug users is still in a relatively early stage. The great geographic variation in seroprevalence rates among IV drug users needs to be understood and incorporated into prevention programs. Evaluation of current AIDS prevention programs aimed at IV drug users is still in a very preliminary stage, and in many communities there may be only a little time left for trying to contain HIV exposure among IV drug users at low levels.

There are also some indications for cautious optimism regarding control of HIV infection among IV drug users. Two factors, the frequency of drug injection and the sharing of injection equipment across friendship groups, have been found to be associated with rapid spread of the virus among IV drug users, suggesting that they receive priority as foci for prevention efforts.

There are also a number of studies showing AIDS risk reduction among IV drug users. The forms of risk reduction that are occurring generally parallel the values and structure of the subculture. The value of getting high is not easily discarded by IV drug users, even those who have entered treatment. Risk reduction through more frequent use of "clean" injection equipment occurs more often than risk reduction through the elimination of drug injection. Risk reduction in terms of reducing the number of persons with whom one will share injection equipment follows the social structure of the subculture: refusing to share injection equipment with strangers and casual acquaintances is more common than refusing to share with sexual partners or close friends.

It should be emphasized that the behavior change among IV drug users observed to date should be characterized as "risk reduction" and not "risk elimination." The amount of behavior associated with transmission of HIV has been reduced, but there undoubtedly still is a high residual level of transmission-related behavior. The present level of behavior change has generally occurred without intensive prevention programming. Presumably, focused efforts on a much larger scale should greatly increase the extent of risk reduction.

The admittedly limited research to date suggests three critical questions with respect to the future transmission of HIV among IV drug users. The first concerns ameliorating the effects of withdrawal on intended risk reduction. The various studies indicate that the acute distress of withdrawal will lead an IV drug user to use whatever injection equipment is readily available, whether or not it is likely to be contaminated. Two strategies would be appropriate for countering the risk-increasing effects of withdrawal. First would be the provision of increased drug abuse treatment, to assist many IV drug users to eliminate drug injection or, for those who are unable to eliminate injecting, to reduce the intensity of injecting to a level less than that associated with withdrawal. The second strategy for ameliorating the effects of withdrawal would be to have sterile injection equipment readily available when IV drug users entered withdrawal. This would require either the widespread distribution of sterile equipment itself or a readily available, fast, and effective method for sterilizing potentially contaminated injection equipment.

The second critical question refers to the connotations of sharing drug injection equipment among close friends. Prior to AIDS, the sharing of injection equipment was perceived as being helpful and expressing solidarity. In order to control the spread of HIV among the group, it may be necessary to redefine the sharing of equipment so that sharing without sterilization between uses is seen as a hostile rather than a friendly act.

The final critical question concerns our ability to divert potential new IV drug users away from starting to inject. If risk reduction among IV drug users does not at least approximate risk elimination, then new IV drug users will be faced with a higher background seroprevalence and will be more likely to become infected quickly. This situation would mean that an increasing percentage of IV drug users would be infected prior to any cessation of IV drug use and that the potential of sexual transmission from IV drug users to persons who do not inject would also accelerate.

REFERENCES

1. U.S. Public Health Service, Centers for Disease Control. AIDS Weekly Surveillance Report, 9 November 1987
2. World Health Organization. WHO Collaborating Center on AIDS. Quarterly Report No. 14. 30 June 1987

3. New York City Department of Public Health, personal communication, 1987

4. Des Jarlais DC, Friedman SR, Strug D: AIDS among intravenous drug users: A sociocultural perspective. In Feldman D, Johnson T (eds.): The Social Dimensions of AIDS: Methods and Theory. New York, Praeger, 1986

5. Agar MH: Ripping and Running: A Formal Ethnography of Urban Heroin Addicts. New York, Seminar Press, 1973

6. Johnson BD, Goldstein PJ, Preble E, et al: Taking Care of Business: The Economics of Crime by Heroin Abusers. Lexington, MA, D.C. Heath and Company, 1985

7. Wikler A: Dynamics of drug dependence: Implications of a conditioning theory for research and treatment. Arch Gen Psychiat 28:611, 1973

8. Des Jarlais DC, Chamberland M, Yancovitz SR, et al: Heterosexual partners: A large risk group for AIDS (letter). Lancet ii:8415, 1984

9. Des Jarlais DC, Wish ED, Friedman SR, et al: Intravenous drug use and the heterosexual transmission of the human immunodeficiency virus: Current trends in New York City. NY State J Med. 87:283, 1987

10. Darrow M: Risk factors among prostitutes. Presented at Workshop on Epidemiological Surveys on AIDS: Epidemiology of HIV Infections in Europe: Spread among Intravenous Drug Users and the Heterosexual Population, Berlin, November 12–14, 1986

11. Van den Hoek JA, Van Zadelhof AW, Goudsmit J, et al: Risk factors for LAV/HTLV-III infection among drug users in Amsterdam. Presented at the 2nd International Conference on AIDS, Paris, June 23–25, 1986

12. Heckmann W: Personal communication, 1987

13. Marmor M, Des Jarlais DC, Cohen H, et al: Risk factors for infection with human immunodeficiency virus among intravenous drug abusers in New York City. AIDS 1:39, 1987

14. Primm: personal communication, 1987

15. Hutchinson M, Craven D, Boston City Hospital: Personal communication.

16. D'Aquila RT, Williams AB, Petersen LR, et al: HIV seroprevalence among Connecticut intravenous drug users in 1986–87: Race/ethnicity as a risk factor for HIV seropositivity. Presented at the III International Conference on AIDS, Washington, D.C., June 1987

17. Loeb L: Personal communication, 1987

18. Ginzburg H: Personal communication, 1987

19. Chaisson RE, Moss AR, Onishi R, et al: Human immunodeficiency virus infection in heterosexual intravenous drug users in San Francisco. Am J Public Health 77:169, 1987

20. Watters JK: Preventing human immunodeficiency virus contagion among intravenous drug users: The impact of street-based education on risk-behavior. Presented at the III International Conference on AIDS, Washington, D.C., 1987

21. Angarano G, Pastore G, Monno L, et al: Rapid spread of HTLV-III infection among drug addicts in Italy. Lancet ii: 1302, 1985

22. Verani P: Seroprevalence among intravenous drug abusers in Italy. Presented at Workshop on Epidemiological Surveys on AIDS: Epidemiology of HIV Infections in Europe Spread Among Intravenous Drug Users and the Heterosexual Population, Berlin, November 12–14, 1986

23. Camprubi J: SIDA: Prevalencia de la infeccion por VIH en los ADVP. Situacion actual y posibilidades de actuacion. Comunidad y Drogas 2:9, 1987

24. Rodrigo JM, Serra MA, Aguilar E, et al: HTLV antibodies in drug addicts in Spain. Lancet ii:157, 1985

25. Hunsmann G, Schneider J, Bayer H: Seroepidemiology of HTLV-III/LAV in the Federal Republic of Germany. Klin Wochenschr 63:233, 1985

26. Schupbach J, Haller O, Vogt M, et al: Antibodies of HTLV-III in Swiss patients with AIDS and pre-AIDS and in groups at risk for AIDS. N Engl J Med 312:265, 1985

27. Adler M: Personal communication, 1987

28. Follett EAC, McIntyre A, O'Donnell B: HTLV-III antibody in drug abusers in the West of Scotland: The Edinburgh connection. Lancet i:446, 1986

29. Novick DM, Kreek MJ, Des Jarlais DC, et al: Abstract of clinical research findings: Therapeutic and historical aspects. In Harris LJ (ed): Problems of Drug Dependence 1985: Proceedings of the 47th Annual Scientific Meeting, The Committee on Problems of Drug Dependence, Inc. NIDA Research Monograph 67, p. 318. Washington, DC, U.S. Government Printing Office, 1985

30. Rex W: Increase of HIV seroprevalence among IVDA in West Berlin prisons since 1982. Presented at Workshop on Epidemiological Surveys on AIDS: Epidemiology of HIV infections in Europe: Spread Among Intravenous Drug Users and the Heterosexual Population, Berlin, November 12–14, 1986

31. Worm AM: Incidence of HIV antibodies in IV drug abusers and prostitutes in Copenhagen. Presented at Workshop on Epidemiological Surveys on AIDS: Epidemiology of HIV Infections in Europe: Spread Among Intravenous Drug Users and the Heterosexual Population, Berlin, November 12–14, 1986

32. Robertson JR, Bucknall ABV, Welsby PD, et al: Epidemic of AIDS related virus (HTLV-III/LAV) infection among intravenous drug users. Br Med J 292:527, 1986

33. Cohen H, Marmor M, Des Jarlais DC, et al: Risk factors for HTLV-III/LAV seropositivity among intravenous drug users. Presented at the International Conference on the Acquired Immune Deficiency Syndrome (AIDS), Atlanta, April 14–17, 1985

34. Weiss SH, Ginzburg HM, Goedert JJ, et al: Risk for HTLV-III exposure and AIDS among parenteral drug abusers in New Jersey. Presented at the 1st International Conference on the Acquired Immune Deficiency Syndrome (AIDS), Atlanta, April 14–17, 1985

35. Schoenbaum EE, Selwyn PA, Klein RS, et al: Prevalence of and risk factors associated with HTLV-III/LAV antibodies among intravenous drug abusers in methadone programs in New York City. Presented at the 2nd International Conference on AIDS, Paris, June 23–25, 1986

36. Chaisson RE: personal communication, 1987

37. Schoenbaum EE, Selwyn PA, Hartel D, et al: HIV seroconversion in intravenous drug abusers: Rate and risk factors. Presented at the III International Conference on AIDS, Washington, D.C., June 1987

38. U.S. Public Health Service: Public Health Service Plan for the Prevention and Control of AIDS and the AIDS virus: Report of the Coolfont Planning Conference, June 4–6, 1986

39. Jackson J, Rotkiewicz L. A coupon program: AIDS education and drug treatment. Presented at the III International Conference on AIDS, Washington, D.C., June 1987

40. Simpson DD, Savage JL, Sells SB: Data Book on Drug Treatment Outcomes: Followup Study of 1969–1972 Admissions to the Drug Abuse Reporting Program (DARP). Institute of Behavioral Research Report 78-10: Fort Worth, Texas Christian University, 1978

41. Friedman SR, Des Jarlais DC, Sotheran JL, et al: AIDS and

self-organization among intravenous drug users. Int J Addict 22:201, 1987

42. Selwyn PA, Cox CP, Feiner C, et al: Knowledge about AIDS and high-risk behavior among intravenous drug abusers in New York City. Presented at Annual Meeting of the American Public Health Association, Washington, DC, September 1985

43. Kleinman PH, Friedman SR, Mauge CE, et al: Beliefs and behaviors regarding AIDS: A survey of street intravenous drug users. Presented at the III International Conference on AIDS, Washington, D.C., June 1987

44. Des Jarlais DC, Friedman SR, Hopkins W: Risk reduction for the acquired immunodeficiency syndrome among intravenous drug users. Ann Intern Med, 103:755, 1985

45. Des Jarlais DC, Hopkins W: Free needles for intravenous drug users at risk for AIDS: Current developments in New York City. N Engl J Med, 103:313, 1985

46. Buning EC, Van Brussel GHA, van Santen G: Amsterdam's drug policy and its implications for controlling needle sharing. R. Battjes (ed): Bethesda, MD, National Institute on Drug Abuse Monograph. (In press)

47. Whyte BM, Dobson AJ, Gold J, and Cooper DA: Epidemiology of AIDS in Australia. Presented at the III International Conference on AIDS, Washington, D.C., June 1987

48. Watters JK, Iura DM, Iura KW: AIDS prevention and education service to intravenous drug users through the Midcity Consortum to Combat AIDS: Administrative report of the first six months, San Francisco, Midcity Consortium, December 1, 1986

49. McAuliffe WE, Doering S, Breer P, et al: An evaluation of using ex-addict outreach workers to educate intravenous drug users about AIDS prevention. Presented at the III International Conference on AIDS, Washington, D.C., June 1987

50. Schaps E, DiBartolo R, Churgin S: Primary Prevention Research: A Review of 127 Program Evaluations. Walnut Creek, California, Pyramid Project, Pacific Institute for Research and Evaluation, 1978

51. Des Jarlais DC, Friedman SR, Casriel C, et al: AIDS and preventing initiation into intravenous (IV) drug use. Psychology and Health 1:179, 1987

52. Buning EC, Coutinho RA, van Brussel GHA, et al: Preventing AIDS in drug addicts in Amsterdam (letter). Lancet, ii:1435, 1986

53. Buning E: Amsterdam's drug policy and the prevention of AIDS. Presented at the Conference on AIDS in the Drug Abuse Community and Heterosexual Transmission, Newark, March 31–April 1, 1986

54. Mauge C: Personal communication, 1987

55. Casadonte P, Des Jarlais DC, Smith T, et al: Psychological and Behavioral Impact of Learning HTLV-III/LAV Antibody Test Results. Presented at the International Conference on Acquired Immunodeficiency Syndrome (AIDS), Paris, June 23–25, 1986

56. Cox CP, Selwyn PA, Schoenbaum EE, et al: Psychological and behavioral consequences of HTLV-III/LAV antibody testing and notification among intravenous drug abusers in a methadone program in New York City. Presented at the International Conference on Acquired Immunodeficiency Syndrome (AIDS), Paris, June 23–25, 1986

57. Marlink RG, Foss B, Swift R, et al: High rate of HTLV-III/LAV exposure in IVDA's from a small-sized city and the failure of specialized methadone maintenance to prevent further drug use. Presented at the III International Conference on AIDS, Washington, D.C., June 1987

58. Friedman SR, Sotheran JL, Abdul-Quader A, et al: The AIDS epidemic among blacks and hispanics. Milbank Q, 65 (suppl 2), 1987

Safety Precautions and Hospital Practices in Dealing with Seropositive Individuals

Kathleen McMahon
M. Glennon Sutterer

25

The human immunodeficiency virus (HIV) has been isolated from blood,[1-3] semen,[4] tears,[5] saliva,[6,7] breast milk,[8] epithelial cells,[9] cerebral and vaginal secretions,[9-11] urine,[7] and brain tissue and cerebrospinal fluid (CSF)[12] of infected persons. Transmission has occurred through sexual contact with infected individuals, infusion of contaminated blood products, sharing of contaminated needles, infected mother-to-child perinatal contact, and rarely, needlestick accidents, and exposure of open skin and mucous membrane to infected blood. At present, the exact method of transmission is unknown. A crucially important fact is that most of these exposures are preventable.

This chapter focuses on the safety precautions that health care institutions and providers can employ to prevent transmission of HIV. It is based on recommendations by the Centers for Disease Control (CDC) and the American Hospital Association. It explains the use of precautions for the HIV seropositive individual and reviews the literature on the risk of HIV transmission to health care workers, the specifics of blood and body fluid precautions, special problems and issues that complicate the situation, and supportive programs that maintain and sustain the underlying goal of prevention of transmission. Also outlined are safety precautions needed for the person with AIDS who has developed an opportunistic infection.

Because of the similarity of transmission of HIV and hepatitis B, hepatitis B precautions are maintained for the HIV seropositive individual. These blood and body fluid precautions rely on the use of protective barriers and attire. Gloves are worn when hand exposure to blood or body fluids is anticipated; masks and protective eye-wear are worn if blood or body fluid splashes to the face and mouth are anticipated. Specimen labels identify the type of precautions indicated. Soiled linens and equipment are separately contained, and blood or body fluid spills are thoroughly disinfected.

Several studies (see Table 25-1) and case reports have been published about the presumptive risk to health care providers for HIV transmission. A review of this literature justifies and supports the recommendations published by the Centers for Disease Control (CDC). In addition, secondary findings and interpretative comments by the researchers are beneficial in evaluating infection control measures. This literature reaffirms that the risk of acquiring HIV through contact with patients or their biologic specimens is rare, but not impossible.

REVIEW OF THE LITERATURE

Health Care Worker Studies

A Report of San Francisco General Hospital Workers

A prospective cohort study of San Francisco General Hospital health care providers[13] involved a pre-test/post-test design. Questionnaires regarding infection control practices and demographics, among other things, were completed by the subjects at the beginning and end of the 10-month study along with HIV testing. In this study, none of the 175 subjects followed through February 1987 have seroconverted to HIV positive despite occupational association with HIV-infected patients and their blood or body fluids. These San Francisco General Hospital workers were drawn from a broad range of functional job categories. Health care workers who identified themselves as being at risk for AIDS through non-occupational high-risk behavior were excluded.

Of primary importance in this study are the inade-

Table 25-1
Risk of HIV Infection Among Health Care Workers

Study	Number Studied	# HIV+	Comments
Gerberding et al (SF, 1987)	175	0	
Hirsch et al (Boston, 1985)	33/39	0/0	
Weiss et al (NY, 1985)	361	9	Six of these seropositives identified themselves being at risk for nonoccupational behaviors. The other three, although not documented seroconversions, could not be ruled out as occupational exposures.
McCray et al (CDC, 1986)	966	2	One occupationally related seroconversion, one unclear.
Kuhls et al (LA, 1986)	390	0	
Henderson et al (NIH, 1986)	531	3	All three seropositives identified themselves to be at risk for HIV infection through nonoccupational behaviors.
Moss et al (SF, 1986)	101	11	Twenty-nine workers identified themselves as at risk because of nonoccupational behaviors. The 11 seropositives found come from this group.

quate infection control precautions reported on the questionnaire by the health care providers. The investigators ranked the infection control precautions reported by the workers as sufficient, inadequate, or excessive, using the standards outlined by the CDC.[14] They found that 56% of the workers used inadequate precautions when dealing with AIDS patients or specimens from AIDS patients. Even poorer practices (63% inadequate) were reported in relation to patients with AIDS-related complex (ARC). The use of excessive precautions was minimal (14% and 10%, respectively).

As noted in the report, the absence of HIV transmission to these health care providers is reassuring and adds significant validation to previous studies of health care workers.

A concern of major proportion is the self-report of inadequate use of protective barriers and attire in this study population. The frequency of the inadequate infection control responses is alarming. In light of the May 1987 CDC report[15] involving three female health care workers presumed to have become HIV-infected during patient care routines, it would be expected that health care workers and institutions are adapting to CDC guidelines in response to this report and the media coverage[16] that it generated.

The report concludes with a reaffirmation of the adequacy of Hepatitis B precautions for AIDS-related infection control first proposed by the CDC five years earlier.[17]

A Report of the National Institutes of Health's Clinical Center Workers

Henderson and colleagues[18] studied 531 health care workers at the NIH's Clinical Center who volunteered to take a questionnaire, with repeat questionnaires each

six months. Details included work history, contact with patients, contact with blood or body fluids, and other demographics. It did not include sexual or drug use history.

These results revealed three HIV-seropositive workers. All three seropositive workers identified themselves as being at risk for HIV due to known high-risk behaviors (i.e., homosexuality, IV drug use). The researchers plan to continue this study for another 4 years.

One of the study's strengths is that viral cultures were also performed on some of the study participants to detect HIV, since a case report of HIV viremia without anti-HIV antibody has been reported in the literature.[19]

A Report of San Francisco General Hospital and the University of California at San Francisco Workers

Moss and associates[20] studied 101 health care workers who were also highly exposed to HIV-infected blood or body fluids. Twenty-nine identified themselves as belonging to a high-risk group. Of these 29, eleven were ELISA positive. None of the other study participants were positive.

The Cooperative Needlestick Surveillance Group and CDC Report

McCray and colleagues[21] reported on the results of a multicenter surveillance project involving 966 health care workers with percutaneous or mucous membrane exposures to the blood or body fluids of AIDS or AIDS-related patients. Enrolled subjects were drawn from a broad range of health occupation categories including nurses, physicians, medical students, laboratory workers, phlebotomists, respiratory therapists and others. Only

2% of the study participants included those with less direct patient or specimen contact. Of the 666 patients to whom they were exposed, 88% fell into the CDC case definition of AIDS, and 12% had an AIDS-related illness.

One case documented an occupationally acquired HIV infection having been seronegative on blood specimens drawn immediately following an exposure, followed by a seropositive blood specimen later.

Another case of HIV seropositivity was difficult to analyze since other risk behaviors or exposures could not be ruled out.

The authors of this study propose that as many as 40% of these 966 occupational exposures could have been minimized or prevented by adequate infection control practices. They conclude with a recommendation that health care workers familiarize themselves with infection control guidelines for HIV.

Of interest, the authors also cite a variable that may complicate the interpretation of research studies on transmission. They limit their findings of risk to contact with CDC-defined AIDS patients, but acknowledge that other HIV-infected persons may have higher levels of circulating T-lymphocytes than CDC-defined AIDS patients and, as such, may pose more of a risk of transmission to workers exposed to their blood or body fluids. More research on the validity of this possibility is needed, but for now, efforts should be directed toward preventing such exposures.

A Report of the Frequency of Seropositivity Among Patients at The Johns Hopkins Hospital Emergency Room

Baker and colleagues[22] undertook their prospective study of HIV seropositivity in persons requiring emergency health care to determine the potential risk to first-response care providers of unsuspected exposure to the virus and to determine whether any readily identifiable patient characteristics could be discerned on presentation to indicate increased likelihood of harboring the virus.

In their 100-day prospective study, undertaken in a critical care area, all patients who underwent any procedure related to the procurement of blood were entered. Two hundred and three specimens from patients were obtained, six of which were confirmed HIV positive by Western blot. Sixty-three patients were excluded because the blood sample was inadequate for testing, but these did not differ significantly from the 203 patients included in the analysis.

Of major interest is their discussion of the relatively uninformed opinion of health care providers about HIV and the potential of occupational exposure. Low risk does not translate into no risk. The authors go on to cite the lack of infection control measures used by health care workers when rendering emergency or resuscitative care to those in need. They argue that gloves and other protective gear need to be used despite the emergency situation.

Of note, there was no outstanding characteristic in pre-identifying a risk of HIV seropositivity. Drug abuse history was not positively correlated. The age group 25–34 had a higher rate of the HIV seropositives (16%), with the highest rate being found in trauma victims of that age group, 19% of whom were seropositive.

Studies are currently under way to determine the HIV seropositivity rate in the general population. The 0.8% prevalence of HIV in the U.S. population[23] previously suggested was lower than that encountered in this Baltimore sample, where a point prevalence of 3% was obtained.

A Report of UCLA Medical Center Workers

Kuhls and associates[24] studied 390 female health care workers in a prospective cohort study. In depth, self-administered questionnaires, limited physical examinations, and laboratory testing at time of intake and at follow-up 9 to 12 months later were performed. The groups with high exposure to AIDS patients and their biologic specimens ($n = 246$), low exposure ($n = 43$), and no exposure ($n = 101$) were categorically similar with respect to age, job description, ethnic background, marital status, and sexual history. Twenty-five of the participants were identified as having needlestick or mucous membrane exposures to AIDS patients or their specimens. None of these female health care workers was found to be HIV seropositive.

A Report of Workers in Medical Centers of Metropolitan Areas

A total of 361 health care personnel volunteers were studied by Weiss and associates.[25] These included 239 interns, residents, and fellows from a single institution with a large AIDS population. Most of these physicians were first and second-year medical or surgical residents, although house staff were from nearly all hospital services. In addition, 39 hospital laboratory workers from the same institution were enrolled. Eighty-three other persons (attending physicians, medical students, physician assistants, nurses, and drug program staff) from several other institutions were also studied. Fifteen percent of the 239 house staff and four (10%) of the 39 laboratory workers gave a history of at least one percutaneous exposure to materials potentially contaminated with the blood of AIDS patients.

There were 6 seropositive individuals among the 23 medical and laboratory workers who identified themselves as already being at risk for HIV due to non-occupational behavior. Three seropositive individuals were found among workers who did not belong to any traditionally recognized high-risk groups. Cases A and B, two female health care workers, had documented parenteral exposures to a patient with AIDS. Case C, a male clinical laboratory worker, had been exposed to pooled platelets. None of these three health care workers had documented seroconversion, nor was complete epidemiologic surveillance data obtained. Consequently, occupationally acquired HIV could not be ruled out.

A Report of Massachusetts General Hospital and New York Medical College Workers

Hirsch and associates[26] studied 30 health care workers with single needlestick injuries from AIDS patients. One worker had her eye splattered with blood from an AIDS patient, and two others had blood contamination from an AIDS patient to an open hand wound. All thirty-three health care workers were seronegative for HIV.

Other at-risk employees were also studied. They included eight pathologists, seven gastroenterologists, two endoscopy nurses, one surgeon, one bronchoscopist, and twenty research scientists and technicians. All of these personnel had been exposed to the blood or body fluids of AIDS or ARC patients while performing their responsibilities. None was seropositive for HIV.

Case Reports: Occupationally-Acquired HIV Infection

The following is a summary of the anecdotal case reports of seroconversion of health care workers presumably due to exposures that occurred during the provision of health care services to HIV-infected persons.

The CDC defines the ideal case for the documentation of seroconversion as follows:

> A health care worker with no identifiable risk factors for AIDS whose serum, obtained within days of the date of a possible occupational exposure, is negative for antibody to HTLV-III/LAV but whose follow-up serum, in the absence of interim exposure to other risk factors, is positive for antibody to HTLV-III/LAV.[27]

Needlestick Exposures

SEROCONVERSION OF A FEMALE HEALTH CARE WORKER AFTER A CONTAMINATED NEEDLESTICK ACCIDENT.[28] During an emergency procedure, this care provider sustained a deep intramuscular needlestick. The large-bore (1.67-mm diameter), visibly contaminated needle and syringe unit had been used on an AIDS patient. The health worker was enrolled in the CDC surveillance study.

After 48 hours, skin tests for mumps and *Candida* were strongly positive. Fourteen days later, fever, chills, myalgias, and arthralgias developed that required hospital admission the following day. She developed a fever to 40.3°C, an enlarged right axillary lymph node, and persistent erythema and induration at the skin test site. Within a few days, she developed a rash on her abdomen; Epstein-Barr virus (EBV) and cytomegalovirus

(CMV) tests were negative. The diagnosis was a viral syndrome of undetermined etiology.

A month later rehospitalization was required for continued abdominal cramping and pain. Because *Clostridium* was detected in her stool, she began oral Vancomycin, which alleviated the symptoms.

Since then she suffered mild, intermittent oral candidiasis, persistent enlargement of a post-cervical lymph node, and transient enlargement of suboccipital and inguinal lymph nodes.

On day 9 after the original needlestick accident, she was HIV seronegative. However, she tested positive on days 184 and 239. Her virus cultures were negative on day 239 as was her husband's HIV test. She does not give a history of other known risk factors.

SEROCONVERSION OF A FEMALE NURSE AFTER A CONTAMINATED NEEDLESTICK INJURY.[29] While resheathing a needle used to draw blood from the arterial line of an AIDS patient, a nurse in Britain accidentally stuck herself. Thirteen days after the injury, she developed a severe flulike illness that included mild sore throat, headache, myalgia, and facial neuralgia. Seventeen days later she developed a rash to her trunk and chest spreading to her neck and face that was not associated with antibiotic use. General malaise persisted with severe arthralgias and pyrexia up to 39°C for 20 days. Generalized lymphadenopathy resolved and she had an uneventful recovery. She tested negative for EBV, CMV, parvovirus and rubella virus.

She was HIV seronegative on day 27 after the injury. On days 49 and 57, she was found to be HIV seropositive. No other risk factors were identified.

SEROCONVERSION OF A FEMALE NURSE AFTER A NEEDLESTICK INJURY.[30] During a thoracentesis performed on a patient with a pleural effusion who had persistent generalized lymphadenopathy and was seropositive for HIV and hepatitis B surface antigen, a nurse suffered a superficial needlestick injury to her finger while recapping a needle contaminated with bloody pleural effusion fluid. She received specific immunoglobulins and hepatitis B vaccine at that time.

Twenty-five days later she developed fatigue, fever and vomiting. On day 26 her fever was 39.4°C. On day 53 she developed an acute anicteric hepatitis. On day 181 CMV, EBV, and hepatitis B and A were negative; her skin test was TB positive.

She was HIV seronegative on days 1 and 13 but seropositive on days 68, 82, and 151. Her serum viral HIV culture was negative on days 103 and 181. Her husband was HIV seronegative on day 110. No other risk factors were determined.

SEROCONVERSION OF A FEMALE NURSING STUDENT AFTER A NEEDLESTICK ACCIDENT.[31] A nursing student pricked the fleshy part of her index finger with a needle used to draw blood from an AIDS patient. There was no apparent injection of blood.

A month later she was HIV seronegative. Subsequently, she developed fever and a rash affecting her face, arms and thorax. Within 4 months, she was HIV seropositive. Her husband was HIV seronegative. No other risk factors were identified.

Non-Needlestick Exposures

SEROCONVERSION OF A HEALTH CARE WORKER/ MOTHER AFTER REPEATED EXPOSURES TO HER YOUNG HIV-SEROPOSITIVE CHILD.[32] An HIV-seronegative mother of a young child was found to be HIV seropositive 3 and 4 months later. The child required extensive nursing care. His HIV seropositivity was traced to a blood transfusion. She did not recall any specific incident, but had ungloved hand contact with the child's blood or body fluids on many occasions. She did not recall having open wounds or cuts, nor did she give a history of washing hands immediately after exposure. The culture of her blood lymphocytes was negative and the child's father was seronegative.

Some of the nursing care activities the mother performed for her child included blood-drawing from an indwelling catheter, removal of peripheral intravenous lines, emptying and maintaining ostomy equipment, insertion of rectal tubes, changing diapers, surgical dressings and nasogastric feeding tubes. She had been working as a paramedic before the child's birth. Her termination of this work preceded the identified HIV-positive blood transfusion the child received.

POSSIBLE SEROCONVERSION OF A WOMAN PROVIDING HOME NURSING CARE TO A PERSON LATER DIAGNOSED AS HAVING AIDS.[33] A woman developed AIDS after she had provided home nonprofessional nursing care to a Ghanian man who was diagnosed as having AIDS at autopsy. The care she provided involved prolonged, frequent skin contact with body secretions and excretions. She recalled having some small cuts on her hands and an exacerbation of chronic eczema. She denied having sexual contact with the patient.

In this case, the timing of seroconversion was untraceable and other risk factors are unknown.

SEROCONVERSION OF FEMALE NURSE AFTER AN INCIDENT INVOLVING SKIN-TO-BLOOD CONTACT WITH A PATIENT LATER FOUND TO HAVE AIDS.[15] During a cardiopulmonary arrest, a nurse applied direct pressure to an arterial line insertion site for about 20 minutes using her index finger. She washed her hands after holding the bleeding site. She was not wearing gloves and may have had chapped hands. She also helped clean up the room after the unsuccessful resuscitation attempt but does not recall any more contact with blood or other body fluids. At post-mortem examination the patient was diagnosed as having AIDS.

Twenty days after the incident, the nurse developed fever, malaise, extreme fatigue, sore throat, nausea, vomiting, diarrhea, a 14-pound weight loss, and gen-

eralized lymphadenopathy. This viral syndrome lasted 3 weeks (day 41). She felt better 9 weeks after the incident and all signs and symptoms had resolved at 6 months.

Eight months before the incident she had donated blood and was found to be HIV seronegative. Sixteen weeks after the cardiopulmonary arrest, she donated blood again and was found to be HIV seropositive.

Her husband was HIV seronegative, as were the other fifteen health care workers involved in the initial cardiopulmonary arrest in the emergency room. No other risk factors were found.

SEROCONVERSION OF A FEMALE PHLEBOTOMIST AFTER AN ACCIDENTAL CONTAMINATED BLOOD SPLASH.[15] While manipulating blood tubes, a phlebotomist was splashed in the face and mouth with blood. She was wearing gloves and glasses to protect herself. She had facial acne but no open wounds. The patient from whom the blood specimens were drawn was suspected of being HIV seropositive.

The phlebotomist was ELISA negative on day 1 and again 8 weeks after the incident. A blood donation 9 months later found her to be HIV seropositive. She recalled a needle scratch sustained about 2 months after the incident. The needle had been used on an intravenous drug user of unknown HIV status.

A co-worker, similarly exposed during the original incident, was HIV seronegative a year later. The phlebotomist does not give a history of sexual activity and no other risk factors were identified.

SEROCONVERSION OF A FEMALE MEDICAL TECHNICIAN AFTER BLOOD SPILL OVER HANDS AND FOREARMS.[15] A medical technician was trouble-shooting apheresis equipment in use on a patient when blood spilled on her hands and forearms. She does not recall any open wounds or having mucous membrane exposure. She had dermatitis on her ear, which she may have touched. She was not wearing gloves. Although the hospital had a policy of testing patients scheduled for apheresis for HIV, this patient had not been tested. The patient was found to be HIV seropositive.

Eight weeks after the incident, the technician developed a flulike illness of fever, myalgia, diarrhea, hives, and a rash on the arms and legs. A physician diagnosed this illness as a viral syndrome. The signs and symptoms resolved over a few weeks.

The technician was HIV seronegative when tested 5 days after the incident and again at 6 weeks. Three months after the incident she was HIV seropositive by ELISA, with Western blot band p24 positive. At four months, bands p24 and gp41 were positive on Western blot.

Her husband was HIV seronegative. She was not found to have other risk factors. More than a year earlier, she had been on corticosteroids for an immunologic disorder. A co-worker similarly exposed during the same accident was seronegative at 3 months.

These case reports of female health care providers should serve as a "call to arms" for all health care workers. Many health care providers can identify with the circumstances of these seroconversions as well as the generalized viral syndrome some of them have experienced. Sensitivity and courage are needed to deal effectively with the fears and worries these case reports generate.

In general, these cases illustrate a few basic tenets: blood or body fluid precautions must be followed in everyday situations, students and non-professional health care deliverers must be informed of prevention methods, and all situations must be evaluated for implementation of infection control practices. Although compassion and understanding are called for, recognizing how difficult it is to change behavior and routinely use protective barriers, change is obviously needed. The number of known seroconversions is quite small, but every effort needs to be made to prevent more of them. Critical review of the case reports reveals an absence of some critical behaviors that could have prevented or minimized the exposures. Health care workers and institutions must construct sound, effective, and coordinated plans to address these issues.

Household Contacts

Research on the risk to household members of an AIDS or ARC patient resoundingly reaffirms the lack of casual transmission. Since in many respects health care workers and fellow patients assume the partial role of "household" contacts for hospitalized HIV seropositive patients, a review of the studies performed on household contacts of AIDS or ARC patients is helpful.

In Fischl and associates'[34] evaluation of household contacts of adults with AIDS, none was seropositive for HIV antibody. These 29 household members had direct contact with the patient, spouse, and children in the household. This included personal contact such as hugging, kissing, and sharing of kitchen and bathroom facilities. Most were directly involved in the care of the adult or child with AIDS or ARC. All of these adult household contacts were clinically as well as immunologically normal. In addition, there was no evidence of horizontal transmission among the 90 HIV seronegative children at entry into Fischl's study. None of the unaffected siblings of children with AIDS or ARC developed or had antibodies to HIV.

Further evidence to support lack of transmission to household contacts comes from the study by Jason and co-workers[35] of hemophiliac AIDS and ARC patients and their household contact. No evidence to support casual transmission was elucidated.

In Redfield and colleagues'[36] study evaluating the degree of intrafamilial transmission of HIV from patients with ARC or AIDS, the spouses and children of a small number of male AIDS or ARC patients were investigated.

None of the older children was HIV-infected and all were clinically normal. This lack of evidence of infection once again suggests that close household contact between parents, children, and siblings is not a significant mode of transmission.

The study by Friedland and associates[37] of 101 nonsexual household contacts of patients with AIDS or the AIDS-related complex who had oral candidiasis also was undertaken to address the issue of transmission. None of the household contacts reported having sexual contact with a patient with AIDS or had any other risk factors for AIDS. The type of contact with the AIDS patients included sharing of household items such as drinking glasses, eating plates, nail clippers, and eating utensils. Contact also involved sharing household facilities such as toilet, bath/shower, kitchen, and beds, and washing items used by the patients, including dishes, bath, toilet, and clothes. The interaction with the patient included hugging, kissing on the cheek, shaking hands, and kissing on the lips. Other less frequent contacts such as helping to bathe, sharing razors, toothbrushes, and sharing clothes were also reported. Despite this close contact, only one of the 101 studied was HIV seropositive. This was a child who had signs and symptoms of HIV infection since infancy and was probably infected perinatally by her mother, who has AIDS. This absence of horizontal transmission of HIV despite close familial contact helps to alleviate the fear of a growing number of household contacts and health care providers. Several other studies have found apparent horizontal transmission of hepatitis B infection in households.[38,39] Therefore, despite the fact that HIV, like hepatitis B, is present in saliva and blood, it is reassuring that horizontal transmission of HIV appears to be minimal to nonexistent in the setting of casual contact.

Conclusions

After reviewing this literature on health care workers, actual case reports and household contacts of HIV-infected persons, it is obvious that some conclusions can be drawn:

- The transmission of HIV is extremely rare but can occur in the delivery of health care services.
- Effective use of infection control procedures can dramatically reduce the number of accidental, occupational exposures.
- Although guidelines were published by the CDC in November 1982, actual behaviors to prevent or minimize the transmission of HIV have not filtered down, and they have not been consistently applied by care providers.
- Health care institutions need to educate their staff and maintain the recommended CDC precautions, complete with monitoring and other interventions.
- Attitudes of health care providers need to be ad-

dressed and altered to promote greater compliance and valuing of infection control behaviors.

- Every person in the health care institution should be approached as if they are HIV seropositive.
- Persons involved in health care but not formally trained or educated in infection control policies and procedures (i.e., family, friends, volunteers) must be taught such procedures. Emphasis should be on the functional risk, not on an official job description or category.
- HIV testing of patients may need to be instituted in certain geographical areas for the identification of risk to health care workers. Careful attention is needed to ensure that an irrational two-tiered medical intervention plan does not develop as a result of this testing and that knowledge of the test result is key to care management.[40]
- Research is needed in the following areas:
    Actual methods of HIV transmission
    Changes in health care workers' attitude and behavior toward infection control
    Prevalence of HIV seropositivity
    Effectiveness of certain barriers (gloves, gowns, goggles) to HIV penetration
    Educational interventions
    Co-factors to infection
    Value of testing patients and staff
    Effectiveness of policy statements
    Requirements for infection control among visitors
    Risk to other health care workers

BLOOD AND BODY FLUID PRECAUTIONS

As noted previously, it is recommended that all patients be approached as potentially infectious.[41] The blood and body fluid precautions described here are appropriate for all patients, not just those known to be HIV seropositive—HIV status cannot be known *a priori*. Furthermore, following such an approach could help prevent the transmission of other blood-borne organisms (e.g., hepatitis B virus, HTLV-I, HTLV-II, HTLV-IV, or HIV II).[42-44]

Persons known or strongly suspected of being HIV seropositive are placed on official precautions (hepatitis). ARC and AIDS patients are also placed on enteric and hepatitis precautions, because of the prevalence of diarrhea in this group. In no way, however, does it negate the need to approach all patients as potentially infectious. This practice is demanded of all health care workers, especially those in certain geographical areas where the virus is suspected of being more prevalent. Health care agencies are in the process of developing universal blood and body fluid safeguards to be used as routine precautions in effect for all patients.[83,84] When fully implemented, these safeguards may replace current hepatitis/enteric precautions or the two systems may

coexist, depending on agency climate, philosophy, and acceptance. At present, most agencies continue to have both systems in place.

Needles and Syringes

1. To prevent injuries, sharp instruments, including needles, syringes, scalpels, piggyback intravenous tubing with attached needles, butterflies, angiocaths, and blood tubes, should be handled with extraordinary care.[14,40]
2. Disposable syringes and needles are strongly preferred. Only leur-lock syringes and one-piece needle-syringe units are to be used to aspirate fluids. The leur-lock connection prevents separation of the needle and syringe during the aspiration process, thereby minimizing risk of aerosolization or inadvertent mucous membrane contamination by the splattering of the contents. The collected fluid can be safely discharged through the needle if desired.
    If reusable syringes are employed, they are decontaminated before reprocessing.[14,17]
3. Needles should not be recapped, purposefully beat, broken, detached from disposable syringes, clipped, or manipulated by hand.[14,17]
4. Cardboard containers should not be used, because they can be easily punctured. Place disposable needles, syringes and other sharp instruments (see no. 1) in puncture-resistant containers located as close as practical to the area in which they were used.[14] If there is a risk of unauthorized access to used needles/ syringes (such as by an intravenous drug abuse patient or visitor), this practice will need to be weighed against the risk of needle injury.[45,46]
5. Whenever possible, health care workers using a sharp instrument should dispose of it themselves. This is especially true during bedside procedures (i.e., thoracentesis, blood gas), because the user of the equipment is more aware of the actual location and amount of used equipment in the tray and does not place another, less-aware care provider at risk.[46]
6. Hospital purchasing departments and equipment review committees should evaluate all new purchases with an eye toward safety and to request proof of requirements needed.

Handwashing

1. Handwashing precedes and follows all patient care activities, even if gloves were worn.
2. Hands are always washed immediately when they become soiled with potentially infectious materials and after leaving the patient's room.
3. Hands are washed thoroughly with soap and water. A liquid soap in a non-refillable container or powdered soap is preferred.[46]
4. An antiseptic or antimicrobial handwashing agent is

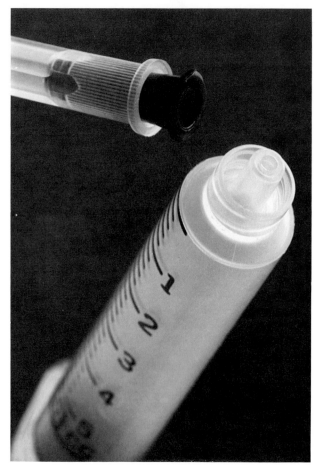

FIG. 25-1. Leur-Lock syringe and needle: This needle locking effect provides a higher level of safety.

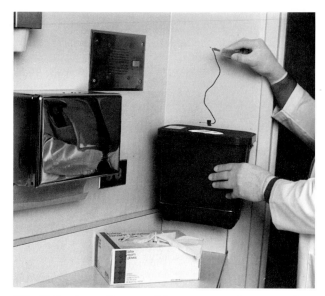

FIG. 25-2. An easily accessible puncture-resistant container for sharp instruments and needles is a sound infection control practice.

to be used by health care personnel before performing an invasive procedure, when caring for patients who are infected or colonized with virulent or epidemiologically significant microorganisms, in the operating room, in newborn nurseries, and in intensive care units. Agents such as povidone-iodine (Betadine) are acceptable.[46] Most health care workers in an oncology setting use antimicrobial scrub solutions because of the immunocompromised patients under their care.

5. Personnel with exudative lesions or weeping dermatitis are not to provide direct services to patients or handle equipment for their use.[47]

Protective Attire

1. As HIV is not transmitted by casual contact, protective attire (gowns, gloves, masks, eye coverings) is not needed unless exposure to blood or body fluids is anticipated.

2. Care is to be provided in such a manner as to minimize the exposure to or formation of infectious aerosols or droplets.[17]

3. Full attention by the health care worker is to be paid to the manipulation of any blood or body fluid while handling it.

Gowns

- The use of disposable gowns is advised if soiling with blood or body fluids is anticipated.
- Additional protection to clothes can be obtained by wearing a disposable plastic apron under the gown.
- Some activities that usually require the use of a gown include changing the bed linen of an incontinent patient, giving care during a vaginal or cesarean delivery or when the patient is not in control of body fluids, such as cardiopulmonary arrest. Gowns are needed during an autopsy.

Gloves

- Gloves are worn when exposure to blood or other body fluids is anticipated.
- Gloves are worn when handling specimens, soiled linen, body fluids, excretions, and secretions as well as surfaces, materials, or objects exposed to them.[17] If the gloves become torn when in use, they should be removed, hands should be washed immediately, and a new pair should be applied.
- Gloves are worn when the health care provider

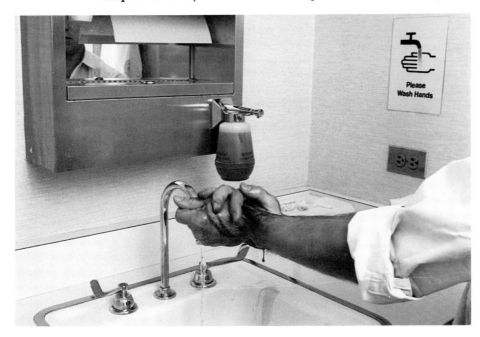

FIG. 25-3. Handwashing remains the first line of defense against the transmission of pathogens.

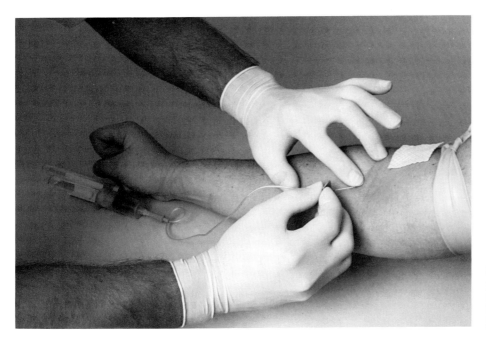

FIG. 25-4. Adjusting to new practices: Adequate preventive measures will require that health care providers change old habits.

has a cut, scratch, or dermatologic lesion of the hands.[14]

- Many health care workers report that latex gloves are generally preferable to vinyl gloves for a number of reasons. They are more comfortable, allow better manual dexterity, conduct heat, and in general have more "give." Vinyl will inhibit the virus but is insufficient for safety in handling chemotherapeutic agents or waste. Therefore, in a cancer care setting, where many patients are receiving chemotherapy, a latex glove is more practical despite the increased cost.

- Some activities that require gloves are venipuncture, invasive procedures, handling blood-soiled items such as placenta, linen, or dressings, emptying bedpans, manipulating specimens, manipulating blood tubes or intravenous lines. Double-gloving is an acceptable practice and has been recommended for autopsies.[48] It has also been used in conjunction with other changes in technique to prevent transmission of HBV during invasive procedures.[49] Usually, however, double-gloving is not necessary.

Masks

- A mask is worn to prevent contamination of the oral mucous membrane by the patient's potentially bloody and infectious respiratory tract secretions.[46]
- A mask is not usually necessary, except when such contact is anticipated.
- Some activities requiring the use of a mask are suctioning, manipulating respiratory therapy equipment, performing invasive procedures that are associated with aerosolization (i.e., autopsy, intubation, and management of major vessel bleeds), caring for a thrombocytopenic patient with poor respiratory secretion hygiene practices, dentistry, and endoscopy.

Eye-Wear/Goggles/Glasses

- Protective eye-wear is not routinely necessary but is used when blood or body fluid splatters to the eyes are anticipated.
- Form-fitting personal eye-wear (glasses) can be used as well as disposable or resterilizable goggles. Disposable protective eye-wear can be used over personal glasses.
- Patient care activities that would routinely call for goggles include those that would require masks.

The justification and rationale for use of protective attire must be discussed with the patients and visitors concerned. They need to have a better understanding of why personnel come into their room "dressed differently" from one another.[46] Their cooperation with infection control practices needs to be elicited.

Sensitive counseling and education will be required to offset the patient's or visitor's potential reaction of feeling unclean or emotionally isolated.[50]

All soiled attire is treated as any other soiled infectious attire.

Resuscitation

1. There has not been a documented case of HIV transmission via mouth-to-mouth resuscitation,[41,51] but in theory a small risk remains.
2. To minimize the need for emergency mouth-to-mouth resuscitation, mouth pieces, resuscitation "ambu" bags, or other ventilation devices are strategically located and available for use in areas where the need for resuscitation is predictable.[14] Some of these areas may include offices, hospital entrances, and areas in close proximity to patient bedsides. A review of the locations of respiratory arrest during the past few years can help institutions to evaluate the need for respiratory equipment.
3. Ambu bags are regularly changed and resterilized twice a week when on stand-by between patients, according to expiration date and when obviously soiled.[52]
4. Full infection control practices are required even though the situation is an emergency.

Food Delivery and Equipment

1. HIV is not casually transmitted, as shown in the previous studies of household contacts. Therefore, meal

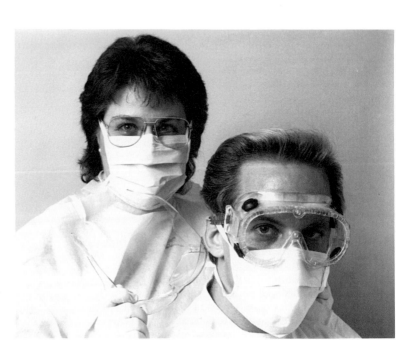

FIG. 25-5. Protective eye-wear: Using eye-wear in conjunction with a mask protects conjunctival, oral, and nasal mucosa from potentially infectious splashes.

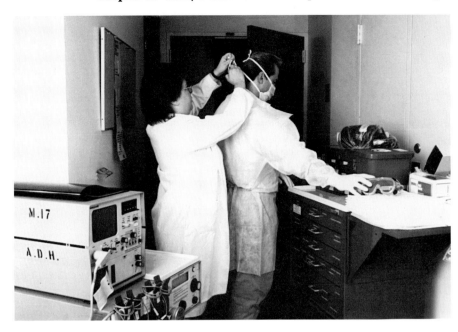

FIG. 25-6. A responsible adjustment in practice: Infection control precautions should not be omitted in an emergency.

trays can be served in a routine manner to HIV seropositive patients without special precautions. HIV seropositive patients on precautions (respiratory, strict) normally receive their meals on disposable equipment.

2. Some hospitals provide disposable trays, dishes, and utensils to HIV-seropositive patients. This is to prevent salivary or blood-borne contamination of any staff member or visitor who removes items from the tray for personal consumption after the patient has eaten. This policy may be needed if efforts to reach and control the food tray "leeches" fail but is not necessary, because dishwashing cycles used in the health care facilities are adequate to decontaminate items.[14,17]

3. Arrangements must be made to have the food tray brought to the patient's bedside and prepared there as needed. Dietary and food service personnel will likely need additional support and education to develop comfort in this area.

4. All food service workers are to follow recommended standards and practices of good personal hygiene and food sanitation. Great care should be taken to avoid injury to hands when preparing food. Should an accident occur that results in food being contaminated with blood, the food is to be discarded.[14]

Blood and Body Fluid Spills

1. All spills of blood and body fluid should be considered potentially infectious and are to be cleaned up immediately.

2. Hospitals should develop and employ an interdepartmental spill containment and clean-up policy.

3. When a spill occurs:

   • Wash hands and don gloves. Wear additional garb as necessary.
   • Contain the spill by demarcating boundaries and placing absorbent material on the spill.
   • Wipe up spill using absorbent material.
   • Dispose of this material in trash identified as infectious waste.
   • Notify housekeeping to respond and appropriately disinfect the area of the spill.

4. Quite a number of agents inactivate the virus. Most of the agents are already routinely used in health care facilities and at higher concentrations than necessary. Germicides that are mycobacteriocidal are preferred because mycobacteria are among the most resistant groups of microorganisms. Germicides that are effective against mycobacterium are also effective against other bacterial or viral pathogens.[14]

5. Most agents already employed by hospitals as sterilants or disinfectants are more than adequate. The following activities and materials inactivate the virus:[53]

   • High or low pH: HIV is susceptible to extremes in pH (pH 1 and 13).
   • Heat: heating to 56°C for ten minutes in the presence of serum.
   • Chemical disinfectants:
     —— 0.3% H_2O_2. (In hospitals, 3% concentrations are routinely used which is more than sufficient).
     —— 50% ethyl alcohol. (In hospitals, 95% concentrations are frequently used, leaving a large margin for safety).
     —— 35% Isopropol alcohol. (Routinely used

concentration unknown. Check the institution's supply).

——— 0.5% paraformaldehyde. (1% concentrations most commonly used).

——— 0.5% Lysol. (3% concentration most commonly used).

——— Household bleach 0.1%. Household bleach is considered to be 5.25% sodium hypochlorite. (In hospitals, 10% concentration is used).

——— 1.0% Nonidet P-40. (0.5% is the common concentration. This needs to be addressed by each hospital).

——— 2.5% Tween-20 is not effective and therefore should not be relied on.

6. Concentration, exposure time, temperature of the solution, and the viral matrix determine inactivation by disinfectants. The conditions of time (2–10 minutes) and temperature (21–25°C) may reasonably apply to many situations in which disinfectants are used.[53] For the most part, the volume used is sufficient to overcome the matrix of the virus.

7. The chemical disinfectants just listed can be applied to dried virus provided that the procedures result in penetration of disinfectant into dried material or cause dissolution/suspension of the virus into disinfectant,[53] as usually does occur in hospital-style cleaning.

8. Solutions should be freshly prepared by the user.

9. Information on specific label claims of commercial germicides can be obtained by writing to: Disinfectants Branch, Office of Pesticides, Environmental Protection Agency, 401 M Street, S.W., Washington D.C. 20460.[14]

Blood and Body Fluid Spills to Clothing

1. All spills are potentially infectious. Efforts should be taken to avoid accidental spills to clothing by using defensive techniques and protective attire such as gowns and laboratory coats.

2. If a spill occurs:

  • Wash hands and don gloves. Avoid contaminating nearby surfaces.
  • Remove the article of clothing and place it in an impervious bag. Don the scrub outfit available in the hospital.
  • Take home and launder separately in a washing machine. Bleach or Lysol may be added to the wash cycle but is not necessary.

Trash and Waste

1. Disposable items used on seropositive individuals should be incinerated or disposed of in accordance with the hospital's policies on infectious wastes. This involves the use of color-coded, waterproof bags, labeling, or both.

2. All trash contaminated with blood or semen should be regarded as potentially infectious and treated as biohazardous material.

3. Double-bagging is necessary if there is contamination by blood or body fluids to the outside of the inner bag.[54]

4. Blood and body fluids can be safely flushed down a toilet or drain connected to a sanitary sewer.[55] Careful attention must be paid not to splatter the waste. Gloves are to be worn. Items that cannot be emptied, such as closed chest drainage systems, are bagged, labeled, and hand carted for waste disposal.

5. Local and state laws regarding the handling of medical waste vary considerably.[56] Practice must be in accordance with health codes, many of which are expected to be revised shortly.

Linens

1. Linens used for patients on precautions are considered potentially infectious. They should be contained, labeled, and handled as biohazardous waste.

2. All *soiled* linens used on any patient should be placed in an impervious laundry bag, preferably hot-water-soluble. Linen is bagged or labeled as biohazardous material.[55]

3. Double-bagging is necessary if the outside of the inner bag is obviously soiled.[55]

4. Gloves should be worn when handling such material. Masks may be required if aerosolization is expected.

5. Hospital laundering procedures provide adequate decontamination of linens.[14] Patients and those caring for them in the home should be instructed that soiled linens are to be washed separately in a washing machine. Bleach or Lysol can be added to the laundry cycle if desired. Consultation with infection control practitioners should be available as needed. Lay persons may contact the National AIDS Hotline operated by the Center for Prevention Services of the CDC for questions regarding infection control in the home.* The telephone number is 1-800-342-AIDS.

Specimens

1. All blood and body fluid specimens collected from patients on precautions, along with the laboratory slip or requisition, should be identified as potentially infectious with special labels. This facilitates appropriate precautions in the handling, collecting, transporting, and study of these specimens. The label need not indicate a diagnosis, for reasons of confidentiality.

2. All blood and body fluid specimens should be considered potentially infectious by the laboratory workers even though the patient may not be on specific precautions.[57]

3. Contamination of the outside of the specimen con-

---

* B. Kohmescher, personal communication, August 1987.

tainer should be wiped off with a disinfectant (See section on Spills).

4. Specimen containers should be placed in clear, impermeable plastic bags (e.g., Zip-lock) to avoid accidental spillage during transport. If the outside of the bag is contaminated with blood or body fluids, a second, outer bag is used. The requisition is then attached.

5. Hospitals using preprinted addressograph plates may want to attach preprinted precaution stickers as appropriate to the isolation or precautions required. This may facilitate interdepartmental communication and labeling of requisitions.[46] In other hospitals, computer systems facilitate the transfer of this information.

Transporting the Patient

1. The test requisition and the patient's name band are labeled with the preprinted precaution sticker. Hospitals with computer systems can facilitate the interdepartmental communication of isolation or precautions through data entered on a system.
2. The patient is wrapped in a clean sheet.
3. The patient need not wear masks, gowns, gloves or other items unless he has another infectious process or is strongly suspected of having one. An example is the use of a mask by a patient highly suspected of having *M. tuberculosis*[58] (or *Pneumocystis carinii* pneumonia [PCP] if other immunocompromised patients are in the patient's vicinity. This practice is controversial, however, with most authorities deeming it unnecessary for PCP). Protective clothing is not required to transport or escort patients.

Patient Care Equipment

1. Reusable, soiled items should be placed in designated, clear, impermeable bags for transporting and processing. These bags are labeled.
2. Disposable items should be placed in pre-determined labeled receptacles for infectious waste.
3. Housekeeping procedures used in hospitals are adequate for cleaning rooms and furniture.[14]
4. Surfaces contaminated with blood or body fluids should be cleaned as soon as possible.
5. Personal items belonging to the patient can be sterilized as needed in central supply. Supplies need to be labeled and arrangements made to retrieve them in a few days at the Security Desk. Items that do not need to be sterilized can be disinfected. Instructions must be given to the patient and his loved ones regarding this process. Items that cannot be disinfected (i.e., drawings) may be discarded or aired in the sun's ray for a few hours.[52] Items do not need special cleaning unless they are soiled with blood or body fluids. Consultation can be provided by infection control practitioners. Patients are encouraged to keep nondisposable personal items brought to the hospital to a minimum.

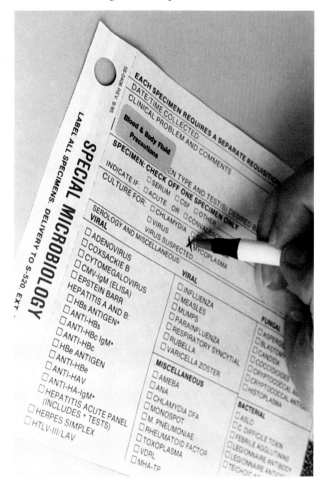

FIG. 25-7. Responsibility and communication are essential: Interdepartmental collaboration is a prerequisite for the prevention of inadvertent exposures. This responsibility starts on an individual level.

Room Assignment

1. Private rooms are not necessary for seropositive individuals unless their personal hygiene is poor, they are not in control of their body fluids, are noncompliant, have altered behavior due to complications, or have other potentially transmittable pathogens.[17,46,54,55,59,60]
2. In general, immunocompromised seropositive patients (ARC or AIDS) do not share rooms with immunosuppressed patients or those infected with potentially transmittable pathogens, especially those transmitted by the airborne route.
3. Grouping or cohorting of AIDS and ARC patients is acceptable if they have the same opportunistic infection.
4. All such decisions need to be made in consultation with an infection control practitioner because of the risk of cross-infection.
5. The minimum of a separate bathroom or commode

is made available for patients with poor hygiene practices or profuse diarrhea and for children.[46]

6. Quality or quantity of health care is not to be dependent on room availability. Care in an open ward such as an ICU or emergency room is acceptable if blood and body fluid precautions can be maintained.
7. Easily identifiable room isolation signs are to be strategically located to provide all workers and visitors information about the type of precaution required.
8. Every effort is made to protect privacy and confidentiality.
9. Special waiting rooms or lounges are not necessary.

Other Services and Areas of the Hospital

All health care workers should follow the precautions outlined in the preceding pages. Additional recommendations for special service areas follow.

LABORATORY SERVICES.[17,54]

1. Mouth pipetting is prohibited. Mechanical pipetting devices must be used for all liquids.
2. Laboratory coats, gowns, or uniforms are worn when working with potentially infectious materials and should be removed before leaving the laboratory.
3. Biological safety cabinets (class II) are used for procedures that have a high potential to generate aerosolizations. These procedures include blending, harvesting infected tissue from animals or embryonated eggs, vigorous mixing, sonicating, and centrifugation.
4. Tissue or serum specimens to be stored must be clearly and permanently labeled as potentially infectious.
5. Laboratory work surfaces are to be cleaned with a suitable disinfectant immediately after spills and at the end of the day.
6. Primary containment devices are used in handling materials that might contain concentrated infectious agents or organisms in greater quantities than expected in clinical settings.
7. Gloves are worn to avoid skin contact with blood, specimens containing blood, blood-soiled items, body fluids, excretions, and secretions as well as surfaces, materials, and objects exposed to them.
8. Public access to the laboratory processing HIV-contaminated substances is restricted under p2 designation. Access is permitted if experiments are not being conducted. The door must be kept closed while work is in progress. Eating, drinking, smoking, and food storage are not allowed.
9. Appropriate precautions must be taken with reagents and controls.
10. The laboratory director is responsible for assessing which biosafety level should be used.
11. Further information on biosafety can be obtained by writing for a copy of the CDC-NIH Biosafety Manual (#01702300167-1), Superintendent of Documents, U.S. Government Printing Office, Washington D.C. 20402. The telephone number is (202) 783-3238. The present cost is $4.

LABORATORY RESEARCH INVOLVING ANIMAL SUBJECTS.[17]

1. Animal cages are decontaminated, preferably by autoclaving, before they are cleaned and washed.
2. Laboratory coats, gowns, or uniforms should be worn by personnel entering rooms housing inoculated animals, consistent with animal BSL-2 practices. Some non-human primates experimentally infected with HIV or other AIDS-related material may bite, throw feces, urinate, or expectorate at humans. Therefore, caregivers must wear coats, protective gloves, coveralls or uniforms, and face shields, as appropriate, to protect their skin and mucous membranes of the eyes, nose, and mouth.
3. Personnel are to wear gloves for all activities involving direct contact with experimental animals, their bedding and cages. Care must be taken to minimize the creation of aerosals or droplets.
4. Necroscopy of animals is performed by personnel wearing gloves and gowns. If aerosolization is anticipated, mask and goggles should also be worn.
5. Some safety equipment and biological safety cabinets may not be available in all clinical laboratories. Assistance should be sought from a microbiology laboratory as needed.

OPHTHALMIC EXAMINATIONS AND PROCEDURES.[54,61]

1. Although HIV has been isolated in tears,[65] conjunctival[62] and corneal tissue,[63] and contact lenses,[64] there is no evidence to date regarding transmission to health care workers by ophthalmic procedures or fittings of contact lenses. While more data is being accumulated, the following precautions are implemented.

- Immediate washing of hands is required by health care workers performing eye examinations or other procedures involving contact with tears. Disposable gloves may be worn and are advisable if there are cuts, scratches, or dermatologic lesions on the hands. Use of other protective gear is not necessary.
- Workers with weeping lesions or other infections of the hands or arms should not perform ophthalmic procedures or examine patients.
- Instruments that come into contact with external surfaces of the eye should be wiped clean and then disinfected by one of the following: a 5- to 10-minute exposure to a fresh solution of 3% hydrogen peroxide; a fresh solution containing 5000 parts per million (5 mg/liter) free available chlorine—a 1/10 dilution of common household bleach (sodium hypochlorite); 70% ethanol; or 70% isopropanol. The device is thoroughly rinsed with tap water and dried before being reused.

- Contact lenses used in trial fittings are to be disinfected between each fitting. Most trial hard lenses can be treated with the standard heat disinfection regimen used for soft lenses (78–80°C for 10 minutes). Hard lens suppliers can inform practitioners which lenses can safely be heat-treated. Commercially available hydrogen peroxide contact lens disinfecting systems currently approved for soft lenses can be used on hard lenses. Hydrogen peroxide preparations containing preservatives should be avoided, because they may discolor the lens. Rigid gas-permeable (RGP) trial fitting lenses can be disinfected using the above hydrogen peroxide disinfection system. RGP lenses may warp if they are heat treated. Soft trial fitting lenses can be disinfected using the same hydrogen peroxide disinfection system. Some soft lenses have also been approved for heat disinfection.
- Bandages or other disposable items contaminated by blood and/or body fluid are treated as infectious waste.

PERINATAL AND NEONATAL CARE[54,65]

1. Because maternal seroconversion may not occur for months after delivery, infection control procedures should be followed during perinatal care of women and their offspring.
2. For high-risk or known seropositive mothers:

- Blood and body fluids of maternal or fetal origin are considered potentially infectious.
- The placenta should not be released for commercial use.
- Protective attire and other actions are taken as previously described.
- Until more information is available, breast feeding should be discouraged for mothers known to be infected with HIV or high-risk mothers whose antibody status is unknown.
- High-risk mothers include intravenous drug users, prostitutes, women from countries where rates of heterosexual transmission are high, and sex partners of known infected bisexual or intravenous drug using men.

OPERATING ROOMS.[54]

1. There is no evidence that HIV infection has occurred from patient to staff or staff to patient. Current infection control practices minimize the risk of transmission of all infectious agents, including HIV. A 1985 report of a surgeon with AIDS who had operated on 400 patients showed no cases of AIDS in patients followed-up during a 2- to 3-year period.[66] Nevertheless, one study[67] showed that approximately 11% of all surgical gloves are perforated during surgery, rendering the surgeon, nurse, or patient liable to a certain risk if their skin is not intact.

2. Separate operating rooms are not necessary. Furthermore, it is not necessary to schedule patients with HIV infections at the end of the day.
3. In addition to the usual sterile dress worn during surgical procedures, protective eyewear should be worn in situations where spattering of blood or body fluids is anticipated.
4. All soiled laundry, trash, or other disposable items are treated as infectious waste.
5. After the procedure, the operating room table should be wiped generously with a 1:10 solution of bleach, which is left on for 10 minutes. The surface is then wiped off with water (prolonged exposure to bleach has a corrosive effect, especially on aluminum).
6. The operating room scheduling desk should be notified in advance by the surgeon in order to prepare protective attire and other infection control measures. The patient's nurse needs to include any information on precautions or isolation in the preoperative check list.

AUTOPSY PRECAUTIONS.

1. As part of routine postmortem nursing care, patients with HIV infection should be identified by appropriate isolation tagging, whether an autopsy is being performed or not. This information is needed by the mortician.
2. Protective gear must be worn by personnel performing or viewing an autopsy. This gear may include eye wear, mask, cap, gown, foot coverings, waterproof apron, and gloves. The CDC has advocated double-gloving while performing autopsies.[48]
3. Methods to minimize the aerosol distribution of infectious agents should be used. An example is the use of a hand saw on bone rather than an electric saw.[54]
4. The deceased and any bagged items for disposal are tagged and wrapped to prevent unwitting exposure of other personnel.
5. After the autopsy, the table, instruments and nondisposable contaminated equipment must be disinfected.
6. Tissue sections should be thoroughly fixed in 10% buffered formalin before trimming for histology. Specimens to be stored and frozen must be clearly and permanently labeled as biohazardous.[54]
7. There have been numerous reports of overcharging and needless precautions by funeral homes in the preparation and presentation of the deceased at wakes, funerals, and burials.* Questions the loved ones may have can be directed to an AIDS advocacy group in the area, such as the Gay Men's Health Crisis, Inc., in the New York area (the Hotline number is (212) 807-6655). Information may also be obtained from the nursing supervisor, social worker, or client representative at the hospital. Instances of abuses or other questionable activities should be brought to

---

* K. Glidden, personal communication, August 27, 1987.

the attention of state departments on human rights or health system management.

TRANSPLANTATION OF TISSUES, ORGANS AND BODY FLUIDS.

1. Members of high-risk groups and those who have engaged in high-risk behaviors or are known HIV seropositive are not to donate blood, tissues, organs, or body fluids.[55,68]
2. The donors of all tissues, organs, blood, and body fluids must be tested for the presence of blood-borne diseases, including HIV. Examples of donations are cornea, skin, sperm, milk, heart, lung, pancreas, liver, bone, kidney, and ova.[55]
3. Educative and counseling services regarding HIV need to be fully available to these persons.

DENTISTRY.[47,69]

1. Obtain a health history from each patient that includes questions about medications, current illnesses, hepatitis, recurrent illnesses, unintentional weight loss, lymphadenopathy, oral soft-tissue lesions, or other infections. A medical consultation may be indicated if a history of active infection or systemic illness is elicited.
2. Gloves must be worn when examining oral lesions. All work should be completed on one person, when possible. Hands are washed and regloved before performing procedures on another patient.
3. Surgical masks and protective eye-wear or chin-length plastic shields must be worn when splashing or spattering of blood or body fluids is likely.
4. Impervious-backed paper, aluminum foil, or clear plastic wrap may be used to cover surfaces (e.g., light handles or x-ray unit heads) that are contaminated by blood or saliva and that are difficult or impossible to disinfect. The coverings should be removed (while dental health care worker's hands are gloved), discarded, and then replaced (after ungloving) with clean material between patients.
5. Careful attention to the minimizing of aerosols or droplets may include the use of rubber dams, high-speed evacuation, and proper patient positioning.
6. Because certain dental procedures may require repeated injections of anesthetic or other medications from a single syringe, it is prudent to place the unsheathed needle onto a "sterile field" instead of recapping the needle between injections. Sterile syringes and fresh solution are used for each patient.
7. Instruments that normally penetrate soft tissue or bone (e.g., forceps, scalpels, bone chisels, scrapers, and surgical burs) should be sterilized after each use. Instruments that come into contact with oral tissues but do not penetrate bone or soft tissues (e.g., amalgam condensers, plastic instruments, and burs) should be sterilized after each use. If sterilization is not possible, high-level disinfection should be achieved.
8. Before cleaning, debris must be removed from the instruments by thoroughly scrubbing with soap and water or detergent, or by using a mechanical device (e.g., an ultrasonic cleaner). Persons involved in cleaning or disinfecting instruments should wear heavy-duty rubber gloves to prevent hand injuries.

- Sterilization: Metal and heat-stable dental instruments should be routinely sterilized between uses by steam under pressure (autoclaving), dry heat, or chemical vapor. The adequacy of sterilization cycles should be verified by the periodic use of spore-testing devices (e.g., weekly for most dental practices). Heat- and steam-sensitive chemical indicators may be used on the outside of each pack to ensure that it has been exposed to a sterilizing cycle.

  Heat-sensitive instruments may require up to 10 hours of exposure in a liquid chemical agent registered by the U.S. Environmental Protection Agency (EPA) as a disinfectant/sterilant. This should be followed by rinsing with sterile water.
- High-level disinfection: This may be accomplished by immersion in boiling water for at least 10 minutes or an EPA-registered disinfectant/ sterilant chemical for the exposure time recommended by the chemical's manufacturer.

9. A chemical germicide registered with the FDA as a hospital disinfectant and having a label claim for mycobactericidal activity is preferred for decontaminating laboratory supplies and equipment. Materials used in the mouth (e.g., impression plates, bite registration, and so on) should be cleaned to remove blood or saliva, especially before polishing and grinding intra-oral devices. Materials, impressions, and intra-oral appliances must be cleaned and disinfected before being handled, adjusted, or sent to a dental laboratory. The same process should be repeated when they return from the laboratory before they are placed in the patient's mouth. Communication between the dental office and the laboratory about this matter is essential. Of note, because of the increasing variety of dental materials, dental health care workers are advised to consult with manufacturers about the stability of specific materials relative to disinfection procedures.
10. Not all equipment can currently receive high-level disinfection or sterilization. The following recommended practices should greatly reduce the risk of disease transmission or viral growth.

- Handpieces that cannot be sterilized or receive high-level disinfection: After using the handpiece, it should be flushed for 20 to 30 seconds, then thoroughly scrubbed with a detergent and water to remove adherent material. It should then be thoroughly washed and wiped with absorbent material saturated with a chemical germicide (FDA-registered "hospital disinfectant" and mycobactericidal). The disinfecting solution must remain in contact with the handpiece for the time specified by the product's manufacturer.

- Ultrasonic scalers and air/water syringes should be treated in a similar manner between patients.
- After disinfection, any chemical residue should be removed by rinsing with sterile water.
- Because water retraction valves may aspirate infective materials back into the handpiece and waterline, check valves should be installed within the dental units to reduce the risk of transfer of infected material. While the magnitude of this risk is not known, it is prudent to allow water to be discharged from the unit for 20 to 30 seconds after completing its use on each patient. This process can be repeated for several minutes at the beginning of each clinic day to flush out bacterial accumulation that may have occurred overnight. Sterile saline or sterile water should be used as a coolant/irrigator while performing surgical procedures involving the cutting of soft tissue or bone.

DIALYSIS TREATMENT.[70]

1. The standard blood or body fluid precautions and disinfection and sterilization strategies already routinely practiced in dialysis centers are adequate to prevent transmission of HIV.
2. The dialyzer and associated blood tubing are disposable. The standard disinfection process for the hemodialysis machine fluid pathways generally consists of using about 500 to 750 ppm of sodium hypochlorite for 30 to 40 minutes or 1.5% to 2% formaldehyde overnight to be sufficient. In addition, several chemical germicides formulated to disinfect dialysis machines are commercially available.
3. Patients infected with HIV can be dialyzed by either hemodialysis or peritoneal dialysis and do not need to be isolated from other patients (refer to room assignment section). The dialyzer may be discarded after each use. Alternatively, centers may have dialyzer-reuse programs in which a specific dialyzer is issued to a specific patient. The dialyzer is removed, cleaned, disinfected, and reused several times on the same patient only. The centers may incorporate HIV-seropositive patients into their protocol. An individual dialyzer must never be used on more than one patient.
4. Of note, dialysis patients can have a false positive ELISA test with negative Western blot due to repeated exposure to blood transfusions and H_9-cell-associated antigens.

CLEANING OF INSTRUMENTS.[14,54]

1. Retroviruses are broadly susceptible to common disinfectants such as alcohols, phenol, formalin, sodium hypochlorite, and glutaraldehyde.[53,71] Exposure of contaminated material to ethylene oxide or autoclaving according to protocols results in sterilization.
2. Refer to blood or body fluids spill section for more detail.
3. HIV or other pathogens may not be eradicated if visibly soiled items are not appropriately cleaned. Specially trained personnel should scrub the instrument with soap and water or a detergent while wearing heavy-duty gloves.
4. All contaminated equipment or instruments should be autoclaved if they can withstand the process.
5. Bronchoscopes, gastroscopes, and other lensed equipment should be sterilized with ethylene oxide or receive high-level disinfection with an agent that is also mycobactericidal. A 2% glutaraldehyde soak for 45 minutes is sufficient for this purpose.[54] Further information can be obtained from the manufacturer. All instruments should be rinsed with sterile water after cleaning. In addition, pieces such as the air insufflatory rubber tubing of the rigid sigmoidoscope should be cleaned using a high-level mycobactericidal disinfectant.
6. Thermometers should be scrubbed after use with soap and water or a detergent to remove any blood or body fluids.[72] They should then be disinfected with alcohol, 2% gluteraldehyde, or another disinfectant. Glass thermometers are changed daily and used for single-patient use. Flexible plastic sheaths are not recommended.[73]

EMPLOYEE CONSIDERATIONS

Pregnant Health Care Workers

Many health care workers have expressed anxiety over the risk to the fetus that HIV infection poses. HIV-infected mothers can pass the virus to their unborn child. All precautions normally taken to prevent the transmission of HIV can safeguard pregnant women. This also applies to women trying to get pregnant. Pregnant health care workers are not known to be at greater risk of contracting HIV infection than nonpregnant health care workers. Because of the potential risk to the child if a pregnant health care worker contracts HIV, these women should be especially familiar with precautions for preventing HIV transmission.[14,55,74,75]

At Memorial Sloan-Kettering Cancer Center, the Employee Health Service department routinely offers employees counseling about biohazardous materials in the workplace. Pregnancy counseling is available.

At some institutions, pregnant employees are not assigned to care for HIV-infected persons or handle blood or body fluids presumed to be so infected. This policy, formal or informal, is in accordance with the long-standing restrictions of pregnant women from other potential occupational exposures, such as radiation therapy, that poses a threat to the fetus.[57,76]

Many patients with AIDS excrete large amounts of CMV. Therefore, it is recommended that pregnant women follow existing policies of infection control to prevent possible CMV exposure.[77] Pregnant women do not provide direct services to patients with CMV pneumonia.

Management of Parenteral and Mucous Membrane Exposures of Health Care Workers

If a health care worker has a parenteral (e.g., needlestick or cut) or mucous membrane (e.g., splash to the eye or mouth) exposure to blood or other body fluids, the source patient should be assessed clinically and epidemiologically to determine the likelihood of HIV infection. If the source patient has AIDS or other evidence of HIV infection, declines testing, or has a positive test, the health care worker should be evaluated clinically and serologically for evidence of HIV infection as soon as possible after the exposure, and, if seronegative, retested after 6 weeks and on a periodic basis thereafter (e.g., 3, 6, and 12 months following exposure) to determine if transmission has occurred. During this follow-up period, especially the first 6–12 weeks, when most infected persons are expected to seroconvert, exposed workers should receive counseling about the risk of infection and follow U.S. Public Health Service recommendations for preventing transmission of AIDS. If the source patient is seronegative and has no other evidence of HIV infection, no further follow-up of the worker is necessary. If the source patient cannot be identified, decisions on appropriate follow-up should be individualized according to the type of exposure and the likelihood that the source patient was infected.[14]

In addition, an incident report needs to be completed by the health care worker, his or her supervisor, and the Health Service department to determine if similar exposures could be prevented by taking certain precautionary actions. At our institution, these employees are referred to the Infectious Disease service for evaluation and follow-up. For reasons connected to insurance, interpersonal relations, job security, confidentiality, and time, some exposed people will refrain from coming forward to seek testing or counseling at their workplace. This may be quite common, as seen in one study,[18] when only 46 of 150 exposed health care workers chose to report their injuries to the occupational medical service.

The health care worker will require instruction and counseling about the possibility of HIV infection and the precautionary measures to take while awaiting the results of the serial blood tests. The content should include a review of blood and body fluid precautions, safer sex practices, and other emotionally laden topics. This service can be offered by the Employee Health Service, the Infectious Disease department, a multidisciplinary AIDS team, or another group as appropriate to the structure of the facility. Strict confidentiality and professionalism is of key importance.

Health care workers who have sustained a needle-stick injury from an HIV-infected patient may be enrolled in the "Health Worker's Surveillance Project" of the CDC. As of October 1, 1987, health care providers who have sustained non-needlestick exposures from HIV-infected patients in the form of splashes of blood to open wounds or mucous membranes may also be entered. Information can be obtained by calling the CDC Hospital Infections Program at (404) 639-1644. An information packet through which the hospital in the program can enroll will be mailed to the infection control practitioner or physician.*

Each institution will need to set guidelines for what is to be done when a non-employee, such as a fireman, policeman, or member of the public, suffers an exposure to a patient. The institution may choose to follow the exposed worker or family member or can refer him to his physician or occupational health center with full cooperation. As yet there are no generally agreed-upon guidelines.

At Memorial Sloan-Kettering Cancer Center, employees who are concerned about previous exposures to HIV incurred during occupational endeavors are formally counseled and educated through the Memorial Information and Testing Program (MIT). This program is staffed by registered nurses and social workers and was developed in conjunction with Psychiatry and Infectious Disease services among others. Those who choose to, can obtain confidential HIV testing. However, it is our experience that the number of employees turning to this service is extremely low. This program is also open to MSKCC patients who received blood products before April 19, 1985 (before HIV-testing of donated blood was available) and their sexual partners and children.

The cost-effectiveness of this and other methods of handling the management of health care worker exposures is as yet unresolved.

Serologic Testing of Patients

Some institutions serving certain areas where the prevalence of HIV infection is high may deem it appropriate to initiate serologic testing of patients. Of course, testing for reasons such as diagnosis or medical management is required. However, testing for reasons of infection control does not necessarily assist in prevention—as noted earlier, one study of health care workers in a geographical area and institution familiar with AIDS patients found inadequate use of infection control procedures.[13] Furthermore, routine testing of patients would not capture those hospitalized for short stays or on an emergency basis.

Despite this, certain procedures, such as apheresis, hemodialysis, peritoneal dialysis, and organ donations,

---

* R Marcus, personal communication, August 27, 1987.

benefit from this testing. This topic is currently a subject of debate, and no consensus has been reached.[40]

Transmission from Health Care Workers to Patients[14]

Although there has been no evidence of HIV-infected health care providers transmitting the infection to patients, the risk does exist in certain circumstances. Transmission could result if the patient has a high degree of trauma that provides a portal of entry (i.e., during invasive procedures) and the provider's blood or serous fluid comes in contact with the patient's tissue.

In light of this possibility, providers who perform invasive procedures such as an operative, obstetric, or dental procedure need to be especially aware of the mode of transmission and methods of prevention by the use of barriers. The CDC defines these invasive procedures as follows:

> An operative procedure is defined as surgical entry into tissues, cavities, organs or repair of major traumatic injuries in an operating or delivery room, emergency department, or outpatient setting, including both physicians' and dentists' offices. An obstetric procedure is defined as a vaginal or cesarean delivery or other invasive obstetric procedure where bleeding may occur. A dental procedure is defined as the manipulation, cutting or removal of any oral or perioral tissues, including tooth structure, where bleeding occurs or the potential for bleeding exists.[47]

Routine precautionary measures are required. These include gloving when touching mucous membranes or nonintact skin of all patients, using barrier precautions when handling the placenta or the infant until blood and amniotic fluid has been removed from the infant's skin, and using extraordinary care to prevent injuries to hands. In addition, no health care worker who has exudative lesions or weeping dermatitis should perform or assist in invasive procedures or other direct patient care activities or handle equipment for patient care. Care providers who have evidence of any illness that may compromise their ability to perform invasive procedures adequately and safely should be evaluated medically to determine whether they are physically and mentally competent to perform invasive procedures.[47]

Serologic testing of health care workers who perform invasive procedures or of patients undergoing such procedures is not recommended.[40] The risk of transmission is low, and the results of such testing would not result in changes in the precautionary activity routinely taken during invasive procedures.

If a patient does become exposed to the blood or serous fluid of a care provider during an invasive procedure, he or she should be informed of the incident, and previous recommendations for management of such exposures should be followed (see the section on the

management of parenteral and mucous membrane exposures of health care workers).

HIV-seropositive care providers with immune defects (especially ARC and AIDS) will need adequate education and counseling about the risk of acquiring other infectious diseases from patients. On a case-by-case basis, the health care worker's personal physician, in conjunction with the employee health service director and possibly the employee's department chief, should determine if the worker can adequately and safely perform patient care responsibilities or suggest changes in work assignment if needed. This conference may also include infection control practitioners. In cases where the individual may jeopardize patient care routines, as in the case of progressive AIDS dementia complex (ADC), this conference should be done in a timely and compassionate way.

Institutional policies concerning requirements such as vaccinating employees with live virus need to be reconsidered also.

Infection Control Management of AIDS-Related Opportunistic Infections

Many AIDS patients develop opportunistic infections. For the most part, these infections are not easily transmissible and present no real threat to care providers or other patients.[58] A full discussion of this aspect of infection control requires more than can be included in this chapter. However, highlights are presented in Table 25-2. (For more details see Chapter 12.)

Education and Quality Assurance

Staff

Many staff members have reacted with anger and anxiety when called upon to care for HIV-seropositive people. Frequently this response is based on fear. A national survey of oncology nurses[78] found that fear was a major response when these nurses were asked what problems they saw in caring for people with HIV disorders. The reasons for this response were varied and included fear of becoming infected or subsequently infecting others in the family (presumably sexual partner and children), AIDS patients' fears of infecting care givers, fear or distrust of hospital administration, and family members' anxiety or fearfulness for the nurse among others. This study also noted that many nurses reported a significant lack of knowledge about disease-specific information, planning for nursing interventions, and treatments (including experimental ones). The survey found that most respondents (82%) reported moderate to extensive knowledge about safety precautions.

Although respondents state that they are knowledgeable regarding safety precautions, their fear response remains high. This suggests that an educational

Table 25-2
Infection Control for Infections in Hospitalized AIDS Patients

Precaution/Isolation*	Infection/Organism	Duration of Precaution/Isolation
Enteric precautions	Salmonellosis, shigellosis	Duration of illness until three consecutive stool cultures taken at least 24 hours apart are negative
	Cryptosporidium	Duration of illness
	Strongyloides	Same as above
	AIDS	Same as above
	Giardiasis, amebiasis	Same as above
Hepatitis precautions	HIV	Duration of illness
	CMV	Same as above
	AIDS	Same as above
	Hepatitis B antigen (HBsAg) positive asymptomatic and symptomatic	Same as above
	Hepatitis A	Until approved by Infectious Disease Service
	Hepatitis non A, non B	Same as above
	Chronic carrier status (*Salmonella, Shigella*)	Consult with Infectious Disease Service
Respiratory precautions	Tuberculosis pulmonary, sputum (positive or suspect) extrapulmonary (open)	Until approved by Infectious Disease Service
	Nocardia (for AIDS patients only)	
	CMV pneumonia	
Strict precautions	Disseminated herpes simplex pneumonia	Duration of illness
	Herpes zoster	Until all lesions are crusted
Wound and skin precautions	Resistant organisms present	Until lesions are completely healed or, if they harbor resistant organisms, until cleared by the Infectious Disease Service
	Draining or purulent wounds	
	Infected or heavily colonized wound	
	Herpes simplex infections	
	Open lesions or eschar	

* All patients are approached as if they are potentially infectious through blood or body fluid contact. This is the cornerstone of universal safeguards.[83]
(Modified from MSKCC Hospital, Infection Control Committee: Infectious Disease Manual. Memorial Sloan-Kettering Cancer Center, January 14, 1987, p 33–43 [unpublished])

program should not just be geared to safety precautions, but should also address the other content areas cited. This approach provides a sense of empowerment and control. These feelings are especially needed when, as frequently seen in our practice, the patients are more knowledgeable about their condition than many health care providers. This uncomfortable position for care providers can lead to self-doubt and avoidance of the "expert" patient.

Surveys of doctors and dentists have also shown a high level of anger, anxiety, or fear, which we would tend to evaluate in the same manner as the nurses' response.

Many hospitals have developed aggressive AIDS education programs for staff. These programs have been successful in minimizing anxiety and providing the staff with this sense of control. These efforts, along with crisis intervention by skilled, knowledgeable and respected hospital personnel, are perhaps the most useful activities to ensure that a hospital continues to function adequately when an AIDS or HIV-seropositive individual is admitted.[55]

Various methods have been used to present such intervention programs. Some authorities have called for the formation of a special AIDS coordinating group with broad educational and support responsibilities within the hospital.[55]

In our experience this approach of forming an "AIDS Task Force" representing every department has been extremely beneficial. Interdepartmental, professional, and nonprofessional concerns and policy development are discussed and agreed upon at this level. Individual members representing a department (usually the chief) then have the responsibility for disseminating this information to their department and for communicating their departments' concerns to others.

In addition, special work groups, such as the testing program and resource utilization group, arise from this coordinating "AIDS Task Force."

Special teams have also been developed to fill the needs of advisors, teachers, supporters, and practitioners. These teams have included infection control practitioners, social workers, psychiatrists, chaplains, nurses, patient representatives, infectious disease experts, per-

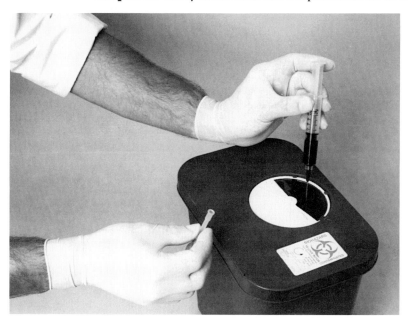

FIG. 25-8. Continued prevalence of needlestick injuries: Despite guidelines, institutions still report many needlestick injuries. Changes in equipment, environment, and behavior need to be re-examined.

sonnel from public relations and other services in the Department of Medicine (notably Immunology, Dermatology, Pulmonary, Neurology) and the Admitting Department.

At MSKCC education is provided to all new employees to the Center. In nursing, programs are maintained in Registered Nurse orientation, inservice education, patient care conferences, and other more formal settings, such as nursing grand rounds. In addition, invaluable standards of care[79] were written and are available on each unit where nurses practice. A copy of the NYC Department of Health AIDS Resource List is on each unit. AIDS content has been incorporated into the housestaff orientation, medical grand rounds, and many other continuing education events.

A multidisciplinary case management group exists to facilitate the provision of care to patients and to work to make the hospital system more amenable to these patients. In addition, at times of perceived crisis or heightened anxiety, experts have provided frequent open sessions for staff to attend and discuss the current issue.[15,16,80] The need for these "open forums" is often related to publication of new information and the level of media coverage it receives. Usually, ongoing AIDS education interventions suffice. Ongoing support groups offer invaluable assistance to staff in their adjustment to current events.*

Integrally related to this, is the oft-discussed advocacy role of health care institutions toward their staff. Many have noted that hospitals' compliance with recommendations from the CDC have been slow to half-hearted. Not all institutions have been lax, however. One

example is the direct mailing of guidelines to their employees by the Harvard Community Health Plan in Boston.† Because of the voluntary nature of these recommendations, the Labor Department's Occupational Safety and Health Administration (OSHA) will be setting standards for protection of health care workers.[81] When these are available, hospitals will be liable for their implementation and could be fined for negligence. This will induce hospital administrators to fully implement education and quality assurance monitoring and follow-up.[82]

Visitors

People coming to the hospital need to be told to avoid contact with blood or body fluid. To this end, educational interventions need to be employed. This program plan may need to involve the public relations department as well.

Signs are routinely posted on isolation or precaution patients' rooms that alert visitors to infection control behaviors. In addition, every sign has a notice to ask for instructions at the nurse's station (a practice not frequently adhered to by visitors).

Visitors and patients can be supplied with a teaching card reviewing infection control and precautions.* In other institutions, interactional video or television teaching techniques may be used. Other strategies, including hospital unit or bedside notices about universal safeguards,[83,84] need to be investigated. By handwashing stations, universal language signs communicate the need to wash hands. Nurses teach visitors and friends prin-

---

* M Feldstein, J Pasacreta, personal communication, August 1987.

† D Gallagher, personal communication, August 26, 1987.

* R Slevin, personal communication, July 1987.

ciples of infection control. This content is incorporated into home care management of the patient. Hospitals are currently investigating the best method to communicate this information to visitors. As repeatedly noted in studies of household contact, HIV transmission is low to non-existent. However, a direct care provider's perception of "casual contact" is frequently quite different from what is understood by those in a non–health care related activity. Because of this, it is necessary to teach our patients' loved ones about blood or body fluid precautions.

REFERENCES

1. Gallo RC, Salahuddin SZ, Popovic M, et al: Frequent detection and isolation of cytopathic retroviruses (HTLV-III) from patients with AIDS and at risk for AIDS. Science 224: 500, 1984

2. Barré-Sinoussi F, Chermann JC, Rey F, et al: Isolation of a T-lymphotropic retrovirus from a patient at risk for acquired immune deficiency syndrome (AIDS). Science 220: 868, 1983

3. Levy JA, Hoffman AD, Kramer SM, et al: Isolation of lymphocytopathic retroviruses from San Francisco patients with AIDS. Science 225:840, 1984

4. Zagury D, Bernard J, Leibowitch J, et al: HTLV-III in cells cultured from semen of two patients with AIDS. Science 226:449, 1984

5. Fujikawa LS, Salahuddin SZ, Palestine AG, et al: Isolation of human T-lymphotropic virus type III from the tears of a patient with the acquired immunodeficiency syndrome. Lancet ii:529, 1985

6. Groopman JE, Salahuddin SZ, Sarngadharan MG, et al: HTLV-III in saliva of people with AIDS-related complex and healthy homosexual men at risk for AIDS. Science 226:447, 1984

7. Levy JA, Kaminsky LS, Morrow WJW, et al: Infection by the retrovirus associated with the acquired immunodeficiency syndrome: Clinical, biological and molecular features. Ann Intern Med 103:694, 1985

8. Thiry L, Sprecher-Goldberger S, Jonckheer T, et al: Isolation of AIDS virus from cell-free breast milk of three healthy virus carriers (letter). Lancet ii:891, 1985

9. Vogt MW, Witt DJ, Craven DE, et al: Isolation patterns of the human immunodeficiency virus from cervical secretions during the menstrual cycle of women at risk for the acquired immunodeficiency syndrome. Ann Int Med 106(3):380, 1987

10. Wofsy CV, Cohen JB, Hauer LB, et al: Isolation of AIDS-associated retrovirus from genital secretions of women with antibodies to the virus. Lancet i:527, 1986

11. Vogt MW, Witt DJ, Craven DE, et al: Isolation of HTLV-III/LAV from cervical secretions of women at risk for AIDS. Lancet i:525, 1986

12. Levy JA, Shimabukuro J, Hollander H, et al: Isolations of AIDS-associated retroviruses from cerebrospinal fluid and brain of patients with neurological symptoms. Lancet ii: 586, 1985

13. Gerberding JL, Bryant-LeBlanc CE, Nelson K, et al: Risk of transmitting the human immunodeficiency virus, cytomegalovirus and hepatitis B virus to health care workers exposed to patients with AIDS and AIDS-related conditions. J Infect Dis 156(1):1, 1987

14. Centers for Disease Control: Summary: Recommendations for preventing transmission of infection with human T-lymphotropic virus type III/lymphadenopathy-associated virus in the workplace. MMWR 34(45):681, 1985

15. Centers for Disease Control: Update: Human immunodeficiency virus infection in health care workers exposed to blood of infected patients. MMWR 36(19):285, 1987

16. Pear R: Three health workers found infected by blood of patients with AIDS. New York Times, pA1, B12, May 20, 1987

17. Centers for Disease Control: Acquired Immune Deficiency Syndrome (AIDS): Precautions for clinical and laboratory staffs. MMWR 31(43):575, 1982

18. Henderson DK, Saah AJ, Zak BJ, et al: Risk of nosocomial infection with human T-cell lymphotropic virus type III/lymphadenopathy-associated virus in a large cohort of intensively exposed health care workers. Ann Intern Med 104(5):644, 1986

19. Salahuddin SZ, Groopman JE, Markham PD, et al: HTLV-III in symptom-free seronegative persons. Lancet ii:1418, 1984

20. Moss A, Osmond D, Bacchetti P, et al: Risk of seroconversion for acquired immunodeficiency syndrome (AIDS) in San Francisco health workers. J Occup Med 28(9):821, 1986

21. McCray E and the Cooperative Needlestick Surveillance Group, Centers for Disease Control. Special Report: Occupational risk of the acquired immunodeficiency syndrome among health care workers. N Engl J Med 314(17): 1127, 1986

22. Baker JL, Kelen GD, Sivertson KT, et al: Unsuspected human immunodeficiency virus in critically ill emergency patients. JAMA, 257(19):2609, 1987

23. Sivak SL, Wormser GP: How common is HTLV-III infection in the United States? N Engl J Med 313:1352, 1985

24. Kuhls TL, Viker S, Parris WB, et al: A prospective cohort study of the occupational risk of AIDS and AIDS-related infections in health care personnel (abstr). Clin Res 343(1):124, 1986

25. Weiss SH, Saxinger WC, Rechtman D, et al: HTLV-III infection among health care workers: Association with needlestick injuries. JAMA 254(15):2089, 1985

26. Hirsch MS, Wormser GP, Schooley RT, et al: Risk of nosocomial infection with human T-cell lymphotropic virus III (HTLV-III). N Engl J Med 312(1):1, 1985

27. Centers for Disease Control: Update: evaluation of HTLV-III/LAV infection in health care personnel—United States. MMWR 34(38):577, 1985

28. Stricof RL, Morse DL: HTLV-III/LAV seroconversion following a deep intramuscular needlestick injury (letter). N Engl J Med 314(17):1115, 1986

29. Anonymous. Needlestick transmission of HTLV-III from a patient infected in Africa. *Lancet* ii:1376, 1984

30. Oksenhendler E, Harzic M, LeRoux J, et al: HIV infection with seroconversion after a superficial needlestick injury to the finger (letter). N Engl J Med 315:582, 1986

31. Neisson-Vernant C, Arfi S, Mathez D, et al: Needlestick HIV seroconversion in a nurse (letter). Lancet ii:814, 1986

32. Centers for Disease Control: Apparent transmission of human T-lymphotrophic virus type III/lymphadenopathy-associated virus from a child to a mother providing health care. MMWR 35(5):76, 1986

33. Grint P, McEvoy M: Two associated cases of the acquired

immune deficiency syndrome (AIDS). PHLS Commun Dis Rep 42:4, 1986

34. Fischl MA, Dickinson GM, Scott GB, et al: Evaluation of heterosexual partner, children and household contacts of adults with AIDS. JAMA 257(5):640, 1987

35. Jason JM, McDougal JS, Dixon G, et al: HTLV-III/LAV antibody and immune status of household contacts and sexual partners of persons with hemophilia. JAMA 255:212, 1986

36. Redfield RR, Markham PD, Salahuddin SZ, et al: Frequent transmission of HTLV-III among spouses of patients with AIDS-related complex and AIDS. JAMA 253(11):1571, 1985

37. Friedland GH, Saltzman BR, Rogers MF, et al: Lack of transmission of HTLV-III/LAV infection to household contacts of patients with AIDS or AIDS-related complex with oral candidiasis. N Engl J Med 314(6):344, 1986

38. Bernier RH, Sampliner R, Gerety R, et al: Hepatitis B infection in households of chronic carriers of hepatitis B surface antigen: Factors associated with prevalence of infection. Am J Epidemiol 116:119, 1982

39. Szmuness W, Price AM, Hirsh RL, et al: Familial clustering of hepatitis B infection. N Engl J Med 289:1162, 1973

40. Centers for Disease Control: Recommended additional guidelines for HIV antibody counseling and testing in the prevention of HIV infection and AIDS. April 30, 1987

41. New York City Department of Health: AIDS Surveillance update (personal communication). New York, May 27, 1987

42. Gerberding JL, Hopewell PC, Kaminsky LS, et al: Transmission of hepatitis B without transmission of AIDS by accidental needlestick. N Engl J Med 312:56, 1985

43. Lane MA, Lettau LA: Transmission of HBV from dental personnel to patients. JADA 110:634, 1985

44. Hadler SC, Sorley DL, Acree KH, et al: An outbreak of hepatitis B in a dental practice. Ann Int Med 95(2):133, 1981

45. Guidelines for facilities treating chemically dependent patients at risk for AIDS or infected by HIV virus. New York, American Medical Society on Alcoholism and Other Drug Dependencies Organization, 1987

46. Leibowitz RE: Infection control measures in institutional settings. In Durham JD, Cohen FL (eds): The Person With AIDS—Nursing Perspectives. New York, Springer, 1987

47. Centers for Disease Control: Recommendations for preventing transmission of infection with human T-lymphotropic virus type III/lymphadenopathy-associated virus during invasive procedures. MMWR 35:221, 1986

48. Centers for Disease Control: Acquired immunodeficiency syndrome (AIDS): Precautions for health care workers and allied professionals. MMWR 32:450, 451, 1983

49. Carl M, Blakey DL, Francis DP, et al: Interruption of hepatitis B transmission by modification of a gynaecologist's surgical technique. Lancet i:731, 1982

50. Zimberg M: Psychosocial isolation. In Brown MH, Kiss ME, Outlaw EM, et al (eds): Standards of Oncology Nursing Practice. New York, John Wiley and Sons, 1986

51. Saviteer SM, White GC, Cohen MS, et al: HTLV-III exposure during cardiopulmonary resuscitation (letter). N Engl J Med 313:1606, 1985

52. Infection Control Committee, Memorial Sloan-Kettering Cancer Center: Infectious Disease Manual. pp 22, 25, 1987 (unpublished)

53. Martin LS, McDougal JS, Loskoski SL: Disinfection and inactivation of the human T-lymphotropic virus type III/lymphadenopathy-associated virus. J Infect Dis 152:400, 1985

54. Conte JE: Infection with human immunodeficiency virus in the hospital: Epidemiology, infection control, and biosafety considerations. Ann Int Med 105:730, 1986

55. Advisory Committee on Infections Within Hospital: Management of HTLV-III/LAV infection in the hospital. Chicago, American Hospital Association, 1986

56. Hanley R: The dangers of dumping medical waste are under scrutiny. New York Times, p B1, B2. August 24, 1987

57. Safai B: Safety precautions for dealing with AIDS. In DeVita VT, Hellman S, Rosenberg SA (eds): AIDS: Etiology, Diagnosis, Treatment, and Prevention. Philadelphia, J. B. Lippincott, 1985

58. Sunderam G, McDonald RJ, Maniatis T, et al: Tuberculosis as a manifestation of the acquired immunodeficiency syndrome (AIDS). JAMA 256:362, 1986

59. Royal College of Nursing AIDS Working Party: Nursing Guidelines on the Management of Patients in Hospital and the Community Suffering from AIDS (2nd report). London, The Royal College of Nursing of the United Kingdom, 1986

60. Kernoff PBA: Annotation: AIDS, infectivity, and health care workers. Br J Haematol, 60:207, 1985

61. Centers for Disease Control: Recommendations for preventing possible transmission of human T-lymphotropic virus type III/lymphadenopathy-associated virus from tears. MMWR 34:533, 1985

62. Fujikawa LS, Salahuddin SZ, Ablashi D, et al: Human T-cell leukemia/lymphotropic virus type III in the conjunctival epithelium of a patient with AIDS. Am J Ophthalmol 100:507, 1985

63. Salahuddin SZ, Palestine AG, Heck E, et al: Isolation of the human T-cell leukemia/lymphotropic virus type III from the cornea. Am J Ophthalmol 101:149, 1986

64. Tervo T, Lahdevirta J, Vaheri A, et al: Recovery of HTLV-III from contact lenses (letter). Lancet i:379, 1986

65. Centers for Disease Control: Recommendation for assisting in the prevention of perinatal transmission of human T-lymphotropic virus type III/lymphadenopathy associated virus and acquired immunodeficiency syndrome. MMWR 34:721, 1985

66. Sacks JJ: AIDS in a surgeon (letter). N Engl J Med 313:1017, 1985

67. Church J, Sanderson P: Surgical glove punctures. J Hosp Infect 1:84, 1980

68. Council on Scientific Affairs, American Medical Association: Autologous Blood Transfusions. JAMA 256:2378, 1986

69. Centers for Disease Control: Recommended infection-control practices for dentistry. MMWR 35:237, 1986

70. Centers for Disease Control: Recommendations for providing dialysis treatment to patients infected with human T-lymphotropic virus type III/lymphadenopathy-associated virus. MMWR 35:376, 1986

71. Klein M, DeForest A: Principles of viral inactivation. In Block SS (ed): Disinfection, Sterilization, and Preservation. Philadelphia, Lea & Febiger, 1983

72. Aseptic handling of thermometers and other equipment for measuring patient temperatures. In Centers for Disease Control: National nosocomial infections study report, Annual Summary 1976. Health, Education, and Welfare Publication (CDC) No. 78-8257. Washington D.C., February 1978

73. Valenti WM, Takacs KM: Infection control and clinical thermometry: Perforation of soft plastic thermometer sheaths during temperature measurement. Am J Infect Control 9:1, 1981

74. Bennett J: AIDS: What precautions do you take in the hospital? AJN 8:952, 1986

75. Scholenberger P: Should pregnant women care for AIDS Patients? Infect Control 6(5):180, 1985

76. Hughes AM, Martin JP, Franks P (eds): AIDS Home Care and Hospice Manual, San Francisco, p 66. San Francisco, AIDS Home Care and Hospice Program, VNA, 1987

77. Balfour CL, Balfour HH: Cytomegalovirus is not an occupational risk for nurses in renal transplant and neonatal units: Results of a prospective surveillance study. JAMA 256:1909, 1986

78. Jacob JL, Grady C, Ostchega Y, et al: National Survey: Assessing the learning needs of oncology nurses in relation to caring for individuals with HIV-related disorders. (Unpublished)

79. McDonnell M, Sevedge K: Acquired immune deficiency syndrome (AIDS). In Brown M, Kiss M, Outlaw EM, Viamontes CM (eds): Standards of Oncology Nursing Practice. New York, John Wiley and Sons, 1986

80. Three caregivers become HIV-antibody positive after blood spills. AJN 87(7):903, 1987

81. Pear R: Health workers to get AIDS protection. New York Times, p A16, Thursday, July 23, 1987

82. Meisenheimer CG (ed): Quality Assurance: A Complete Guide to Effective Programs. Rockville MD, Aspen Systems, 1985

83. CDC: Recommendations for Prevention of HIV Transmission in Health Care Settings. MMWR 36(25):15, 1987

84. Department of Labor/Department of Health and Human Services: Joint Advisory Notice: HBV/HIV. Federal register 52(210):41818, 1987

Screening and Testing Asymptomatic Persons for HIV Infection

James R. Allen

26

Although the first commercial tests to detect antibody to human immunodeficiency virus (HIV) were not licensed and made commercially available until the spring of 1985, experimental and prototype tests had been in use in the United States for almost 2 years. Much of the work in identifying the HTLV-III and LAV strains of HIV as the probable cause of acquired immunodeficiency syndrome (AIDS) was dependent on reliable tests to detect antibodies in the serum of patients to the viruses being isolated. Once the viruses had been identified, other investigators rapidly began submitting serum specimens for testing or participated in clinical trials with developmental versions of the commercial tests to begin to link together the diverse clinical manifestations suspected of being associated with AIDS and to elucidate the asymptomatic phase of infection. From the earliest days that these tests were available to investigators, the unique medical and social aspects of AIDS resulted in searching discussions about the ethics of antibody testing, the requirements for specific informed consent, the need for confidentiality about test results, and the obligation to inform persons whose serum was tested of the results.

The HIV antibody tests were specifically licensed by the Food and Drug Administration (FDA) for use in testing donated units of blood and plasma. Even before the tests were licensed, however, steps were taken to ensure that tests would be available through "alternate test sites" so that persons who believed they were at risk of infection and wished to be tested could do so without donating blood. Subsequently, the Public Health Service published a series of recommendations for preventing further spread of HIV in which antibody testing was an important element as an adjunct to counseling and education. Less than a year after the first tests were licensed, the Department of Defense decided to screen all recruit applicants for HIV antibody and not to accept any applicant whose positive screening test

was validated by other tests such as the Western blot. This decision was subsequently extended to testing of all active duty military persons, and others such as the Job Corps and the Department of State for various reasons have reached similar decisions about testing applicants or persons in selected positions.

Of greater concern, many persons and groups have continued to exert pressure for broad-based screening of selected populations or even of the entire population to detect persons who are infected. Most of these suggestions have emanated from persons not familiar with the public health bases of screening programs and the implications of testing. This chapter will review the bases of screening for HIV infection and will discuss the context in which testing for antibody is useful for prevention of further spread of infection and potential problems with screening and testing programs.

PRINCIPLES OF SCREENING FOR MEDICAL PROBLEMS

Definitions

The terms *screening* and *testing* often are used interchangeably, although each has discrete connotations. *Screening* generally means the use of a test or procedure on a population of persons who are generally healthy to identify those with a particular condition or predisposition that is still asymptomatic or has not yet been recognized. Persons who have a positive screening test are usually referred for or provided with more definitive diagnostic procedures or follow-up. Screening may be performed under voluntary or mandatory conditions and may be applied systematically or nonuniformly to entire populations or selected target populations. In contrast, *testing* generally implies that the test or procedure is used for an individual person regardless of whether the person is symptomatic or not and whether the test is recommended by a health-care provider or requested by the individual being tested.

The concepts are not always clearly separated, however. For example, a clinic for treatment of sexually transmitted diseases (STDs) may be funded by a health department to screen all persons seen at the clinic for HIV antibody and all women for asymptomatic gonorrhea or a family planning clinic may be funded to screen all women with a Papanicolaou smear to detect early cervical carcinoma. Persons attending these clinics would be offered the tests on an individual basis as part of the screening program, but would have the opportunity to decline to be tested if they wished.

Purposes and Types of Screening Programs

The first widespread use of medical screening in the United States occurred just before and during World War II to detect asymptomatic persons with syphilis and tuberculosis. The intent was to refer those who tested positive for treatment to curtail further spread of infection and to initiate therapy at a point in the disease process when treatment was expected to be more effective. Subsequently, screening programs for asymptomatic diabetes and hypertension were established, and persons found through screening to be positive were referred for careful follow-up in an attempt to ameliorate disease progression.

The early efforts at screening were quickly expanded. Today, cancer screening programs are aimed at early detection and definitive treatment, while screening of newborns for phenylketonuria (PKU) or hypothyroidism shortly after birth identifies those who are affected so that they can be placed on a phenylalanine-restricted diet or treated with thyroid supplements to avoid the severe mental retardation that otherwise would result. Screening programs for Tay-Sachs disease have been successful because reliable tests to detect the heterozygous carrier state and for prenatal diagnosis of an affected fetus are both available. Adult couples in selected populations with a high prevalence of the gene causing Tay-Sachs disease can be screened for the carrier state; if both parents are affected, they can be counseled about the risks of an affected child and about family planning and prenatal diagnosis. Efforts to establish similar screening programs for other genetic disorders such as sickle cell anemia have been less well accepted. Multiphasic screening programs of various types also have been used in the United States for more than 30 years with variable success; many of the components of these screening programs attempt to identify risk factors (e.g., high cholesterol or total lipids) correlated with potentially preventable diseases or conditions and to encourage the individual to modify these through treatment or changes in lifestyle.

Several important conclusions can be reached by studying the types of screening programs that have been implemented: Only a few have been implemented on a national or statewide basis, although some have been made widely available for populations in target areas. Participation in most is voluntary; only a few, such as the screening of newborns for PKU, are required by law. Most provide a specific benefit for the person being screened, whether it is early diagnosis of a condition amenable to definitive therapy (cervical carcinoma in situ, syphilis, tuberculosis), improved therapy and management of a chronic condition (hypertension, diabetes), or genetic counseling and options during pregnancy. Virtually all the screening programs are conducted in the context of health care delivery (although in a variety of settings, including the workplace); none has a social control overtone. Although many of the diseases or conditions for which screening is available are frightening to the individual and potentially disabling or life-threatening, none has the current psychological impact of a diagnosis of HIV infection (often mistakenly assumed to be a diagnosis of AIDS) and none has the potential for overt discrimination and social disruption that a diagnosis of HIV infection does.

Public Health Considerations for Screening Programs

Once a definite purpose or outcome has been established for a screening program, a number of program characteristics must be evaluated and resolved before initiating the program. Of primary concern are the operating characteristics of the screening test(s) that will be used: The sensitivity and specificity of the test(s) and the availability and characteristics of supplemental procedures to be used for validation or definitive diagnosis. Other considerations include the availability of special facilities or requirements for collecting specimens or performing the test.

Of equal importance is the designation of the target populations to be screened and the estimated prevalence of the condition or disease in the target populations. Associated considerations include the ability to reach the target populations effectively and to provide the range of services required to support the screening efforts.

These two major factors—the tests and the target populations—then need to be considered together: Given the sensitivity and specificity of the tests and the estimated prevalence of the condition, the predictive values of positive and negative tests should be calculated and the impact or consequences for the individual and the program of both false-positive and false-negative tests carefully considered. Resources and facilities should be available before the program starts to handle the evaluation and counseling of persons with potentially false-positive tests. Adverse consequences of the screening program or the test(s), whether physical, psychological, social, or economic, also must be considered and potential problems resolved before the program is undertaken.

Finally, provisions should be made from the outset to evaluate the impact of the screening program in terms of projected outcomes, costs, benefits, and adverse effects. This need for evaluation is particularly important for new programs or those that are incorporating new technology. A corollary to program evaluation is the desirability of using data from justified screening programs to enhance our knowledge of a condition or disease problem within the legal and ethical limitations imposed by the type of informed consent obtained and restrictions on disclosure of personal medical information.

Ethical Considerations for Screening Programs

As discussed briefly above, the adverse consequences of a proposed screening program must be carefully considered. Bayer and his colleagues at The Hastings Center have provided a comprehensive ethical framework for evaluating proposed screening programs based on the fundamental principles of respect for all persons, the harm principle (limiting a person's liberty to pursue objectives or make choices that will harm others), beneficence (acting on behalf of the interests and welfare of others), and justice (equitable distribution of the burdens and benefits of particular actions). Although they recognize that these ethical principles at times conflict with each other and that any individual situation may be difficult to resolve, they use them to establish seven prerequisites that "constitute the threshold requirements for ethical acceptability" of screening programs (Table 26-1).

PROGRAM CONSIDERATIONS: HIV ANTIBODY TEST PERFORMANCE

Significance of HIV Antibody

Several studies since the first publications describing isolation of the HTLV-III strain of HIV have showed that most of those infected with HIV develop antibody against the virus and remain chronically infected with the virus. Relatively few studies have been able to document adequately the time from initiation of infection with HIV to seroconversion, but in those that have, most persons have seroconverted between 2 and 4 months after infection. These studies establish the basis for using HIV antibody as a marker for current and chronic infection with the virus. The long-term implications of HIV infection are also significant. For some, the infection will be active and progressive; for others, it may be latent for a highly variable period of time. Current experience from prospective natural history cohort studies suggests that the longer the duration of infection with HIV, the higher the probability of immunologic abnormalities and clinical evidence of HIV infection.

Table 26-1
Prerequisites for Ethical Screening Programs

1. The purpose of the screening must be ethically acceptable.
2. The means to be used in the screening program and the intended use of the information must be appropriate for accomplishing the purpose.
3. High-quality laboratory services must be used.
4. Individuals must be notified that screening will take place.
5. Individuals who are screened have a right to be informed about the results.
6. Sensitive and supportive counseling programs must be available before and after screening to interpret the results, whether they are positive or negative.
7. The confidentiality of screened individuals must be protected.

(Bayer R, Levine C, Wolf SM: HIV antibody screening: An ethical framework for evaluating proposed programs. JAMA 256:1768, 1986)

Sensitivity and Specificity of HIV Screening Tests

An ideal screening test would be capable of identifying all persons who have the condition being studied (in this case, HIV infection) and of excluding all persons who do not have the condition. The ability of a test to identify those who are affected is termed *sensitivity,* which is the probability (usually expressed as a percentage) that a test result will be positive if infection is present. The ability of a test to exclude those who are not affected is termed *specificity,* which is the probability (also usually expressed as a percentage) that a test result will be negative if infection is *not* present.

The sensitivity and specificity of a test for HIV antibody describe the ability of the test to separate the infected and uninfected populations. The sensitivity and specificity of a given test are primarily determined by the intrinsic characteristics of the test (which includes the potential for technical laboratory error) and the decision point. For a given test, these values vary inversely depending on the level at which the decision point for a positive test is set. Although the sensitivity and specificity of a test are considered fixed, in actual practice they are also influenced (usually decreased) by the quality of the laboratory performing the tests and by any special characteristics of the population being tested.

The HIV antibody tests used for initial testing (or screening) in the United States are enzyme immunoassays (EIA or ELISA) using disrupted whole virus antigen. The test kits of the various manufacturers licensed by the FDA to produce and sell EIA HIV-antibody test kits in the United States vary somewhat in design and characteristics, but all are comparable in test performance.

According to the FDA, virtually all the licensed tests have been refined and improved since being introduced; both the sensitivity and the specificity for the currently licensed EIA tests are estimated to be greater than 99% given optimal laboratory conditions. The actual performance sensitivity of the tests, however, varies with both the precision of the laboratory performing the test and the incidence of new infections in the population being tested. This value is estimated to be 97% to 98%.

To increase the specificity of the test results and reduce the probability of laboratory error and inadvertent results, manufacturers have instructed laboratories using the test to perform a sequence of tests for specimens that have an initially reactive (potentially positive) test result. Based on the results of testing more than 10 million blood donors in the United States, the calculated specificity of a repeatedly reactive EIA test is 99.7% (false-positive rate of 0.3%). Given the medical and social significance of the results of this test, however, even this degree of specificity is not high enough, and so there is a need for a supplemental or validation test.

Performance of HIV Validation Procedures

In the United States the supplemental or validation test used most often is a Western blot test, although radioimmunoprecipitation assays and fluorescent antibody assays also are used by some laboratories. The potential problems in interpreting and using Western blot tests for validation have been highlighted. Under the best of circumstances, however, the joint false-positive rate of the EIA and Western blot tests is less than 0.001% (<1 per 100,000 persons tested).

Only one manufacturer is currently licensed to market Western blot test kits in the United States to validate HIV-antibody screening tests; this test has a sensitivity and specificity comparable to the best of the EIA test kits. When the manufacturer's strict criteria are used for interpreting the test results, the probability of a false-positive result is extremely remote. However, some persons with reactive EIA tests who are tested with this Western blot will have a nonspecific pattern on the blot that cannot be interpreted adequately. A person recently infected with HIV may show an equivocal Western blot pattern; repeating the test on a second specimen obtained 3 to 6 months after the initial specimen shows progression of the blot pattern to one that is positive. Conversely, for a person who is not infected with HIV but has an initially equivocal blot pattern, this equivocal pattern usually will persist when a second specimen is obtained and tested 3 to 6 months later.

False Positives, False Negatives, and Predictive Values of Tests

The proportion of test results expected to be false positive or false negative in a specified population is summarized in the concept of predictive value. The predic-

tive value of a positive test is the probability, usually expressed as a percentage, that the person will be affected if the test result is positive, while the predictive value of a negative test is the probability that the person will not be affected if the test result is negative. Predictive value, therefore, measures how well a test performs in a given population.

Unlike sensitivity and specificity (which are relatively fixed for a given test), the predictive values change, often dramatically, with the prevalence of the condition in the population being tested. As a result, if the prevalence of the condition is low (for example 0.2%) in a population being tested, the performance of a test that is 98% sensitive and 99% specific appears suboptimal because the proportion of reactive tests that are false positive is high and the predictive value of a positive test is correspondingly low (Table 26-2). Using the same test in a population in which the prevalence of infection is 100 times higher, however, gives quite different results, with the predictive value of a positive test being 96.1% and the predictive value of a negative test being 99.5%.

With a low prevalence of infection in the population being tested, increasing the specificity of the test to near-perfect levels is still not sufficient to provide a high predictive value. If the specificity of the test in the first example were 99.9%, the predictive value positive would only increase to 66.2%. Retesting those persons who have a positive test from the initial screening with a second procedure (preferably one that uses a different process to give truly independent results), increases the predictive value of a positive test from 16.4% after the first test to 97.5% after the second test, given a specificity of the second test of 99.5% (Table 26-3). This is the reason it is critically important not to accept and use the results of a screening procedure alone to notify a person about HIV infection status; the test results must be validated with a supplemental test of high specificity conducted by a laboratory with impeccable performance standards.

EVALUATION OF POSSIBLE HIV ANTIBODY SCREENING PROGRAMS

Rationale for HIV Antibody Screening Programs

The rationale for HIV antibody screening programs is to identify persons infected with HIV. Although many possible reasons exist for wanting to know who is infected, the predominant public health concern is for prevention: Persons who are infected with HIV are capable of transmitting their infection to others and need to be educated about the lifestyle changes necessary to prevent infecting others, and persons who are at risk but not infected need to be educated about ways to avoid infection. Testing persons for HIV antibody through the screening program, therefore, becomes a way to target specific educational programs to induce behavior

Table 26-2
*Predictive Value of a Repeatedly Reactive Screening Test for Asymptomatic
Infection in Two Hypothetical Populations*

Assumptions: Test sensitivity: 98.0%.
　　　　　　Test specificity: 99.0%.

A. *Prevalence of infection in population 0.2%*

| Test Result | Actual Condition | | Totals | | Predictive Value |
	Infected	Not Infected	Number	Percent	
Reactive	196	998	1,194	1.2%	16.4%
Nonreactive	4	98,802	98,806	98.8%	99.99%
TOTALS	200	99,800	100,000	100.0%	

B. *Prevalence of infection in population 20%*

| Test Result | Actual Condition | | Totals | | Predictive Value |
	Infected	Not Infected	Number	Percent	
Reactive	19,600	800	20,400	20.4%	96.1%
Nonreactive	400	79,200	79,600	79.6%	99.5%
TOTALS	20,000	80,000	100,000	100.0%	

Table 26-3
*Impact of a Second, Highly Specific (Confirmatory) Test on the Final Predictive
Value of Test Results*

Assumptions: Sensitivity of the confirmatory test: 100%
　　　　　　Confirmatory test method is independent of the screening test
　　　　　　Prevalence of infection in the unscreened population: 0.2%

| Specificity of Test (%) | Number Tested | Number with Reactive Test | | Predictive Value |
		Infected	Not Infected	
Screening test:　99.0	100,000	196	998	16.4%
Confirmatory test: 99.0	1,194*	196	10	95.1%
99.5	1,194	196	5	97.5%
99.8	1,194	196	2	99.0%
99.9	1,194	196	1	99.5%

* The number tested using the confirmatory test (n = 1,194) is the number from the screening test
procedure who had a repeatedly reactive test, 196 of whom were truly infected and 998 of whom
were not infected.

changes that will minimize or eliminate risk of HIV infection or transmission.

The concern of many persons who are at risk of HIV infection, however, is that these tests will be used for other purposes. Transmission of HIV from one person to another occurs most frequently through sexual contacts (male homosexual or heterosexual) or through sharing of blood-contaminated needles and syringes for injection of drugs. Although transmission of infection primarily occurs through contacts that are voluntary and not coerced, the overt fear that accompanies the public understanding of AIDS has resulted in numerous suggestions about the need to control spread of HIV through the use of quarantine or other restrictions of persons who are infected. Also, since persons infected with HIV are at high risk of premature death from AIDS or associated conditions, health and life insurance companies, others responsible for the costs of medical care, and some employers, who do not want to incur expenses for training programs or disruption in the workplace caused by employees who become ill or die, all may justify HIV antibody testing for their own purposes.

Mandatory Screening of Blood and Organ Donors

The most frequent use of HIV antibody screening is the mandatory testing for persons who wish to donate blood or plasma in the United States and many other countries of the world. Similarly, persons who donate sperm, organs, or tissues all should be tested for HIV antibody before donation or use of the material. The purpose of these screening programs, obviously, is prevention through assuring that blood, sperm, tissues, or organs that may have infectious virus are not transfused or given to another person. In general, persons who donate blood or plasma are requested to read an informational pamphlet that describes antibody testing, answer a series of medical history questions, and sign a consent to donate (and to be tested). Donors are notified about validated positive test results and are invited to undergo counseling and to be referred for additional evaluation and follow-up. The procedure for organ and tissue donation from a living donor should be as complete, but the process may not be as highly organized. The issue of informed consent for antibody testing for cadaver donors and the question about whom to notify, if anyone, about a validated positive test have not been fully resolved.

Other Mandatory HIV Antibody Screening Programs

HIV antibody screening is mandatory for military recruit applicants and active duty military in the United States or for those who wish to participate in certain other programs, such as the Job Corps or the foreign service. The rationale for these programs varies. In the military, the reasons are that infected persons may be immunosuppressed and should not receive live virus vaccines, be deployed to areas of the world where medical care is suboptimal and they may be exposed to a variety of new pathogens, or be in a situation where they may be asked to provide blood for an emergency transfusion. State Department personnel are concerned about similar issues, but also about diplomatic sensitivities. Supporters of these screening programs note that it is not required for any person to join or participate in any of these programs; to do so is voluntary and the screening is not truly mandatory. Consent to undergo testing is obtained from the applicant after the process is explained, but the extent to which the applicants to many of these programs truly understand the explanation about risk factors or the implications of a positive test has not been evaluated.

From a public health perspective, mandatory screening of large segments of the population will not control the epidemic of HIV infection; it will, however, result in expenditure of an enormous effort and large sums of money. Most persons in the United States are at low risk of infection. The prevalence of infection among the highly selected population of blood donors is only a few per 10,000, while among the less highly selected population of military recruit applicants it is 1.5 per 1,000 (1.6 per 1,000 among males and 0.6 per 1,000 among females). Screening the population to detect a few persons who are infected and providing them with intensive counseling about prevention of transmission is not likely to be cost effective even if it could be accomplished. Most of the effort would be placed on the screening program and relatively little on the counseling program to change the behavior patterns that result in transmission. Such a program would not identify those persons who are at risk but not yet infected, and so would not encourage them to change behaviors to avoid infection in the future. In addition, to be even partially successful the program would need to be repeated periodically so that newly infected persons could be identified and counseled.

A more general education program for the population without the antibody screening would provide information to those who are at risk without the difficulties and problems associated with obtaining and testing serum specimens from a large population; those who have been at risk can be encouraged during the educational program to seek voluntary counseling and testing through other sources. Criteria have been proposed to assess the types of populations or situations in which a mandatory screening program could be successful.

HIV Antibody Screening in Correctional Systems

Instituting routine HIV antibody counseling and testing programs for asymptomatic seropositive persons presents an enormous challenge to correctional systems, but one that is being adopted with increasing frequency. The basic justification is the fact that many inmates have a history of intravenous (IV) drug abuse and that sexual activity and drug usage by the inmates continue to occur after incarceration. One estimate is that as many as 5% to 10% of the inmates of national and state prisons may be HIV infected, with this population heavily skewed toward inmates from states where infection in IV drug abusers has been common.

A variety of programs have been established; many only test inmates who are ill, while a few have instituted mandatory screening programs for inmates, primarily at the time of admission to or discharge from the system. Among the important issues to be addressed are the right of the inmate to prior information and/or consent about being tested; confidentiality and management of the test results, including the level of access of facility staff to the results; notification of spouses and sexual partners; and housing policies. These programs have not been in place for a sufficient period to allow evaluation and assessment of their utility at preventing further spread of HIV within the correctional system. Most facilities segregate or provide special facilities only for inmates with signs or symptoms of infection or a diagnosis of AIDS; it is too early to determine the future pattern in providing segregated facilities or areas for inmates who are seropositive to try to prevent subsequent transmission. The type of educational programs about AIDS and HIV infection that will be provided is also undetermined. Placing all the emphasis on screening and failing to acknowledge and develop programs to prevent transmission through sexual behavior and IV drug abuse in correctional facilities will not solve the problems that currently exist.

SPECIFIC RECOMMENDATIONS FOR HIV ANTIBODY COUNSELING AND TESTING PROGRAMS

Establishing Public Health Priorities for Counseling and Testing

Comparison of the relative effectiveness of counseling and testing for different populations demonstrates a wide range in the number and proportion of persons who would be found infected with HIV and could benefit from counseling programs. Programs that offer counseling and HIV antibody testing to homosexual men, IV drug abusers, persons with hemophilia, the sex partners or needle-sharing partners of these persons, and STD clinic patients will provide the most effective services. Persons in these groups would benefit most from prevention information since they are most likely to be exposed or to be infected already.

Programs for counseling and testing pregnant patients in high-prevalence areas also are likely to be effective at reaching women who already are infected or who may continue to be at risk of infection if they do not follow recommendations to minimize exposure. Since it is preferable to reach women who are at risk before they become infected, or before they become pregnant if already infected, counseling and testing in settings where family planning services are offered is also likely to be effective. Priority decisions about programs for women receiving family planning services and their sex partners should be based on the local prevalence and patterns of HIV infection. Implementing programs in areas with a low prevalence of infection in women will not reach many who are at risk.

Premarital counseling and HIV antibody testing will have highly variable success at reaching persons who are at risk of infection. Most persons at highest risk of infection are already sexually active and often become pregnant before marriage or do not plan to be in a marriage relationship. In areas with a low prevalence of infection (e.g., less than 0.005%), premarital counseling and testing programs are likely to reach few persons who are infected.

Public Health Service Recommendations for HIV Antibody Counseling and Testing

The Public Health Service has published specific recommendations for HIV antibody counseling and testing that provide a broad-based approach to reaching the persons at highest risk of HIV infection. In these recommendations, the term "routine counseling and testing" is defined as a policy to provide these services to all clients after informing them that testing will be done. Except where testing is required by law, individuals have the right to decline to be tested without being denied health care or other services.

Persons Who May Have Sexually Transmitted Disease

All persons seeking treatment for a sexually transmitted disease, in all health-care settings, including the offices of private physicians, should routinely be counseled and tested for HIV antibody.

IV Drug Abusers

All persons seeking treatment for IV drug abuse or who have a history of IV drug abuse should routinely be counseled and tested for HIV antibody. Medical professionals in all health-care settings, including prison clinics, should seek a history of IV drug abuse from patients and be aware of its implications for HIV infection. In addition, state and local health policy makers should address the following issues about availability of drug-abuse treatment programs: (1) Treatment programs for IV substance abusers should be sufficiently available that anyone seeking assistance can be entered promptly and encouraged to alter the behavior that places him or her and others at risk of HIV infection. (2) Outreach programs for persons who are IV drug abusers should be undertaken to increase their knowledge of AIDS and ways to prevent HIV infection, to encourage them to obtain HIV antibody counseling and testing, and to persuade them to be treated for substance abuse.

Persons Who Consider Themselves at Risk

All those who consider themselves at risk of HIV infection for whatever reason should be counseled and offered testing for HIV antibody.

Women of Childbearing Age Who Are at Risk

All women of childbearing age with identifiable risks for HIV infection should routinely be counseled and tested for HIV antibody, regardless of the health-care setting. Each encounter between a health-care provider and women at risk or their sex partners is an opportunity to reach them with information and education about AIDS and prevention of HIV infection. Women with identifiable risks for HIV infection include those who have used IV drugs; have engaged in prostitution; have had sex partners who are infected or who are at risk of infection because they are IV drug abusers, bisexual, or hemophiliacs; are living in communities or were born in countries where there is a known or suspected high prevalence of infection among women; have received a transfusion before blood was being screened for HIV antibody but after HIV infection occurred in the United States (e.g. between 1978 and 1985). Educating and testing these women before they become pregnant maximizes their opportunities to avoid pregnancy and subsequent intrauterine or perinatal infection of their newborn (30–50% of the infants born to HIV-infected women also will be infected).

All pregnant women at risk of HIV infection should routinely be counseled and tested for HIV antibody. The identification of HIV-infected pregnant women as early in pregnancy as possible is important to ensure appropriate medical care for the pregnant women, to plan medical care for their infants, and to provide counseling about family planning, future pregnancies, and the risk of sexual transmission of HIV to others.

All women seeking family planning services who are at risk of HIV infection should routinely be counseled about AIDS and HIV infection and tested for HIV antibody. Decisions about the need for counseling and testing programs in a community should be based on the best available estimates of the prevalence of HIV infection and the demographic variables of infection.

Persons Planning Marriage

All persons considering marriage should be given information about AIDS, HIV infection, and the availability of counseling and testing for HIV antibody. Decisions about instituting routine or mandatory premarital testing for HIV antibody should be based on the likely cost-effectiveness of such testing in preventing further spread of the infection, taking into account area prevalence and other factors. For example, premarital testing in an area with a prevalence of HIV infection as low as 0.1% among those getting married may be cost effective if reaching an infected person through testing can prevent subsequent transmission to the spouse or pregnancy in a woman who is infected.

Persons Undergoing Medical Evaluation or Treatment

Tests for HIV antibody have diagnostic utility in the evaluation of patients with selected clinical signs and symptoms such as generalized lymphadenopathy; unexplained dementia; chronic unexplained fever or diarrhea; unexplained weight loss; or diseases such as tuberculosis and sexually transmitted disease, generalized herpes, and chronic candidiasis.

Since persons infected with both HIV and the tubercle bacillus are at high risk of severe clinical tuberculosis, all patients with tuberculosis should routinely be counseled and tested for HIV antibody. Guidelines for managing patients with both HIV and tuberculous infection have been published.

The risk of HIV infection from transfusions of blood or blood components from 1978 to 1985 was greatest for persons who received large numbers of units and who received blood collected from areas with a high incidence of AIDS. Persons who have this increased risk should be counseled about the potential risk of HIV infection and should be offered antibody testing.

Persons Admitted to Hospitals

Hospitals, in conjunction with state/local health departments, should periodically determine the prevalence of HIV infections in the age groups at highest risk of infection. Consideration should be given to routine counseling and testing in those age groups in which HIV antibody prevalence is deemed to be high. The many considerations and potential difficulties of implementing this type of program have been reviewed.

Persons in Correctional Systems

Correctional systems should undertake studies of counseling and HIV antibody testing of inmates at admission and discharge from the system to examine the utility of such counseling in preventing further transmission of HIV and the implications of the testing programs. Federal prisons have been instructed to implement testing of all prisoners upon entering and leaving the prison system.

Prostitutes

Male and female prostitutes should be counseled and tested and made aware of the risks of HIV infection to themselves and others. Prostitutes who test positive for HIV antibodies should be instructed to discontinue the practice of prostitution. Local or state jurisdictions should adopt procedures to ensure that those instructions are followed.

Partner Notification/Contact Tracing

Sex partners and those who share needles with HIV-infected persons are at risk of HIV infection and should routinely be counseled and tested for HIV antibody. Persons who test positive for HIV antibodies should be instructed in how to notify their partners and to refer them for counseling and testing. If they are unwilling to notify their partner(s) or if it cannot be assured that their partners will seek counseling, physicians or health department personnel should take steps to ensure that the partners are notified, using confidential procedures.

Confidentiality and Antidiscrimination Considerations

The ability of health departments, hospitals, and other health-care providers and institutions to ensure confidentiality of patient information, and the public's confidence in that ability, are crucial to efforts to increase the number of persons being counseled and tested for HIV infection. Moreover, to ensure broad participation in the counseling and testing programs, it is of equal or greater importance that the public perceive that persons found to be positive will not be subject to inappropriate discrimination.

Every reasonable effort should be made to improve confidentiality of test results. The confidentiality of related records can be improved by a careful review of actual record-keeping practices and by assessing the degree to which these records can be protected under applicable state law. State laws should be examined, and strengthened when necessary. Because of the wide scope of "need-to-know" situations, because of the possibility of inappropriate disclosures, and because of the established practice of records-release authorization procedures, it is recognized that there is no perfect solution to confidentiality problems in all situations. Whether disclosures of HIV testing information are deliberate, inadvertent, or simply unavoidable, public health officials need to carefully consider ways to reduce the harmful impact of such disclosures.

Public health prevention policy to reduce the transmission of HIV can be furthered by an expanded program of counseling and testing for HIV antibody, but the extent to which these programs are successful depends on the level of participation. Persons are more likely to participate in counseling and testing programs if they believe that they will not experience negative consequences in areas such as employment, school admission, housing, and medical services should they test positive. There is no known medical reason to avoid an infected person in these and ordinary social situations, since the cumulative evidence is strong that HIV is not spread through casual contact. It is essential to the success of counseling and testing programs that persons who are tested for HIV are not subjected to inappropriate discrimination.

AIDS Control in Africa

Daniel Zagury
Zirimwabagangabo Lurhuma

27

AIDS and HIV infection now confront humanity with a global problem and not just a specific challenge to African, European, Australian, or American societies. An estimated 5 to 10 million persons worldwide may currently be infected with the human immunodeficiency virus (HIV). Infection with HIV is likely to be present, at least to some extent, in virtually every country. As of mid-September 1987, over 60,000 AIDS cases had been officially reported to the World Health Organization (WHO) from 124 countries (Table 27-1). AIDS affects both the developing and the industrialized world, and since AIDS knows no social, political, economic, or cultural borders, efforts at the national and international level must be unified. Prevention efforts cannot wait for a vaccine or therapeutic breakthroughs. A global strategy for AIDS prevention incorporates the concept that no country will be able to stop HIV until it is stopped in all countries.

AIDS AND HIV INFECTION IN AFRICA

Discovery

The first African cases of acquired immunodeficiency syndrome were reported in Europe in 1983–1984.[1,2,3] In the following years, a description of the epidemiology of infection with LAV/HTLV-III (as HIV was then termed) in Africa emerged from a series of studies.[4,5,6,7,8,9,10,11] Firm conclusions about the history of HIV infection in Africa, its origin, and its actual prevalence can only be inferred from the available evidence. However, the existing data are compatible with HIV infection being absent or at low levels in Africa until the mid to late 1970s. Changes in morbidity or mortality patterns (e.g., cryptococcal meningitis,[12] Kaposi's sarcoma,[4] and life-threatening chronic enteropathic illnesses[10]) occurring at that time were retrospectively identifiable as AIDS-related. In fact, within the frame of available knowledge, the AIDS epidemic in Africa appears to coincide with the American and Haitian epidemic.[13]

Magnitude of the Epidemic

The geographic scope and intensity of HIV infection in Africa has been difficult to assess with accuracy because of limited infectious disease surveillance and laboratory serodiagnostic facilities and lack of a widely accepted and practical clinical case definition. (The CDC/WHO definition[14] requires sophisticated laboratory support for diagnosis of opportunistic infections and malignancies). Nevertheless, it appears that Central Africa and adjacent areas of East, West, and Southern Africa are currently most severely affected by HIV, while populations thus far studied in most of West and Southern Africa[15] have less evidence of HIV infection.

HIV is now being detected in areas of Africa previously thought to be free of the infection[16]; however, with few exceptions, recent introduction of the virus cannot be distinguished from recent recognition of awareness of the problem. It appears likely that one to several million Africans may already be infected with HIV, and a substantial number of AIDS cases are expected from this pool of infected persons. It is noteworthy that more recently, in 1986, another human retrovirus generating immunodeficiency (HIV2) has been found mainly in West Africa (Guinea-Bissau, Cap Verde, Senegal, Ivory Coast, etc.).[17] At the present time, the second AIDS virus seems less widely disseminated than HIV1.

Descriptive Epidemiology

Surveillance data from several areas demonstrate that the sex ratio of African AIDS patients is approximately 1:1.[4,7–11] In Kinshasa, the mean age of AIDS patients is

Table 27-1
Summary of AIDS Cases Reported to WHO by 16th September 1987

Continent	No. Cases	No. Countries/ Territories Reporting:		
		To WHO	Zero Cases	1 or More Cases
Africa	5,814	44	9	35
Americas	46,456	44	4	40
Asia	195	25	7	18
Europe	7,082	28	1	27
Oceania	635	6	3	3
TOTAL	60,182	147	24	123

Source: WHO, Geneva, September 1987

34 years, and nearly 90% of all cases occur in patients between 20 and 49 years of age.[7] Seroepidemiologic studies of healthy populations in Kinshasa have shown a bimodal age-specific curve (Fig. 27-1). A first prevalence peak was observed among infants of whom approximately 8% were seropositive, comparing with only 1% to 2% among healthy children 1 to 14 years of age. The second peak (8% prevalence) occurred among adolescents and young adults (16–29 years of age).

Differences in AIDS prevalence between urban and rural areas have been noted in several countries. Although in a few instances (e.g., Uganda), HIV infection appears to be mainly a rural or small-town phenomenon,[10] in general the cities appear to be predominantly affected (Rwanda[11] and Zaire[7,9]). Similarly, variations in HIV infection rates according to socioeconomic status have been reported.[19]

Transmission

The basic modes of HIV transmission worldwide are hematologic, sexual, and perinatal. In sub-Saharan Africa, blood contamination proceeds from transfusions,[7,13,20,21] intravenous (IV) injections of medicine with nonsterile syringes or needles in some dispensaries, and possibly ritual practices such as scarifications with shared instruments.[7] Heterosexual intercourse is the major mode of transmission. Finally, perinatal infection is also important and well-documented.[22,23]

There is no evidence to support the existence of other modes of HIV transmission in Africa, such as casual contact. The rate of seropositivity did not differ significantly between nonspousal household members of 46 AIDS cases and household members of 43 seronegative age- and sex-matched persons.[23] Clusters of HIV infection in households are readily explainable by sexual or perinatal transmission. In addition, the absence of HIV infections among expatriates with no personal risk factors (sexual or parenteral) and living in HIV epidemic areas* further suggests that HIV is not transmitted by casual contacts in Africa.[24]

Available data also argue against insects as a mode of HIV transmission in Africa.[25] Age- and sex-specific seroprevalence data do not suggest a vectorborne disease. The lack of increased infection risks for household contacts living and sleeping in close proximity to AIDS cases suggests that insect transmission over short distances is unlikely.[23] HIV infections among expatriates living in epidemic areas are readily attributable to classic risk factors. In one well-studied area of Central Africa, the geographic distributions of malaria and HIV infections were found to be substantially different.† The possibility of a mechanical transmission by insect vectors such as mosquitoes seems remote, given the relatively small quantities of HIV in the blood of infected persons.[25]

Clinical Characteristics

In Africa, most individuals learn that they are HIV positive either through specialized medical consultations or through screening during hospitalization for symptoms often not related to AIDS. Thus, most infected people are unaware of their condition. As in Western countries, the large majority of Africa's infected people are asymptomatic carriers. Individuals may present with the typical signs of AIDS as defined by CDC/WHO, which are directly related to HIV infection and characterized by opportunistic infections or Kaposi's sarcoma. More often, the patient has a series of associated symptoms, which were defined as diagnostic of African AIDS at the WHO conference in Bangui (October 1985). The clinical diagnosis of African AIDS requires at least two major symptoms, such as weight loss, recurrent diarrhea, persistent fever, and at least one additional complication such as herpes zoster, prurigo, or candidiasis. The "slim" disease described in Uganda[26] is often observed in African AIDS.

In a study on patients hospitalized during the first semester of 1985 at the University clinic of Kinshasa,[27] two conclusions relevant to AIDS in Africa could be drawn. On one hand, chronic immune activation by endemic agents may contribute to immunodeficiency and speed up AIDS manifestations with opportunistic infections, Kaposi's sarcoma, or AIDS-related complex as described by CDC/WHO. On the other hand, concomitant HIV infection that increases the immune T cell defect may enhance clinical manifestations not included in the first CDC definition of specific endemic infections, such as tuberculosis,[28,29] malaria,[30] or malignant diseases such as chronic B cell leukemia.

* P. Piot, personal communication

† J. M. Mann, unpublished observations

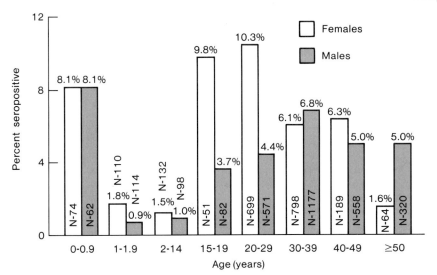

FIG. 27-1. HIV seroprevalence rates among 5099 healthy persons by age in Kinshasa, Zaire, 1984–1985. Sample population consisted of 2982 men and 2117 women. Positive patients had sera that were repeatedly reactive on a commercially available ELISA and were Western blot–positive. In age groups 16 to 19 years and 20 to 29 years, seroprevalence rates were significantly higher in women (10.3%) than men (4.3%). For 50 to 59 years of age, seroprevalence rates were significantly higher in men (5.0%) than women (1.6%).

AFRICAN BACKGROUND RELEVANT TO AIDS CONTROL

Sociocultural Considerations

To discuss control of AIDS in Africa, one must realize that the African continent is an enormous conglomerate of widely varying people. "Africans" were once divided into thousands of units—each tribe complete and virtually independent, each with its own internal government, religion, customs, language, and way of life. They were influenced by outside factors, such as Arab traders, colonial governments, and Western religions. Generally, tribal lines are muted today, especially in large cities, but they are still important. It would be presumptuous to categorize all Africans as the same. This work is therefore based on perceived trends that are shared by Central, West, South, and East African societies.

Today's African population centers consist of villages and urban areas to which people have migrated. Travel was intensified by decolonization and easier transportation, which opened up exchanges between villages and cities. Urban dwellers were entire families or single people temporarily separated from their families who had moved for economic reasons. In the context of sexual behavior, they are still conditioned by their traditions but are also influenced by Western ideas and modern commodities.

A variety of sociocultural attitudes in Africa will strongly influence AIDS and its control. The following description is provided only as a generalization in order to illustrate some of the factors to be considered in discussing AIDS prevention and control. The first concerns conceptions of groups and individuals. In contrast to Westerners, Africans generally give preference to groups and group members as opposed to individuals. Second, procreation is vitally important in African cultures. Life events may be viewed as having two parts that act in-terdependently: the natural (physical) and the spiritual. Spiritual forces are the underlying reason for physical results. Thus, illness is considered to have a supernatural base.[31-33] Finally, the body may be viewed as a machine with biologic fluids such as blood in a constant turnover that is equilibrated by taking in nutrients and voiding sweat, urine, and feces; this concept underlies the use of purges and blood-letting.[34] These principles are basic in the understanding of family, sex, ritual, and health behavior in relation to AIDS control.

Procreation aiming at the proliferation of the group is often the reference for both marriage and sexual intercourse. Since membership in the group prevails, marriage may be seen as a relationship between the two groups that goes beyond the two individuals concerned.[35] Thus, in Bantu societies, extraconjugal intercourse within the group may not be considered as adulterous. For example, on becoming a widow in Zambia, a woman may ask men of her husband's group to have intercourse with her to expel the husband's ghost from her body.[36] Having children may be both a duty toward the group and a means of personal status and promotion. For instance, the Samo society of the Ivory Coast requires a woman to have a child as proof of her fertility before she gets married. In the pursuit of increased fertility, Africans encourage conditions favoring procreation. These include traditional aphrodisiacs (ingested or applied locally), dances, and meticulous body care, such as baths, ointments, make-up, and elaborate hair-styles. In contrast, condoms are often rejected in Africa as both anti-procreative and as an unnatural intermediary measure.*

Homosexuality is not developed and is virtually negligible as a factor of HIV transmission. However, parenteral HIV infection may occur through traditional practices, such as tattoos and scarifications, that identify

---

* Dr. Okware, personal communication

the person's position (sex, age, marital status), and by circumcision performed with shared and nonsterile instruments. In addition, traditional practices in many societies prescribe blood-letting, blood-exchange, or the local use of blood and blood by-products to heal wounds. Western medicine, which is an adjunct to traditional cures, adds the risk of contaminated blood transfusions and unsterile needles, both important sources of HIV infection.

Education and Information

Education includes informal channels; knowledge is most of all empirically acquired and complemented by the words of influential people (elders, soothsayers and religious leaders, village chiefs, and government officials) and stories passed by word of mouth.[37] In addition, formal education has been generalized since Independence, for girls as well as boys. The Media have a growing influence in relaying information and education. This process is linked to the recent expansion in communication facilities, including magazines, books, printed materials, comics, radio, television clips, movie theaters, and cartoons in the cities, and at least radio in the country. News is avidly sought; an isolated villager may buy a radio and batteries with his first extra cash. In cities a well-to-do family may place their T.V. outside in the yard to share with the neighbors. The mass media could be a powerful tool for AIDS related communication. Figure 27-2 presents a portion of a comic on AIDS edited by the Zairian Ministry of Public Health that emphasizes both the concept of interdependent physical and spiritual forces and nonexclusive sexual behaviour.

IMMUNIZATION AND TREATMENT PROGRAMS IN ZAIRE

The promotion of medical action in infected people is important for several reasons. First, it would tend to banalize AIDS to a common sexually transmissible disease and would suppress both the stigmatizing of infected people and the perception that we are in the midst of a 20th century plague. Second, antiviral treatment of AIDS patients and infected individuals would restrict epidemiologic spread. Finally, and perhaps most important, the availability of treatments should prompt voluntary testing and the subsequent identification of HIV-infected people. This could limit the epidemic spread currently caused by unawareness of infection. A progress report of the Franco-Zairian action developed in Kinshasa is described in this section.

The need for medical action to control AIDS in Zaire prompted us to set up in Kinshasa, within the framework of a Franco-Zairian cooperation, a therapeutic and prophylactic program supervised by the University Clinic of Kinshasa (Lurhuma), the Institut National de Re-

cherche Biomédicale in Kinshasa (Salaün) and the Laboratoire de Physiologie Cellulaire de l'Université P. & M. Curie in Paris (Zagury). This program, which was based on the activation of immune defenses against HIV or HIV-infected cells, was supported by Zairian authorities and had the consent of the Zairian ethics committee.

Rationale

Cytopathogenic studies performed in collaboration with Gallo[38] demonstrated that infected T cells produce virus only after immune activation. As a consequence, released virions infect a new round of virgin T cells that promote viral dissemination in the organism and thus produce AIDS. If viral cell propagation is to be blocked, infected cells must be destroyed by immune defenses before the production of virus.

Immune response against HIV infection, as against other viral infection, may be triggered either by direct signals from virions or viral products through epitopes in their tertiary configuration or by membrane signals from infected cells that are formed by a major histocompatibility complex (MHC) product associated with a viral stretch (oligopeptide) in its native configuration.[39] The direct signals trigger a direct humoral response through antibody receptors at the B-cell surface, yielding antibodies only against the immunizing HIV strain and not against other strains.[40] Infected cell membrane signals, on the other hand may trigger, through receptors at the cell surface, a cell-mediated immunity that presumptively acts against different HIV strains (i.e., is group specific). Cell-mediated immunity yields an effector response formed both by generation of killer T cells against infected cells and by enhancement of anti-HIV antibody secretion by T-dependent B cells. Indeed T-cell receptors have a broader specificity for antigen recognition than do antibodies, and cell-mediated immunity should be more limited by allelic restriction due to the MHC component of its signal than by HIV subtype diversity. These considerations prompted us to determine experimental conditions to amplify antigenic viral cell membrane signals and induce cell-mediated immunity aimed at destroying infected cells before they release virions. In addition, production of antibodies by T-dependent B cells should neutralize free virions in both already infected and noninfected individuals.

Cell-surface viral signals do not exist in infected cells at a resting stage but are expressed after immune activation and before viral production. This immunogenic phase prior to viral release, which is crucial for immune reaction against HIV to occur both at its afferent and effector phase, unfortunately does not last long in infected human T cells.* Therefore our strategy was to amplify these antigenic viral cell membrane signals, and several procedures have been used to accomplish this.

* I. Desportes, manuscript in preparation

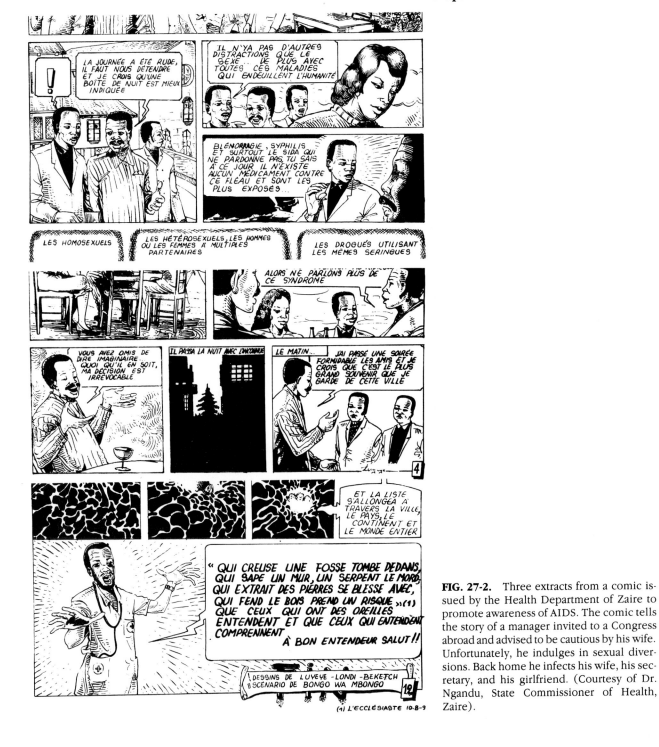

FIG. 27-2. Three extracts from a comic issued by the Health Department of Zaire to promote awareness of AIDS. The comic tells the story of a manager invited to a Congress abroad and advised to be cautious by his wife. Unfortunately, he indulges in sexual diversions. Back home he infects his wife, his secretary, and his girlfriend. (Courtesy of Dr. Ngandu, State Commissioner of Health, Zaire).

HIV *env* gp 160 Determinant Used as Immunogenic Signal

To amplify cell membrane gp 160 determinant signals, we have used two immunization procedures. The first mode of immunization was based on priming with a live vaccinia recombinant virus (VR), whose genome carries HIV gp 160 *env* gene. VR was prepared through genetic engineering first by B. Moss, who used the WHR vaccinia strain,[41] then by George Beaud who, with Moss's technology, used a Lister strain (a non-neurotropic vaccinia strain kindly donated by Dr. Pourquier, Montpel-

Table 27-2
Cell-Mediated Immunity Against HIV Infection

Stimulated PBL Origin	Time Following Immunization (Days)*	Proliferative Index† Against HIV			IL2 Receptor Positive Cells (%)‡		
		No Virus	B	RF	No Virus	B	RF
N1–(BR)	—	1	<2	<2	<3	<3	<3
N2–(MF)	—	1	<2	<2	<3	<3	<3
DZ	63	1	26	8	<3	14	10
	110	1	60	22	ND	ND	ND
	120	1	40	16	<3	20	12

PBL, peripheral blood lymphocytes; B, HIV1 strain HTLV III-B; RF, HIV1 strain HTLV III-RF; N1(BR), N2-MF, Non immunized healthy controls; DZ, immunized individual; VR, recombinant vaccinia expressing gp 160
* Immunization protocol : Day 0   : Vr priming
                      Day 100 : Inoculation with autologous Vr infected and paraformaldehyde fixed cells.
† Proliferative index is measured by the mean results of triplicate samples divided by the control values (no virus).
‡ IL2 receptor positive cells were identified by indirect IFA, after incubation with TAC MAb.

lier, France). Cells infected by VR express at the cell surface HIV gp 160 *env* proteins, which represent antigenic signals to trigger cell-mediated immunity.

The second procedure was based on immunization with massive doses of HIV (HTLV-IIIB strain) or VR-infected autologous blood cells that had previously been fixed by paraformaldehyde (1% in PBS at 4°C for 4 minutes). In these preparations, 20% to 50% of cells express HIV gp 160 *env* antigens as detected by indirect immunofluorescence. In addition, these fixed cells, even though not alive, are still immunogenic since they stimulate autologous fresh PBL in vitro, as detected both by proliferation and by cell-mediated cytotoxicity assays.†

In the near future, other procedures using gp 160 determinant signals to trigger cell-mediated immunity against HIV, not yet tested in primates, might represent a second generation of antigenic preparations, to be tested for priming and boost. These procedures are based on the use of non-lived immunogenic compounds, such as the T1 and T2 peptides prepared by J. Berzovsky[42] or the tuftsinilated HIV gp 160 *env* protein prepared by M. Feldman and S. Waksall from insect cells infected with a bacula virus construct.

In vivo Safety and Immunogenicity

Preliminary experiments using the first two immunizing procedures were performed on cercopithecus, baboons, and chimps as indicated in Table 27-2. After administration of VR as well as HIV- or VR-infected cells, whether subsequently fixed or not, no clinical manifestations (fever or digestive, respiratory or nervous disorders) were found; only local pustules, 0.5 cm to 1 cm in diameter, were observed after VR scarifications. In addition, Western blot analysis showed evidence of antibodies against HIV proteins in sera from treated monkeys.

† M. Fouchard, unpublished results

Progress Report for AIDS Vaccine

There is today no vaccine available against AIDS. However, researchers worldwide are trying to engineer a vaccine, which could ultimately eradicate HIV infection as vaccinia eradicated smallpox. Along this line, the vaccine program designed at Kinshasa by the Franco-Zairian group consisted of promoting a group-specific cell-mediated immunity against HIV by using gp 160 viral cell membrane signals, as described above. We report here the results, some not yet published, of this vaccine program, which entails several successive phases.

Choice of Subjects

The first series of volunteers consisted of DZ, one of the promoters of this program, and 10 Zairians who entered the program in November 1986. BG, a French collaborator living at Kinshasa, joined this group in January 1987. These 12 subjects had all previously been vaccinated against smallpox, were all HIV seronegative, and had normal T4 cell counts and in vitro production of interleukin-2 (IL-2) upon phytohemagglutinin activation of their fresh blood mononuclear cells. Thereafter, two new series of seronegative healthy volunteers, consisting of 27 French cooperants and 12 Zairians, joined the program.

Priming

In the first group of 12, we were prompted to use VR as primer because live vaccinia is known to trigger a cell-mediated immunity and to present a negligible risk for vaccine complications in previously vaccinated, HIV seronegative, non-immunodeficient individuals. In the later series, 28 other volunteers were also primed with VR and a further 9 received the gp 160 antigen mixed with either an oil (6 subjects) or a water-soluble adjuvant (1 control). The gp 160 antigen was purified from VR-infected mammalian cell cultures.

Boosting

Within the first series, we resorted to four different preparations as boosters:

- autologous cells infected with VR and subsequently fixed (injected into DZ)
- VR used by scarification for four volunteers
- Pgp 120 peptide purified from cultured cells infected with VR; this peptide, which reacts against monoclonal antibody against gp 120, was administered to six individuals
- purified cell membrane fraction from autologous cells infected in vitro with VR (injected into BG). These membranes were purified in collaboration with A. Amar Costesec (Bruxelles) according to the procedure previously described.[43]

In the subsequent series, some VR-primed individuals were boosted with one or another of these preparations, but the majority received purified gp 160 antigen either in water or mixed with a mineral oil adjuvant.

Follow-up

The four protocols used for the 12 individuals of the first group all induced an immune reaction against HIV, with cell-mediated immunity identified both by proliferation of fresh PBL stimulated by ultraviolet-irradiated virus[44,45] and by specific antibody detected by Western blot and/or neutralizing activity against different strains of HIV.[46] However, individuals boosted with either VR or Pgp 120 expressed a relatively low titer of serum antibody neutralizing against the two strains of HIV (B and RF) distant from each other by 1000 nucleotides.[47] Subject BG, who had received purified infected cell membranes as a booster, exhibited high titers of neutralizing antibody for a short period after the boost. By contrast, DZ, who was boosted with fixed infected cells, presented a high cell-mediated immunity response for both B and RF strains (Table 27-2) and long-lasting high titers of serum Ab neutralizing against both HIV

strains (i.e., group specific) (Table 27-3). We concluded from these data that the protocol used for DZ yielded an optimal group-specific immune reaction against HIV, with titers of antibodies (Fig. 27-3A) neutralizing in vitro infection of T cells by widely divergent HIV strains. In addition, DZ has exhibited an anamnestic T-cell response 300 days after priming, showing a strong delayed-type hypersensitivity skin reaction against intradermally injected purified gp 160. Also, DZ was challenged with purified gp 160 (100 μg in PBS) injected intramuscularly. As early as 7 days afterward, high levels of both cell-mediated immunity against B and RF strains and serum antibodies detected by Western blot were demonstrated.

The high level of immune response against different strains of HIV and the anamnestic response observed after 10 months allow us to consider the DZ protocol as a prototype of AIDS vaccine, which might protect in vivo as it does in vitro against HIV infection. This "candidate vaccine" protocol using fixed infected cells as booster would not, however, be appropriate for a large-scale trial.

A more readily usable booster system capable of promoting a similar group-specific immune reaction against HIV would be a pertinent candidate vaccine for a large-scale trial. To this purpose, purified gp 160 antigen either mixed with an adjuvant or alone in water, injected as a booster after priming, is being tested in the new series of volunteers.

Whichever protocol will fulfil the requirements of a good candidate vaccine—that is, yield a group-specific anamnestic response against HIV with evidence of both cell-mediated immunity and neutralizing antibodies in vitro—it will have to be tested in the field. This will be done in two different ways: HIV challenge in appropriate primates and large-scale volunteer human trials.

Challenging Primates with HIV

Experiments are now being conducted in collaboration with Dr. P. Fishinger and P. Nara to test whether the only candidate vaccine available—the one used for

Table 27-3
Immunization Against HIV D.Z. Serum Antibody Analysis

Day	Immunization	Neutralizing AB		Western Blot		
		B	RF	gp160	gp120	gp41
0		0	0	−	−	−
40	Vr	40	0	−	−	−
63		42	0	−	−	−
102	Fixed Vr-infected autologous cells					
110		108	94	−	−	−
120		108	70	++	+	−
160		108	108	ND	ND	ND
171		108	108	++	+	+
178		108	108	++	+	+

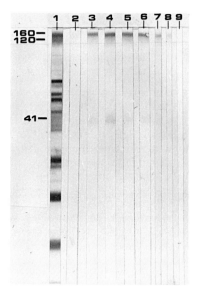

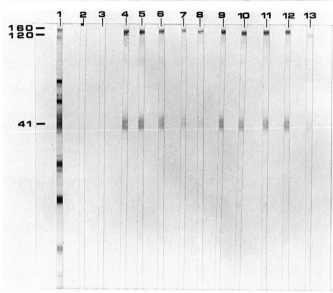

FIG. 27-3. Western blot analysis of DZ serum. (A) lane 1 = AIDS serum control; lane 2 = after priming; lane 3–7 = 10–70 days after boost; lanes 8 & 9 = 90 & 100 days after boost. (B) Culture of clones from EBV transformed cells from DZ, 70 days after boost. Clones 17 and 18 expressed HIV gp 160 Ab. (C) Subclones of clone 18. Most of these monoclonal cultures expressed Ab against gp 160 and gp 41.

DZ—is protective against infection in chimpanzees. Challenge of these immunized chimps is done by IP HIV injections, according to guidelines set up by Dr. P. Fishinger's group at Frederick, a procedure which yields 100% in vivo infection.

We are also attempting to set up a protocol using HIV-2 in African cercopithecus or cercocebus. These animals, easier to obtain and manipulate, could represent an alternative animal model to chimps relevant for viral challenge, if indeed they can be regularly infected.

Large-Scale Clinical Trials

Large-scale clinical trials eventually will be required to demonstrate protection against infection. This phase implies the participation of an uninfected population of volunteers who have a high risk of natural infection. This population would be divided into two groups, one getting wild vaccinia (placebo), the second receiving the candidate vaccine. The efficiency of the HIV vaccine would be made apparent by comparing the incidence of infections in the two groups.

To prepare this assay, in cooperation with Doctors Nzangolo and Dechazal, we have screened various population subsets in Zaire for HIV infection. Among the four groups tested, we found a medically well-monitored subset with a high rate of natural infection. Before the clinical trial can start, however, we have to make the candidate vaccine(s) and protocol available for a large number of individuals. Such a trial also requires the full endorsement of local authorities and will have to be done in conformity and with the help of WHO.

Progress Report on Active Immunotherapy in AIDS

Two patients were treated in July, 1986, and eight others in December, 1986. All the patients presented clinical manifestations of African AIDS with biological characteristics of immune defect, i.e. a T4 cell count less than 300, a T4/T8 ratio less than 0.5, and a much lower than normal production of PHA-induced IL-2 by blood mononuclear cells. These patients received injections of $2 \times 10^{7-8}$ fixed autologous cells massively infected by HIV or by a vaccinia recombinant (RV). Cells were given one-third intravenously and two-thirds subcutaneously about every 3 months.

Though clinical benefit cannot be unequivocally asserted as of 10 months, most of the patients have gained weight (2–10 kg) and recovered their social and professional activities. Although T4 cell numbers were not restored to normal, the immune system has functionally improved, as assessed by IL-2 production. In addition, specific cell-mediated cytotoxicity against autologous infected cells was found in two cases.*

These preliminary results showed that active immunization specifically directed against HIV infection was at least innocuous. More documented data are required, however, before conclusions can be drawn on whether specific immunization against HIV infection should be applied for ARC and early AIDS patients, as an alternative or adjuvant therapy for chemotherapy, or even, as suggested by Salk, as a preventive procedure against AIDS in non-immunodeficient HIV carriers.[48]

Progress Report for Offspring Prevention

The final Franco-Zairian project is adoptive immunotherapy to protect offspring of infected women. This program contains three successive steps: preparation of purified antibodies that neutralize HIV virus, animal testing for side effects and protection against infection, and inoculation of mothers and newborns with analysis of effective protection by follow-up. We are currently at stage 1. Indeed, we have already prepared monoclonal antibody against HIV from EBV-transformed B cells from DZ† (Fig. 27-3*B*).

WHO PROGRAM FOR AIDS CONTROL IN AFRICA

Because the WHO has the responsibility to direct and coordinate international health, it has been given the mandate to lead the global fight against AIDS. Thus, in November 1986, the Director-General of WHO announced that WHO was dedicating itself to global AIDS control with the same energy and commitment that characterized the global smallpox eradication program. On 1st February 1987, the WHO Special Program on AIDS (SPA) was created as the architect of and vehicle for the global AIDS strategy. In May 1987, the 40th World Health Assembly declared AIDS to be a "worldwide emergency" and endorsed SPA and the global strategy. The SPA has designed the global strategy, has raised the necessary funds to begin implementing this strategy, and toward this effort has marshalled the support of every nation.

Objectives

The Global AIDS strategy has three major objectives:

- To prevent HIV transmission
- To take care of HIV-infected persons (to reduce morbidity and mortality associated with HIV-infections); the care of HIV-infected persons is not limited to medical management or to AIDS or AIDS-Related Complex (ARC) patients. Combatting discrimination against HIV-infected persons is as vital to the global strategy as provision of medical care.

---

* R. Cheynier, personal communication

† C. Desgranges et al., manuscript in preparation

- To unify national and international AIDS control efforts.

General Concepts

The principal components of the global AIDS strategy are:

- Comprehensive national AIDS prevention and control programs
- Strong international leadership, coordination, and cooperation

Every country will need a strong and committed national AIDS program. The major components of such a program have been developed, and are described below. International leadership, coordination, and cooperation are essential for effective utilization of resources, to minimize duplication, and to ensure rapid and widespread sharing of critical information.

National AIDS Program Plans

Administrative Framework

POLITICAL WILLINGNESS TO CONFRONT THE AIDS PROBLEM. Until a government is prepared to speak openly about the national HIV/AIDS situation, an effective national program is not possible. Now that approximately three-quarters of all countries in the world have reported at least some AIDS cases to WHO, the perceived stigma associated with reporting the existence of AIDS should disappear.

CREATION OF A NATIONAL AIDS COMMITTEE. A National AIDS Committee must be formed, including in its membership representatives of the health and broad social sectors involved in AIDS. In addition to health professionals, the educational, informational/media, women's and children's groups and the economic/planning sectors of government must be represented. Important nongovernmental and private voluntary organizations should also be represented. In many countries, the Committee is created either under the Ministry of Health or under an Inter-Ministry arrangement. The Committee is also advisory to a Ministry (Health) and Inter-Ministry Group (Cabinet Committee), or to the Chief Executive of government. The Committee is responsible, in the first instance, for initial assessment and planning of the national AIDS program.

DEVELOPMENT AND ADOPTION OF A NATIONAL AIDS PLAN. A comprehensive, written plan is essential, for it serves to organize, prioritize, and rationalize the use of national and external resources. A written plan for a 3- to 5-year period (medium-term plan) is required for this purpose. The process through which the plan is developed is critical, for it must involve the many groups in the community whose support and understanding will be required for implementation of the plan.

Prerequisites to Execution of National Programs

INITIAL EPIDEMIOLOGIC AND RESOURCE ASSESSMENTS. Until fundamental information about the scope and extent of HIV infection and AIDS is known, it will be difficult to plan rationally. In addition, baseline information about HIV seroprevalence will be critical to assess the impact of intervention strategies. In many areas, preliminary serosurveys have already been conducted. However, these surveys usually involved readily available, perhaps unrepresentative, population samples. For example, patients at sexually transmitted disease clinics or hospitalized patients are often included in such surveys. Although these surveys are useful to establish the presence of HIV in the community and to gauge its approximate extent, more systematic and less biased sample selection is required. In order to assist in assessing HIV seroprevalence, SPA has developed a model methodology, based on cluster sampling techniques, which is now undergoing field evaluation. Similarly, an assessment of available resources (human, financial, and material) for AIDS prevention and control is needed. These two surveys form the basis for planning initial interventions and development of a national AIDS plan.

EPIDEMIOLOGIC SURVEILLANCE. AIDS may provide the impetus for developing or strengthening a national disease surveillance and reporting system. In many countries, surveillance of AIDS cases is underway. In any surveillance system, the problem of case definition must be resolved. When evaluated in at least one HIV-endemic area of Central Africa, the African AIDS definition (Bangui definition) was highly specific but had low sensitivity. Therefore CDC has revised its case definition, and this recent revision (1987) has been adopted as the CDC/WHO definition. Surveillance based on HIV seroprevalence is preferred, for several reasons. First, ascertainment of AIDS cases is subject to major bias. Second, AIDS cases reflect the epidemiology of several years earlier, rather than the current situation. Third, HIV seroprevalence, if determined in an acceptable manner, will permit periodic comparisons—of great importance to program evaluation.

LOGISTICAL ORGANIZATION. In-country laboratory capability should be sufficient for diagnostic, testing, and screening purposes. Existing laboratories should be strengthened; existing laboratory staff should be trained. The development of newer laboratory tests (i.e., dot ELISA, agglutination) that are more robust and easier to perform in field conditions should help assure widespread use of first-line screening methods.

EDUCATIONAL PROGRAMS FOR HEALTH WORKERS. Health workers at all levels must be informed and educated about HIV and AIDS. This education should focus on diagnosis and management of HIV infection, prevention of iatrogenic HIV transmission, protection of the health care worker, and information/education for clients.

General Prevention Programs

Prevention programs are linked to the three modes of HIV transmission: sex, blood, and mother-to-child.

PREVENTING SEXUAL TRANSMISSION. Ultimately, preventing sexual transmission requires education. The general public and designated subgroups (including adolescents, sexually active persons with multiple partners, prostitutes) must be informed about HIV transmission and its prevention. The objective of this education is to produce sustained behavioral changes regarding numbers of sexual partners, choice of sexual partners, sexual acts, and use of condoms. The development of a national educational program on AIDS is vital, to ensure consistency, accuracy, and widespread delivery of key information and messages on HIV prevention. The National AIDS Committee often creates a subcommittee on education that designs and oversees implementation of the national educational effort. Public health communication requires a long-term commitment. Although a coordinated program may be divided into sequential phases, called "campaigns," which intensify activities during selected periods, public health communication is not limited to a single campaign. Among the key steps in developing a national educational strategy are the following:

- Identifying the potential target audiences and segmenting these audiences on the basis of country-specific variables including sex, age, literacy level, socioeconomic status
- Selecting primary and secondary target audiences (primary = key targets on the basis of risk status; secondary = persons who provide essential support for primary target audience acceptance, such as decision-makers)
- Determining specific, measurable educational objectives based on intended changes in behavior
- Selecting appropriate educational strategies (mass media, pamphlets, person-to-person)
- Determining the specific context of the messages (focus on key benefits and motivations for target audience behavior change)
- Determining the character and content of specific strategies (message "tone," positioning of the issue, phrases and symbols, images)
- Selecting the "channels" for implementing each program strategy (mass media, interpersonal, traditional media, churches, other)

Finally, the development and implementation of a national educational strategy should not be viewed as a rigid sequence leading to a single campaign. The education process will be prolonged, and strategies will need to be revised and modified over time in the light of experience and changing needs.

PREVENTING BLOOD TRANSMISSION. Several measures may be required, depending upon the epidemiological situation.

BLOOD TRANSFUSIONS. The existing strategies for reducing the risk of transfusing HIV-contaminated blood include reducing the use of blood for transfusion, epidemiological/clinically based donor deferral, and screening of blood for HIV contamination.

Reducing the need for blood transfusions may be important. It involves strategies to prevent or otherwise treat conditions that may lead to a need for transfusion (e.g., automobile accidents (via safety programs), anemia during pregnancy) and a careful review of transfusion practices and policies to eliminate unnecessary transfusions. In particular, practices such as giving a single unit of blood prior to surgery should be reviewed.

Donor deferral policies are based on the elimination of "higher risk" persons from blood donation. Risk may be determined epidemiologically (homosexual/bisexual men, prostitutes) or clinically (current health; unexplained lymphadenopathy). Donor deferral programs have been successful in areas (North America, Europe) where HIV infection has been relatively well confined to persons with identifiable risk factors (homosexual or bisexual men, intravenous drug users). However, in areas characterized by heterosexual transmission (Africa, Haiti), donor deferral on epidemiologic criteria has generally not been successful. In one study in Central Africa, application of epidemiologic criteria capable of reducing the risk of accepting an HIV-infected donor by 80% required exclusion (denial) of approximately two-thirds of prospective donors.

Blood donor screening is important, with or without efforts to reduce the number of transfusions and donor deferral programs. In contrast to educational efforts, which at least initially may produce uncertain benefits, the screening of blood for HIV contamination immediately prevents HIV transmission. Screening technology has been simplified so that rapid, reliable blood screening methods can be made widely available. However, no screening technology removes the need for careful training, protection of laboratory reagents, quality control, and meticulous laboratory record-keeping. In addition, the personal and public health consequences of HIV infection mandate that pre- and post-screening counseling be developed.

BLOOD PRODUCTS. Factors VIII and IX have been associated with HIV transmission to persons with hemophilia. Fortunately, neither immune serum globulin prepared using the cold ethanol fractionation method nor albumin have been implicated in HIV transmission. It is essential that clotting factors for persons with hemophilia be prepared according to currently accepted methods judged HIV-virucidal. In addition, use of HIV-screened blood for production of clotting factors provides an additional margin of safety.

INJECTIONS—INTRAVENOUS DRUG ABUSERS.   Clearly, the prevention of intravenous drug abuse is the optimal strategy, followed by treatment of existing users. However, efforts must also be directed to helping existing users (who lack access to treatment or who do not wish to be treated) to avoid HIV infection. Tactics include increasing the availability of sterile needles and syringes and educating users about simple rules to avoid infection (e.g., not sharing equipment; sterilization methods).

INJECTIONS—MEDICAL AND TRADITIONAL.   The re-use of any skin-piercing instrument or other instrument that may become contaminated with blood creates a potential hazard for HIV transmission. Problems arise within the modern medical system as well as for traditional healers and for various cosmetic and ritual practices. First, injections are often over-prescribed, as a result of the beliefs and preferences of both provider and consumer. Then, in general, the principles of sterilization are not widely applied unless specific informational/educational efforts have been undertaken. For needles and syringes, two basic approaches are possible: strict use of single-use equipment, with prompt and careful destruction, to avoid both accidental injuries and re-use; or reusable syringes and needles, with strict adherence to cleaning and sterilizing practices.

Fortunately, HIV is not hard to inactivate, and practices sufficient to protect against hepatitis B virus (HBV) are entirely sufficient against HIV. However, education of providers may not be sufficient; education of consumers to request alternatives to injection or at least to ensure use of sterile injection equipment may be vital.

ORGAN DONATION.   To prevent HIV transmission by way of donated organs the donor must be tested.

PREVENTING PERINATAL TRANSMISSION.   The ideal way to prevent perinatal transmission is to prevent infection of childbearing age women altogether. The second method is for all HIV-infected women to avoid pregnancy, at least until the risk factors associated with perinatal transmission are clarified. In this context, HIV screening programs among women of childbearing age who are considered to be at higher risk may be suggested. HIV-infected women should be offered a safe, effective, and convenient method for contraception, along with counseling and strong social support, as personal and social pressures to conceive may be intense. Despite these efforts, pregnant women may be infected with HIV either before or during pregnancy. Available data suggest that 25% to 50% of children of infected women will be perinatally infected. Perinatal infection may occur in utero, co-natally (during birth, as with hepatitis B), or after birth. Limited experience suggests that HIV may be transmitted through breast milk, although the contribution of breast-feeding to overall perinatal transmission is thought to be minimal. The natural history of perinatally acquired HIV infection is not yet well-documented, but HIV-infected infants are clearly at risk of HIV-related clinical illness and death during the first year of life, and beyond. Programs to screen already pregnant women (prenatal clinics) should take into account the extensive counseling and social support required by pregnant women found to be HIV-seropositive. Finally, in the postnatal period, HIV-infected women should receive counseling and support for the adoption of acceptable contraceptive methods.

Specific National Programs to Reduce the Morbidity and Mortality Associated with HIV Infection (To Take Care of HIV-Infected Persons)

A national AIDS program is not complete unless provision is made for the care of all HIV-infected persons. Clearly, needs for counseling, social support, and medical care vary according to the clinical status of the infected person. Asymptomatic HIV-infected persons may experience higher levels of anxiety related to their infection than patients with clinical AIDS. The uncertain prognosis, fears that minor symptoms may herald the onset of AIDS or ARC, and the need to adopt lifestyle changes to protect oneself and others creates enormous pressures. To this burden is often added concern about, or management of, discrimination and exclusion. HIV-infected persons experiencing symptoms of HIV-associated disease require medical support, which may be quite expensive. Direct medical care costs for ARC or AIDS patients in the developing world have not yet been determined, but AIDS patients will utilize considerable diagnostic, therapeutic, and medical care resources. Decisions about use of limited supplies of therapeutic agents to treat opportunistic infections in persons with AIDS may be required. Throughout the world, strategies for medical management, adapted to resource constraints and social practices, must be developed. In addition to focusing services on HIV-infected persons, a national strategy to prevent discrimination and exclusion of HIV-infected persons is essential. Information and education about HIV infection is vital, for society must understand and accept that HIV-infected persons do not create a random or uncontrollable risk for transmission. On the one hand, AIDS must be banalized as a new sexually transmitted disease, and on the other hand, HIV-infected persons must not be victims of stigmatization and seen as "the others," but as a part of "ourselves." The challenge of fighting against prejudices based on fear and ignorance is great.

Evaluation

Evaluation of national AIDS programs is vital, not only to preserve and maximize limited resources but to discover how HIV prevention can best be achieved. Therefore, careful evaluation of education efforts should not only attempt to examine self-reported changes in knowledge, attitudes, and behavior, but also determine directly the impact of knowledge on rates of HIV infection. In addition to educational programs, the value of a series of strategic decisions must be assessed, including the impact of counseling (or different counseling methods) in achieving sustained behavior change among HIV-infected persons; the value of testing as an adjunct to behavior change in higher-risk persons; and the usefulness of contact follow-up for sexual partners of infected persons.

Only by carefully and dispassionately examining the impact of prevention strategies will we learn how best, and at least cost, to prevent HIV infection. Therefore, the importance of evaluation extends beyond national borders; the lessons learned in any country may be valuable for global efforts.

Progress to Date: National Programs

As of mid-September 1987, over 100 countries had formed national AIDS committees. Over 90 countries around the world had entered into collaboration with the Special Program on AIDS for support to national AIDS programs. The Special Program has provided over 250 technical support missions, involving epidemiologists, laboratory specialists, planners, educators, and other health professionals. Urgent support had been provided to countries to start the work of AIDS control without delay. Fifty countries had developed written plans for AIDS prevention and control at the national level. Five countries (Uganda, Kenya, Tanzania, Rwanda, and Ethiopia) had developed medium-term (3- to 5-year) national AIDS plans, which were adopted by the government and which served as the basis for in-country meetings. These meetings, organized in collaboration with WHO, resulted in mobilization of sufficient resources for the implementation of these programs. At government request, WHO staff are being assigned to these countries to strengthen the national AIDS program further. Thus, national programs are being rapidly established throughout the world with the technical and financial support of the Special Program. When national AIDS plans are implemented, the Special Program will be closely involved in monitoring and evaluating their effectiveness. Finally, support from the Special Program will continue to be provided as the national programs evolve and new needs become apparent.

Global Activities of WHO

In addition to supporting national AIDS programs, the WHO Special Program on AIDS provides global leadership to ensure international coordination and cooperation. The three elements of global leadership are strategy, science, and resource.

Strategic Leadership

WHO works to articulate principles for AIDS prevention and control, for consideration by the World Health Assembly. For example, WHO Resolution 40.26 (15 May 1987) states, inter alia: "the transmission of AIDS can be prevented . . . information is an essential element in all control of AIDS . . . every individual has a responsibility," and ". . . information and education on the modes of transmission as well as the assurance and use of safe blood and blood products, and sterile practices in invasive procedures, are still the measures available that can limit the further spread of AIDS." In addition to general principles, the Special Program develops guidelines, consensus statements, and prototypes and models. For example, guidelines have been written for HIV screening programs, sterilization and disinfection practices, and educational strategies for HIV prevention. Consensus statements have been developed on HIV and international travel, HIV and breastfeeding, and HIV and childhood immunization. Finally, prototypes or models have been developed in the following areas: educational materials; seroprevalence methodology; surveys for knowledge, attitude, and behavior.

Scientific Coordination and Collaboration

The scientific work to master AIDS, like the disease itself, is now firmly and irrevocably international. In AIDS, there really can no longer be any such thing as purely local or even purely national research. These international links must be strengthened, and WHO, with its principles of objectivity, neutrality, open exchange, and consensus, can play a powerful facilitating and stimulating role in this area. Examples of WHO's work include the creation of a AIDS reagent project—a world bank for the collection, characterization, and exchange of viruses and other key reagents. In the field of social and behavioral research, WHO has identified several priorities, including cross-cultural studies of perception of, and attitudes towards AIDS, counseling practices, risk behaviors, and impact of AIDS on social structures, especially families. The global AIDS data bank at WHO is an example of information exchange at the international level. Finally, international collaboration and coordination will be required to bring drug and vaccine development from initial concepts to final field evaluation. Looking to the future, WHO is working to ensure that the fruits of international research—drugs and vaccines—will be made available to the entire world.

Resource Leadership

Two major tasks inherent in global AIDS control are mobilization and coordination of international resources. Resource mobilization is required at the national and international levels. At the national level, the national AIDS plan serves as the key document for considering resource allocation as well as for external support of a national program. At the international level, it is essential that the resources dedicated to AIDS control supplement resources already targeted to major, existing health programs such as childhood immunization and diarrheal disease control. One critical issue in mobilizing resources is whether any additional resources for the health sector can be generated. AIDS may provide an opportunity to demonstrate why health deserves a larger portion of national resources. Coordination of resources at the international level requires commitment to common goals, strategy, and coordinating mechanisms. The Special Program is providing these mechanisms at the national, regional, and global levels. Nevertheless, the challenge of coordination is great, and innovative approaches will be required to ensure both short-term and long-term resource coordination against AIDS.

In summary, at the global level, WHO's Special Program on AIDS is providing strategic leadership, developing consensus, coordinating scientific research, exchanging information, and mobilizing and coordinating resources for global AIDS control.

CONCLUSION

AIDS was first recognized only six years ago; as a result of an extraordinary effort of the medical and scientific international community, we have within a few years determined the clinical manifestations associated with this disease in the different parts of the world, identified the causal agent, defined its modes of transmission, delineated its worldwide epidemic profile, and characterized the biology of the virus. Researchers are experimenting with preventive (vaccine) and therapeutic (chemotherapy and/or immunotherapy) cures against AIDS, as illustrated by the Franco-Zaïrian program. Although the development and evaluation of these treatments is not complete, we know enough now to prevent the spread of HIV infection by appropriate prophylactic and educative measures. This would require that each country, according to its sociocultural background, take a set of locally specific actions conceived and enforced by national authorities. The need for such operations in the fight against a worldwide dissemination of AIDS has prompted WHO to promote and coordinate national AIDS programs.

The success of these programs, be they medical, prophylactic or educational, implies enormous efforts: dedication, solidarity, creativity, investment, full international cooperation, and consciousness that AIDS is a global challenge for humans that will not be overcome anywhere unless it is solved everywhere.

The section concerning the WHO program has been written thanks to documentation kindly supplied by Dr. Jonathan Mann, Director of the WHO special program on AIDS. The authors also thank Professor Ngandu, Minister of Health in Zaire, for providing us with educational documents related to AIDS and acknowledge the generous contribution of the following scientists: J. Leibovitch (Hôpital Raymond Poincaré, Garches, France); A. G. Saimot (Institut de Médecine et d'Epidémiologie tropicale, Hôpital Claude Bernard, Paris, France); M. Bekombo and R. Hamayon (Laboratoire d'Ethnologie et de Sociologie Comparative, Université de Paris, France); D. Messinger and J. J. Salaun (Institut National de Recherches Biomédicales, Kinshasa, Zaire) and R. C. Gallo (National Cancer Institute, Bethesda, Md, USA).

This work was partly supported by the Association for Cancer Research (ARC, Villejuif, France) and the U.S. Army (Contract N'DAMD 17866284).

REFERENCES

1. Brunet JB, Bouvet E, Chaperon J, et al: Acquired immunodeficiency syndrome in France. Lancet i:700, 1983
2. Clumeck N, Mascart-Lemone F, De Maulbeuge J, et al: Acquired immunodeficiency syndrome in black Africans. Lancet i:642, 1983
3. Katlama C, Leport C, Matheron S, et al: Acquired immunodeficiency syndrome (AIDS) in Africans. Ann Soc Belge Med Trop 64:379, 1984
4. Bayley AC: Aggressive Kaposi's sarcoma in Zambia 1983. Lancet i:1318, 1984
5. Kreiss JK, Koech D, Plummer EA, et al: AIDS virus infection in Nairobi prostitutes: Spread of the epidemic to East Africa. New Engl J Med 314:414, 1986
6. Lyons SF, Shoub BD, Mc Gillivray GM, et al: Lack of evidence of HTLV-III endemicity in Southern Africa. New Engl J Med 312:1257, 1985
7. Mann JM, Francis H, Quinn T, et al: Surveillance for AIDS in a central African city: Kinshasa, Zaire. JAMA 255:3255, 1986
8. Odio W, Kapita B, Bendi N, et al: Le syndrome d'immunodeficience acquise (SIDA) a Kinshasa (Zaire): Observations cliniques et epidemiologiques. Ann Soc Belges Med Trop 65:357, 1985
9. Piot P, Quinn TC, Taelman H, et al: Acquired immunodeficiency syndrome in a heterosexual population in Zaire. Lancet ii:65, 1984
10. Serwadda D, Muserwa RD, Sewankambo NK, et al: Slim disease: A new disease in Uganda and its association with HTLV-III infection. Lancet ii:849, 1985
11. Van de Perre P, Rouvroy D, Lepage P, et al: Acquired immunodeficiency syndrome in Rwanda. Lancet 62, 1984
12. Van de Pitte J, Verwilghen R, Zachee P: AIDS and cryptococcosis (Zaire, 1977). Lancet i:925, 1983
13. Curran JW, Robert-Guroff M, Van de Perre P, et al: Seroepidemiological studies of HTLV-III antibody prevalence among selected groups of heterosexual Africans. JAMA 254:2599, 1985
14. World Health Organization: Acquired immunodeficiency syndrome WHO/CDC case definition for AIDS. Weekly Epidem Rec 10:69, 1986
15. Sher RS: Serological studies in Southern Africa (abstract). Presented at International Symposium on African AIDS. Brussels, November 22/23, 1985
16. M'Boup S, Prince-Devid M, Boye CS, et al: Serological ev-

idence that HTLV-III is present in Senegal, West Africa (abstract). Presented at International Symposium on African AIDS, Brussels, November 22/23, 1985

17. Clavel F, Guetard D, Brun-Vezinet F, et al: Isolation of a new human retrovirus from West African patients with AIDS. Science 233:343, 1986

18. Quinn TC, Mann JM, Curran JW, Piot P: AIDS in Africa: An epidemiological paradigm. Science 234:955, 1986

19. Biggar RJ: The AIDS problem in Africa. Lancet i:79, 1986

20. Clumeck N, Robert-Guroff M, Van de Perre P, et al: seroepidemiological studies of HTLV-III antibody prevalence among selected group of heterosexual Africans. JAMA 254:2599, 1985

21. Izzia KW, Lepira B, Kayembe M, et al: Syndrome d'immunodeficiencie acquise et drepanocytose homozygote a propos d'une observation Zairoise. Ann Soc Belge Med Trop 64:391, 1984

22. Centers for Disease Control: Recommendation for assisting the prevention of perinatal transmission of human T-lymphotropic virus type III/lymphadenopathy-associated virus and acquired immunodeficiency syndrome. MMWR 34:721, 1985

23. Mann JM, Quinn TC, Francis H, et al: Prevalence of HTLV-III/LAV in household contacts of confirmed AIDS patients and controls in Kinshasa, Zaire. JAMA 256:3099, 1986

24. Mann JM, Francis H, Quinn TC, et al: HTLV-III/LAV seroprevalence among hospital workers in Kinshasa (Zaire). JAMA 255:3255, 1986

25. Zuckerman AJ: AIDS and insects. Br Med J 292:1094, 1986

26. Serwadda D, Mugerwa RD, Servan NK, et al: Slim disease: a new disease in Uganda and its association with HTLV-III infection. Lancet ii:849, 1983

27. Laure F, Leonard R, Zagury D, Gallo RC, et al: Genomic diversity of Zairian HIV isolates: Biological characteristics and clinical manifestation of HIV infection. AIDS Research and Human Retrovirus 3(4):343, 1987

28. Nzila N, Mann JM, Francis H, et al: LAV/HTLV-III seroprevalence among tuberculosis patients in Zaire (abstract). Presented at the Second International AIDS Conference, Paris, June 23/25, 1986

29. Pitchenik AE, Cole C, Russell BW, et al: Tuberculosis, atypical mycobacterium and the acquired immunodeficiency syndrome among Haitian and non-Haitian patients in South Florida. Ann Intern Med 101:641, 1985

30. Biggar RJ, Gigase PL, Melbye M, et al: ELISA HTLV retrovirus antibody reactivity associated with malaria and immune complexes in healthy Africans. Lancet ii:520, 1985

31. Zempleni A: la maladie et ses causes. L'Ethnographie 96–97, LXXXI, 13–44, 1985

32. Janzen JM, Prins G: Causality and classification in African medicine and health. Soc Science Medi, 15B:3, 1981

33. Horton R: African traditional thought and Western Science. Africa, 37(1):50, 32(2):155, 1967

34. Buhan C, Kanga Essiben E: la Mystique du Corps. Paris, l'Harmattan, 1986

35. Radcliffe-Brown AR, Ford D: African systems of kinship and marriage. London, Oxford University Press, 1950

36. Moyo D: Fighting AIDS in Africa. Africasia, 41:54, 1987

37. Bekombo M, Houseman M, De Sales A, et al: L'institution Scolaire et l'Education Traditionnelle en Afrique. Paris, Unesco, 1978

38. Zagury D, Bernard J, Leonard R, et al: Long term cultures of HTLV-III infected T cells: A model of cytopathology of T-cell depletion in AIDS. Science 231:850, 1986

39. Unanue ER, Allen PM, Kurt-Jones EA, et al: Molecular nature of T cell recognition of antigen in immune regulation. In Feldman M, Mitchison NA (eds): Humana Press, 225–230, 1985

40. Putney SD, Matthews TJ, Robey WG, et al: HTLV-III/LAV neutralizing antibodies to an *E. coli*–produced fragment of the virus envelope. Science, 234:1392, 1986

41. Chakrabarti S, Robert-Guroff M, Wong-Staal F, et al: B-expression of the HTLV-III envelope gene by a recombinant vaccinia virus. Nature 320:535, 1986

42. Margalit H, Spouge JL, Berzovsky J, et al: Prediction of immunodominant helper T cell antigenic sites from the primary sequence. J Immunol 138:2213, 1987

43. Beaufay M, Amar-Costesec A, Thines-Sempoux D, et al: Analytical study of microsomes and isolated subcellular membranes from rat liver. J Cell Biol 61:213–231, 1974

44. Zarling JM, Morton W, Moran PA, et al: T-cell responses to human AIDS virus in macaques immunized with recombinant vaccinia viruses. Nature 323:344, 1986

45. Zagury D, Leonard R, Fouchard M, et al: Immunization against AIDS in humans. Nature 326:249–250, 1987

46. Robert-Guroff M, Brown M, Gallo RC: HTLV-III neutralizing antibodies in patients with AIDS and AIDS related complex. Nature 316:72–74, 1985

47. Hahn BH, Gonda MA, Shaw GM, et al: Genomic diversity of the acquired immunodeficiency syndrome virus HTLV-III: Different viruses exhibit greatest divergence in their envelope genes. Proc Nat Acad Science (USA) 82:4813, 1985

48. Salk J: Prospects for the control of AIDS by immunizing seropositive individuals. Nature 327:473, 1987

Reflections on the Mobilization of a National Effort to Control AIDS

Edward N. Brandt, Jr.

28

The first cases of what is now known as acquired immune deficiency syndrome, or AIDS, were reported to the Centers for Disease Control from Los Angeles in the spring of 1981. Five cases were then described in the June 6, 1981, issue of *Morbidity and Mortality Weekly Report.* These five were young homosexual men with an immune deficiency of no identifiable cause and *Pneumocystis carinii* pneumonia. Earlier there had been reports of young men with similar characteristics who had Kaposi's sarcoma. In the summer of 1981, it became clear that these reports were related. Investigation of this outbreak, like that of all sudden outbreaks of disease, became the responsibility of the United States Public Health Service (USPHS).

THE UNITED STATES PUBLIC HEALTH SERVICE

The USPHS was established in 1789 by a one-page Act of Congress entitled "An Act For The Relief of Sick and Disabled Seamen." Signed by President John Adams, this act had as its stated purpose the provision of care to merchant seamen, but its underlying objective was to prevent the importation of infectious diseases from other countries. In the nearly two hundred years since, the USPHS Act has grown to nearly 1000 pages, with a concomitant increase in the responsibilities of the USPHS. In 1981, the USPHS had about 55,000 employees and a budget of nearly $10 billion, operated more than 60 hospitals, and had responsibilities ranging over the entire spectrum of public health activities from basic biomedical research through primary, secondary, and tertiary health care to epidemiology, disease surveillance, and others. Much of its work is accomplished through cooperative and collaborative activities with academic institutions, state governments, and industry. Its record of accomplishment has led to a proud organization staffed with competent, dedicated professionals.

When AIDS was first described, the USPHS consisted of six functioning agencies: The National Institutes of Health (NIH), Alcohol, Drug Abuse and Mental Health Administration (ADAMHA), Centers for Disease Control (CDC), Food and Drug Administration (FDA), Health Services Administration (HSA), and Health Resources Administration (HRA); and the Office of the Assistant Secretary for Health (OASH) consisting of the Office of the Surgeon General, administrative and policy development offices, and three national centers: Health Statistics (NCHS), Health Care Technology (NCHCT), and Health Services Research (NCHSR). Subsequently, the HSA and HRA were merged into the Health Services and Resources Administration (HRSA) and the NCHCT was abolished with its responsibilities reassigned. The Assistant Secretary for Health (ASH) heads the USPHS and is appointed by the President with Senate confirmation.

Each of the USPHS agencies has its own mission, but there is overlap in functions. Furthermore, each has its own constituency, again with overlap. This structure has resulted in a tradition of independence in activities that has led to criticism during the AIDS epidemic. In addition, the agencies are staffed with proud, competent professionals who work hard and are highly mission-oriented. Hence, personal ambitions and rivalries arise on occasion, leading to public disagreements. Similar comments are true of the constituencies, especially academic scientists, and this, too, leads to public criticism and frequent questioning of motivation.

EPIDEMICS

The control of epidemics depends on a number of actions, some of which occur simultaneously. These steps include recognition of the outbreak, surveillance of cases, identification of persons at risk and risk factors, identification of the causal and contributing factors, and, finally, prevention of further cases by preventive or therapeutic actions. With complex illnesses such as AIDS and the resultant complexities of the work required for control, two activities are essential—coordination and communication. It is important that work not be unnecessarily duplicated and that everyone working on the epidemic be aware of the findings of others to avoid unnecessary activities. Traditionally, such communication is accomplished by publication in scientific journals; however, this process requires 9 to 12 months after manuscripts are written and submitted, a very long time with a serious illness like AIDS. Furthermore, the rapid rate of new developments can also make this method too slow. Not only is timely communication essential among scientists, it is also important to keep practicing health care workers, the public, and elected officials informed to avoid warranted concerns and fears.

THE USPHS RESPONSE

After receipt of the first reports of AIDS cases, the CDC assumed primary responsibility for tracking the epidemic. A group was established to investigate each reported case in conjunction with state health authorities. Soon thereafter, the NIH began admitting people with AIDS to the Clinical Center for intensive study of the pathology, symptomatology, and possible etiologies. In September, 1981, the National Cancer Institute held an invited workshop in which 54 scientists and physicians discussed the outbreak of Kaposi's sarcoma. As the number of reported cases increased, the etiologic possibilities began to narrow. For example, in June of 1982, the first cases in hemophiliacs appeared, and in late 1982, a case resulting from blood transfusion came to light. This transmission by blood narrowed the range of possible agents to an infectious or other transmissible agent. The infectious organism hypothesis was stronger, since it was clear that AIDS was transmitted sexually as well as by blood.

By the end of 1982, a Coordinating Committee was established in the USPHS. It was composed of senior officials of the various agencies and chaired by one from the CDC. The primary purpose of the committee was to facilitate communication, with better coordination to result from each of the members of the committee reporting back to key personnel in his or her agency. This committee operated until 1984, when it was replaced by the Executive Committee on AIDS composed of the Agency Heads and chaired by the ASH.

At the same time, the Public Affairs office developed material for public release. It is of interest to note the lack of interest in AIDS displayed by the public media except for those in the San Francisco area, where the bulk of the cases had originated.

The beginning of 1983 saw a number of problems. The safety of the blood supply had become a public concern, and numerous theories about the origin of the disease had arisen. The blood supply issue was the more controversial aspect. For example, the public was saying, "Insure our safety if blood is required." The blood banks were asking for simplicity in any protective steps, and specifically, that they not be assigned some sort of enforcement role in denying donors. Finally, the gay community was urging that the guidelines not lead to further discrimination against their membership. The FDA is the agency responsible for protecting the safety of the blood supply. In March 1983, after meetings with the CDC and the National Heart, Lung and Blood Institute (NHLBI), the FDA released guidelines calling for voluntary deferral by blood donors who had reason to believe that they were at risk of AIDS.

During the latter half of 1982 and early 1983, research efforts at the NIH and in academic centers was progressing. Most types of infectious agents were being evaluated as possible causes of immune deficiency. In May, 1983, two articles appeared in *Science* suggesting retroviruses as possible etiologic agents. Then on April 23, 1984, in one of the largest press conferences ever held by the Department of Health and Human Services, the findings of Dr. Robert Gallo and his associates were announced. One of the major accomplishments was the development of the blood test for the detection of antibodies. With this discovery, it was now possible to measure the extent of the epidemic and to define the pathogenesis of AIDS. In addition, investigations of therapeutic options could be narrowed down to those with antiviral effects and the characteristics of the causal virus studied.

SOCIETAL REACTIONS

Complicating the already complex scientific investigations were the reactions of the public. The fears and anxieties generated by AIDS led to doubts about the adequacy and efficacy of the scientific efforts. Furthermore, in 1983, there was national attention to some cases—one in particular—of scientific misconduct. This led to even greater doubts as some used this to question much of the scientific advance. The credibility of the USPHS, its stock-in-trade, was being questioned. The April, 1984, press conference did much to quiet those concerns.

The overall societal reaction was fear. AIDS is a fatal illness that is transmitted primarily by sexual activity and by intravenous drug abuse. Both of these are controversial in American society. Fear leads to irrational behavior, and when it is coupled with sexual activity, the outcome is accentuated. The results included bus drivers in San Francisco wearing masks and gloves, children being denied attendance at school or even church, and other such acts. Although understandable, such behavior was inconsistent with the knowledge of the disease, and was a manifestation of the disbelief of the public. It became clear that public education had not kept pace with the accumulating knowledge. Even today that gap has not yet been bridged, although local service groups are making significant headway.

Another factor contributing to the public's concern was the natural tendency of scientists to be precise. Most people were not reassured by statements that were not absolute. Furthermore, legitimate scientific disagreements were magnified to the point of suggesting that the scientific community did not really understand how AIDS was spread. Even today, isolated reports of people who apparently do not fit the usual risk characteristics receive a great deal of media attention, thereby stimulating doubt. It is not clear how to deal effectively with this problem, but it must be understood.

DISCUSSION

The USPHS has dealt effectively with many epidemics. Consider toxic shock syndrome, Legionnaire's disease, and numerous gastrointestinal infections. However, all of these have been limited in their scope and were associated with factors largely outside the control of the affected individuals. AIDS is clearly different in almost all respects. The fundamental issue is: How is the United States to deal with epidemics of the magnitude of AIDS in the future?

The public health and scientific activities in the United States are dispersed widely and operate under many different authorities. There is no central authority, and therefore mobilization of scientific talent depends largely on persuasion. For example, it is necessary to convince the scientific community of the existence of a problem that needs their attention and efforts. With AIDS, the response has been overwhelming and the results effective, but time is required to get the scientific community mobilized and ready to attack the problem.

In addition, if scientists are to make maximum use of their talents and efforts, they must be informed, again emphasizing the need for a good communication system. This prevents their wasting time and effort following leads already shown to be unproductive and wasting their efforts on unnecessary duplication of research.

In my view, the following steps are required to mobilize to fight an epidemic.

1. The problem must be identified, including its potential scope and severity.
2. The complexity of the issues must be defined. That necessitates some early understanding of the epi-demiology of the illness, including the risk factors and methods of transmission.
3. A plan of action must be developed. In general, the initial plan will be vague, and will largely indicate directions for research. With AIDS, the initial plan was to explore three possible causes—infectious, chemical (due to the relatively common use of "poppers" by affected persons), and the slim possibility of some aspect of homosexual behavior. As knowledge accumulates, the plan can become more detailed.
4. Mechanisms for coordinating the total effort must be developed. Such mechanisms cannot be proscriptive or they are doomed to failure. Rather, they must be directed toward facilitating work that will lead to advances. It is important to remember that most scientific advances occur slowly as data accumulate, but it is individual scientists or groups who gain enough insight to see an answer. No formula or rigid plan will ensure that that insight occurs. Coordination of science includes communication of new information as it develops. In particular, it is essential that the scientific journals assist in such communication. Most of the major journals did so during the AIDS epidemic by speeding up their review process and permitting public disclosure after the decision had been made to print the findings.
5. Steps must be taken to keep the public informed and to assure them that progress is being made to protect their health. That assurance must be accompanied by necessary actions without compromising their fundamental rights and freedoms. The education should include the facts about how science advances—not by a series of "breakthroughs" but by a sequence of steps, each of which leads to improved understanding. It is important to emphasize that 1983 was a year of great advances in AIDS; yet, it was also the darkest period of public concerns and fears. One reasonable explanation is that there were no significant "breakthroughs" to convince the public that progress was being made. One contributing factor was probably that many scientists committed to solving this problem were frustrated, and that frustration was seen as evidence of lack of progress.

Coordinating the efforts of independent, brilliant, competitive scientists is not a simple task. Scientists are convinced that their line of research is very important or they would not be pursuing it. If peer reviewers do not agree, many scientists air their grievances. That is certainly acceptable behavior in U.S. society, and it must be tolerated and explained to the public. Coordination becomes easier with more knowledge, but with AIDS, even that has not been entirely effective. The leadership of the USPHS is the key element in this endeavor. Its credibility with the public, elected officials and the scientific community must be preserved.

SUMMARY

The history of AIDS is one of great scientific achievements made with unbelievable speed. It is also one of dedicated work in laboratories, clinics, and communities. Indeed, the scientific progress is so extensive that the debates have largely shifted to other spheres, such as health care access and reimbursement.

Many lessons have been learned from the AIDS epidemic; one of the most critical is the importance of a strong basic science research program. Without the accumulated basic knowledge brought to bear on the problem, we would have been powerless to deal with AIDS. That fact must be communicated to the public and to elected officials. A second important lesson is that the scientific apparatus of the United States is capable of responding effectively to health threats, and has done so. Finally, the importance of timely, factual communication that leads to understanding of all elements of our society has been reinforced.

Appendix: Recommendations for Prevention of HIV Transmission in Health-Care Settings:

Morbidity and Mortality Weekly Report
36(2S), August 21, 1987

INTRODUCTION

Human immunodeficiency virus (HIV), the virus that causes acquired immunodeficiency syndrome (AIDS), is transmitted through sexual contact and exposure to infected blood or blood components and perinatally from mother to neonate. HIV has been isolated from blood, semen, vaginal secretions, saliva, tears, breast milk, cerebrospinal fluid, amniotic fluid, and urine and is likely to be isolated from other body fluids, secretions, and excretions. However, epidemiologic evidence has implicated only blood, semen, vaginal secretions, and possibly breast milk in transmission.

The increasing prevalence of HIV increases the risk that health-care workers will be exposed to blood from patients infected with HIV, especially when blood and body-fluid precautions are not followed for all patients. Thus, this document emphasizes the need for health-care workers to consider *all* patients as potentially infected with HIV and/or other blood-borne pathogens and to adhere rigorously to infection-control precautions for minimizing the risk of exposure to blood and body fluids of all patients.

The recommendations contained in this document consolidate and update CDC recommendations published earlier for preventing HIV transmission in health-care settings: precautions for clinical and laboratory staffs[1] and precautions for health-care workers and allied professionals[2]; recommendations for preventing HIV transmission in the workplace[3] and during invasive procedures[4]; recommendations for preventing possible transmission of HIV from tears[5]; and recommendations for providing dialysis treatment for HIV-infected patients.[6] These recommendations also update portions of the "Guideline for Isolation Precautions in Hospitals"[7] and reemphasize some of the recommendations contained in "Infection Control Practices for Dentistry."[8] The recommendations contained in this document have been developed for use in health-care settings and emphasize the need to treat blood and other body fluids from *all* patients as potentially infective. These same prudent precautions also should be taken in other settings in which persons may be exposed to blood or other body fluids.

DEFINITION OF HEALTH-CARE WORKERS

Health-care workers are defined as persons, including students and trainees, whose activities involve contact with patients or with blood or other body fluids from patients in a health-care setting.

HEALTH-CARE WORKERS WITH AIDS

As of July 10, 1987, a total of 1,875 (5.8%) of 32,395 adults with AIDS, who had been reported to the CDC national surveillance system and for whom occupational information was available, reported being employed in a health-care or clinical laboratory setting. In comparison, 6.8 million persons—representing 5.6% of the U.S. labor force—were employed in health services. Of the health-care workers with AIDS, 95% have been reported to exhibit high-risk behavior; for the remaining 5%, the means of HIV acquisition was undetermined. Health-care workers with AIDS were significantly more likely than other workers to have an undetermined risk (5% versus 3%, respectively). For both health-care workers and non-health-care workers with AIDS, the proportion with an undetermined risk has not increased since 1982.

AIDS patients initially reported as not belonging to recognized risk groups are investigated by state and local health departments to determine whether possible risk factors exist. Of all health-care workers with AIDS reported to CDC who were initially characterized as not having an identified risk and for whom follow-up information was available, 66% have been reclassified because risk factors were identified or because the patient was found not to meet the surveillance case definition for AIDS. Of the 87 health-care workers currently categorized as having no identifiable risk, information is incomplete on 16 (18%) because of death or refusal to be interviewed; 38 (44%) are still being investigated. The remaining 33 (38%) health-care workers were interviewed or had other follow-up information available. The occupations of these 33 were as follows: five physicians (15%), three of whom were surgeons; one dentist (3%); three nurses (9%); nine nursing assistants (27%); seven housekeeping or maintenance workers (21%); three clinical laboratory technicians (9%); one therapist (3%); and four others who did not have contact with patients (12%). Although 15 of these 33 health-care workers reported parenteral and/or other non-needlestick exposure to blood or body fluids from patients in the 10 years preceding their diagnosis of AIDS, none of these exposures involved a patient with AIDS or known HIV infection.

RISK TO HEALTH-CARE WORKERS OF ACQUIRING HIV IN HEALTH-CARE SETTINGS

Health-care workers with documented percutaneous or mucous-membrane exposures to blood or body fluids of HIV-infected patients have been prospectively evaluated to determine the risk of infection after such exposures. As of June 30, 1987, 883 health-care workers have been tested for antibody to HIV in an ongoing surveillance project conducted by CDC.[9] Of these, 708 (80%) had percutaneous exposures to blood, and 175 (20%) had a mucous membrane or an open wound contaminated by blood or body fluid. Of 396 health-care workers, each of whom had only a convalescent-phase serum sample obtained and tested ≥90 days post-exposure, one—for whom heterosexual transmission could not be ruled out—was seropositive for HIV antibody. For 425 additional health-care workers, both acute- and convalescent-phase serum samples were obtained and tested; none of 74 health-care workers with nonpercutaneous exposures seroconverted, and three (0.9%) of 351 with percutaneous exposures seroconverted. None of these three health-care workers had other documented risk factors for infection.

Two other prospective studies to assess the risk of nosocomial acquisition of HIV infection for health-care workers are ongoing in the United States. As of April 30, 1987, 332 health-care workers with a total of 453 needlestick or mucous-membrane exposures to the blood or other body fluids of HIV-infected patients were tested for HIV antibody at the National Institutes of Health.[10] These exposed workers included 103 with needlestick injuries and 229 with mucous-membrane exposures; none had seroconverted. A similar study at the University of California of 129 health-care workers with documented needlestick injuries or mucous-membrane exposures to blood or other body fluids from patients with HIV infection has not identified any seroconversions.[11] Results of a prospective study in the United Kingdom identified no evidence of transmission among 150 health-care workers with parenteral or mucous-membrane exposures to blood or other body fluids, secretions, or excretions from patients with HIV infection.[12]

In addition to health-care workers enrolled in prospective studies, eight persons who provided care to infected patients and denied other risk factors have been reported to have acquired HIV infection. Three of these health-care workers had needlestick exposures to blood from infected patients.[13-15] Two were persons who provided nursing care to infected persons; although neither sustained a needlestick, both had extensive contact with blood or other body fluids, and neither observed recommended barrier precautions.[16,17] The other three were health-care workers with non-needlestick exposures to blood from infected patients.[18] Although the exact route of transmission for these last three infections is not known, all three persons had direct contact of their skin with blood from infected patients, all had skin lesions that may have been contaminated by blood, and one also had a mucous-membrane exposure.

A total of 1,231 dentists and hygienists, many of whom practiced in areas with many AIDS cases, participated in a study to determine the prevalence of antibody to HIV; one dentist (0.1%) had HIV antibody. Although no exposure to a known HIV-infected person could be documented, epidemiologic investigation did not identify any other risk factor for infection. The infected dentist, who also had a history of sustaining needlestick injuries and trauma to his hands, did not routinely wear gloves when providing dental care.[19]

PRECAUTIONS TO PREVENT TRANSMISSION OF HIV

Universal Precautions

Since medical history and examination cannot reliably identify all patients infected with HIV or other blood-borne pathogens, blood and body-fluid precautions should be consistently used for *all* patients. This approach, previously recommended by CDC,[3,4] and referred to as "universal blood and body-fluid precautions" or "universal precautions," should be used in the care of *all* patients, especially including those in emergency-care settings in which the risk of blood exposure is increased and the infection status of the patient is usually unknown.[20]

1. All health-care workers should routinely use appropriate barrier precautions to prevent skin and mucous-membrane exposure when contact with blood or other body fluids of any patient is anticipated. Gloves should be worn for touching blood and body fluids, mucous membranes, or non-intact skin of all patients, for handling items or surfaces soiled with blood or body fluids, and for performing venipuncture and other vascular access procedures. Gloves should be changed after contact with each patient. Masks and protective eyewear or face shields should be worn during procedures that are likely to generate droplets of blood or other body fluids to prevent exposure of mucous membranes of the mouth, nose, and eyes. Gowns or aprons should be worn during procedures that are likely to generate splashes of blood or other body fluids.

2. Hands and other skin surfaces should be washed immediately and thoroughly if contaminated with blood or other body fluids. Hands should be washed immediately after gloves are removed.

3. All health-care workers should take precautions to prevent injuries caused by needles, scalpels, and other sharp instruments or devices during procedures; when cleaning used instruments; during disposal of used needles; and when handling sharp instruments after procedures. To prevent needlestick injuries, needles should not be recapped, purposely bent or broken by hand, removed from disposable syringes, or otherwise manipulated by hand. After they are used, disposable syringes and needles, scalpel blades, and other sharp items should be placed in puncture-resistant containers for disposal; the puncture-resistant containers should be located as close as practical to the use area. Large-bore reusable needles should be placed in a puncture-resistant container for transport to the reprocessing area.

4. Although saliva has not been implicated in HIV transmission, to minimize the need for emergency mouth-to-mouth resuscitation, mouthpieces, resuscitation bags, or other ventilation devices should be available for use in areas in which the need for resuscitation is predictable.

5. Health-care workers who have exudative lesions or weeping dermatitis should refrain from all direct patient care and from handling patient-care equipment until the condition resolves.

6. Pregnant health-care workers are not known to be at greater risk of contracting HIV infection than health-care workers who are not pregnant; however, if a health-care worker develops HIV infection during pregnancy, the infant is at risk of infection resulting from perinatal transmission. Because of this risk, pregnant health-care workers should be especially familiar with and strictly adhere to precautions to minimize the risk of HIV transmission.

Implementation of universal blood and body-fluid precautions for *all* patients eliminates the need for use of the isolation category of "Blood and Body Fluid Precautions" previously recommended by CDC[7] for patients known or suspected to be infected with blood-borne pathogens. Isolation precautions (e.g., enteric, "AFB"[7]) should be used as necessary if associated conditions, such as infectious diarrhea or tuberculosis, are diagnosed or suspected.

Precautions for Invasive Procedures

In this document, an invasive procedure is defined as surgical entry into tissues, cavities, or organs or repair of major traumatic injuries (1) in an operating or delivery room, emergency department, or outpatient setting, including both physicians' and dentists' offices; (2) cardiac catheterization and angiographic procedures; (3) a vaginal or cesarean delivery or other invasive obstetric procedure during which bleeding may occur; or (4) the manipulation, cutting, or removal of any oral or perioral tissues, including tooth structure, during which bleeding occurs or the potential for bleeding exists. The universal blood and body-fluid precautions listed above, combined with the precautions listed below, should be the minimum precautions for *all* such invasive procedures.

1. All health-care workers who participate in invasive procedures must routinely use appropriate barrier precautions to prevent skin and mucous-membrane contact with blood and other body fluids of all patients. Gloves and surgical masks must be worn for all invasive procedures. Protective eyewear or face shields should be worn for procedures that commonly result in the generation of droplets, splashing of blood or other body fluids, or the generation of bone chips. Gowns or aprons made of materials that provide an effective barrier should be worn during invasive procedures that are likely to result in the splashing of blood or other body fluids. All health-care workers who perform or assist in vaginal or cesarean deliveries should wear gloves and gowns when handling the placenta or the infant until blood and amniotic fluid have been removed from the infant's skin and should wear gloves during post-delivery care of the umbilical cord.

2. If a glove is torn or a needlestick or other injury occurs, the glove should be removed and a new glove used as promptly as patient safety permits; the needle or instrument involved in the incident should also be removed from the sterile field.

Precautions for Dentistry*

Blood, saliva, and gingival fluid from *all* dental patients should be considered infective. Special emphasis should

---

* General infection-control precautions are more specifically addressed in previous recommendations for infection-control practices for dentistry.[8]

be placed on the following precautions for preventing transmission of blood-borne pathogens in dental practice in both institutional and non-institutional settings.

1. In addition to wearing gloves for contact with oral mucous membranes of all patients, all dental workers should wear surgical masks and protective eyewear or chin-length plastic face shields during dental procedures in which splashing or spattering of blood, saliva, or gingival fluids is likely. Rubber dams, high-speed evacuation, and proper patient positioning, when appropriate, should be utilized to minimize generation of droplets and spatter.
2. Handpieces should be sterilized after use with each patient, since blood, saliva, or gingival fluid of patients may be aspirated into the handpiece or waterline. Handpieces that cannot be sterilized should at least be flushed, the outside surface cleaned and wiped with a suitable chemical germicide, and then rinsed. Handpieces should be flushed at the beginning of the day and after use with each patient. Manufacturers' recommendations should be followed for use and maintenance of waterlines and check valves and for flushing of handpieces. The same precautions should be used for ultrasonic scalers and air/water syringes.
3. Blood and saliva should be thoroughly and carefully cleaned from material that has been used in the mouth (e.g., impression materials, bite registration), especially before polishing and grinding intra-oral devices. Contaminated materials, impressions, and intra-oral devices should also be cleaned and disinfected before being handled in the dental laboratory and before they are placed in the patient's mouth. Because of the increasing variety of dental materials used intra-orally, dental workers should consult with manufacturers as to the stability of specific materials when using disinfection procedures.
4. Dental equipment and surfaces that are difficult to disinfect (e.g., light handles or X-ray-unit heads) and that may become contaminated should be wrapped with impervious-backed paper, aluminum foil, or clear plastic wrap. The coverings should be removed and discarded, and clean coverings should be put in place after use with each patient.

Precautions for Autopsies or Morticians' Services

In addition to the universal blood and body-fluid precautions listed above, the following precautions should be used by persons performing postmortem procedures:

1. All persons performing or assisting in postmortem procedures should wear gloves, masks, protective eyewear, gowns, and waterproof aprons.
2. Instruments and surfaces contaminated during post-

mortem procedures should be decontaminated with an appropriate chemical germicide.

Precautions for Dialysis

Patients with end-stage renal disease who are undergoing maintenance dialysis and who have HIV infection can be dialyzed in hospital-based or free-standing dialysis units using conventional infection-control precautions.[21] Universal blood and body-fluid precautions should be used when dialyzing *all* patients.

Strategies for disinfecting the dialysis fluid pathways of the hemodialysis machine are targeted to control bacterial contamination and generally consist of using 500–750 parts per million (ppm) of sodium hypochlorite (household bleach) for 30–40 minutes or 1.5%–2.0% formaldehyde overnight. In addition, several chemical germicides formulated to disinfect dialysis machines are commercially available. None of these protocols or procedures need to be changed for dialyzing patients infected with HIV.

Patients infected with HIV can be dialyzed by either hemodialysis or peritoneal dialysis and do not need to be isolated from other patients. The type of dialysis treatment (i.e., hemodialysis or peritoneal dialysis) should be based on the needs of the patient. The dialyzer may be discarded after each use. Alternatively, centers that reuse dialyzers—i.e., a specific single-use dialyzer is issued to a specific patient, removed, cleaned, disinfected, and reused several times on the same patient only—may include HIV-infected patients in the dialyzer-reuse program. An individual dialyzer must never be used on more than one patient.

Precautions for Laboratories†

Blood and other body fluids from *all* patients should be considered infective. To supplement the universal blood and body-fluid precautions listed above, the following precautions are recommended for health-care workers in clinical laboratories.

1. All specimens of blood and body fluids should be put in a well-constructed container with a secure lid to prevent leaking during transport. Care should be taken when collecting each specimen to avoid contaminating the outside of the container and of the laboratory form accompanying the specimen.
2. All persons processing blood and body-fluid specimens (e.g., removing tops from vacuum tubes) should wear gloves. Masks and protective eyewear should be worn if mucous-membrane contact with blood or body fluids is anticipated. Gloves should

---

† Additional precautions for research and industrial laboratories are addressed elsewhere.[22,23]

be changed and hands washed after completion of specimen processing.

3. For routine procedures, such as histologic and pathologic studies or microbiologic culturing, a biological safety cabinet is not necessary. However, bio logical safety cabinets (Class I or II) should be used whenever procedures are conducted that have a high potential for generating droplets. These include activities such as blending, sonicating, and vigorous mixing.

4. Mechanical pipetting devices should be used for manipulating all liquids in the laboratory. Mouth pipetting must not be done.

5. Use of needles and syringes should be limited to situations in which there is no alternative, and the recommendations for preventing injuries with needles outlined under universal precautions should be followed.

6. Laboratory work surfaces should be decontaminated with an appropriate chemical germicide after a spill of blood or other body fluids and when work activities are completed.

7. Contaminated materials used in laboratory tests should be decontaminated before reprocessing or be placed in bags and disposed of in accordance with institutional policies for disposal of infective waste.[24]

8. Scientific equipment that has been contaminated with blood or other body fluids should be decontaminated and cleaned before being repaired in the laboratory or transported to the manufacturer.

9. All persons should wash their hands after completing laboratory activities and should remove protective clothing before leaving the laboratory.

Implementation of universal blood and body-fluid precautions for *all* patients eliminates the need for warning labels on specimens since blood and other body fluids from all patients should be considered infective.

ENVIRONMENTAL CONSIDERATIONS FOR HIV TRANSMISSION

No environmentally mediated mode of HIV transmission has been documented. Nevertheless, the precautions described below should be taken routinely in the care of *all* patients.

Sterilization and Disinfection

Standard sterilization and disinfection procedures for patient-care equipment currently recommended for use[25,26] in a variety of health-care settings—including hospitals, medical and dental clinics and offices, hemodialysis centers, emergency-care facilities, and long-term nursing-care facilities—are adequate to sterilize or disinfect instruments, devices, or other items contaminated with blood or other body fluids from persons infected with blood-borne pathogens including HIV.[21,23]

Instruments or devices that enter sterile tissue or the vascular system of any patient or through which blood flows should be sterilized before reuse. Devices or items that contact intact mucous membranes should be sterilized or receive high-level disinfection, a procedure that kills vegetative organisms and viruses but not necessarily large numbers of bacterial spores. Chemical germicides that are registered with the U.S. Environmental Protection Agency (EPA) as "sterilants" may be used either for sterilization or for high-level disinfection depending on contact time.

Contact lenses used in trial fittings should be disinfected after each fitting by using a hydrogen peroxide contact lens disinfecting system or, if compatible, with heat (78°C–80°C [172.4°F–176.0°F]) for 10 minutes.

Medical devices or instruments that require sterilization or disinfection should be thoroughly cleaned before being exposed to the germicide, and the manufacturer's instructions for the use of the germicide should be followed. Further, it is important that the manufacturer's specifications for compatibility of the medical device with chemical germicides be closely followed. Information on specific label claims of commercial germicides can be obtained by writing to the Disinfectants Branch, Office of Pesticides, Environmental Protection Agency, 401 M Street, SW, Washington, D.C. 20460.

Studies have shown that HIV is inactivated rapidly after being exposed to commonly used chemical germicides at concentrations that are much lower than used in practice.[27-30] Embalming fluids are similar to the types of chemical germicides that have been tested and found to completely inactivate HIV. In addition to commercially available chemical germicides, a solution of sodium hypochlorite (household bleach) prepared daily is an inexpensive and effective germicide. Concentrations ranging from approximately 500 ppm (1:100 dilution of household bleach) sodium hypochlorite to 5,000 ppm (1:10 dilution of household bleach) are effective depending on the amount of organic material (e.g., blood, mucus) present on the surface to be cleaned and disinfected. Commercially available chemical germicides may be more compatible with certain medical devices that might be corroded by repeated exposure to sodium hypochlorite, especially to the 1:10 dilution.

Survival of HIV in the Environment

The most extensive study on the survival of HIV after drying involved greatly concentrated HIV samples, i.e., 10 million tissue-culture infectious doses per milliliter.[31] This concentration is at least 100,000 times greater than that typically found in the blood or serum of patients with HIV infection. HIV was detectable by tissue-culture techniques 1–3 days after drying, but the rate of inactivation was rapid. Studies performed at CDC have also shown that drying HIV causes a rapid (within several hours) 1–2 log (90%–99%) reduction in HIV concentration. In tissue-culture fluid, cell-free HIV could be detected up to 15 days at room temperature, up to 11 days at 37°C (98.6°F), and up to 1 day if the HIV was cell-associated.

When considered in the context of environmental conditions in health-care facilities, these results do not require any changes in currently recommended sterilization, disinfection, or housekeeping strategies. When medical devices are contaminated with blood or other body fluids, existing recommendations include the cleaning of these instruments, followed by disinfection or sterilization, depending on the type of medical device. These protocols assume "worst-case" conditions of extreme virologic and microbiologic contamination, and whether viruses have been inactivated after drying plays no role in formulating these strategies. Consequently, no changes in published procedures for cleaning, disinfecting, or sterilizing need to be made.

Housekeeping

Environmental surfaces such as walls, floors, and other surfaces are not associated with transmission of infections to patients or health-care workers. Therefore, extraordinary attempts to disinfect or sterilize these environmental surfaces are not necessary. However, cleaning and removal of soil should be done routinely.

Cleaning schedules and methods vary according to the area of the hospital or institution, type of surface to be cleaned, and the amount and type of soil present. Horizontal surfaces (e.g., bedside tables and hard-surfaced flooring) in patient-care areas are usually cleaned on a regular basis, when soiling or spills occur, and when a patient is discharged. Cleaning of walls, blinds, and curtains is recommended only if they are visibly soiled. Disinfectant fogging is an unsatisfactory method of decontaminating air and surfaces and is not recommended.

Disinfectant-detergent formulations registered by EPA can be used for cleaning environmental surfaces, but the actual physical removal of microorganisms by scrubbing is probably at least as important as any antimicrobial effect of the cleaning agent used. Therefore, cost, safety, and acceptability by housekeepers can be the main criteria for selecting any such registered agent. The manufacturers' instructions for appropriate use should be followed.

Cleaning and Decontaminating Spills of Blood or Other Body Fluids

Chemical germicides that are approved for use as "hospital disinfectants" and are tuberculocidal when used at recommended dilutions can be used to decontaminate spills of blood and other body fluids. Strategies for decontaminating spills of blood and other body fluids in a patient-care setting are different than for spills of cultures or other materials in clinical, public health, or research laboratories. In patient-care areas, visible material should first be removed and then the area should be decontaminated. With large spills of cultured or concentrated infectious agents in the laboratory, the contaminated area should be flooded with a liquid germicide before cleaning, then decontaminated with fresh germicidal chemical. In both settings, gloves should be worn during the cleaning and decontaminating procedures.

Laundry

Although soiled linen has been identified as a source of large numbers of certain pathogenic microorganisms, the risk of actual disease transmission is negligible. Rather than rigid procedures and specifications, hygienic and common-sense storage and processing of clean and soiled linen are recommended.[26] Soiled linen should be handled as little as possible and with minimum agitation to prevent gross microbial contamination of the air and of persons handling the linen. All soiled linen should be bagged at the location where it was used; it should not be sorted or rinsed in patient-care areas. Linen soiled with blood or body fluids should be placed and transported in bags that prevent leakage. If hot water is used, linen should be washed with detergent in water at least 71°C (160°F) for 25 minutes. If low-temperature (≤70°C [158°F]) laundry cycles are used, chemicals suitable for low-temperature washing at proper use concentration should be used.

Infective Waste

There is no epidemiologic evidence to suggest that most hospital waste is any more infective than residential waste. Moreover, there is no epidemiologic evidence that hospital waste has caused disease in the community as a result of improper disposal. Therefore, identifying wastes for which special precautions are indicated is largely a matter of judgment about the relative risk of disease transmission. The most practical approach to the management of infective waste is to identify those wastes with the potential for causing infection during handling and disposal and for which some special precautions appear prudent. Hospital wastes for which special precautions appear prudent include microbiology laboratory waste, pathology waste, and blood specimens or blood products. While any item that has had contact with blood, exudates, or secretions may be potentially infective, it is not usually considered practical or necessary to treat all such waste as infective.[23,26] Infective waste, in general, should either be incinerated or should be autoclaved before disposal in a sanitary landfill. Bulk blood, suctioned fluids, excretions, and secretions may be carefully poured down a drain connected to a sanitary sewer. Sanitary sewers may also be used to dispose of other infectious wastes capable of being ground and flushed into the sewer.

IMPLEMENTATION OF RECOMMENDED PRECAUTIONS

Employers of health-care workers should ensure that policies exist for:

1. Initial orientation and continuing education and training of all health-care workers—including students and trainees—on the epidemiology, modes of transmission, and prevention of HIV and other blood-borne infections and the need for routine use of universal blood and body-fluid precautions for *all* patients.
2. Provision of equipment and supplies necessary to minimize the risk of infection with HIV and other blood-borne pathogens.
3. Monitoring adherence to recommended protective measures. When monitoring reveals a failure to follow recommended precautions, counseling, education, and/or re-training should be provided, and, if necessary, appropriate disciplinary action should be considered.

Professional associations and labor organizations, through continuing education efforts, should emphasize the need for health-care workers to follow recommended precautions.

SEROLOGIC TESTING FOR HIV INFECTION

Background

A person is identified as infected with HIV when a sequence of tests, starting with repeated enzyme immunoassays (EIA) and including a Western blot or similar, more specific assay, are repeatedly reactive. Persons infected with HIV usually develop antibody against the virus within 6–12 weeks after infection.

The sensitivity of the currently licensed EIA tests is at least 99% when they are performed under optimal laboratory conditions on serum specimens from persons infected for ≥12 weeks. Optimal laboratory conditions include the use of reliable reagents, provision of continuing education of personnel, quality control of procedures, and participation in performance-evaluation programs. Given this performance, the probability of a false-negative test is remote except during the first several weeks after infection, before detectable antibody is present. The proportion of infected persons with a false-negative test attributed to absence of antibody in the early stages of infection is dependent on both the incidence and prevalence of HIV infection in a population (Table A-1).

The specificity of the currently licensed EIA tests is approximately 99% when repeatedly reactive tests are considered. Repeat testing of initially reactive specimens by EIA is required to reduce the likelihood of laboratory error. To increase further the specificity of serologic tests, laboratories must use a supplemental test, most often the Western blot, to validate repeatedly reactive EIA results. Under optimal laboratory conditions, the sensitivity of the Western blot test is comparable to or greater than that of a repeatedly reactive EIA, and the Western blot is highly specific when strict criteria are used to interpret the test results. The testing sequence of a repeatedly reactive EIA and a positive Western blot test is highly predictive of HIV infection, even in a population with a low prevalence of infection (Table A-2). If the Western blot test result is indeterminant, the testing sequence is considered equivocal for HIV infection. When this occurs, the Western blot test should be repeated on the same serum sample, and, if still indeterminant, the testing sequence should be repeated on a sample collected 3–6 months later. Use of other supplemental tests may aid in interpreting of results on samples that are persistently indeterminant by Western blot.

Testing of Patients

Previous CDC recommendations have emphasized the value of HIV serologic testing of patients for: (1) man-

Table A-1
Estimated Annual Number of Patients Infected With HIV Not Detected by HIV-Antibody Testing in a Hypothetical Hospital With 10,000 Admissions/Year*

Beginning Prevalence of HIV Infection (%)	Annual Incidence of HIV Infection (%)	Approximate Number of HIV-Infected Patients	Approximate Number of HIV-Infected Patients Not Detected
5.0	1.0	550	17–18
5.0	0.5	525	11–12
1.0	0.2	110	3–4
1.0	0.1	105	2–3
0.1	0.02	11	0–1
0.1	0.01	11	0–1

* The estimates are based on the following assumptions: 1) the sensitivity of the screening test is 99% (i.e., 99% of HIV-infected persons with antibody will be detected); 2) persons infected with HIV will not develop detectable antibody (seroconvert) until 6 weeks (1.5 months) after infection; 3) new infections occur at an equal rate throughout the year; 4) calculations of the number of HIV-infected persons in the patient population are based on the mid-year prevalence, which is the beginning prevalence plus half the annual incidence of infections.

Table A-2
*Predictive Value of Positive HIV-Antibody Tests
in Hypothetical Populations With Different
Prevalences of Infection*

	Prevalence of Infection (%)	Predictive Value of Positive Test (%)*
Repeatedly reactive enzyme immunoassay (EIA)†	0.2	28.41
	2.0	80.16
	20.0	98.02
Repeatedly reactive EIA followed by positive Western blot (WB)§	0.2	99.75
	2.0	99.97
	20.0	99.99

* Proportion of persons with positive test results who are actually infected
  with HIV.
† Assumes EIA sensitivity of 99.0% and specificity of 99.5%.
§ Assumes WB sensitivity of 99.0% and specificity of 99.9%.

agement of parenteral or mucous-membrane exposures
of health-care workers, (2) patient diagnosis and management, and (3) counseling and serologic testing to
prevent and control HIV transmission in the community.
In addition, more recent recommendations have stated
that hospitals, in conjunction with state and local health
departments, should periodically determine the prevalence of HIV infection among patients from age groups
at highest risk of infection.[32]

Adherence to universal blood and body-fluid precautions recommended for the care of all patients will
minimize the risk of transmission of HIV and other
blood-borne pathogens from patients to health-care
workers. The utility of routine HIV serologic testing of
patients as an adjunct to universal precautions is unknown. Results of such testing may not be available in
emergency or outpatient settings. In addition, some recently infected patients will not have detectable antibody to HIV (see Table A-1).

Personnel in some hospitals have advocated serologic testing of patients in settings in which exposure
of health-care workers to large amounts of patients'
blood may be anticipated. Specific patients for whom
serologic testing has been advocated include those undergoing major operative procedures and those undergoing treatment in critical-care units, especially if they
have conditions involving uncontrolled bleeding. Decisions regarding the need to establish testing programs
for patients should be made by physicians or individual
institutions. In addition, when deemed appropriate,
testing of individual patients may be performed on
agreement between the patient and the physician providing care.

In addition to the universal precautions recommended for all patients, certain additional precautions
for the care of HIV-infected patients undergoing major
surgical operations have been proposed by personnel

in some hospitals. For example, surgical procedures on
an HIV-infected patient might be altered so that hand-
to-hand passing of sharp instruments would be eliminated; stapling instruments rather than hand-suturing
equipment might be used to perform tissue approxi-
mation; electrocautery devices rather than scalpels might
be used as cutting instruments; and, even though uncomfortable, gowns that totally prevent seepage of blood
onto the skin of members of the operative team might
be worn. While such modifications might further minimize the risk of HIV infection for members of the operative team, some of these techniques could result in
prolongation of operative time and could potentially
have an adverse effect on the patient.

Testing programs, if developed, should include the
following principles:

- Obtaining consent for testing.
- Informing patients of test results, and providing
  counseling for seropositive patients by properly
  trained persons.
- Assuring that confidentiality safeguards are in place
  to limit knowledge of test results to those directly
  involved in the care of infected patients or as required
  by law.
- Assuring that identification of infected patients will
  not result in denial of needed care or provision of
  suboptimal care.
- Evaluating prospectively (1) the efficacy of the program in reducing the incidence of parenteral, mucous-membrane, or significant cutaneous exposures
  of health-care workers to the blood or other body
  fluids of HIV-infected patients and (2) the effect of
  modified procedures on patients.

Testing of Health-Care Workers

Although transmission of HIV from infected health-care
workers to patients has not been reported, transmission
during invasive procedures remains a possibility. Transmission of hepatitis B virus (HBV)—a blood-borne
agent with a considerably greater potential for nosocomial spread—from health-care workers to patients has
been documented. Such transmission has occurred in
situations (e.g., oral and gynecologic surgery) in which
health-care workers, when tested, had very high concentrations of HBV in their blood (at least 100 million
infectious virus particles per milliliter, a concentration
much higher than occurs with HIV infection), and the
health-care workers sustained a puncture wound while
performing invasive procedures or had exudative or
weeping lesions or microlacerations that allowed virus
to contaminate instruments or open wounds of patients.[33,34]

The hepatitis B experience indicates that only those
health-care workers who perform certain types of invasive procedures have transmitted HBV to patients.
Adherence to recommendations in this document will

minimize the risk of transmission of HIV and other blood-borne pathogens from health-care workers to patients during invasive procedures. Since transmission of HIV from infected health-care workers performing invasive procedures to their patients has not been reported and would be expected to occur only very rarely, if at all, the utility of routine testing of such health-care workers to prevent transmission of HIV cannot be assessed. If consideration is given to developing a serologic testing program for health-care workers who perform invasive procedures, the frequency of testing, as well as the issues of consent, confidentiality, and consequences of test results—as previously outlined for testing programs for patients—must be addressed.

MANAGEMENT OF INFECTED HEALTH-CARE WORKERS

Health-care workers with impaired immune systems resulting from HIV infection or other causes are at increased risk of acquiring or experiencing serious complications of infectious disease. Of particular concern is the risk of severe infection following exposure to patients with infectious diseases that are easily transmitted if appropriate precautions are not taken (e.g., measles, varicella). Any health-care worker with an impaired immune system should be counseled about the potential risk associated with taking care of patients with any transmissible infection and should continue to follow existing recommendations for infection control to minimize risk of exposure to other infectious agents.[7,35] Recommendations of the Immunization Practices Advisory Committee (ACIP) and institutional policies concerning requirements for vaccinating health-care workers with live-virus vaccines (e.g., measles, rubella) should also be considered.

The question of whether workers infected with HIV—especially those who perform invasive procedures—can adequately and safely be allowed to perform patient-care duties or whether their work assignments should be changed must be determined on an individual basis. These decisions should be made by the health-care worker's personal physician(s) in conjunction with the medical directors and personnel health service staff of the employing institution or hospital.

MANAGEMENT OF EXPOSURES

If a health-care worker has a parenteral (e.g., needlestick or cut) or mucous-membrane (e.g., splash to the eye or mouth) exposure to blood or other body fluids or has a cutaneous exposure involving large amounts of blood or prolonged contact with blood—especially when the exposed skin is chapped, abraded, or afflicted with dermatitis—the source patient should be informed of the incident and tested for serologic evidence of HIV infection after consent is obtained. Policies should be de-

veloped for testing source patients in situations in which consent cannot be obtained (e.g., an unconscious patient).

If the source patient has AIDS, is positive for HIV antibody, or refuses the test, the health-care worker should be counseled regarding the risk of infection and evaluated clinically and serologically for evidence of HIV infection as soon as possible after the exposure. The health-care worker should be advised to report and seek medical evaluation for any acute febrile illness that occurs within 12 weeks after the exposure. Such an illness—particularly one characterized by fever, rash, or lymphadenopathy—may be indicative of recent HIV infection. Seronegative health-care workers should be retested 6 weeks post-exposure and on a periodic basis thereafter (e.g., 12 weeks and 6 months after exposure) to determine whether transmission has occurred. During this follow-up period—especially the first 6–12 weeks after exposure, when most infected persons are expected to seroconvert—exposed health-care workers should follow U.S. Public Health Service (PHS) recommendations for preventing transmission of HIV.[36,37]

No further follow-up of a health-care worker exposed to infection as described above is necessary if the source patient is seronegative unless the source patient is at high risk of HIV infection. In the latter case, a subsequent specimen (e.g., 12 weeks following exposure) may be obtained from the health-care worker for antibody testing. If the source patient cannot be identified, decisions regarding appropriate follow-up should be individualized. Serologic testing should be available to all health-care workers who are concerned that they may have been infected with HIV.

If a patient has a parenteral or mucous-membrane exposure to blood or other body fluid of a health-care worker, the patient should be informed of the incident, and the same procedure outlined above for management of exposures should be followed for both the source health-care worker and the exposed patient.

REFERENCES

1. CDC: Acquired immunodeficiency syndrome (AIDS): Precautions for clinical and laboratory staffs. MMWR 31: 577, 1982
2. CDC: Acquired immunodeficiency syndrome (AIDS): Precautions for health-care workers and allied professionals. MMWR 32:450, 1983
3. CDC: Recommendations for preventing transmission of infection with human T-lymphotropic virus type III/lymphadenopathy-associated virus in the workplace. MMWR 34:681, 1985
4. CDC: Recommendations for preventing transmission of infection with human T-lymphotropic virus type III/lymphadenopathy-associated virus during invasive procedures. MMWR 35:221, 1986
5. CDC: Recommendations for preventing possible transmission of human T-lymphotropic virus type III/lymphadenopathy-associated virus from tears. MMWR 34:533, 1985

6. CDC: Recommendations for providing dialysis treatment to patients infected with human T-lymphotropic virus type III/lymphadenopathy-associated virus infection. MMWR 35:376, 1986

7. Garner JS, Simmons, BP: Guideline for isolation precautions in hospitals. Infect Control 4(suppl):245, 1983

8. CDC: Recommended infection control practices for dentistry. MMWR 35:237, 1986

9. McCray E,: The Cooperative Needlestick Surveillance Group: Occupational risk of the acquired immunodeficiency syndrome among health care workers. N Engl J Med 314:1127, 1986

10. Henderson DK, Saah AJ, Zak BJ, et al: Risk of nosocomial infection with human T-cell lymphotropic virus type III/lymphadenopathy-associated virus in a large cohort of intensively exposed health care workers. Ann Intern Med 104:644, 1986

11. Gerberding JL, Bryant-LeBlanc CE, Nelson K, et al: Risk of transmitting the human immunodeficiency virus, cytomegalovirus, and hepatitis B virus to health care workers exposed to patients with AIDS and AIDS-related conditions. J Infect Dis 156:1, 1987

12. McEvoy M, Porter K, Mortimer P, et al: Prospective study of clinical, laboratory, and ancillary staff with accidental exposures to blood or other body fluids from patients infected with HIV. Br Med J 294:1595, 1987

13. Anonymous. Needlestick transmission of HTLV-III from a patient infected in Africa. Lancet ii:1376, 1984

14. Oksenhendler E, Harzic M, Le Roux JM, et al: HIV infection with seroconversion after a superficial needlestick injury to the finger. N Engl J Med 315:582, 1986

15. Neisson-Vernant C, Arfi S, Mathez D, et al: Needlestick HIV seroconversion in a nurse. Lancet ii:814, 1986

16. Grint P, McEvoy M: Two associated cases of the acquired immune deficiency syndrome (AIDS). PHLS Commun Dis Rep 42:4, 1985

17. CDC: Apparent transmission of human T-lymphotropic virus type III/lymphadenopathy-associated virus from a child to a mother providing health care. MMWR 35:76, 1986

18. CDC. Update: Human immunodeficiency virus infections in health-care workers exposed to blood of infected patients. MMWR 36:285, 1987

19. Kline RS, Phelan J, Friedland GH, et al: Low occupational risk for HIV infection for dental professionals [Abstract]. In: Abstracts from the III International Conference on AIDS, 1–5 June 1985. Washington, DC: 155

20. Baker JL, Kelen GD, Sivertson KT, Quinn TC: Unsuspected human immunodeficiency virus in critically ill emergency patients. JAMA 257:2609, 1987

21. Favero MS: Dialysis-associated diseases and their control. In Bennett JV, Brachman PS (eds): Hospital Infections. Boston, Little, Brown and Company, 267, 1985

22. Richardson JH, Barkley WE (eds): Biosafety in microbiological and biomedical laboratories, 1984. Washington, DC, US Department of Health and Human Services, Public Health Service, HHS publication no. (CDC) 84-8395

23. CDC: Human T-lymphotropic virus type III/lymphadenopathy-associated virus: Agent summary statement. MMWR 35:540, 1986

24. Environmental Protection Agency: EPA guide for infectious waste management. Washington, DC, U.S. Environmental Protection Agency, May 1986 (Publication no. EPA/530-SW-86-014)

25. Favero MS: Sterilization, disinfection, and antisepsis in the hospital. In Manual of Clinical Microbiology. 4th ed. Washington, DC: American Society for Microbiology, 129, 1985

26. Garner JS, Favero MS: Guideline for handwashing and hospital environmental control, 1985. Atlanta, Public Health Service, Centers for Disease Control. HHS publication no. 99–1117, 1985

27. Spire B, Montagnier L, Barré-Sinoussi F, Chermann JC: Inactivation of lymphadenopathy associated virus by chemical disinfectants. Lancet 2:899, 1984

28. Martin LS, McDougal JS, Loskoski SL: Disinfection and inactivation of the human T lymphotropic virus type III/lymphadenopathy-associated virus. J Infect Dis 152:400, 1985

29. McDougal JS, Martin LS, Cort SP, et al: Thermal inactivation of the acquired immunodeficiency syndrome virus-III/lymphadenopathy-associated virus, with special reference to antihemophilic factor. J Clin Invest 76:875, 1985

30. Spire B, Barré-Sinoussi F, Dormont D, et al: Inactivation of lymphadenopathy-associated virus by heat, gamma rays, and ultraviolet light. Lancet i:188, 1985

31. Resnik L, Veren K, Salahuddin SZ, et al: Stability and inactivation of HTLV-III/LAV under clinical and laboratory environments. JAMA 255:1887, 1986

32. CDC: Public Health Service (PHS) guidelines for counseling and antibody testing to prevent HIV infection and AIDS. MMWR 3:509, 1987

33. Kane MA, Lettau LA: Transmission of HBV from dental personnel to patients. J Am Dent Assoc 110:634, 1985

34. Lettau LA, Smith JD, Williams D, et al: Transmission of hepatitis B with resultant restriction of surgical practice. JAMA 255:934, 1986

35. Williams WW: Guideline for infection control in hospital personnel. Infect Control 4(suppl):326, 1983

36. CDC: Prevention of acquired immune deficiency syndrome (AIDS): Report of inter-agency recommendations. MMWR 32:101, 1983

37. CDC: Provisional Public Health Service inter-agency recommendations for screening donated blood and plasma for antibody to the virus causing acquired immunodeficiency syndrome. MMWR 34:1, 1985

INDEX

ISBN 0-397-50892-1

90000

9 780397 508921